Cerebrovascular Surgery
Volume II

Cerebrovascular Surgery

Volume II

Edited by
Jack M. Fein and Eugene S. Flamm

With 201 Illustrations in 286 Parts

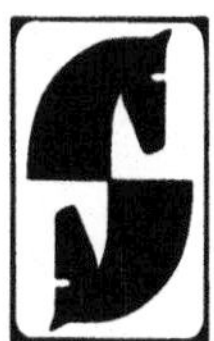

Springer Science+Business Media, LLC

JACK M. FEIN, M.D.
Department of Neurological Surgery, Albert Einstein College of Medicine, 1300 Morris Park Avenue, Bronx, NY 10461 USA

EUGENE S. FLAMM, M.D.
Department of Neurosurgery, New York University, 550 First Avenue, New York, NY 10016 USA

Library of Congress Catalog in Publication Data
Main entry under title:
Cerebrovascular surgery.
Includes bibliographies and index.
1. Cerebrovascular disease--Surgery. I. Fein, Jack M.
II. Flamm, Eugene S. [DNLM: 1. Cerebrovascular Disorders
--surgery. WL 355 C4138]
RD594.2.C49. 1984. 617'.481. 84-13869

ISBN 978-1-4612-9532-7 ISBN 978-1-4612-5032-6 (eBook)
DOI 10.1007/978-1-4612-5032-6

Originally published by Springer-Verlag New York Inc.
Softcover reprint of the hardcover 1st edition 1985

Typeset by Bi-Comp, Inc., York, Pennsylvania.

9 8 7 6 5 4 3 2 1

Dedicated to our children
Shari Fein
Andrew and Douglas Flamm

Foreword

Considerable impetus was given to the study and understanding of cerebrovascular anatomy by Thomas Willis and his contemporaries in the seventeenth century, yet almost two hundred years were to pass before further significant advances were made in this field. Then, from the mid-nineteenth century onwards, the dark ages of cerebrovascular research gradually lifted through the efforts of such workers as Luschka, Heubner, and Windle, whose pioneering anatomical studies formed the basis of the present-day understanding of the morphology of the cerebral circulation. The turn of the century saw an increasing influence of the early neurologists in describing anatomy of cerebral vessels in relation to their areas of distribution and to the production of focal deficits through specific vascular lesions and anomalies. Later still, Padget and others made important observations concerning phylogenetic and developmental aspects of the cerebral circulation.

These anatomical and clinical studies were remarkable enough but the real breakthrough in investigating cerebral pathophysiology and in devising appropriate corrective neurosurgical procedures had to await the remarkable advances in technology of the past fifty years. These began with the advent of cerebral angiography with all its subsequent refinements and progress has been accelerated through establishing noninvasive Doppler and high resolution ultrasound imaging techniques, methods for the accurate measurement of cerebral blood flow, CT scanning, PET scanning, and, most recently, imaging and metabolic NMR scanning. Also the electron microscope has facilitated investigation into the structural changes in brain blood vessels in various pathological conditions such as hemorrhagic stroke, cerebral infarction, and hypertension. In line with these numerous technical advances the number of investigations into CNS function carried out by neurosurgeons, neurologists, neuropathologists, physiologists, biochemists, and cell biologists has blossomed.

In contrast, cerebrovascular surgery might be considered still to be in its infancy. Early successes and advances in operative technique owed much to the individual brilliance and surgical expertise of surgeons such as Cushing and Dandy. Although cerebral arterial aneurysms have been operated upon directly for almost fifty years, and carotid occlusive disease since the 1950s, it is only in the past fifteen years that the introduction of the operating microscope, microtechniques, bipolar coagulation, and improved neuroanesthesia has brought about generally acceptable results for most surgeons in these fields.

In spite of the overall development of neuroscience on such a massive scale, we have to ask ourselves just how big are the steps we have taken in the understanding of cerebrovascular disease? Are we really that much nearer to knowing the true relationships of hypertension and cerebral arteriosclerosis, the development of aneurysms and AVMs, carotid occlusive disease, and the etiology and proper treatment of stroke and cerebral vasospasm? We are forced to admit that our therapeutic successes are still severely limited.

The present-day worker in almost every discipline of neuroscience is constantly assailed by steadily increasing numbers of scientific papers, journals, and monographs on his own and allied subjects. Their relevance and relative merits become increasingly difficult to discern in the context of what has gone before and what is currently acceptable theory.

These four volumes form a truly encyclopedic review of all aspects of cerebrovascular disease and its treatment yet remain uncluttered by irrelevant detail and yield so much more than simple lists of facts for reference. They present not only a remarkable perspective and clear review of what has been achieved so far in investigation and treatment of each subject considered, but each section reflects also a sensible and balanced opinion of current thinking in the field with some indication as to which direction we should next take.

I feel that the authors have achieved their aim in presenting these books not simply as reference volumes but in affording the discerning reader with an opportunity to open his mind to new perspectives which may thus stimulate further improvements in the understanding and treatment of cerebrovascular disease.

M. G. Yaşargil

Preface

In the last decade, cerebrovascular surgery has emerged as a distinct subspecialty within neurological surgery. Given the variety of diseases which involve the cerebral circulation and the large number of patients affected, cerebrovascular disorders are an important public health problem. A number of neurosurgeons now devote a major portion of their time to the study and treatment of these problems. Several centers of excellence have developed worldwide and a variety of innovative surgical approaches to these problems have been proposed. Clinical and basic research has widened the cerebrovascular horizon. There have been major advances in our understanding of the pathophysiology of ischemia, subarachnoid hemorrhage, vasospasm and the hypertensive vasculopathies. Noninvasive imaging techniques such as digital subtraction angiography and quantitative metabolic and hemodynamic studies are becoming more important clinically. Intraoperative monitoring techniques have been refined and microvascular surgery is now a way of life for many surgeons. Many of these advances are described in journal publications, topical monographs and symposium proceedings. With the growth of interest and concentration in this surgical subspecialty, however, there is a need for a more comprehensive treatment of cerebrovascular surgery.

Cerebrovascular operations require precise surgical skills. These skills are an amalgam of technical facility, knowledge, judgment, experience, and discipline. All four volumes of *Cerebrovascular Surgery* describe technical innovations which have been found useful through trial and error. They provide the fundamental concepts and facts which should form the basis for surgical judgments.

The experience required to formulate a logical surgical plan and the discipline required to carry it through to completion is difficult to describe. Given the variety of approaches to the various cerebrovascular disorders, we felt that this should be a multiauthored work. By pooling such a fund of knowledge the reader is given the opportunity for a broad education in cerebrovascular surgery.

Cerebrovascular surgery cannot be carried out in a vacuum. A sophisticated appreciation of the heart as a pump and the brain as a functional organ are requisite ingredients. Volume I was therefore designed to address these issues and to provide the reader with the insights into the anatomy and physiology of the cerebral circulation. Since microsurgery has become an important component in the treatment of all cerebrovascular disorders, the concluding chapters in volume I describe the fundamental principles, instrumentation, and techniques utilized in microvascular surgery. This volume describes the specific management of patients with cerebrovascular occlusive disease. Volume III describes the surgery of arterial aneurysm. Volume IV completes the series with a description of the surgical treatment of arteriovenous malformations, spontaneous hematomas, and surgery of the sagittal sinus.

The editors would like to acknowledge the efforts of the senior surgeons and their staff who participated in this effort. These individuals will undoubtedly continue to provide the creative leadership needed to reduce the morbidity and mortality due to cerebrovascular disease.

JACK M. FEIN
EUGENE S. FLAMM

Contents of Volume II

Contents of Volume I

Contents of Volume III

Contents of Volume IV

Contributors to Volume II

Moustapha Abou-Samra, M.D.
Neurosurgeon, 100 Brent Street, Ventura, California 93003 USA

Henry J. M. Barnett, M.D.
Chairman, Department of Neurological Sciences, University of Western Ontario, University Hospital, London, Ontario N6A 5A5, Canada

George L. Bohmfalk, M.D.
Clinical Instructor, Division of Neurosurgery, University of Texas Health Science Center, San Antonio, Texas 78284 USA

Willis E. Brown, Jr., M.D.
Associate Professor, Division of Neurosurgery, University of Texas Health Science Center, San Antonio, Texas 78284 USA

Robert Coté, M.D., F.R.C.P.
Assistant Professor, Department of Neurology and Neurosurgery, McGill University, Assistant Physician, Montreal General Hospital, Montreal, Quebec H3G 1A4, Canada

Humberto M. Cravioto, M.D.
Professor of Neuropathology, New York University School of Medicine, New York, New York 10016 USA

Michael E. DeBakey, M.D.
Chancellor of Baylor College of Medicine and Chairman of Department of Surgery, Director of the Heart and Blood Vessel Research and Demonstration Center, Baylor College of Medicine and the Methodist Hospital, Houston, Texas 77030 USA

Bennett M. Derby, M.D.
Professor of Clinical Neurology and Clinical Pathology, New York University School of Medicine, New York, New York 10016 USA

Jack M. Fein, M.D.
Department of Neurological Surgery, Albert Einstein College of Medicine, Bronx, New York 10461 USA

Mark J. Goldman, M.D.
Department of Radiology, Montefiore Medical Center, Bronx, New York 10467 USA

Hajime Handa, M.D.
Professor and Director of Neurosurgery, Kyoto University Medical School, Sakyo-ku, Kyoto 607, Japan

Norman E. Leeds, M.D.
Department of Radiology, Albert Einstein College of Medicine, Director of Neuroradiology Section, Montefiore Hospital and Medical Center, Bronx, New York 10467 USA

C. W. McCormick, M.D.
Dalhousie University Faculty of Medicine, Sir Charles Tupper Medical Building, Halifax, Nova Scotia, B3H 4H7, Canada

Chikao Nagashima, M.D., Dr. med. Sc.
Director and Chairman, Department of Neurological Surgery, Saitama Medical School, Director of Neurological Surgery, Saitama Medical School Hospital, Moro, Saitama-ken, Japan

George P. Noon, M.D.
Cora and Webb Madding Department of Surgery, Baylor College of Medicine, Houston, Texas 77030 USA

Robert G. Ojemann, M.D.
Department of Neurosurgery, Massachusetts General Hospital, Harvard Medical School, Boston, Massachusetts 02114 USA

Takehiko Okuno, M.D.
Department of Pediatrics, Kyoto University Hospital, Sakyo-ku, Kyoto 606, Japan

David G. Piepgras, M.D.
Department of Neurosurgery, Mayo Medical School, Rochester, Minnesota 55901 USA

Charles G. Rob, M.D.
Uniformed Services University of The Health Sciences, Bethesda, Maryland, Professor of Surgery, School of Medicine, East Carolina University, Greenville, North Carolina 27834 USA

Jim L. Story, M.D.
Professor and Head, Division of Neurosurgery, University of Texas Health Science Center, San Antonio, Texas 78284 USA

Thoralf M. Sundt, Jr., M.D.
Chairman of the Department of Neurologic Surgery, Mayo Clinic, Rochester, Minnesota 55905 USA

Waro Taki, M.D.
Instructor of Neurosurgery, Kyoto University Hospital, Sakyo-ku, Kyoto 606, Japan

Sen Yamagata, M.D.
Instructor of Neurosurgery, Kyoto University Hospital, Sakyo-ku, Kyoto 606, Japan

Yasuhiro Yonekawa, M.D.
Associate Professor of Neurosurgery, Department of Neurosurgery, Kyoto University Hospital, Sakyo-ku, Kyoto 606, Japan

Robert D. Zimmerman, M.D.
Associate Professor of Clinical Radiology, Cornell University Medical School, Associate Attending in Radiology, New York Hospital, New York, New York 10021 USA

Contributors to Volumes I–IV

Abou-Samra, M. *Vol. II, Ch. 7*
Ackerman, R. H. *Vol. I, Ch. 8*
Alksne, J. F. *Vol. III, Ch. 11*
Apfelbaum, R. I. *Vol. I, Ch. 12*
Astrup, J. *Vol. I, Ch. 4*
Barnett, H. J. M. *Vol. II, Ch. 3*
Bohmfalk, G. L. *Vol. II, Ch. 7*
Bowie, E. J. W. *Vol. I, Ch. 5*
Brackett, C. E. *Vol. III, Ch. 19*
Brisman, R. *Vol. III, Ch. 16*
Brown, W. E., Jr. *Vol. II, Ch. 7*
Buncke, H. J. *Vol. I, Ch. 13*
Byrd, S. E. *Vol. I, Ch. 2*
Chater, N. *Vol. I, Ch. 13*
Choi, I-S. *Vol. I, Ch. 3*
Chou, S. N. *Vol. III, Ch. 12*
Corbaz, J-M. *Vol. I, Ch. 2*
Coté, R. *Vol. II, Ch. 3*
Cottrell, J. E. *Vol. I, Ch. 9*
Cravioto, H. M. *Vol. II, Ch. 14*
DeBakey, M. E. *Vol. II, Ch. 6*
Debrun, G. *Vol. IV, Ch. 8*
Derby, B. M. *Vol. II, Ch. 14*
Dujovny, M. *Vol. III, Ch. 17*
Erickson, D. L. *Vol. III, Ch. 12*
Faria, M. A. *Vol. III, Ch. 6*
Fein, J. M. *Vol. I, Ch. 1, 6, 10, 14; Vol. II, Ch. 5, 8; Vol. III, Ch. 5, 8, 9*
Flamm, E. S. *Vol. III, Ch. 4, 9, 10*
Fleischer, A. S. *Vol. III, Ch. 6*
Frishman, W. H. *Vol. I, Ch. 6*
Fujii, K. *Vol. III, Ch. 1*
Gamache, F. W. *Vol. IV, Ch. 3*
George, A. E. *Vol. I, Ch. 3*
Goldman, M. J. *Vol. II, Ch. 2*
Gouaze, A. *Vol. I, Ch. 2*
Guidetti, B. *Vol. III, Ch. 7*
Handa, H. *Vol. II, Ch. 10, 13; Vol. III, Ch. 15; Vol. IV, Ch. 4*
Hilal, S. K. *Vol. IV, Ch. 5*
Ishikawa, M. *Vol. III, Ch. 15*
Jane, J. A. *Vol. III, Ch. 2*
Karanjia, P. N. *Vol. I, Ch. 7*
Kirschner, M. *Vol. I, Ch. 6*
Kossovsky, N. *Vol. III, Ch. 17*
Kossowsky, R. *Vol. III, Ch. 17*
Kricheff, I. I. *Vol. III, Ch. 3*
Laha, R. K. *Vol. III, Ch. 17*
Lassen, N. A. *Vol. I, Ch. 4*
Leeds, N. E. *Vol. II, Ch. 1, 2*
Lin, J. P. *Vol. III, Ch. 3*
Malis, L. I. *Vol. I, Ch. 11*
McCormick, C. W. *Vol. II, Ch. 3*
McCormick, W. F. *Vol. IV, Ch. 1*
Michelsen, W. J. *Vol. IV, Ch. 5*
Mizukami, M. *Vol. IV, Ch. 9*
Moritake, K. *Vol. IV, Ch. 4*
Nagashima, C. *Vol. II, Ch. 12*

Nelson, D. *Vol. III, Ch. 17*
Newfield, P. *Vol. I, Ch. 9*
Nicole, S. *Vol. III, Ch. 7*
Noon, G. P. *Vol. II, Ch. 6*
O'Boynick, P. *Vol. III, Ch. 19*
Ojemann, R. G. *Vol. II, Ch. 11; Vol. III, Ch. 18*
Okuno, T. *Vol. II, Ch. 13*
Olinger, R. *Vol. I, Ch. 14*
Ommaya, A. K. *Vol. IV, Ch. 7*
Owen, C. A. *Vol. I, Ch. 5*
Patterson, R. *Vol. IV, Ch. 3*
Peardon Donaghy, R. M. *Vol. IV, Ch. 12*
Perlin, A. *Vol. III, Ch. 17*
Perlmutter, D. *Vol. III, Ch. 1*
Piepgras, D. G. *Vol. II, Ch. 9*
Reinmuth, O. M. *Vol. I, Ch. 7*
Rhoton, A. L., Jr. *Vol. III, Ch. 1*
Richardson, A. E. *Vol. III, Ch. 2*
Rob, C. G. *Vol. II, Ch. 4*
Saeki, N. *Vol. III, Ch. 1*
Salamon, G. *Vol. I, Ch. 2*
Samson, D. *Vol. III, Ch. 13*
Shapiro, K. *Vol. III, Ch. 14*
Stein, B. M. *Vol. IV, Ch. 2*
Steiner, L. *Vol. IV, Ch. 6*
Story, J. L. *Vol. II, Ch. 7*
Sundt, T. M., Jr. *Vol. II, Ch. 9*
Sypert, G. W. *Vol. IV, Ch. 10, 11*
Szabo, Z. *Vol. I, Ch. 13*
Taki, W. *Vol. II, Ch. 10*
Tindall, G. T. *Vol. III, Ch. 6*
Wackenhut, N. *Vol. III, Ch. 17*
Winn, H. R. *Vol. III, Ch. 2*
Yamagata, S. *Vol. II, Ch. 10*
Yaşargil, M. G. *Foreword*
Yoneda, S. *Vol. III, Ch. 15*
Yonekawa, Y. *Vol. II, Ch. 13*
Zeal, A. *Vol. III, Ch. 1*
Zimmerman, R. D. *Vol. II, Ch. 1, 2,*

1

Neuroradiology of Cerebrovascular Disease

Norman E. Leeds and Robert D. Zimmerman

Introduction

Stroke is a common cause of death and morbidity in the United States. Surgical techniques are now readily available to correct the stenosis or wall irregularity by endarterectomy. Bypass procedures provide an alternative route for circulation to an ischemic intracranial region from the external to the internal carotid or vertebral circulations.

Angiographic equipment and techniques have been improved so that it is now possible to examine, extracranial and intracranial vessels safely and in detail. This also applies to elderly patients.[56]

In this institution, criteria modified from Kerber et al,[29] for angiographic investigation in the patient with atherosclerosis includes (1) transient ischemic attack, (2) suspected stroke, (3) clinical recovery following a stroke, (4) stroke in a young patient, (5) asymptomatic carotid bruit on preoperative workup prior to coronary artery or peripheral artery surgery, (6) patient with ischemia or stroke considered as a candidate for vascular bypass, and (7) miscellaneous other presentations.

The most common abnormality affecting an artery is atherosclerosis.[30] Atherosclerotic plaque is usually circumferential but may occur only along one wall. The plaques may cause arterial narrowing. Crawford et al[11] demonstrated that the degree of constriction and the length of the stenotic segment are two important factors that result in hemodynamic changes. An ulcerated or roughened plaque may act as a source of emboli[1,15,30,31,60,64] or can be the site of development of an intraluminal thrombus.[52] Kishore et al[31] pointed out the frequency of cerebral emboli from ulcerated or roughened plaques, and Roberson et al[52] demonstrated the frequent occurrence of an intraluminal thrombus in many of these cases. Recognition of the intravascular thrombus is important in these cases, as it can be easily overlooked.

Method of Investigation

Kerber et al[29] recently described their technique for evaluation of the patient with suspected extracranial vascular disease. The examination did not include the aortic arch except when selective vascular injections did not explain the symptoms or when a subclavian steal syndrome was suspected. We prefer to begin the examination of the patient with suspected extracranial vascular disease with an arch study to exclude the possibility of severe stenoses at the origin of the right or left common carotid artery or tight long-segment stenosis of common and/or internal carotid artery with reduced intracranial flow. In either of these instances, selective arterial injections may be avoided since an increase in complications may occur owing to potential arterial damage or cerebral anoxia due to reduced flow. The arch study also serves as a "road map" in planning the remainder of the angiographic examination in patients who have extremely tortuous vascular anatomy.

In our examination, for these reasons, an arch study in the right posterior oblique projection is performed first, with an 6.8 French catheter, using 66 cc of contrast (76% Renografin) injected at a flow of 25 cc/s. The films are then carefully reviewed prior to continuing the examination (Fig. 1.1). After analyzing the first set of roentgenograms of the arch, the following choices are available: (1) examine the arch in the opposite oblique, (2) discontinue the examination, (3) proceed to selective injections of the common carotid arteries, and (4) examine intracranial vessels following an arch injection.[16]

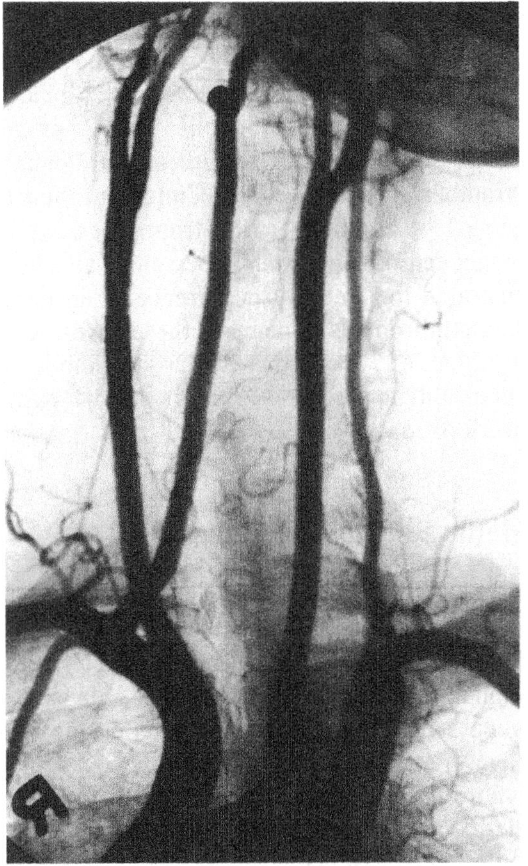

Figure 1.1. Normal aortic arch injection in right posterior oblique projection.

In the patient with stenosis at the common carotid artery origin (Figs. 1.2, 1.3) or with significant long stenoses at the carotid bifurcation, with reduced intracranial flow, the examination may be discontinued after the opposite oblique injection, because of the potential risk of catheterization of proximal stenotic lesions in these patients. If these possibilities are eliminated, one then usually proceeds to selective opacification of the common carotid arteries, beginning with the affected side. The extracranial common carotid artery bifurcation is visualized to advantage on selective injection (Fig. 1.4). Often the common carotid artery (Fig. 1.5) or carotid bifurcation are poorly visualized on an arch study but can be optimally visualized on selective common carotid artery injections (Figs. 1.6, 1.7). We prefer to keep the number of contrast injections to a minimum in the patient with cerebrovascular disease bearing in mind the inherent risk of repeated injections. Circulation time is usually prolonged in patients with cerebrovascular disease, and "contact time" of contrast, accounts for an increased incidence of complications.[4] A lateral view of the neck is obtained to evaluate the extracranial carotid bifurcation and also the petrosal segment. A simultaneous anterior-posterior projection is obtained in the Caldwell projection which includes the extracranial carotid bifurcation and will project the middle cerebral artery into the orbit. This will visualize the proximal segment of the middle cerebral artery as projected in the orbit. (Fig. 1.8). The opposite common carotid artery is always examined since atherosclerosis is frequently diffuse, and the asymptomatic opposite side may be affected in many cases (Fig. 1.9).

The roentgenographic examination should include the following: (1) the origin of the arteries arising from the aortic arch (Fig. 1.1); (2) the carotid bifurcation extracranially, in an optimum projection, to exclude stenotic, ulcerated (Figs. 1.6, 1.7), or roughened plaques (Fig. 1.10) or thrombus within the proximal internal carotid artery (Fig. 1.11); (3) the distal internal carotid artery, including petrous and cavernous segments (Fig. 1.12); (4) the intracranial vessels to exclude focal, regional, or diffuse disease, hyperemic areas, zones of abnormal circula-

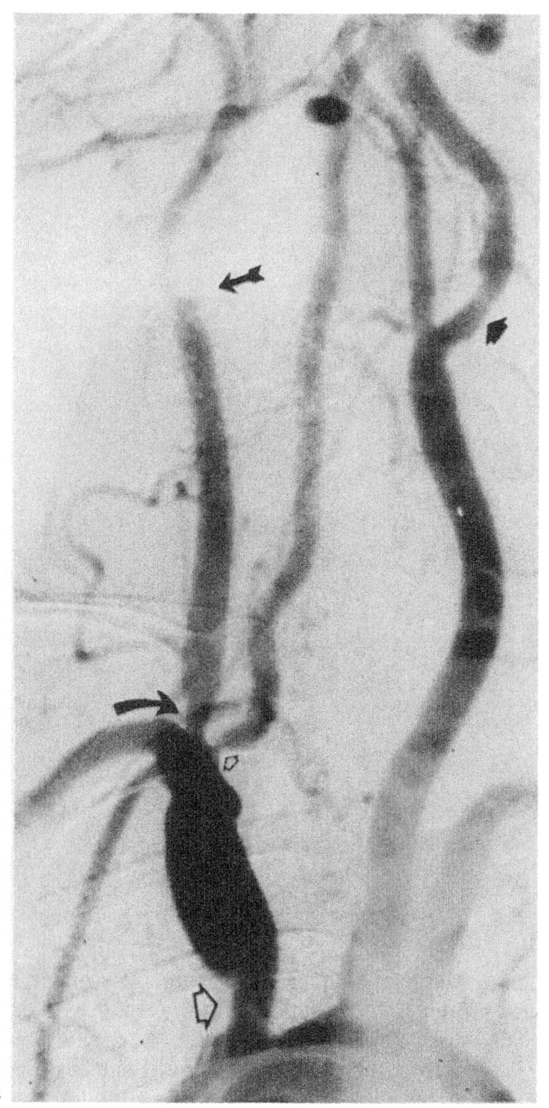

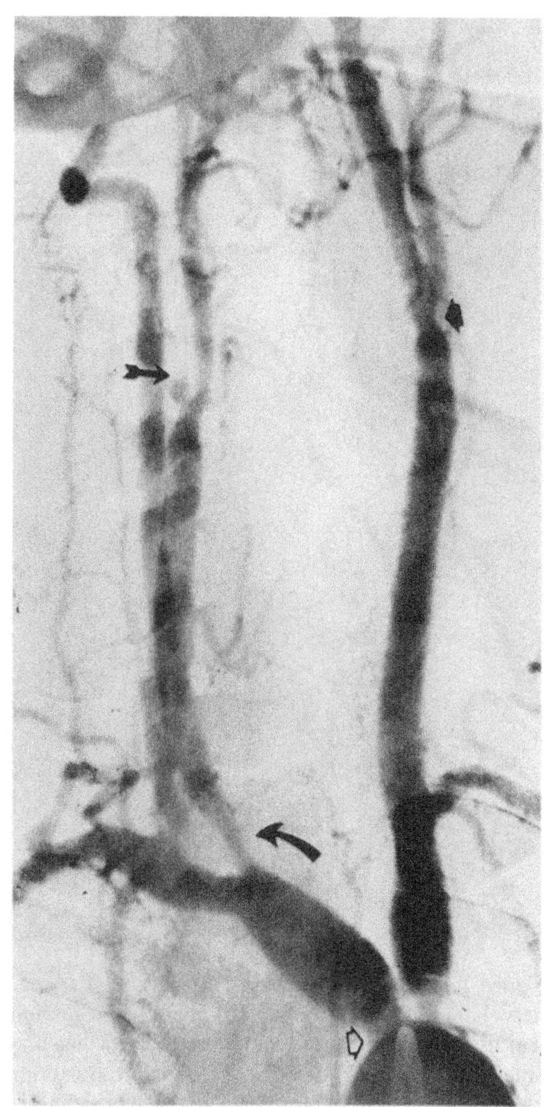

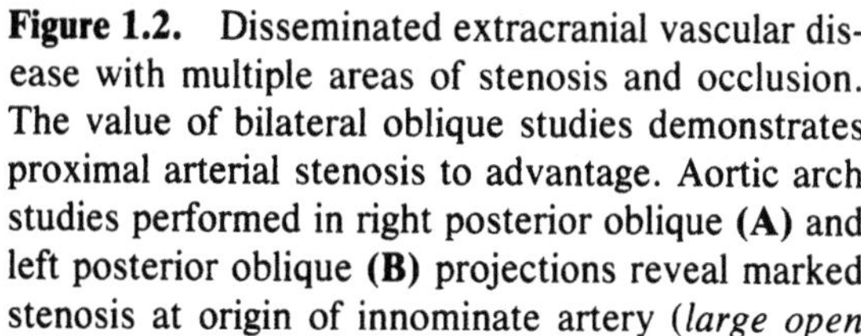

Figure 1.2. Disseminated extracranial vascular disease with multiple areas of stenosis and occlusion. The value of bilateral oblique studies demonstrates proximal arterial stenosis to advantage. Aortic arch studies performed in right posterior oblique **(A)** and left posterior oblique **(B)** projections reveal marked stenosis at origin of innominate artery (*large open arrow*) and proximal right common (*curved arrow*) and left internal carotid arteries (*arrowhead*). Proximal stenosis of left internal carotid artery is observed in **B** (*curved arrow*) and is not as well seen in **A**. Occlusion of proximal right internal carotid artery (*arrow*) and complete occlusion of left vertebral artery are also present.

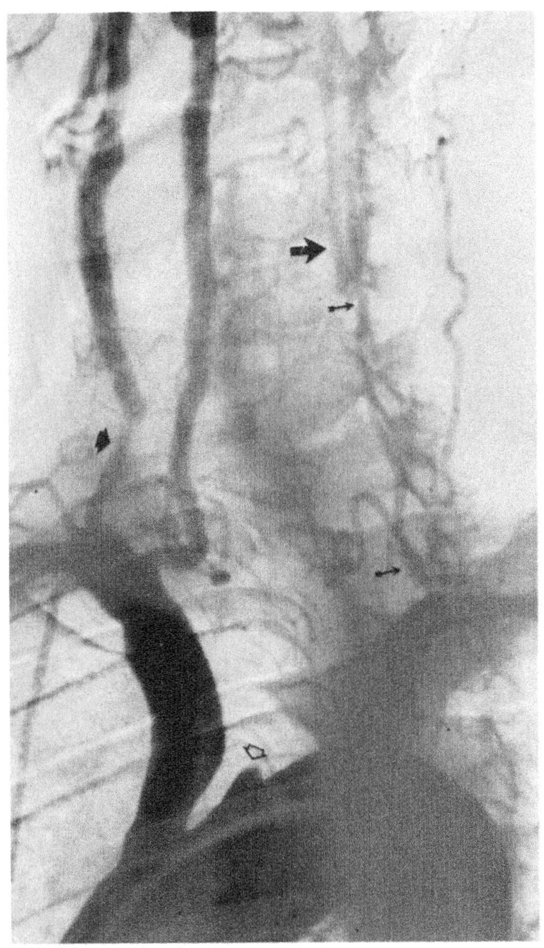

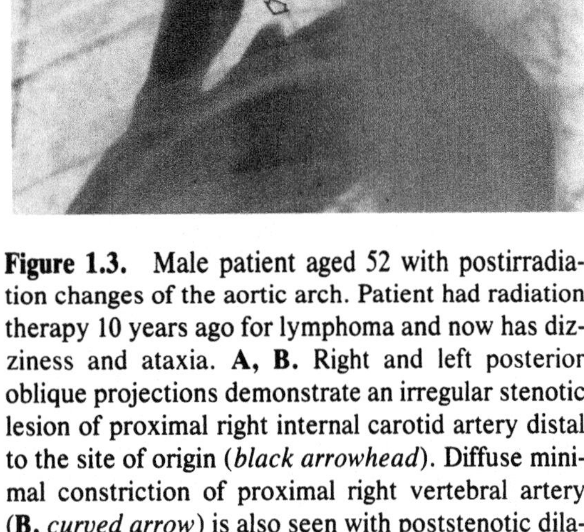

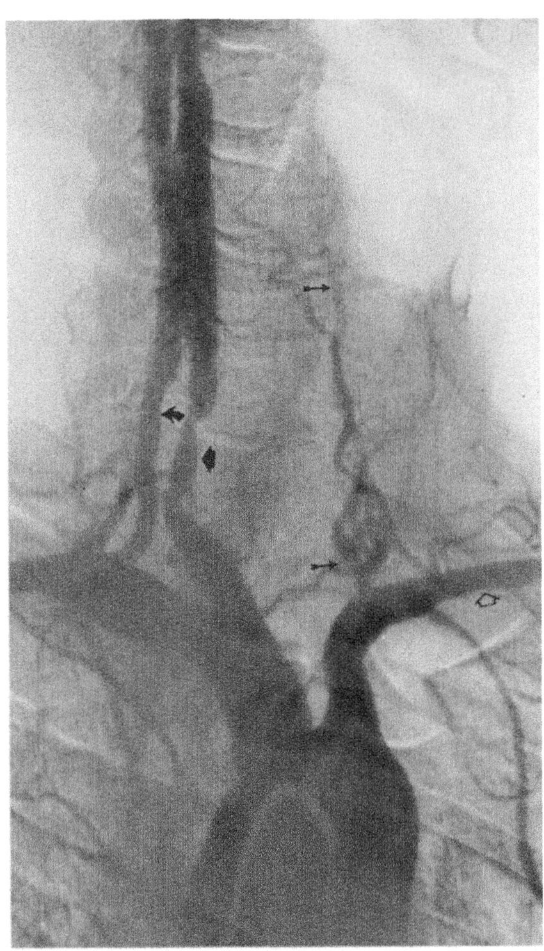

A B

Figure 1.3. Male patient aged 52 with postirradiation changes of the aortic arch. Patient had radiation therapy 10 years ago for lymphoma and now has dizziness and ataxia. **A, B.** Right and left posterior oblique projections demonstrate an irregular stenotic lesion of proximal right internal carotid artery distal to the site of origin (*black arrowhead*). Diffuse minimal constriction of proximal right vertebral artery (**B,** *curved arrow*) is also seen with poststenotic dilatation. Marginal plaque of the innominate artery is also present. The left common carotid artery is occluded just beyond its site of origin (**A,** *open arrowhead*). Left vertebral is occluded at its site of origin and reformed via cervical collaterals (*small arrow*) adjacent to C5 (**A,** *large arrow*), A long stenotic lesion of the subclavian artery is also seen (**B,** *open arrowhead*).

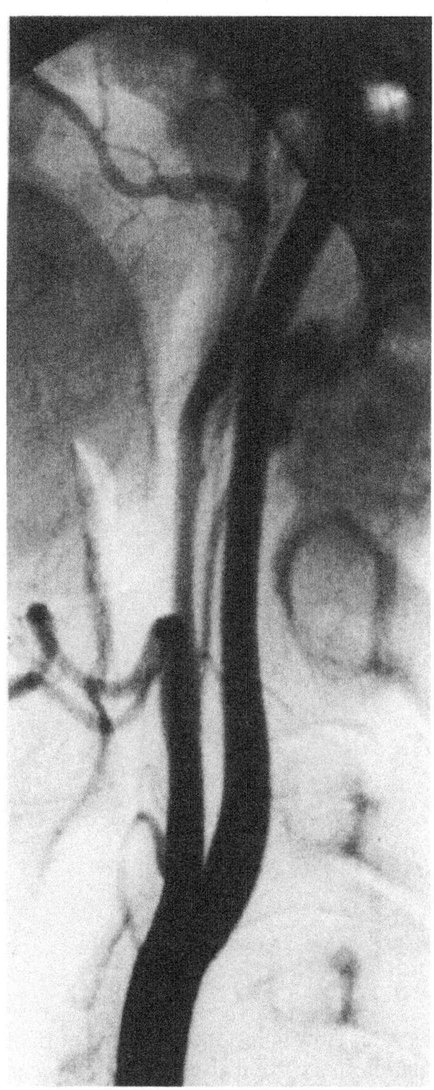

Figure 1.4. Normal selective left common carotid artery injection.

tion, early filling veins, and the presence or absence of collateral channels. In patients with disease of the carotid bifurcation (Figs. 1.13, 1.14) or the distal internal carotid artery, a reduced lumen or "string sign" may occur.[26]

In patients with diseased femoral arteries or in high-risk patients in whom femoral catheterization might be contraindicated, an axillary or brachial angiogram with visualization of the aortic arch and subsequent opacification of intracranial vessels may be performed. A 17- or 18-gauge thin-wall needle is inserted into the brachial artery at the antecubital fossa. In each injection a total of 50 cc of contrast material is injected at a rate of 25 to 35 cc/sec. This type of examination affords excellent visualization of the right common carotid and internal carotid arteries, extracranially and intracranially as well as the right vertebral and innominate arteries.

The left common carotid artery may be examined by utilizing countercurrent injections retrograde into the left common carotid artery. The artery is punctured by an 18-gauge Teflon-sheathed needle retrograde into the left common carotid artery. After the satisfactory needle puncture, the Teflon needle is advanced down the common carotid artery, and a scout film is obtained to check the position of the needle within the arterial lumen. Two contrast injections are then obtained. The first is of the aortic arch to observe the origin of the left common carotid artery and extracranial bifurcation. The second injection is made to observe the intracranial internal carotid artery with biplane examination (Fig. 1.15).

The injection of the aortic arch and neck is made with a total of 18 cc of iodinated contrast at a rate of 12 cc/sec, and the neck and head examination is performed with an injection of 18 cc of contrast at 10 cc.sec.

The advantages of this technique are that the artery is punctured below the possible diseased carotid bifurcation and that since the injection is made in this retrograde manner, the contrast bolus that eventually is directed intracranially arrives in a physiologic state. This technique allows contrast to mix with blood within the common carotid artery, and this mixture is carried by the normal arterial pressure present. With the femoral technique, the catheter is placed within the common carotid artery and the contrast bolus is introduced by an artificial pressure induced by the pressure of the mechanical injector used.

A recent technologic advance, digital intravenous angiography,[8] promises to aid in the evaluation of patients with cerebrovascular disease. Utilizing this technique, the fluoroscopic image is converted to a digital signal. This digitized information can then be put through a host of computerized manipulations, in particular, electronic subtraction with logarithmic density enhancement, edge enhancement, and image smoothing. These techniques produce a dramatic improvement in visualization of intra-

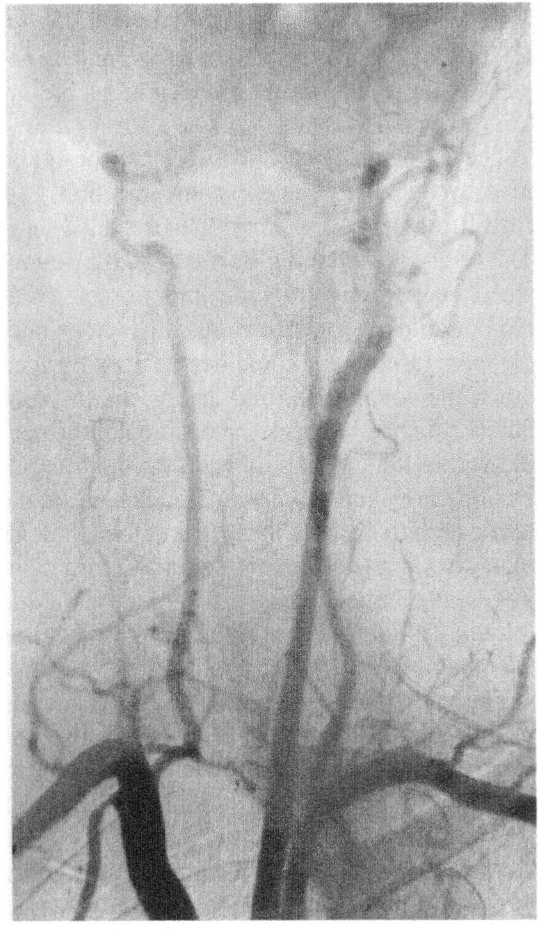
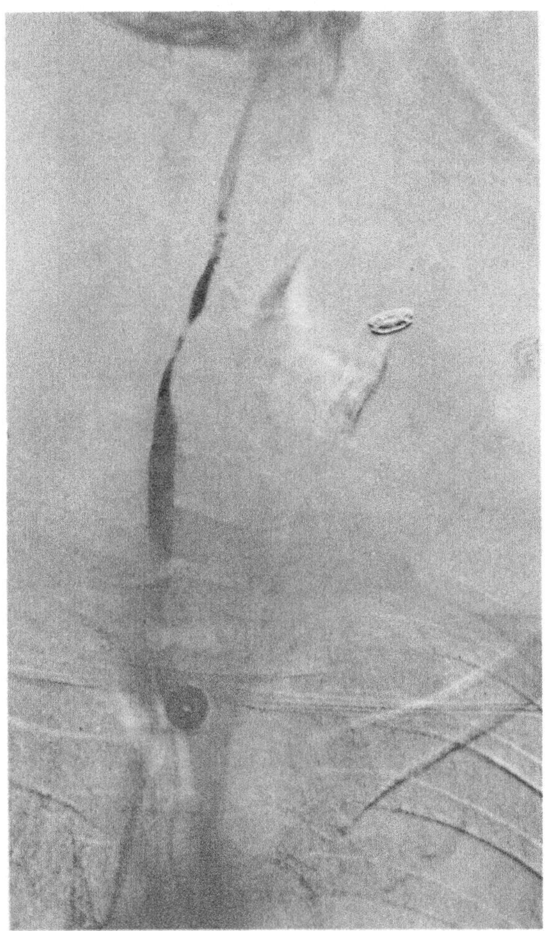

Figure 1.5. Patient with TIA and left hemiparesis. **A.** Aortic arch examination demonstrates markedly slow filling of right common carotid artery which is not well seen on this examination. **B.** Selective oblique injection of right common carotid artery demonstrates slow filling and emptying of right common and internal carotid arteries. Marked segmental stenosis and irregularity of carotid bifurcation and proximal internal carotid artery are present. The external carotid artery is occluded at the bifurcation.

vascular contrast material. Using the standard angiographic techniques, a concentration of 40% to 50% contrast material must be obtained for good visualization of vascular structures, whereas with digitalized flurography, images of similar quality may be obtained with only 2% to 3% contrast concentration. This concentration of contrast material may be obtained with an intravenous (rather than intra-arterial) injection. Thus, with digital fluorography, high-quality aortic arch angiography may be obtained following power injection of a large bolus of contrast material into the subclavian vein or superior vena cava. The use of an intravenous route produces a much less invasive and therefore less dangerous study, which in most instances can be performed on an outpatient basis. This procedure is replacing arch angiography in those patients in whom selective catheterization of individual vessels is felt to be unnecessary. Digital intravenous fluorography would therefore be of value in assessing several problems, including the following: (1) the effect of surgical and/or medical therapy on cerebrovascular atherosclerosis; (2) as a screening procedure for patients with minimal clinical evidence of cerebrovascular disease (e.g., asymptomatic bruits), especially in patients in whom other surgical procedures, such as cardiac surgery are contemplated; (3) the evaluation of patients in whom intra-arterial angiography is contraindicated because of the pa-

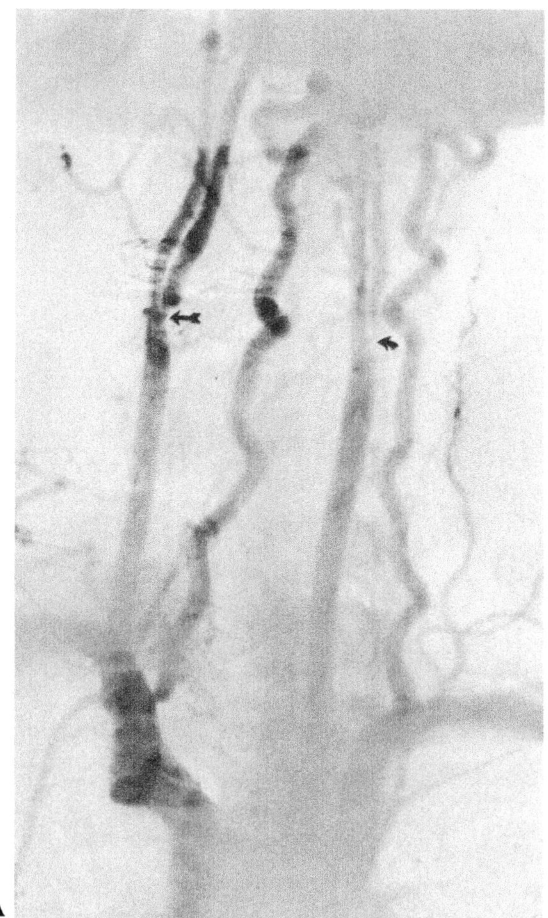

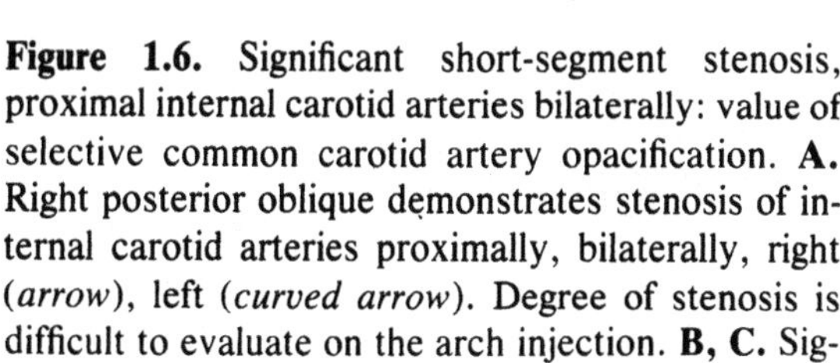

Figure 1.6. Significant short-segment stenosis, proximal internal carotid arteries bilaterally: value of selective common carotid artery opacification. **A.** Right posterior oblique demonstrates stenosis of internal carotid arteries proximally, bilaterally, right (*arrow*), left (*curved arrow*). Degree of stenosis is difficult to evaluate on the arch injection. **B, C.** Significant short-segment stenosis of proximal internal carotid arteries is observed beginning at the carotid bifurcation. A marked degree of stenosis is evident on these lateral projections (*right arrow* and *left curved arrow*) and not easily appreciated in the aortic arch examination **(A).**

tient's medical status, (e.g., elderly patients with systemic disease) or of patients with known severe diffuse atherosclerotic disease.

Complications of Angiography

Complication rates currently have been reduced. In a series reported by Huckman et al[27] comparing transfemoral catheter examinations to direct puncture techniques, the incidence of serious complications were less than 0.5% and ranged generally from 0.18% to 0.28%. Transient neurologic complications varied from 2.1% to 3.6% in these patients. Mani et al[46] reviewed 5,000 cases examined with transfemoral catheterization only. Permanent complications were 0.1% and were similar in both nontraining and training hospitals. Transient complications in the same series performed in hospitals training radiologists were 3.9% and in nontraining hospitals, 0.9%. Mani and Eisenberg,[44] further evaluating complications in these same cases relative to the disease process, reported complications of 1.2% to 1.9% in patients examined for cerebrovascular disease, trauma, subarachnoid hemorrhage, and after neurosurgical procedures. An incidence of less than 0.36% was

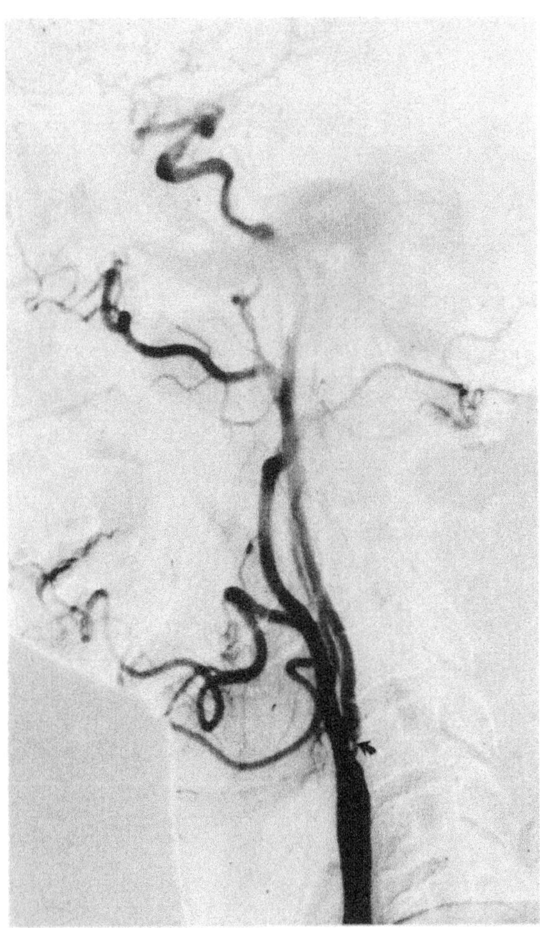

Figure 1.6. C.

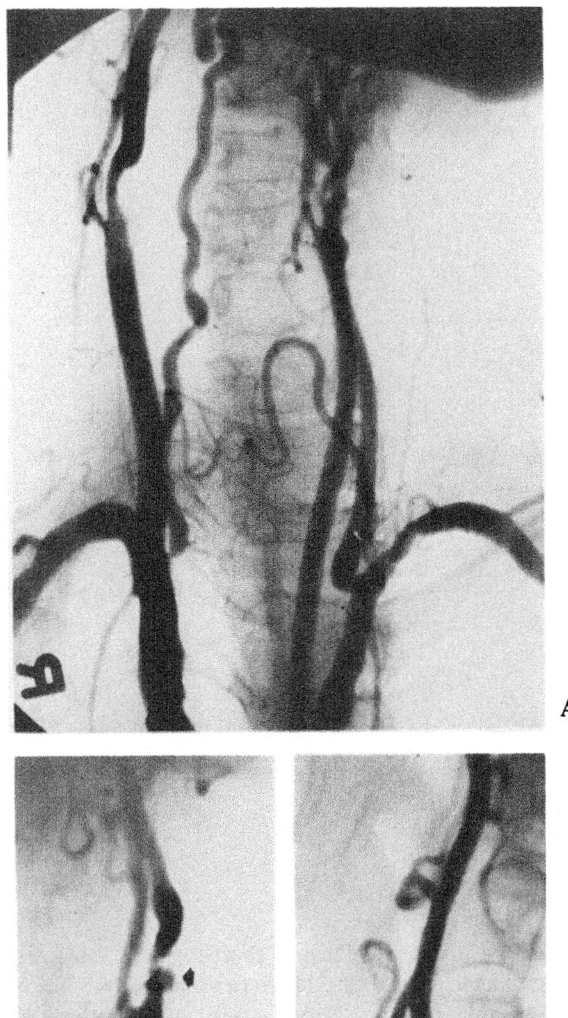

A

B C

Figure 1.7. Patient with diffuse extracranial and intracranial cerebrovascular disease. The advantages of selective injection for evaluation of the carotid bifurcation as opposed to arch injection is observed. **A.** Right posterior oblique study demonstrated diffuse extracranial vascular disease with atherosclerotic plaques in the innominate artery, both subclavian arteries, and at the origin of the right vertebral artery. Stenotic lesions of both proximal internal carotid arteries are seen. Ulceration, however, is not identified with certainty, and evaluation of bifurcation is limited. **B, C.** Left common carotid artery injection, arterial phase, demonstrates diffuse stenotic lesion affecting carotid bifurcation and proximal internal carotid over 1 cm, with a posterior lateral ulceration (*arrowhead*).

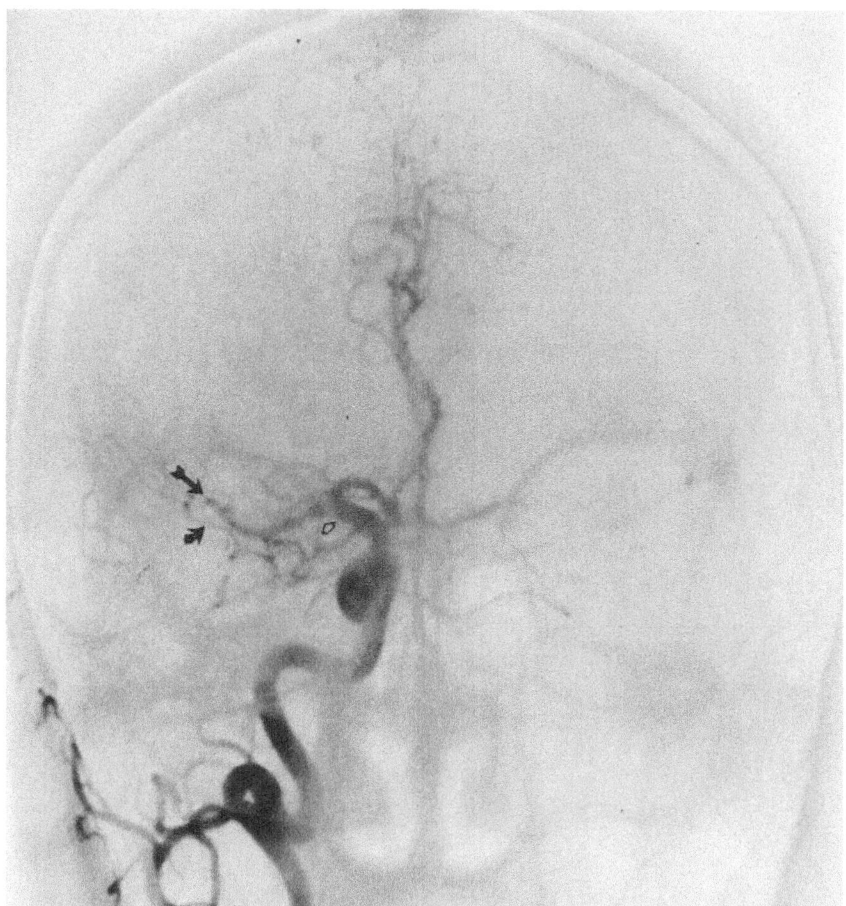

Figure 1.8. Middle cerebral artery occlusion. **A.** On the right common carotid artery injection, abrupt occlusion of horizontal segment of middle cerebral artery (*large arrow*) is identified in the Caldwell projection. A temporal branch of the middle cerebral artery (*curved arrow*) is opacified since it arises from the more proximal portion of the middle cerebral artery (*open arrowhead*). **B.** Left common carotid artery injection demonstrates collateral filling of right middle cerebral artery (*black arrowheads*) from leptomeningeal collaterals from the right anterior cerebral artery. Note the normal middle cerebral artery on the left common carotid artery injection in the Caldwell projection.

found in patients with tumor, seizure, and headache. In another paper, these authors[45] evaluated the effects of the number of arteries injected, patient age, contrast material used, and duration of procedure as an effect on complications. Duration of procedures greater than 80 minutes was an important factor, particularly in patients over 60 years old with cerebrovascular disease or tumor. Volume of contrast seemed to be important only if the agents contained sodium. The number of arteries injected did not appear to be an important factor.

The complication rate, therefore, in the current modes used are significantly low if reasonable care and skill are used.[43] One should be particularly careful in examining the patient with cerebrovascular disease or diffuse intracranial diseases involving brain parenchyma or blood vessels, since prolonged circulation time with added contact time of contrast increases patient risk.[4] The use of anticoagulants in the saline solution for flushing the artery is also necessary to reduce emboli. Prolonged examinations should be avoided, and after a reasonable period of examination time, the study should be discontinued. Remember, there is always another day!

Another important point is that in the interval between each injection into an artery, a reasonable delay is necessary to permit parenchymal

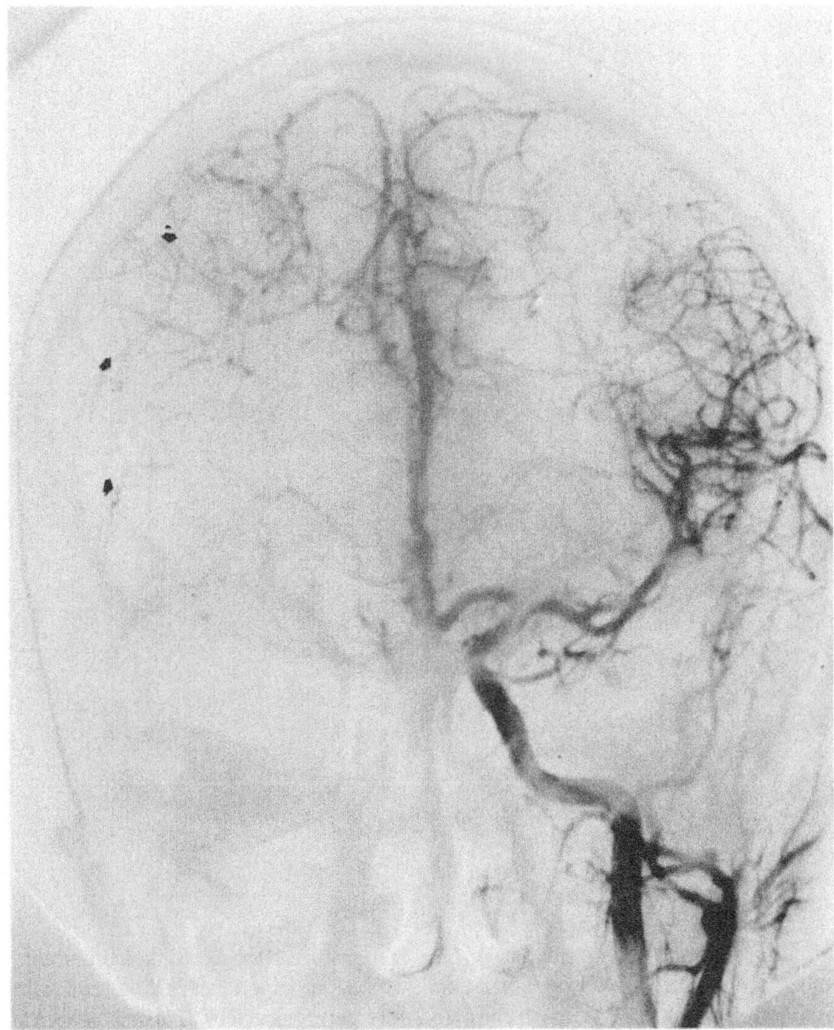

Fig. 1.8B

recovery from the previous injection. If sequential examinations of the same artery are performed without a suitable delay of up to 10 minutes, complications may occur.

Atherosclerotic Cerebrovascular Disease

Plain roentgenograms may reveal the presence of calcification as a consequence of damage to the intima in an atherosclerotic plaque. The identification of calcium in the cervical region may be a clue to the presence of extracranial vascular disease, although calcification may often be found in ansymptomatic patients.

Stenosis of the common or internal carotid artery that is hemodynamically significant may result in reduction of blood flow to the brain. The arterial caliber may also be reduced by a plaque in the distal internal carotid artery.[26] In the patient with significant stenosis of the common carotid artery, the external carotid artery may fill prior to or coincident with the internal carotid artery[26] (Fig. 1.21). The most common site of vascular disease is at the bifurcation of the common carotid artery or proximal internal carotid artery in 85% of cases.[22] Disease affecting the proximal portion of the common carotid artery is uncommon. In those exceptional cases, selective opacification of the affected common carotid artery should be avoided and

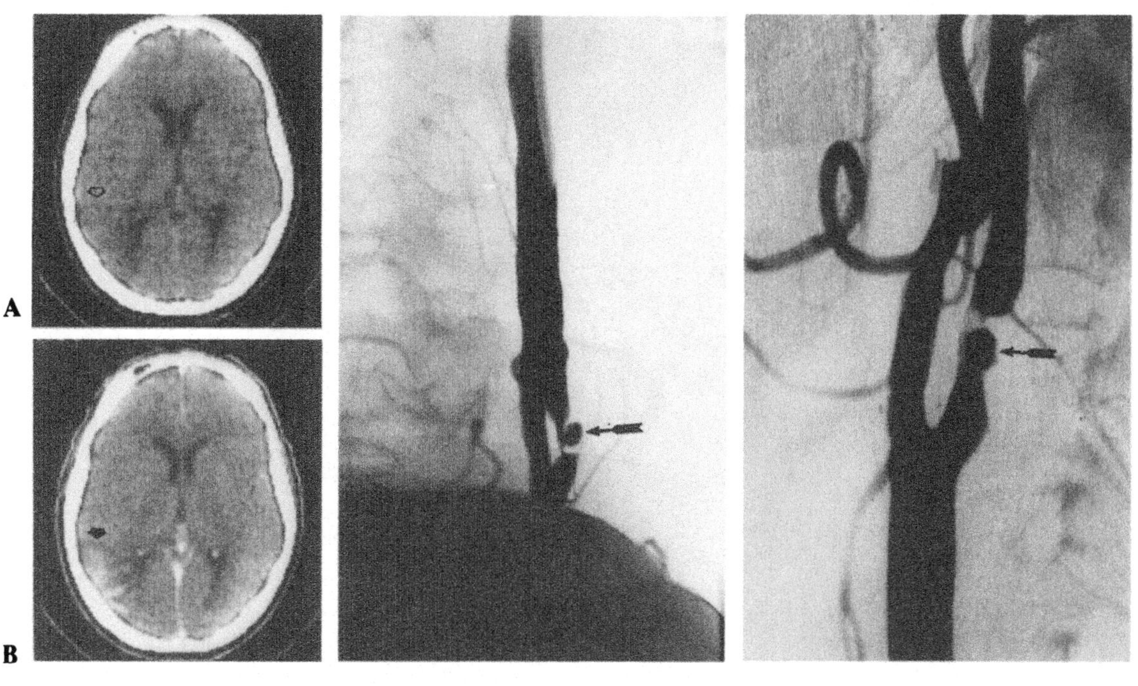

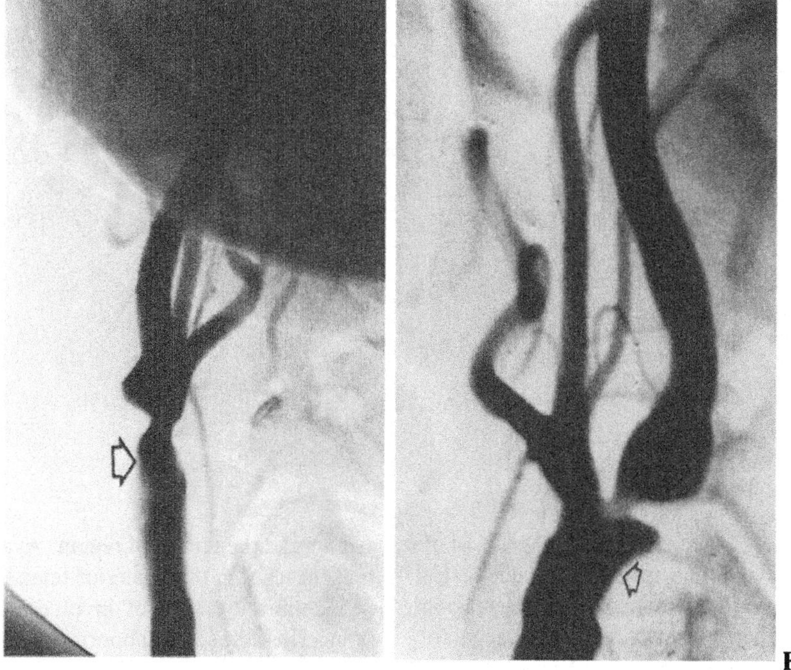

Figure 1.9. Patient with transient weakness of the right arm and leg. Serial CT scans demonstrated persistent left gyral blush and cortical enhancement, suggesting a cerebral infarct. The lesion was persistent so it was necessary to exclude lymphoma or neoplasm. **A.** Noncontrast CT scan demonstrates mixed density lesion in left posterior parietal region (*open arrowhead*) with minimal compression of the atrium and occipital horn. **B.** Similar section after contrast opacification demonstrates a cortical and gyral blush in left posterior parietal region (*closed arrowhead*). These findings are rather characteristic of a zone of hyperperfusion with a loss of cerebral autoregulation. **C, D.** 98% stenosis of proximal left internal carotid artery is demonstrated with a large ulcerated plaque (*arrow*). **E, F.** On the asymptomatic right side, plaque is observed along posterior lateral wall of the distal common carotid artery (*open arrow-*

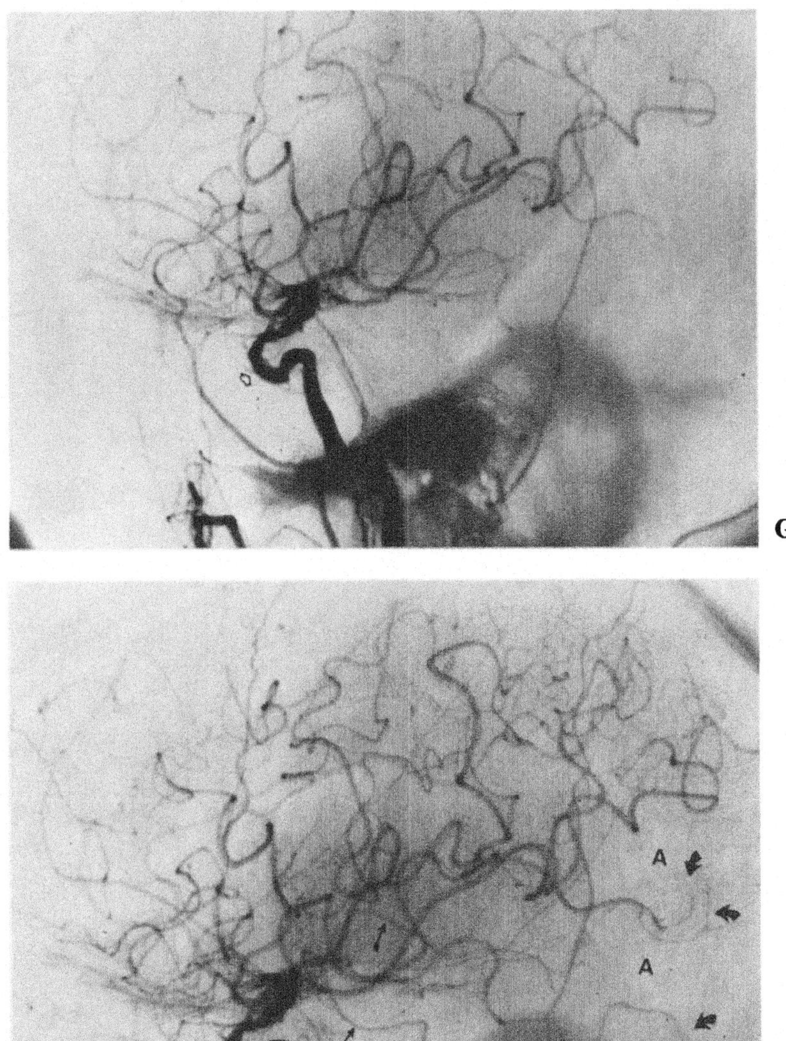

head) and a short segment, 85% stenosis, of the proximal internal carotid artery is observed. **G.** Lateral projection, left common carotid arteriogram, early arterial phase, shows arterial irregularity within cavernous carotid artery segment (*open arrowhead*). **H.** One second later, in the midarterial phase, stretching and spreading of midtemporal arterial branches is observed (*arrows*). This is due to swelling in the temporal region. Avascular zones are present also, in the posterior temporoparietal region **(A)** confirming area of involvement noted on CT scan. These vascular abnormalities are probably on the basis of emboli (*curved arrows*). **I.** In the intermediate phase, overlying the upper portion of the avascular zone **(A),** hypervascularity is observed **(V)** **Fig. 1.9I** see next page.

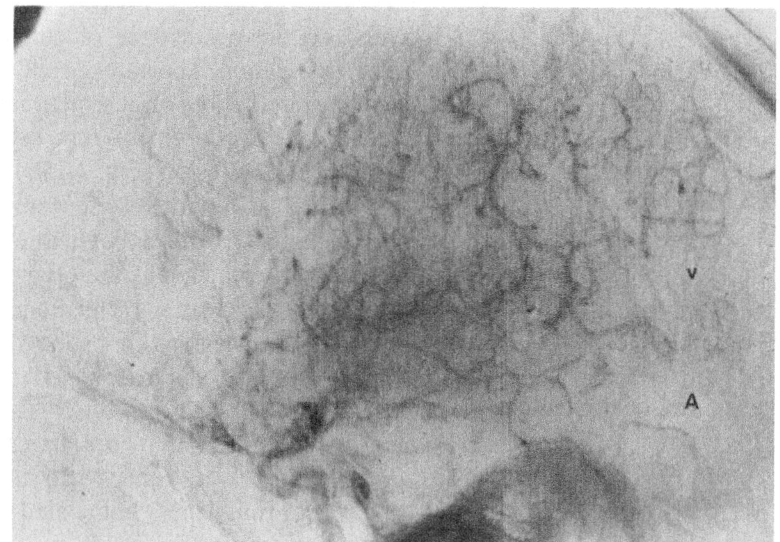

Fig. 1.9I

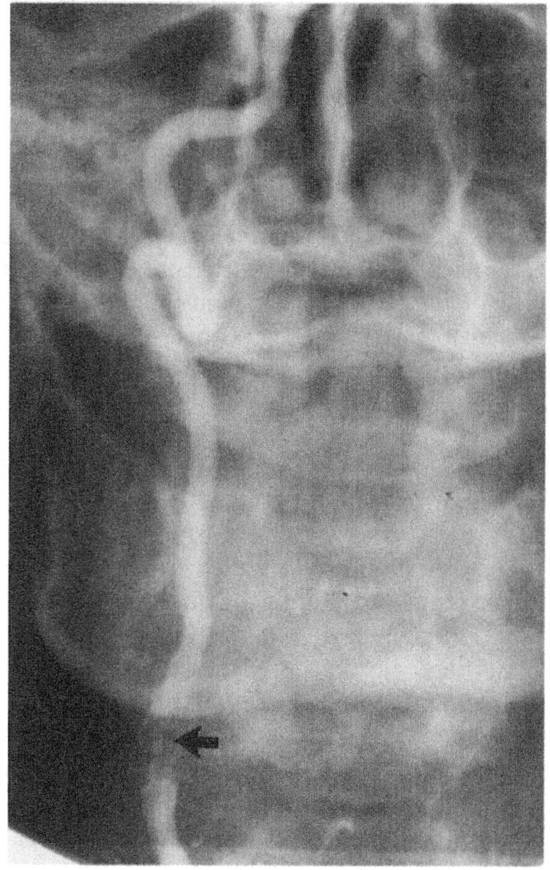

A

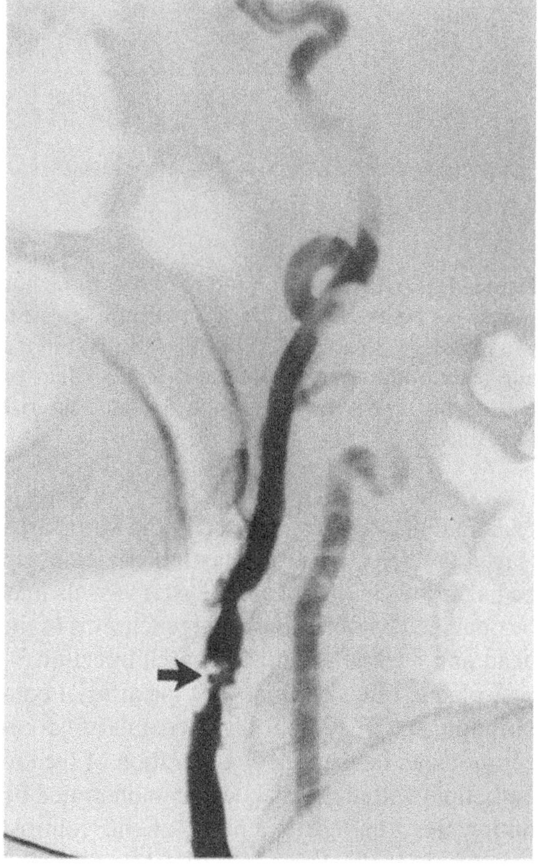

B

Figure 1.10. Patient with irregular stenotic plaque within carotid artery which simulates ulceration. **A, B.** Right common carotid arteriogram demonstrates a marked constriction with superimposed nodular collections of contrast that do not project beyond the vessel wall and are therefore considered to be trapped in crevices within a roughened plaque, rather than true ulceration. This was confirmed at surgery.

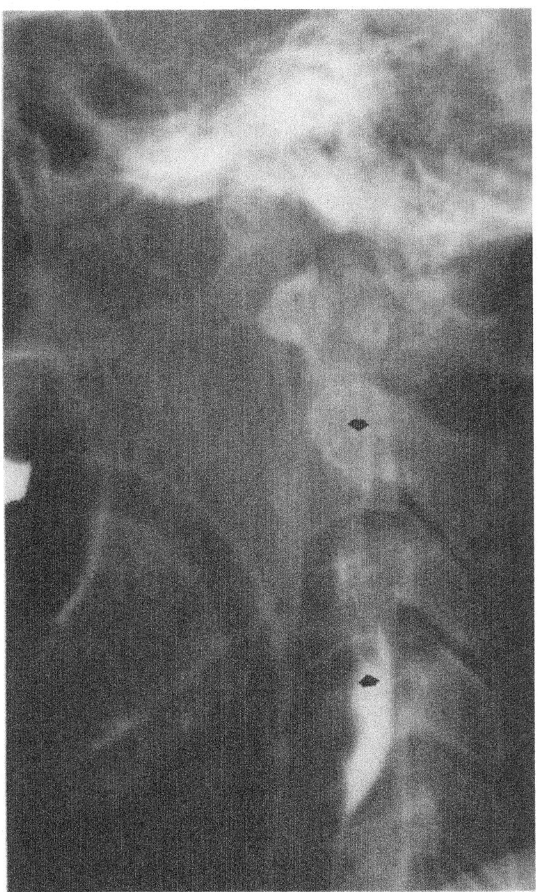

Figure 1.11. Presence of intra-arterial thrombus should not be overlooked. In this patient a low density is observed partially outlined by contrast in the internal carotid artery at the level of C2-3 (*closed arrowheads*), which represents an intra-arterial thrombus.

examination should be limited to the aortic arch (Fig. 1.2). Selective arterial catheterization can be hazardous in these cases. Distal vessels may be opacified by obtaining roentgenograms of the head and neck after an aortic arch injection.[16]

A plaque often accounts for the arterial constriction, and frequently slight irregularity or ulceration can be identified. Ulceration of the endothelium within the plaque is demonstrated by noting the apparent extension of the contrast beyond the luminal margin during arteriography (Fig. 1.9C,D).[30,42] The most common location for an ulcerated plaque is the common carotid artery bifurcation, although infrequently ulceration has been observed at other sites.[31] According to Kishore et al,[31] ulcerated or roughened plaques are more likely to cause neurologic symptoms than smooth plaques. The reasons for this are the occurrence of emboli due to platelet aggregation. The latter result from damage to the endothelium or basement membrane, while atherosclerotic emboli can escape from the surface of the lesion (Fig. 1.15B).

In a study of 177 patients with transient ischemic attacks (TIA) the radiographic diagnosis of stenosis or occlusion at the cervical carotid bufurcation was made. A correlation was found between smooth lesions in patients with less than 50% stenosis and roughened plaques in those with greater constrictions.[20] The correlation of the interpretation by the surgeon and the neuroradiologist was good when the lesions were larger or roughened, but tended to be poor with minimal lesions.[20]

Fields and Lemac[19] demonstrated that 79% of patients with TIA had a lesion on the appropriate side. The majority of patients who developed stroke had hypertension or cardiac symptoms. Sixty percent of the patients with TIA had no further symptoms during the follow-up period.

Edwards et al[13] reviewed the cerebral angiograms of a series of patients operated on for TIA or cerebral infarction. The insensitivity of cerebral angiography is pointed out in that of 20 ulcers identified at surgery, only 12 were identified angiographically, and, conversely, of 30 patients with ulcers not present at surgery, 17 patients were diagnosed as having ulcerations at the time of angiography. In these false positive cases at surgery, the authors observed intramural hemorrhage and subintimal hematomas[14] in 10 cases as the cause of radiographic defect.

Stenosis at the origin of the vertebral artery is often recognized. Rarely the distal vertebral artery is affected.

Martin et al[47] demonstrated the frequency of extracranial vascular disease in 100 consecutive patients over aged 50 examined post mortem. Forty patients had at least one vessel with greater than 50% stenosis; 11 patients had occlusions of at least one vessel; and in three patients, two or more vessels were affected. Whisnant et al,[63] reviewing the same 100 cases, demonstrated that in patients with marked cervical carotid artery stenosis, 71% had cerebral ischemic symptoms, while 30% were asymptomatic. Symptomatic patients had more severe

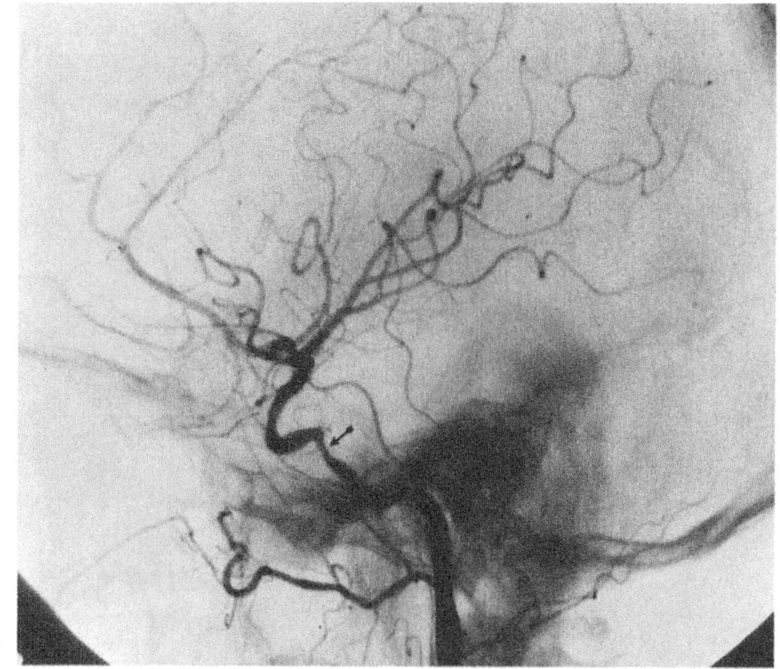

A

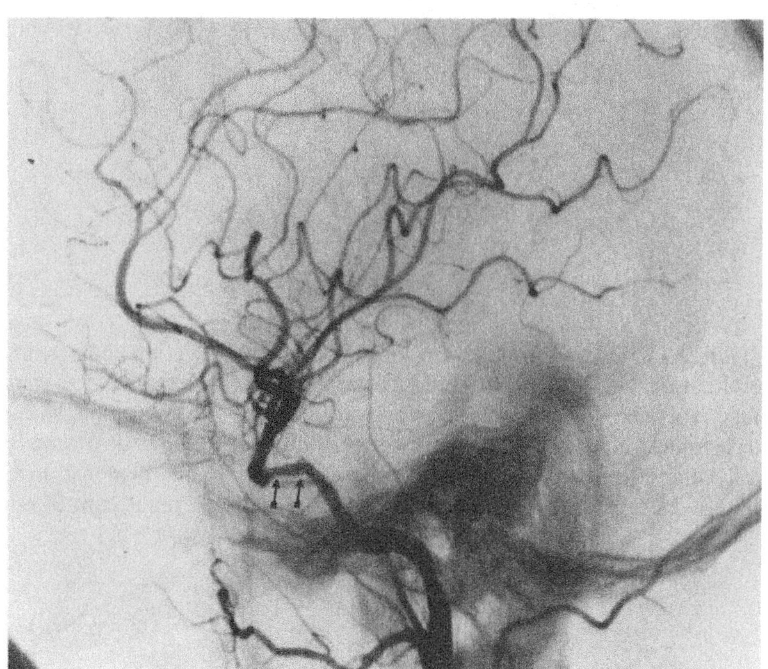

B

Figure 1.12. Cavernous carotid disease in a 38-year-old female patient with diabetes and TIA. Lateral projections after right and left common carotid artery injections demonstrate focal atherosclerotic narrowing of both cavernous carotid arteries (*arrows*).

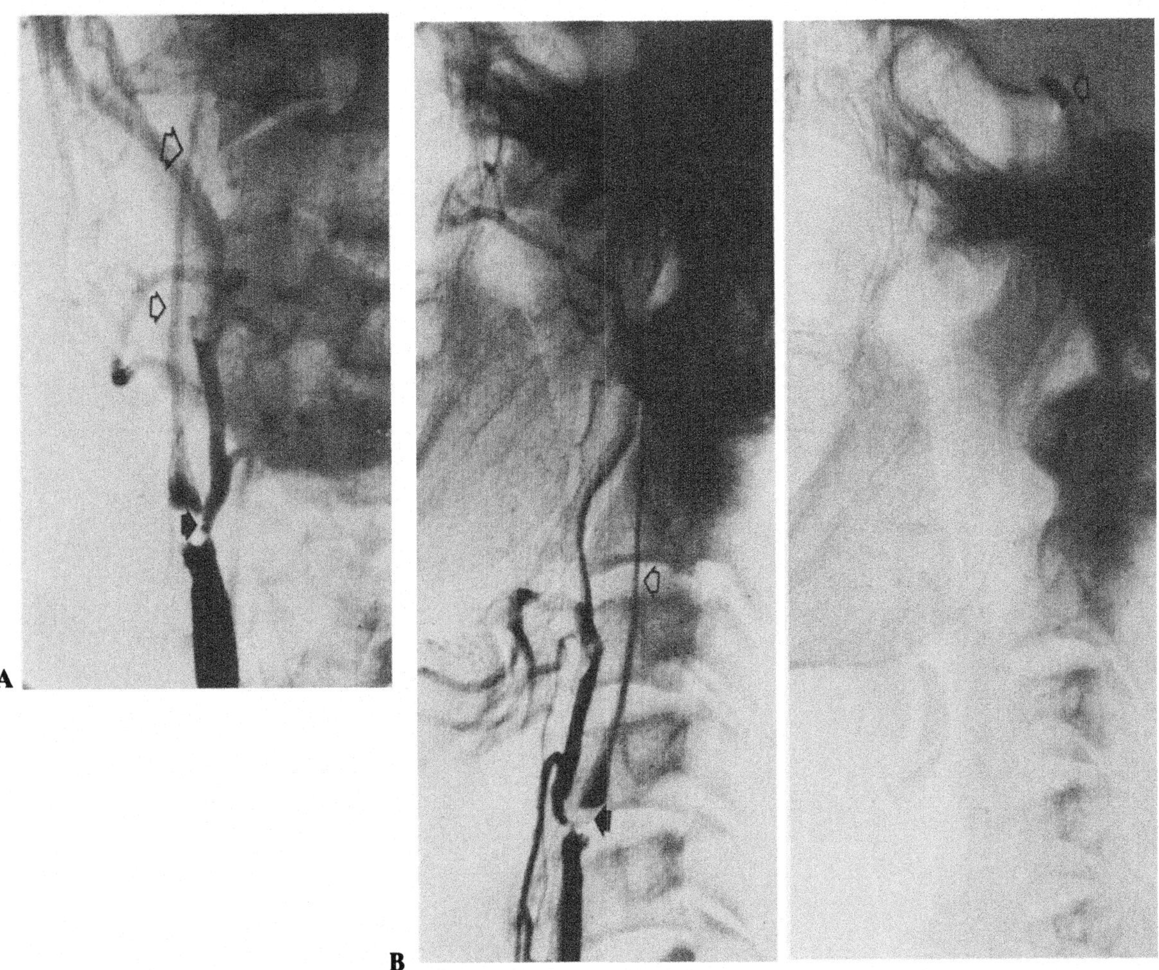

Figure 1.13. Patient with severe stenosis of carotid bifurcation with delayed filling of internal carotid artery. The internal carotid artery is patent. **A, B.** Anterior posterior, and lateral projections of the neck following injection of the right common carotid artery reveal a 95% stenosis affecting the carotid bifurcation and proximal internal and external carotid arteries (*closed arrowheads*). A string sign indicating slow runoff within the internal carotid is observed (*open arrowheads*). **C.** A lateral film at the end of 12 sec demonstrates delayed opacification of the cavernous carotid artery (*open arrowhead*).

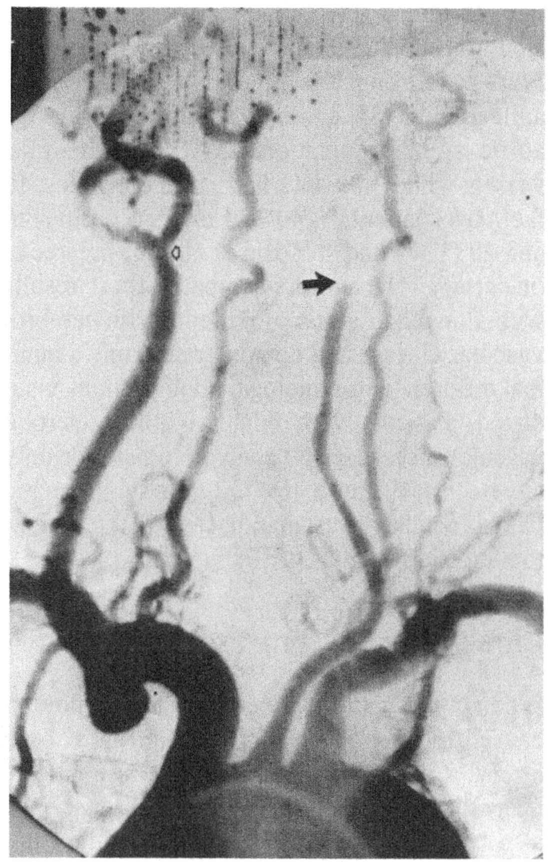

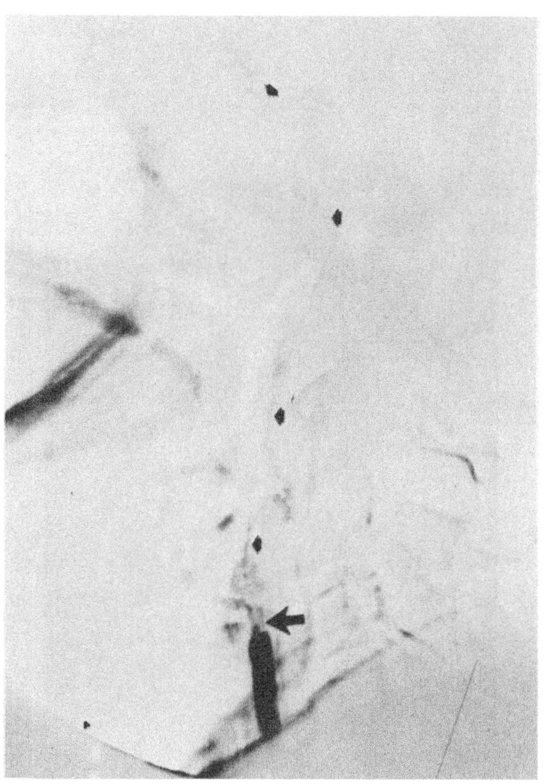

Figure 1.14. Slow flow in internal carotid artery beginning at carotid bifurcation. The patient is an 81-year-old female with intermittent TIAs over a 3-yr period with speech arrest. Two years prior to admission, the patient had a right hemiparesis with aphasia, which virtually resolved. Then, two days prior to admission, the patient developed transient aphasia over 2 hr. The internal carotid is ribbonlike from the internal carotid origin to the cavernous carotid because of poor runoff. **A.** The aortic arch examination demonstrates minimal stenotic plaque along the medial wall of the right carotid artery bifurcation (*open arrowhead*). On the left, severe narrowing of the common carotid artery, just below the bifurcation (*arrow*) is present. **B.** Left common carotid artery injection in the midarterial phase demonstrates delayed emptying of common carotid artery with constriction and arterial irregularity at the bifurcation (*arrow*). The internal carotid above the bifurcation is seen as a string and is opacified to the level of the carotid siphon (*arrowheads*). This suggests a poor runoff due to a stenotic plaque below or possibly a stenotic plaque or occlusion distal to the carotid siphon.

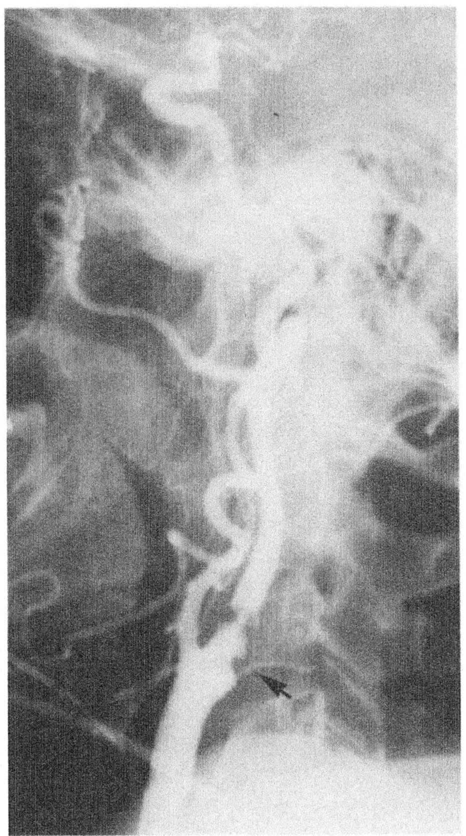
A

B

intracranial disease. Cervical carotid arterial stenosis or occlusion were not necessarily related to the patients' complaints.[63] This conclusion was substantiated by a study performed by Faris et al[17] on 43 asymptomatic prisoners examined clinically and by arch aortography. On aortic arch examinations, 54% had abnormal vessels while only 46% had normal arteries. In fact, two patients (4%) had arterial occlusion, and 20 (23%) had stenosis of 50% or greater of one artery. The authors compared these results with a matched group of patients with cerebrovascular disease and demonstrated only a minimal difference in radiologic abnormalities visualized. Patients with bilateral atherosclerotic vascular disease may be asymptomatic or only have a bruit (Fig. 1.16). Often a symptomatic patient will have vascular disease on the asymptomatic side (Fig. 1.9 E,F).

Intracranial Cerebrovascular Disease

When a reduction in cerebral blood flow is caused by involvement of the internal carotid artery, a bypass or shunting procedure may be necessary (Fig. 1.12). Segmental disease may also be identified in the proximal middle cerebral artery proximal to the trifurcation, at the trifurcation, or affecting one or major distal branches (Figs. 1.8, 1.17). Occlusion or severe stenosis of the proximal anterior cerebral artery is rare.

Intracranial vascular disease may be focal, multifocal, or disseminated. The vascular pat-

Figure 1.15. Retrograde left carotid arteriogram with ulceration of internal carotid and radiologic evidence of emboli. The patient developed no symptoms despite radiologic observations of emboli on arteriogram. **A.** Retrograde left carotid anteriogram demonstrates marked constriction of internal carotid with an ulcer situated posteriorly (*arrow*) below the constriction. Good filling is noted above the area of stenosis. **B.** Lateral projection, intermediate phase; delayed emptying of a convexity middle cerebral artery is noted, probably as a result of embolic material from atheromatous ulcer within the neck. (Reprinted with permission from *Neuroradiology;* Burrows and Leeds, 1981, Churchill Livingstone Inc.)

terns are often mixed with arterial irregularity, stenosis, and/or occlusion. Intracranial vascular disease as a result of atherosclerotic disease may be difficult to discriminate from other forms of arterial involvement. One must look for the presence of the characteristic notchlike defect usually identified along one wall (Fig. 1.18). The identification of this arterial defect should enable one to establish a diagnosis of atherosclerotic vascular disease. The plaque may be circumferential and involve short or long segments and be multiple. In these instances, histologic diagnosis may be difficult.[18]

In intracranial vascular disease, in addition to the arterial plaques or stenosis, vasodilatation due to hypoxia[39] may occur. In addition, various hemodynamic changes can be identified. These include delayed arterial emptying due to reduced flow as a result of arterial stenosis. In some cases, a paucity or absence of arteries may be observed as a result of arterial occlusion. Collateral channels may be identified. In some instances a zone of increased vascularity may be identified as a consequence of a profusion of collateral channels in the area,[36] or as a result of hyperperfusion.[39] A variety of vascular patterns characteristic of intracranial occlusions in childhood as described by Hilal et al[23,24] may also be identified in adults. These include basal arterial occlusion without telangiectasia, basal occlusion with telangiectasia (Moya Moya disease), primary distal branch occlusion, and small artery disease.

Luxury Perfusion

Lassen[32] in 1966 described the concept of "luxury perfusion," which described a zone of increased cerebral flow as a result of a loss in cerebral autoregulation. The loss of cerebral autoregulation is the result of an accumulation of acid metabolites and carbon dioxide. Leeds and Goldberg[39] called this localized derangement of cerebral blood flow as recognized during cerebral angiography "hyperperfusion." This aberration is recognized as a process in evolution and varies with time. The abnormality occurs as a result of parenchymal damage, vascular changes, or both. The vascular patterns which are seen are related to the time after injury.

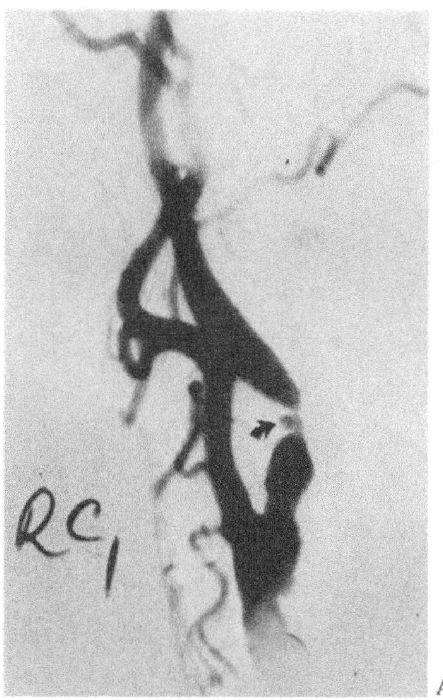

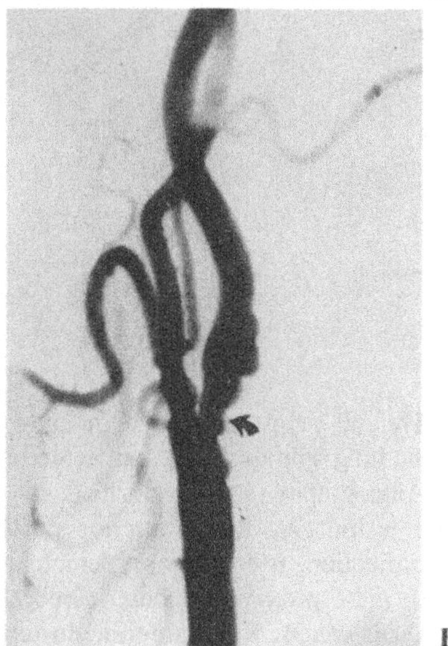

Figure 1.16. Asymptomatic patient with carotid bruit, bilateral extracranial vascular disease with marked stenosis and ulceration on right, and multiple ulcers with minimal stenosis on left. **A.** Right lateral carotid arteriogram demonstrates evidence of circumferential stenosis involving proximal internal carotid artery over 4 mm. The artery then dilates slightly. Approximately 2 cm above the bifurcation, a short segment of marked stenosis is seen with an ulcer projecting anteriorly (*curved arrow*) **B.** Left lateral carotid arteriogram shows slight stenosis with numerous ulcerations along posterior wall of common carotid and internal carotid arteries with one of the ulcerations marked by a *curved arrow*.

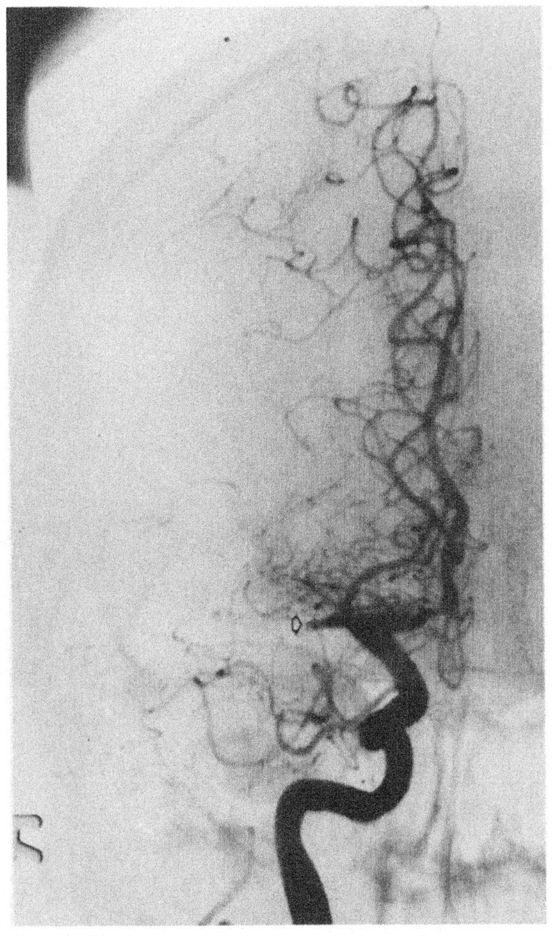

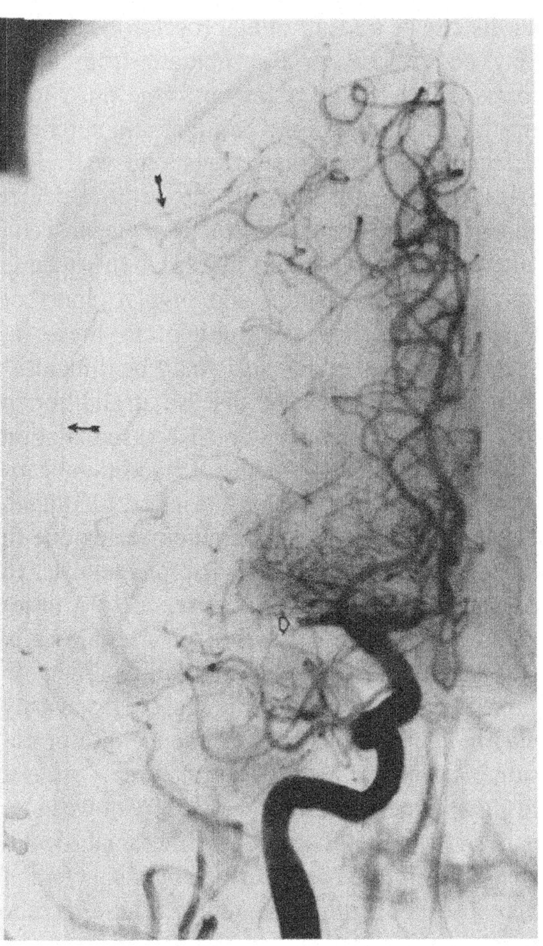

Figure 1.17. 60-Year-old male with known carcinoma of the lung who developed an acute left hemiparesis. Angiography was performed to exclude metastatic lesion. **A.** Right anterior posterior in Caldwell projection, arterial phase, demonstrates occlusion of right proximal middle cerebral artery (*open arrowhead*). **B.** Right anterior posterior projection, 2 sec later, again demonstrates middle cerebral occlusion (*open arrowhead*) with leptomeningeal collaterals (*arrows*) from anterior cerebral artery to middle cerebral artery. **C:** Right lateral projection, arterial phase, demonstrates middle cerebral occlusion with retrograde filling of middle cerebral artery via leptomeningeal collaterals from the anterior cerebral artery (*arrows*). An enlarged posterior lateral choroidal artery branch (*curved arrow*) of the posterior cerebral artery is also acting as a collateral.

The initial angiographic pattern[39] seen in the first seven to ten days is a stippled perivascular blush that represents dilatation of second- and third-order penetrating cortical arteries with or without an early filling vein. The early filling vein is denser than neighboring veins as a result of the open capillary bed due to the loss of cerebral autoregulation (Fig. 1.19).

The significant difference in increased density of the premature filling vein aids in distinguishing the benign process present from a neoplasm. As time passes, the hypervascular zone fades and the early filling vein fills later so that by three to six weeks, the abnormal zone may have a normal configuration. The abnormal vascular pattern is not observed within a vascular

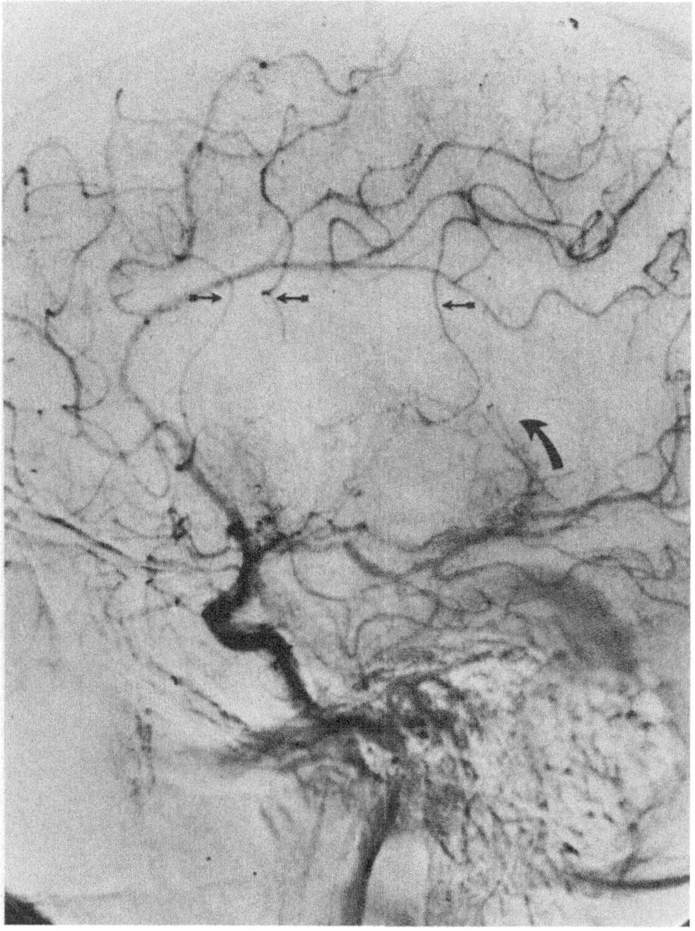

Fig. 1.17C

occlusion, but is present at the margin of the lesion.

The features that aid in distinguishing a "hyperperfusion stain" from a "neoplastic" stain are[39]

1. mass or shift is minimal
2. early filling veins identified are normal regional draining veins and are often significantly denser than neighboring veins
3. a time-course pattern is recognized
4. location of lesion limited to zones of cortical grey matter, superficial or deep (cortical surface, basal ganglia, and island of Reil).

A variety of pathologic lesions may affect blood vessels and can cause stenosis, occlusion, or aneurysm formation (Table 1.1).

The abnormalities identified are often similar since the artery affected can respond in only a limited number of ways, and differentiation of

Table 1.1. Arterial vascular disease in children and adults.

Hypertension
Diabetes mellitus
Collagen vascular disease
Intracranial arteritis
Infectious disease
Trauma
Neuroectodermal dysplasias (phakomatosis)
Cardiac origin
Drug abuse
Hematologic disorders
Metabolic disorders
Neoplasms
Radiation therapy
Undetermined origin
Basal arterial occlusion without telangiectasia
Basal occlusion with telangiectasia
Nontraumatic stenosis of the cervical internal carotid artery in children

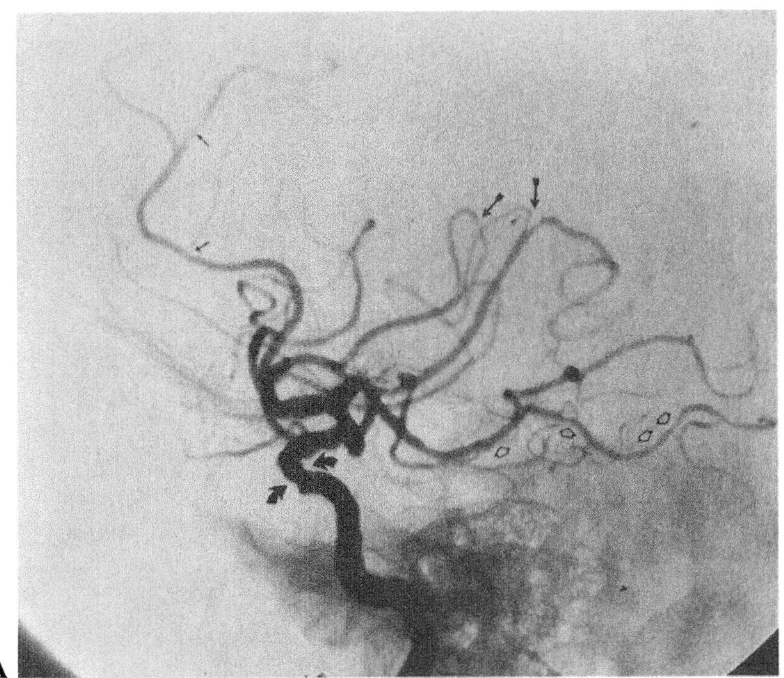

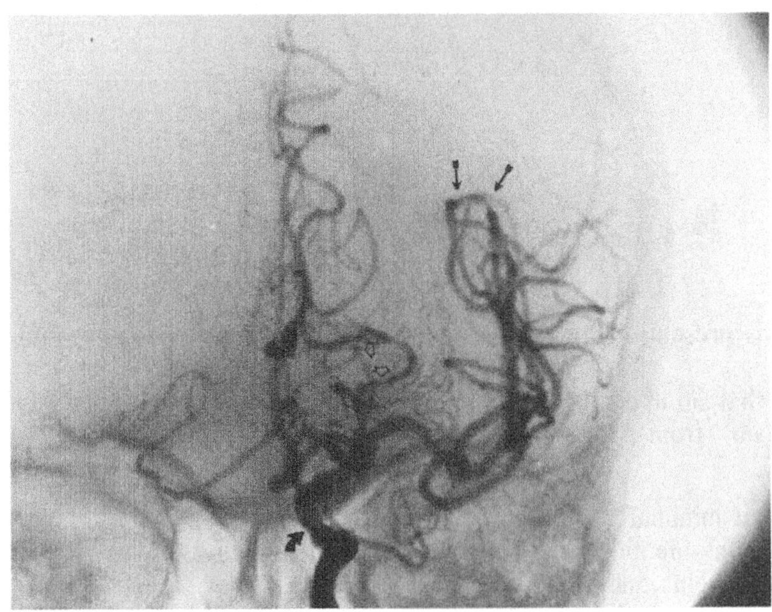

Figure 1.18. Patient with diffuse intracranial atherosclerosis. Common carotid artery injections in this patient with left cerebral TIAs demonstrate atherosclerotic involvement of the cavernous carotid artery (*curved arrows*), bilaterally. Aside from this typical location of atherosclerotic change, there is extensive involvement of the anterior cerebral artery distribution (*small arrows*), middle cerebral artery distribution (*large arrows*), and posterior cerebral artery distributions (*open arrows*). Note the atherosclerosis produces eccentric bitelike defects in the vessel, often at site of bifurcation. This is well demonstrated in **(A, B)** left common carotid arteriogram, where a large plaque is present at the bifurcation of the pericallosal artery into a large callosomarginal (*lower small arrow*) and small distal pericallosal branch. In this case, the most severe involvement is in both posterior cerebral artery distributions (*open arrowheads*) whereas middle cerebral artery involvement is more severe on the right (**C,** *larger arrows*).

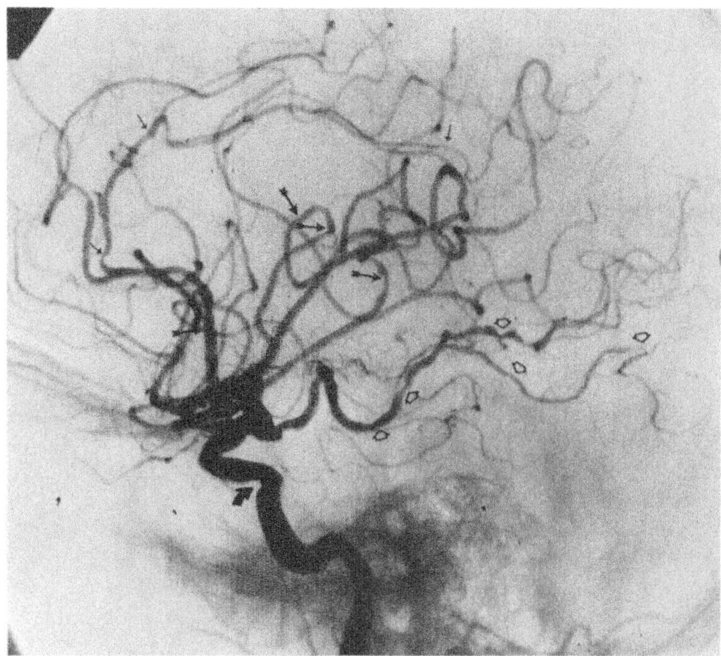

Fig. 1.18C

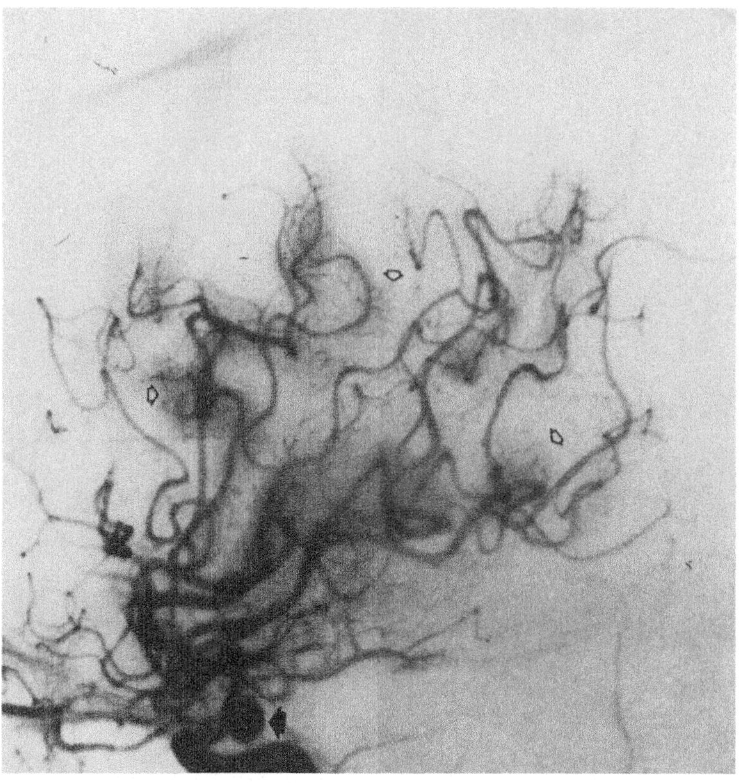

A

Figure 1.19. Patient with posterior communicating artery aneurysm with subarachnoid bleed and spasm who developed cerebral infarct. **A.** Left common carotid arteriogram, lateral projection, midarterial phase. A posterior communicating artery aneurysm is seen (*arrowhead*). Diffuse perivascular blush (hyperemic zone) is observed overlying middle cerebral artery distribution (*open arrowheads*). **B, C.** In the intermediate phase and early venous phase, dense, premature-filling veins are observed (*arrows*) draining the hyperemic zone (*open arrowheads*).

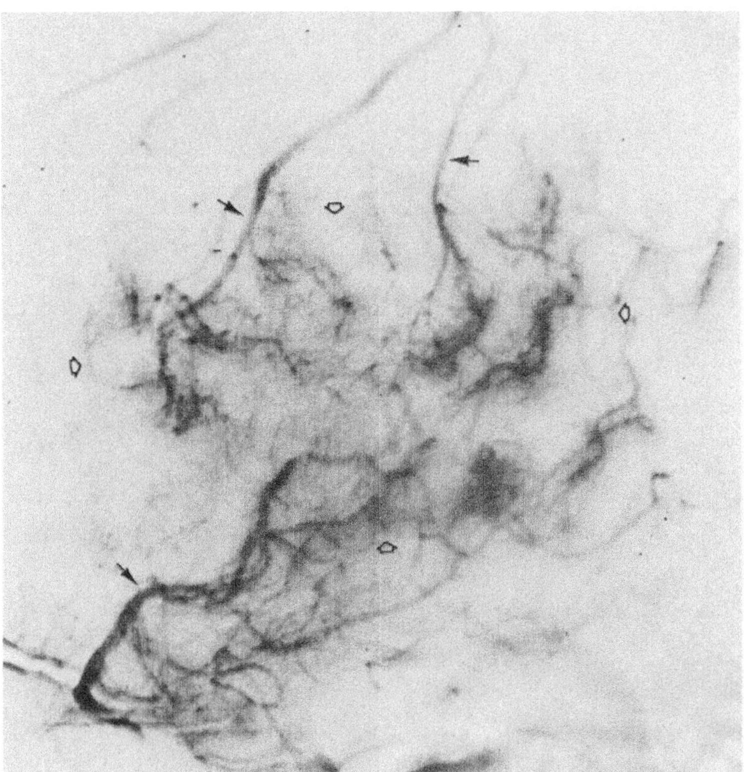

Fig. 1.19B

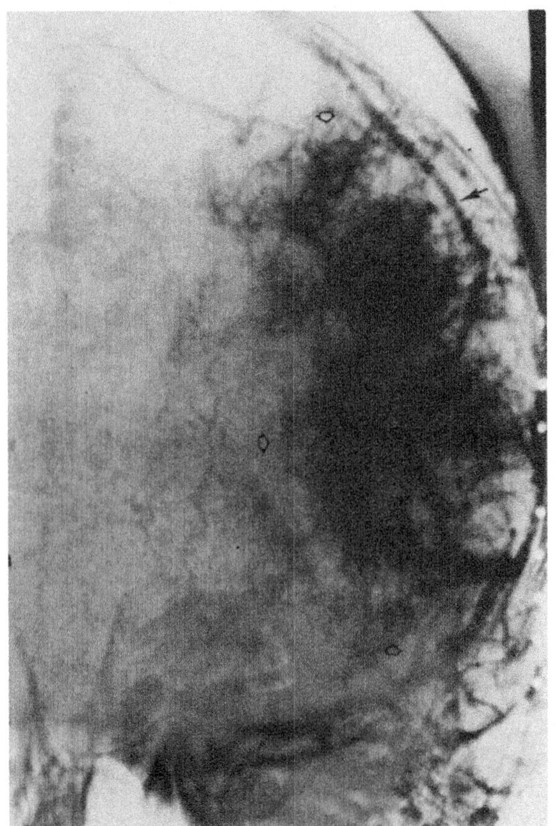

Fig. 1.19C

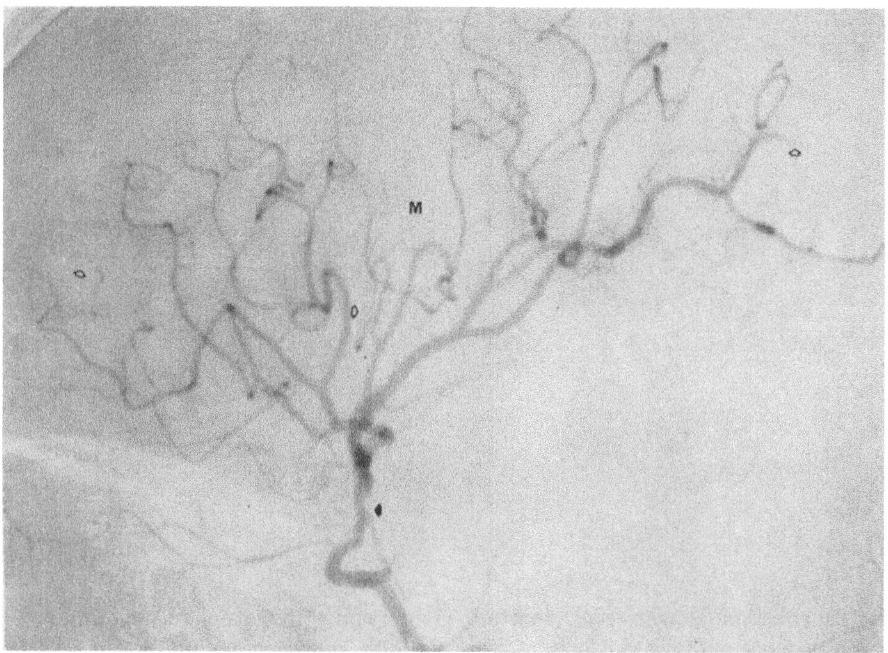

Figure 1.20. Patient with pyogenic meningitis, with involvement of supraclinoid internal carotid artery and intracranial arterial branches. Lateral projection, arterial phase, demonstrates constriction and irregularity of the supraclinoid internal carotid artery (*closed arrowhead*). Disseminated intracranial arterial irregularity and occlusions are seen (*open arrowheads*). A focal avascular zone is observed in the rolandic region, which is probably the result of arterial occlusion and swelling (*M*). All the changes manifested are the result of meningeal involvement by an inflammatory process resulting in involvement of basal and peripheral arteries.

the various processes is dependent on the age of patient, the clinical presentation and data. In some cases angiographic or computed tomography (CT) abnormalities may be specific.

Infectious Lesions

In the patient with meningitis, clinical presentation and laboratory data are often helpful.[12] Arterial involvement may be seen at the base (Fig. 1.20), or over the surface of the brain,[38] or both. Arterial lesions may be focal, multifocal, or disseminated. Arterial irregularity, stenosis, occlusion, or aneurysm may be visualized. In patients with tuberculous meningitis or pneumococcal meningitis, basal arteries are involved with occasional peripheral arterial involvement. In patients with *Hemophilus influenzae* meningitis, convexity arteries are more commonly involved, and subdural effusions can be identified.[38] In addition to arterial wall involvement, one can identify zones of hyperperfusion, collateral channels, or venous thrombosis.[38]

In the patient with encephalitis, no abnormality may be identified, or more likely, multifocal or diffuse vasoconstriction or vasodilatation (of surface ateries) may be visualized.

In intracerebral or epidural abscess, arterial wall changes in proximity to the collection of pus may be identified.[28,38] Subacute bacterial endocarditis may cause arterial irregularity, occlusion, or aneurysm.

Cranial arteritis[18] is an entity that is difficult to prove as the patients often survive the insult and no specific diagnostic tests are available. The majority of patients affected are young, from infancy to young adults. The vessels predominantly involved are larger vessels, including the internal carotid artery above the bifurcation, and major vessels at the base. Convexity vessels may be involved.[23,55,59] The lesions are usually smooth and may be focal, multifocal, or

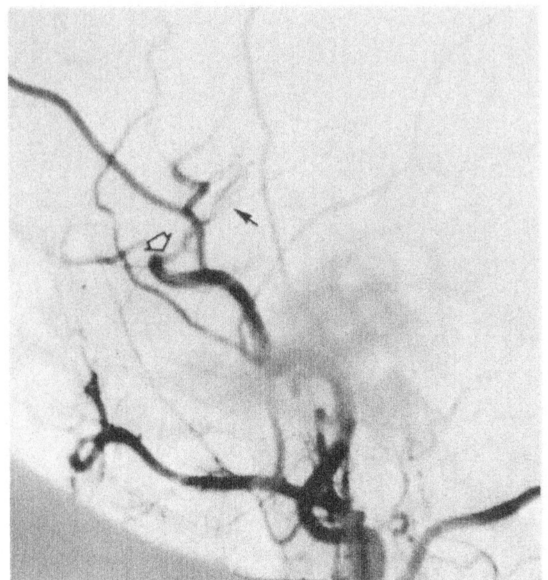

A

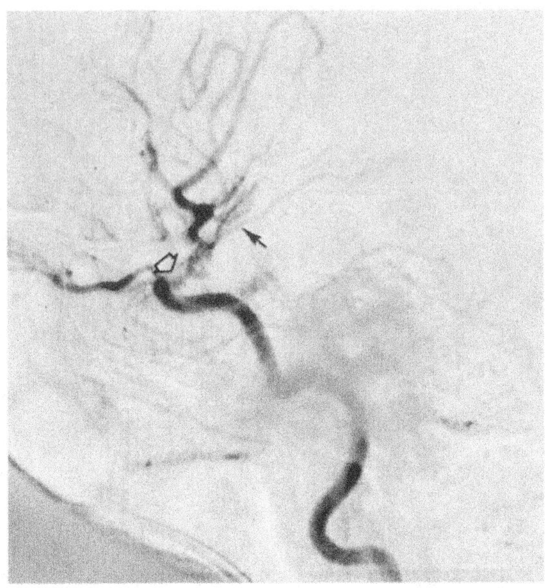

B

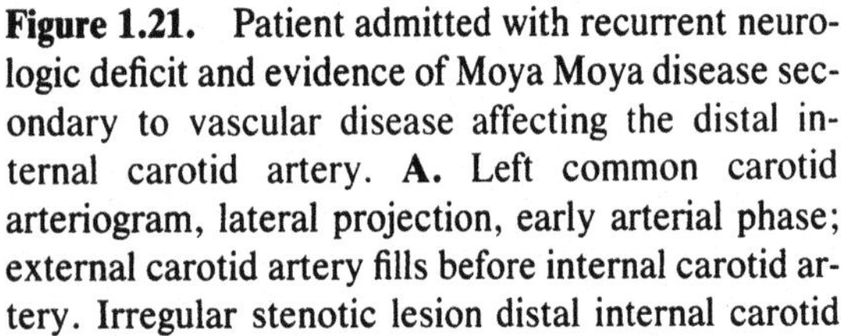

Figure 1.21. Patient admitted with recurrent neurologic deficit and evidence of Moya Moya disease secondary to vascular disease affecting the distal internal carotid artery. **A.** Left common carotid arteriogram, lateral projection, early arterial phase; external carotid artery fills before internal carotid artery. Irregular stenotic lesion distal internal carotid artery just above ophthalamic artery (*open arrowhead*). Telangiectatic blush at base is seen (*arrow*). **B.** Two seconds later, stenosis (*open arrowhead*) and basal telangiectatic blush (*arrow*) are still present due to slow flow. The middle cerebral artery is partially visualized.

disseminated. This entity is most commonly called Moya Moya when basal stenosis or occlusion occurs with a profusion of basal collaterals[23,48,59] (Fig. 1.21).

Collagen Vascular Disease

These lesions are similar to those seen with cranial arteritis, with involvement of extracranial, internal carotid, basal arteries or convexity branches.[18]

The arterial changes, in lupus erythematosus, include single or multiple vascular occlusions due to emboli,[6] or just diffuse cranial arteritis (Fig. 1.22). Peripheral aneurysms have been observed in patients with lupus erythematosus, periarteritis nodosa, and temporal (giant) arteritis.[18] Beading of blood vessels may be identified owing to contiguous segments of narrowing and dilatation.[6] Venous occlusions occur along or in combination with arterial disease.[6,18]

Hypertension

While the angiogram may be normal, a variety of changes may be identified in the patient with hypertension. Cole and Yates[10] and Ross Russel[53] demonstrated the selective involvement of the lenticulostriate arteries. Microaneurysms were demonstrated in 46 of 100 brains examined by Cole and Yates.[10] Leeds and Goldberg,[37] utilizing magnification angiography, demonstrated the following arterial changes in the lenticulostriate arteries: elongation, luminal irregularity, decrease in number, occlusion, dilatation, tortuosity, and microaneurysms (Fig. 1.23). Hemorrhage occurs often in the ganglionic region as a result of the microaneurysms and severe disease in the lenticulostriate arteries.

As a result of the hypertension, the following complications may develop: hypertensive encephalopathy, subarachnoid hemorrhage or intracerebral bleed, and a loss in cerebral autoregulation with resultant luxury perfusion

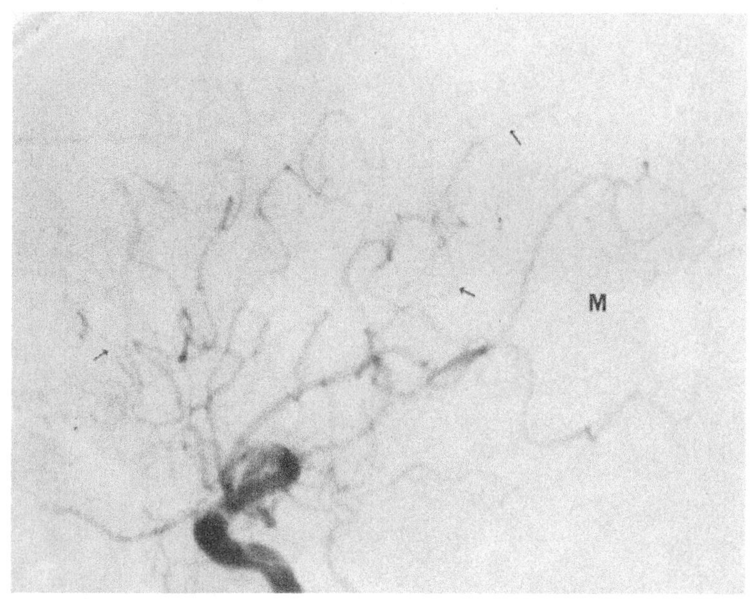

Figure 1.22. Patient with lupus erythematosus and intracranial vasculopathy. A left common carotid arteriogram demonstrates disseminated arterial irregularity and constrictions (*arrows*) affecting second-order branches of middle cerebral artery. A focal area of infarction with edema is observed as a result of the vasculopathy (*M*).

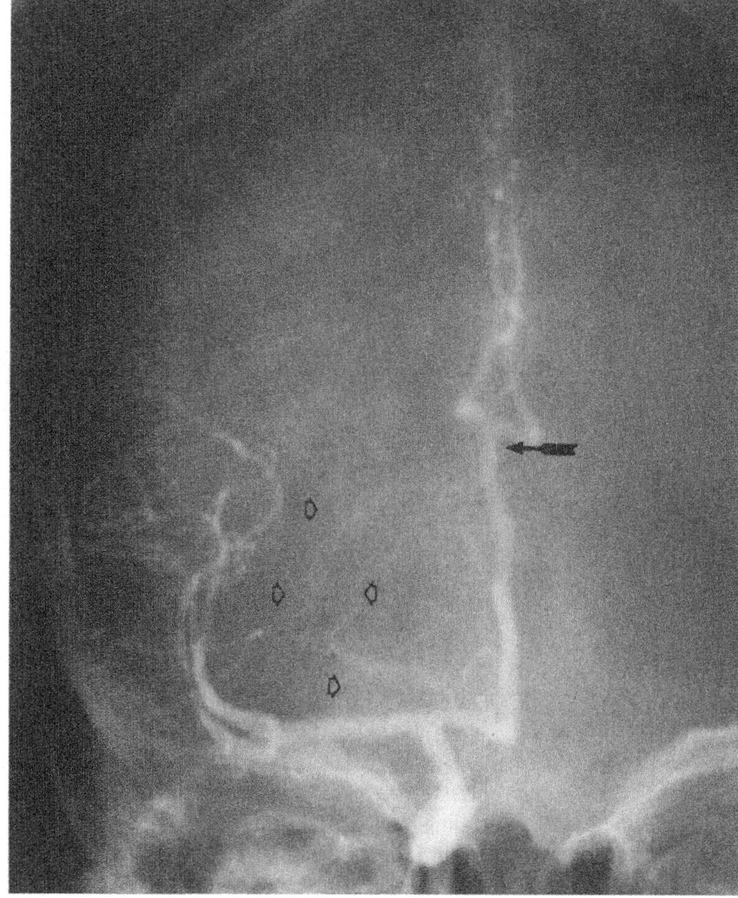

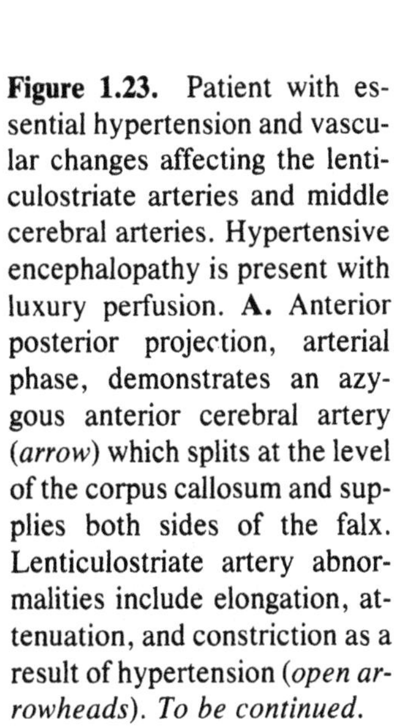

Figure 1.23. Patient with essential hypertension and vascular changes affecting the lenticulostriate arteries and middle cerebral arteries. Hypertensive encephalopathy is present with luxury perfusion. **A.** Anterior posterior projection, arterial phase, demonstrates an azygous anterior cerebral artery (*arrow*) which splits at the level of the corpus callosum and supplies both sides of the falx. Lenticulostriate artery abnormalities include elongation, attenuation, and constriction as a result of hypertension (*open arrowheads*). *To be continued.*

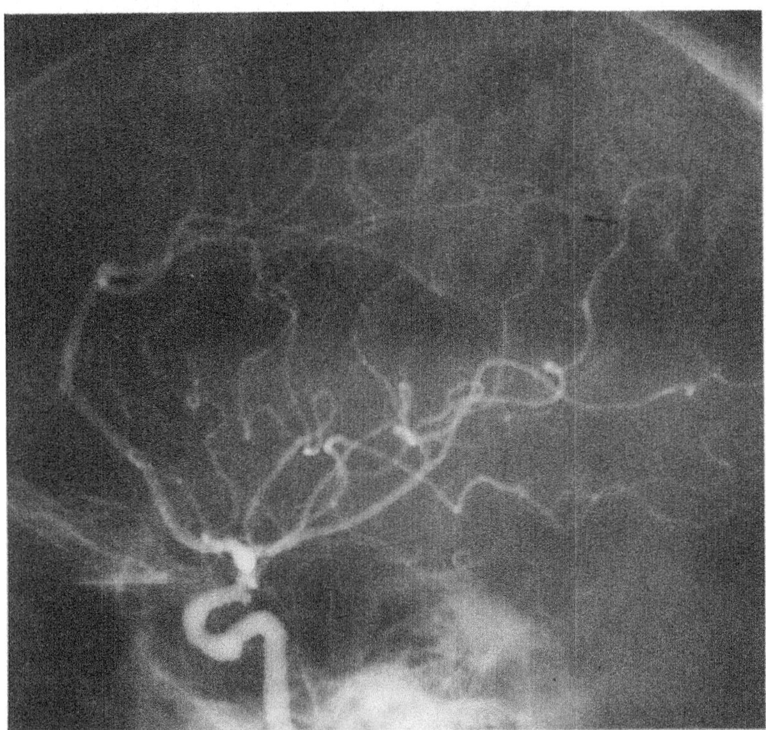

B. Lateral projection, arterial phase, diffuse constriction of convexity branches of the middle cerebral are noted (*arrows*). **C.** Lateral projection, arterial phase. 0.5 sec later, demonstrates arterial constrictions (*arrows*) and also a zone of increased vascularity (*open arrowhead*).

Fig. 1.23 B

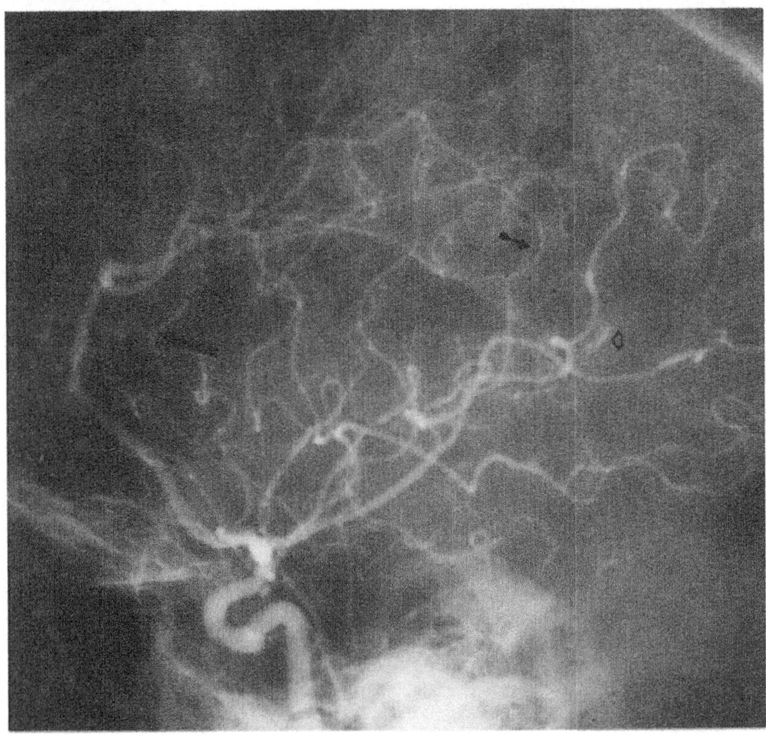

Fig. 1.23 C

Figure 1.23. **D.** 0.5 sec later, the zone of increased vascularity becomes denser (*open arrowhead*) and represents premature venous filling (*closed arrow*). Faint opacification now leading from this area represents early filling of the vein of Labbe (*closed arrowheads*). **E.** One second later, the venous phase, the prematurely opacified vein of Labbe is denser (*closed thick arrowheads*) than other neighboring veins. This represents luxury perfusion with premature venous filling as a consequence of the patient's hypertensive encephalopathy.

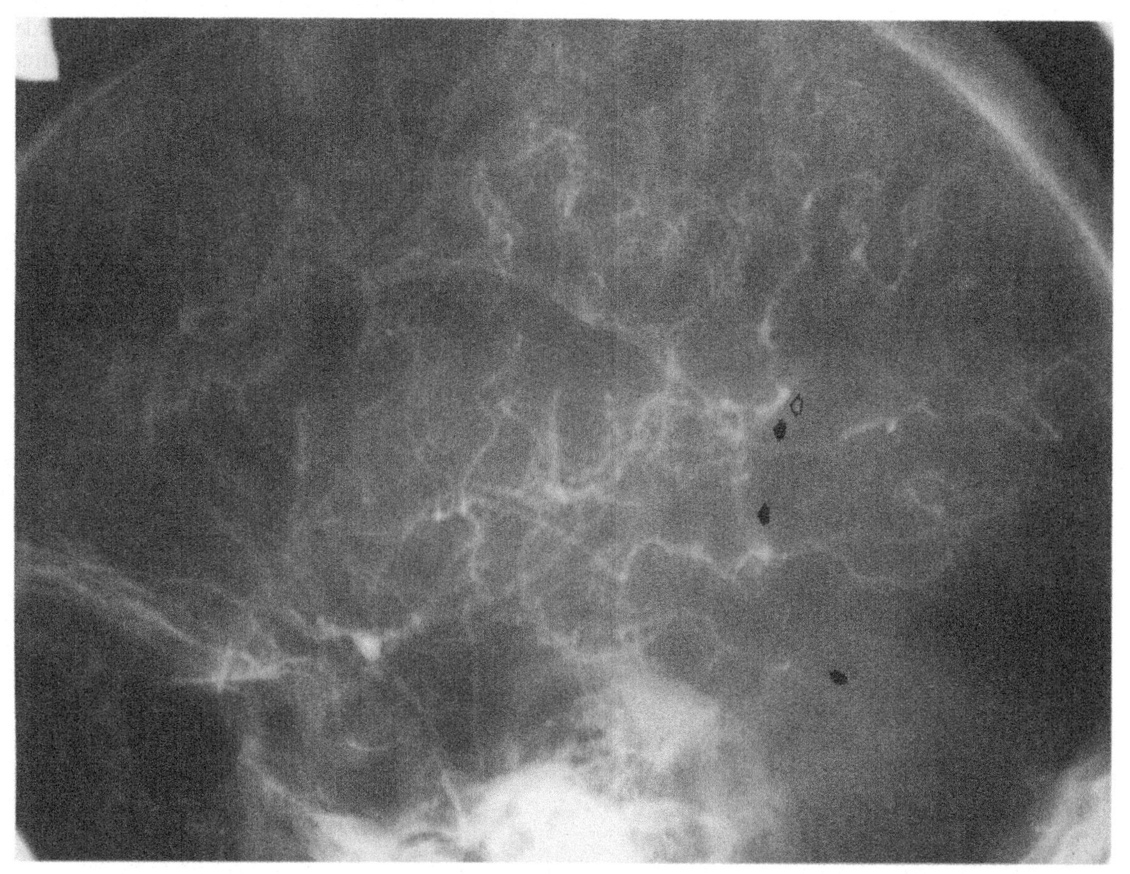
D

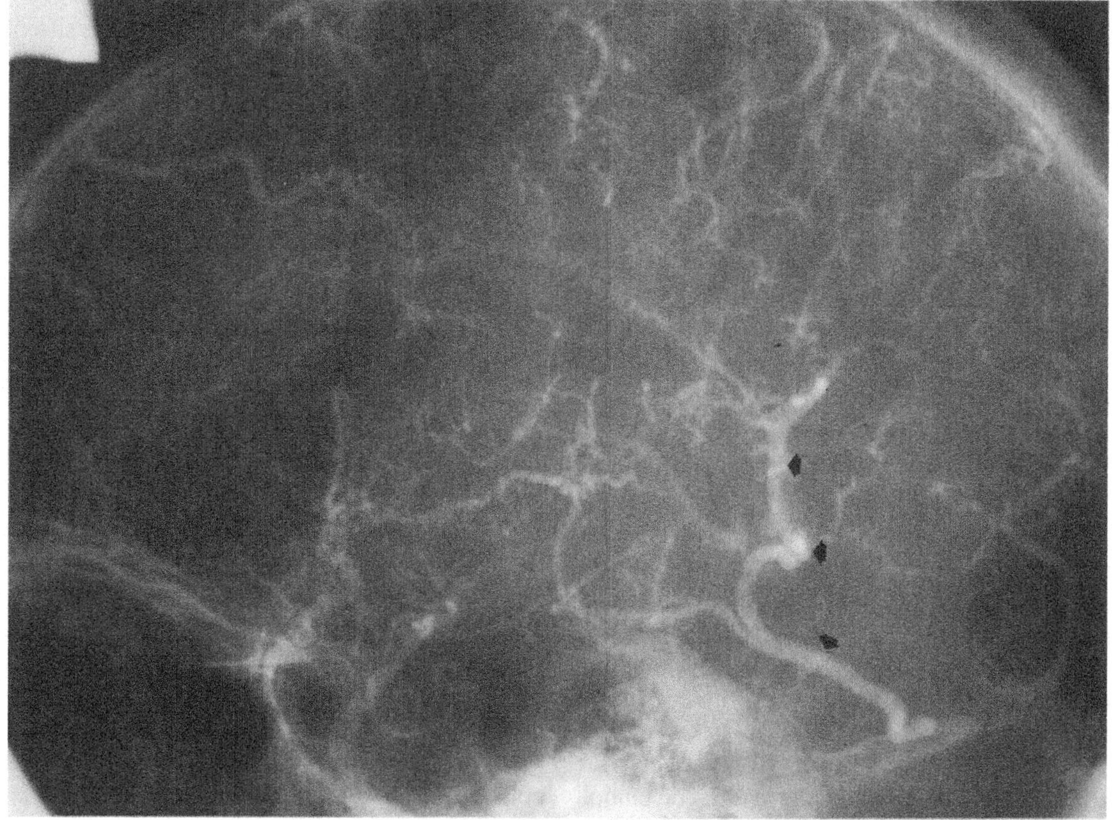
E

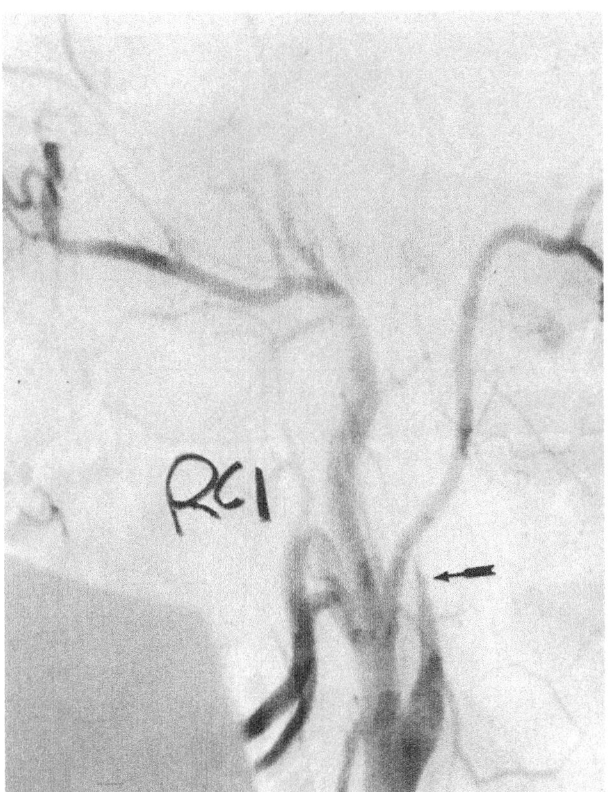

Figure 1.24. Traumatic occlusion of right internal carotid artery in 17-year-old male with acute onset of left hemiparesis after acute trauma to neck. A tapered occlusion of the internal carotid artery is seen distal to the carotid artery bifurcation (*arrow*). (Reprinted with permission from *Neuroradiology;* Burrows and Leeds, 1981, Churchill Livingstone Inc.)

(hyperperfusion)[32,39] (Fig. 1.23). In such cases vasoconstriction may be secondary to subarachnoid bleeding and vasospasm or to cerebral edema.

Trauma

Damage directly to the internal carotid artery or as a result of compression due to soft-tissue swelling or hemorrhage may occur from blunt or nonpenetrating trauma to the neck. The arterial constriction or occlusion that occurs is similar to the appearance of atherosclerotic vascular disease (Fig. 1.24).

Dissecting aneurysms often occur in the cervical carotid artery at the level of C1-2 but may also be observed more distally (Fig. 1.25). Stenosis of the internal carotid artery occurs in some cases because of medial or subintimal hemorrhage. If the intima is disrupted a false aneurysm or false channel will be observed. These lesions may resolve spontaneously. A complication may be the formation of emboli due to wall damage or turbulence at the site of the lesion.

In patients with elevated intracranial pressure, reduced or absent flow in the internal carotid artery occurs, simulating a carotid occlusion[6] (Fig. 1.26).

Neoplastic Vasculopathy and Radiation Vasculopathy

Vasoconstriction or dilatation may occur in the vicinity of the neoplasm[35,40,57] or of diffuse vascular changes in neoplasm simulating a vascular process[41] (Fig. 1.27).

The usual cause of the vascular abnormality is arterial wall involvement by the neoplasm.[40] Ridley and Cavanaugh[50] suggested, as another mechanism, perivascular cuffing due to lymphocyte infiltration of the brain parenchyma as a result of a breakdown in the hosts immune mechanism.

Lymphoma and leukemia may cause arterial constriction at the base, simulating inflamma-

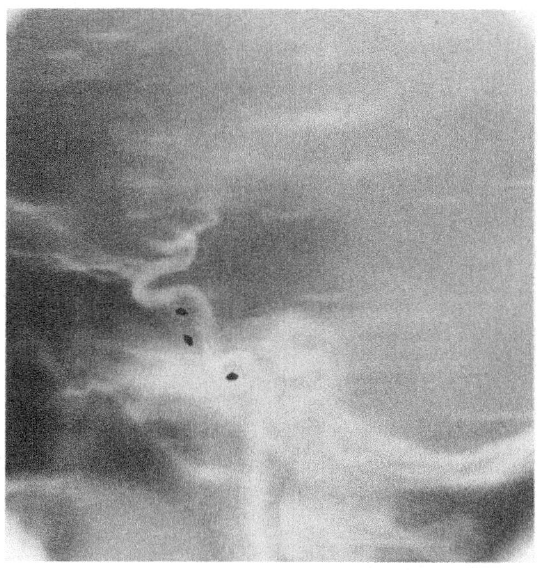

A

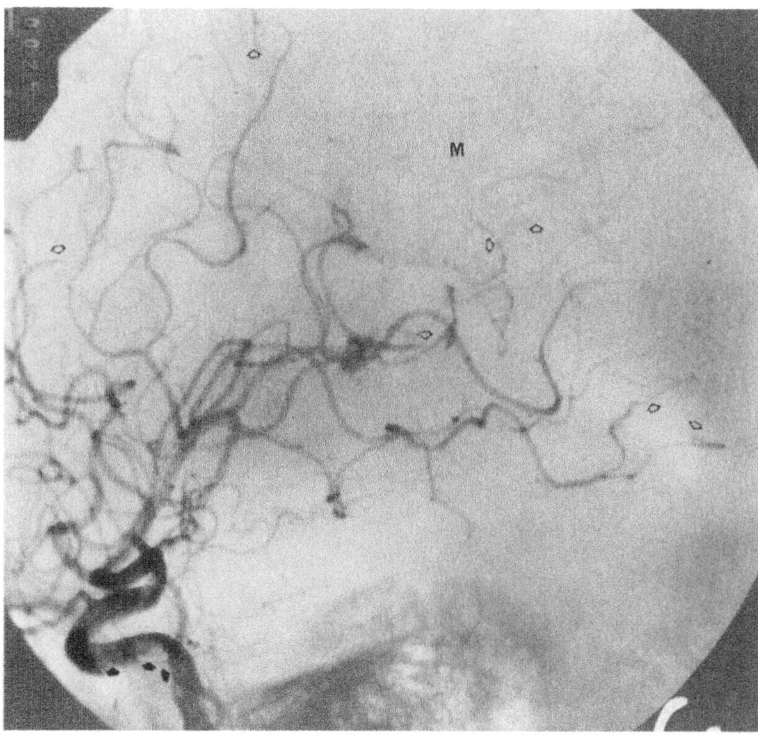

B

Figure 1.25. Patient with dissection of internal carotid artery affecting the petrous portion and proximal cavernous segment, with this dissection being the site of origin of multiple intracranial emboli. **A.** Lateral projection, arterial phase, angiotomography demonstrates arterial irregularity due to intimal involvement with a question of filling defects in the vascular lumen (*closed arrowheads*) affecting the petrous and proximal cavernous portion of the internal carotid artery. **B.** Lateral projection in arterial phase again demonstrates luminal irregularity of internal carotid artery within the petrous and cavernous segments (*closed arrowheads*). In addition, intracranially, multiple sites of occlusion and arterial irregularity are seen (*open arrowheads*). A large avascular zone is observed in the posterior frontoparietal region (*M*).

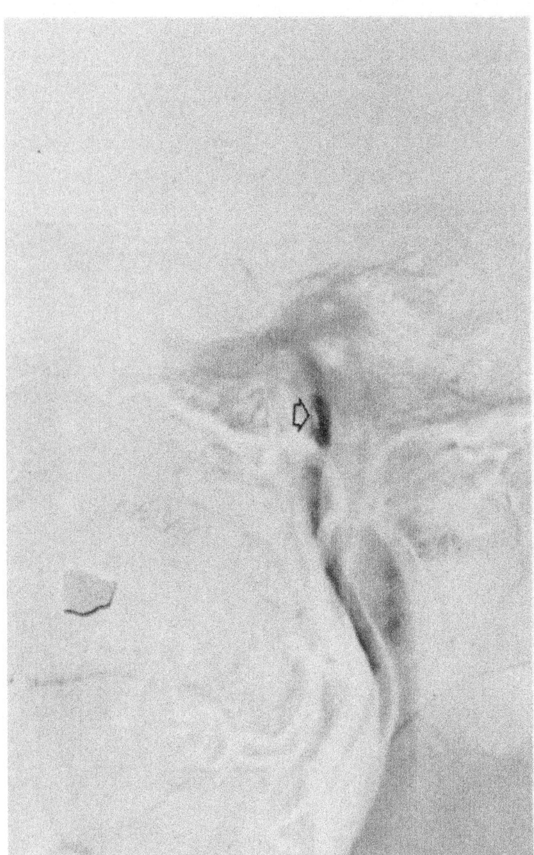

Figure 1.26. Demonstration of brain death with no intracranial perfusion. At the end of 12 sec contrast opacification of the internal carotid artery is only to the petrous segment of the internal carotid artery (*open arrowhead*). No intracranial filling is observed. The vessel overlying the calvarium represents opacification of external carotid branches. This is an example of no intracranial flow after a long duration.

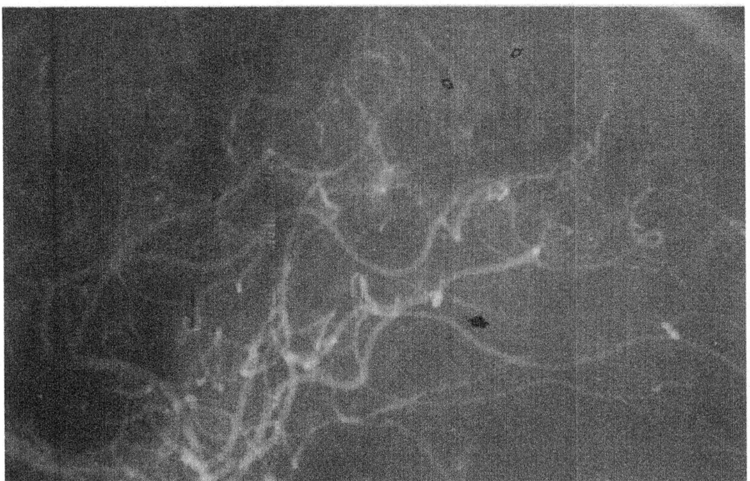

Figure 1.27. Patient with glioblastoma with arterial irregularity and occlusion. Lateral left common carotid arteriogram demonstrates stretching and spreading of middle cerebral artery branches in watershed region (*open arrowheads*). Arterial irregularity of another branch of the middle cerebral artery is seen with thrombus within the artery (*closed arrowhead*) in posterior temporoparietal region. Draping of temporal branches posteriorly is also seen. Two disparate lesions were thought to be present in the posterior frontoparietal region and in the posterior temporoparietal region. At surgery the lesions were contiguous and represented a glioblastoma multiforme accounting for the arterial changes identified. (Reprinted with permission from *Neuroradiology;* Burrows and Leeds, 1981, Churchill Livingstone Inc.)

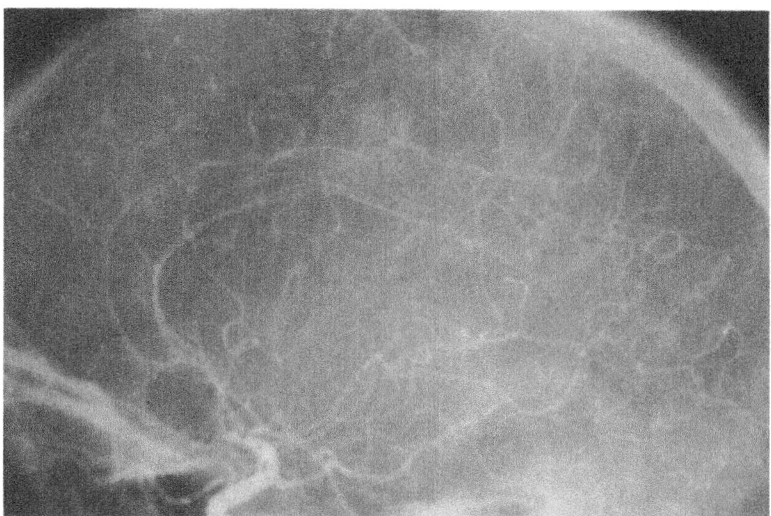

Figure 1.28. Patient with carcinomatous meningitis with diffuse vasculopathy. Lateral carotid arteriogram, arterial phase, demonstrates diffuse constriction affecting almost all the anterior and middle cerebral artery branches as a result of meningeal infiltration in this patient with carcinoma of the breast. (Reprinted with permission from *Neuroradiology;* Burrows and Leeds, 1981, Churchill Livingstone Inc.)

tory lesions. When diffuse meningeal involvement is present with lymphoma, leukemia, or metastasis, disseminated arterial constriction may be present[33] (Fig. 1.28). Radiation therapy may result in arterial stenosis or occlusion two to seven years after therapy, or it may be seen as early as six months after treatment[6] (Fig. 1.29).

Drug-Abuse Patients

Arterial changes are often identified in the patient with drug addiction. The vascular patterns visualized include stenosis, occlusion, and peripheral aneurysms[54] (Fig. 1.30). It is difficult to pinpoint the cause of the angiographic changes. Factors responsible for the arterial changes may include the drug, the vehicle used, introduced contaminated material, trauma, and sensitivity reactions to materials injected.[54] In the drug-abuse patient taking amphetamines, Citron et al[9] demonstrated pathologic changes in blood vessels similar to those in patients with a necrotizing angiitis. This supports the possibility of an autoimmune or hyperimmune process.

Vascular Abnormalities Related to the Use of Contraceptive Drugs

In England, Bickerstaff[3] observed an increased incidence of stroke in young female patients taking oral contraceptives. Prior to the pill, two to three young women with strokes were seen per year in his catchment area. Following introduction of the pill, eight to nine cases per year were identified. This represents a statistically significant increase in the number of cases.

The vascular changes include occlusion of the internal carotid artery or basal arteries and occlusion of luminal changes in convexity arteries.[2]

Fibromuscular Dysplasia

Fibromuscular dysplasia (FMD) affects the extracranial carotid arteries predominantly and infrequently affects the intracranial branches. FMD is most often encountered in the midsegment of the cervical carotid artery adjacent to C-2.[25] The configuration identified during angiography is that of corrugations with contiguous,

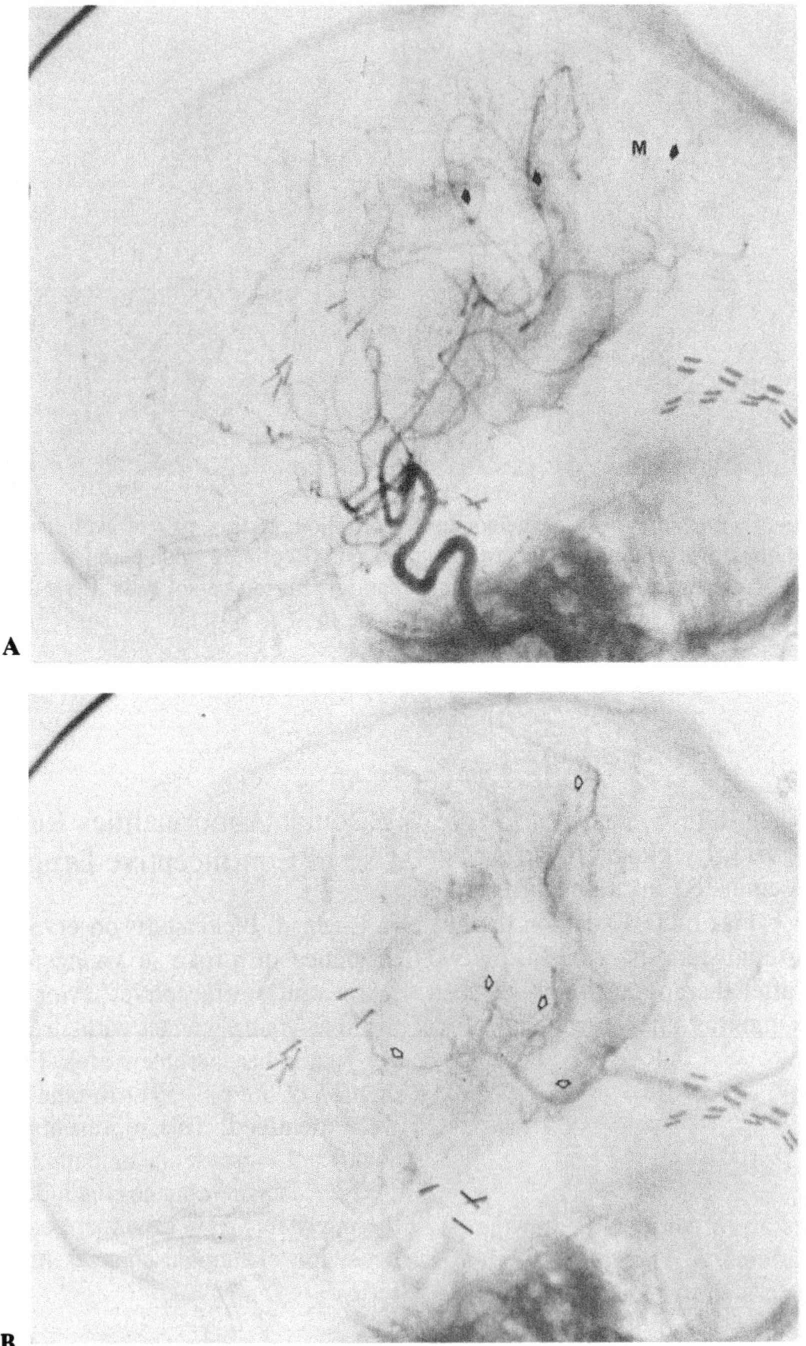

Figure 1.29. Child with astrocytoma, removed 2 yr previously and treated with radiation. Now has radiation arteritis with luxury perfusion. **A.** Lateral projection, arterial phase demonstrates diffuse constriction of proximal branches of middle cerebral artery in the region of the silver clips. Separation of branches is noted. Dilatation of post rolandic convexity arterial branches has occurred (*arrowheads*) and an avascular mass is observed in the posterior parietal region (*M*) due to cerebral swelling. **B.** One and one-half seconds later, in the intermediate phase, premature filling of superficial veins (*open arrowheads*) that drain into the superior sagittal sinus and inferiorly into the vein of Labbe (*open arrowheads*) are noted.

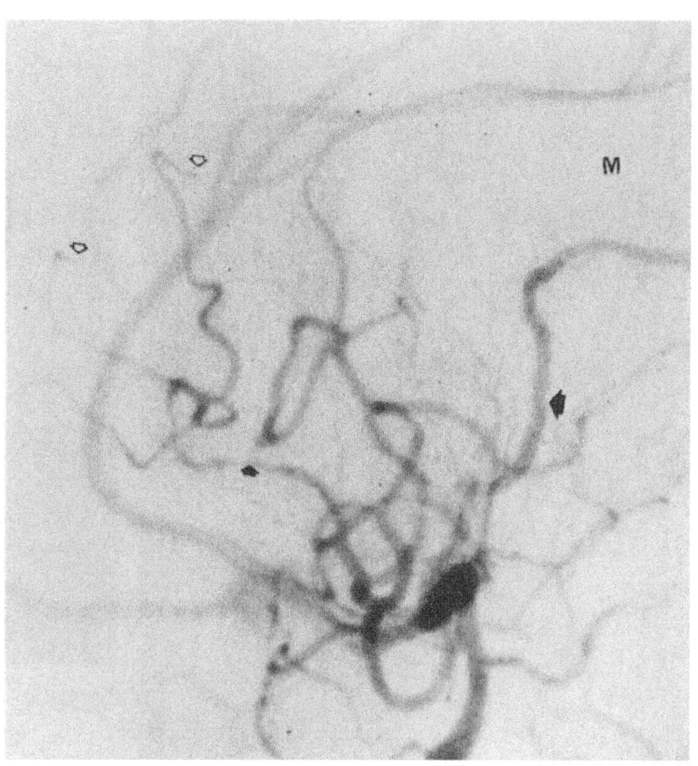

Figure 1.30. 13-Year-old male with history of drug abuse and disseminated intracranial vascular disease. **A.** Lateral projection, left common carotid arteriogram in early arterial phase, demonstrates diffuse arterial constrictions (*small closed arrowhead*). Vasodilatation is also noted (*large arrowhead*) and an avascular area is observed as a result of vascular occlusion (*M*). Arterial occlusion can also be identified (*small open arrows*). **B.** Anterior posterior projection, arterial phase, demonstrates vascular constrictions (*small closed arrowhead*) and occlusions (*small open arrowhead*). In addition, as a consequence of disseminated vascular disease, lenticulostriate artery dilatation (*large arrows*) has occurred to provide satisfactory flow to the ganglionic structures.

A

narrow or dilated segments (Fig. 1.31). The pattern in FMD must be differentiated from "standing waves" (a normal, transient finding due to spasm). FMD produces areas of true luminal dilatation alternating with areas of narrowing, whereas standing waves produce only narrowing. Infrequently, a long stenotic portion of the internal carotid artery above the bifurcation is seen (Fig. 1.32). The string of beads configuration is observed infrequently affecting the extracranial vertebral artery or the internal carotid artery as it enters the foramen lacerum or within the anterior or middle cerebral arteries.[65]

The lesions are found more commonly in females than in males and only rarely have pathologic examinations been performed. According to Houser et al,[25] the pathologic changes have been limited to medial fibroplasia as opposed to the various types observed within the renal arteries.

As a result of caliber changes within the artery, turbulence may occur and emboli may be formed. Since the arterial wall may be weakened in the development of the lesion, aneurysm formation is possible. Carotid cavernous fistulas may result when the lesion affects the cavernous carotid artery.[66]

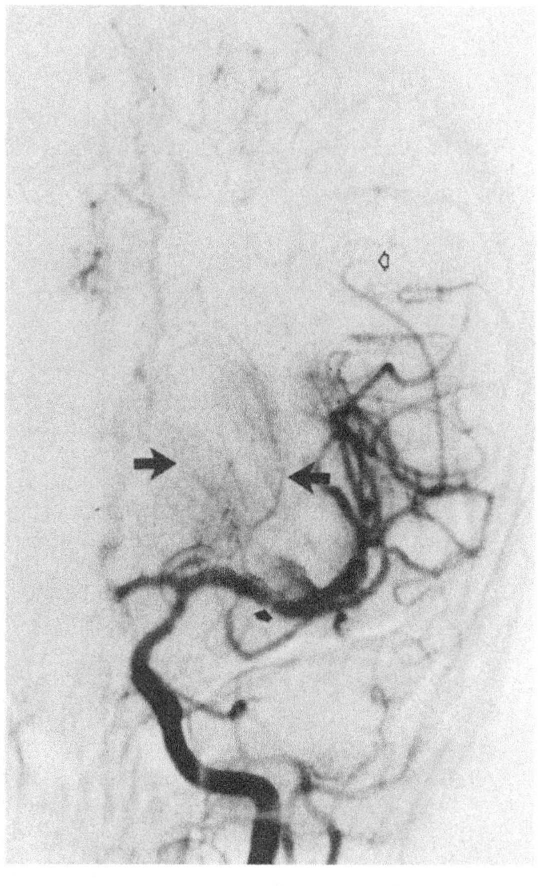

B

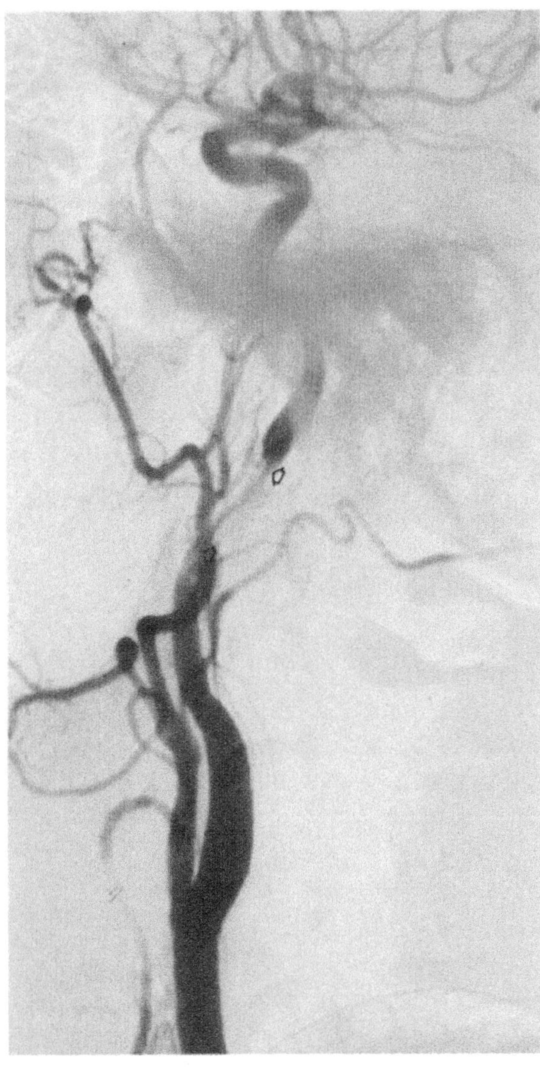
A

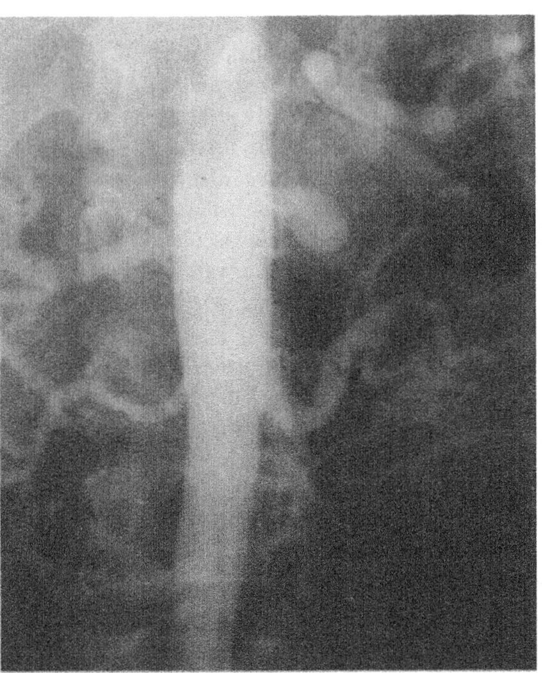
B

Figure 1.31. Fibromuscular dysplasia affecting internal carotid and left renal artery. **A.** Left common carotid arteriogram, arterial phase, demonstrates segmental constriction of midportion of the internal carotid artery (*arrowheads*) in proximity to C-2. No other abnormality is seen. **B.** Abdominal anteriogram demonstrates corrugated appearance of the left renal artery (*arrowhead*). (Published with permission from *Neuroradiology;* Burrows and Leeds, 1981, Churchill Livingstone Inc.)

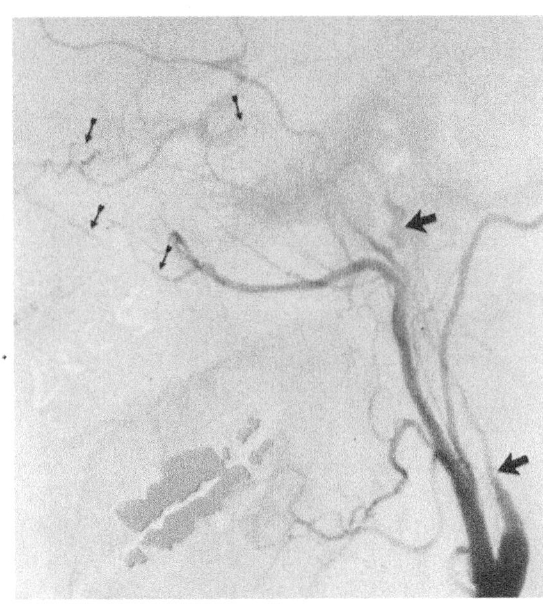

◁

Figure 1.32. Young female patient with fibromuscular dysplasia. Presented with TIA and right hemiparesis. Lateral projection, left common carotid arteriogram at 2 sec, demonstrates to advantage the marked constriction of internal carotid artery beginning at 2 cm. above carotid bifurcation (*large arrows*). Localized dilatation of internal carotid artery is seen at the level of C1 (*upper arrow*). Segmental arterial dilatation beyond distal segment of constriction and location suggests the diagnosis of fibromuscular dysplasia. The internal maxillary artery, via collateral channels, fills the ophthalmic artery, which then opacifies the internal carotid artery to the level of the cavernous carotid artery (*small arrows*). (Reprinted with permission from *Neuroradiology;* Burrows and Leeds, 1981, Churchill Livingstone Inc.)

Takayasu's Arteritis

This unusual form of arteritis is observed primarily in adolescent females and is identified at the origins of the major vessels. Skip areas are common. Long or short stenoses are observed affecting branches of the aortic arch and the carotid bifurcation. The disease is primarily extracranial, but intracranial involvement has been identified.

Collateral Channels

The most significant collateral channel is the circle of Willis. This permits free communication at the base of the brain between right and left carotid arteries and between the carotid and vertebral arteries.

Only about one half of the population have a normal circle of Willis.[51] In the remaining patients a variety of patterns of communication are present.

Transdural collateral channels may be extensive (Fig. 1.33). These include collateral channels from the internal maxillary artery to the ophthalamic artery via ethmoidal and frontal branches (Figs. 1.32, 1.34) and from the middle meningeal artery to the artery of the inferior cavernous sinus to the cavernous segment of the internal carotid artery. Communications also exist between the external occipital artery and cervical muscular arterial branches of the vertebral artery so that a communication in either direction exists, depending on pressure changes within the system.

Leptomeningeal collaterals represent the free communication over the surface between the anterior, middle, and posterior cerebral arteries (Figs. 1.8, 1.17, 1.35).[61] These communications are pressure-related and will serve as a communication between any of the systems, depending on the site of interruption. The collateral channels will open immediately.

Other channels of communication that may occur include proliferation of small vessels (Figs. 1.21)[23,36,59] at the base, when the distal internal carotid artery is interrupted. These vessels can act as collateral channels and should not suggest the presence of a neoplasm.[36,59]

The lenticulostriate arteries may communicate with either the anterior or middle cerebral artery.[6] In some instances a distal telangiectatic blush in the brain may be identified when medullary arteries dilate to serve as collateral channels (Fig. 1.36).[6]

In basilar artery occlusion, the collateral supply can come from leptomeningeal collaterals to the posterior cerebral artery and then to the basilar artery or from the superior cerebellar artery (SCA), retrograde to the posterior-inferior cerebellar (PICA) or visa versa from the PICA to the SCA, depending on the flow patterns.[34]

Collateral channels can provide an effective circulation, with the patient having no signs of vascular insufficiency. In other cases, despite the presence of large collateral channels, the patient may have ischemic symptoms.

Computed Tomography and Radionuclide Imaging in Stroke

The detection rate for ischemic stroke is similar for CT and radioisotope scanning at approximately 60%.[7] The CT scan is more effective than the radioisotope scan in discriminating between ischemic and hemorrhagic lesions. On the other hand, dynamic studies with radioisotopes are more effective than CT in the investigation of the patient with stenosis of extracranial vessels or TIA.[5] CT scans are effective in demonstrating sites of involvement and are most advantageous 7 to 11 days after the ictus.[7] The CT scan can be evaluated by relating the low-density lesion to the arterial area of supply.

1. holo-hemispheric (internal carotid) (Fig. 1.37)
2. cortical orientation on surface (middle cerebral) (Fig. 1.38)
3. deep cortical structures (lenticulostriate arteries)
4. a combination of superficial and deep cortical involvement (middle cerebral artery and lenticulostriate arteries) (Fig. 1.39)
5. confined to distribution of anterior cerebral artery (Fig. 1.40)
6. confined to distribution of posterior cerebral artery (Fig. 1.41)
7. posterior fossa distribution with or without posterior cerebral involvement (Fig. 1.42)
8. nonspecific changes, e.g., focal dilatation of ventricle, ill-defined low-density zone or focal dilatation of cortical sulci (Fig. 1.38C)

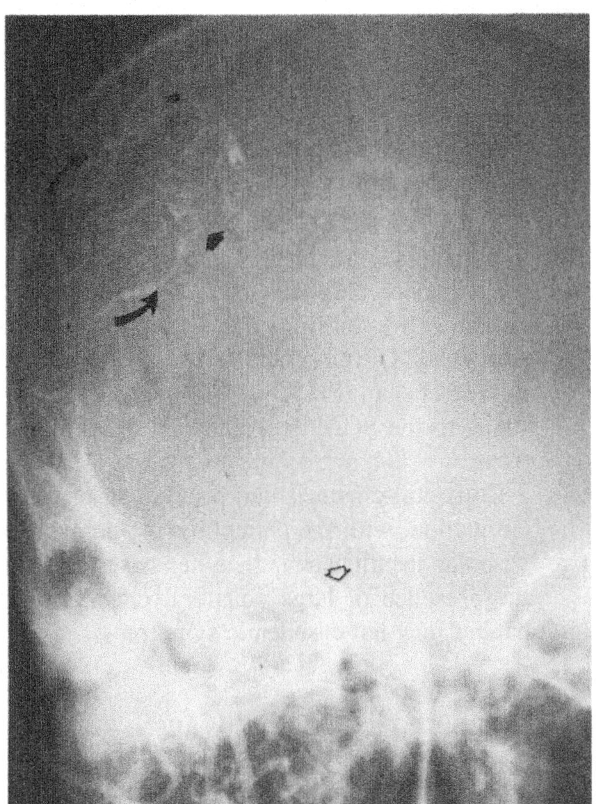

A

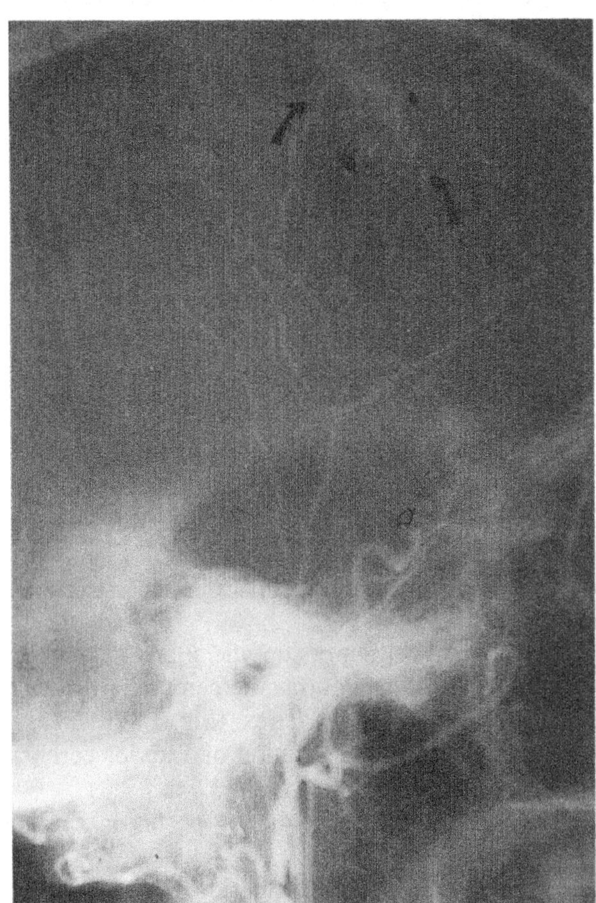

B

Figure 1.33. Patient with vascular occlusion, with Moya Moya disease and hemorrhage from dilated arterialized capillaries, which resulted in cerebral hemorrhage and patient's eventual demise. **A, B.** Cuplike occlusion of internal carotid artery is observed at the level of the anterior clinoid (*open arrowhead*). Dilated penetrating middle meningeal arteries are seen which are serving as collaterals to middle cerebral artery by penetrating the dura (*curved arrows*). Hypervascular blush due to dilatation of these transdural collateral vessels (*closed arrowheads*) is observed. (Reprinted with permission from *Neuroradiology;* Burrows and Leeds, 1981, Churchill Livingstone Inc.)

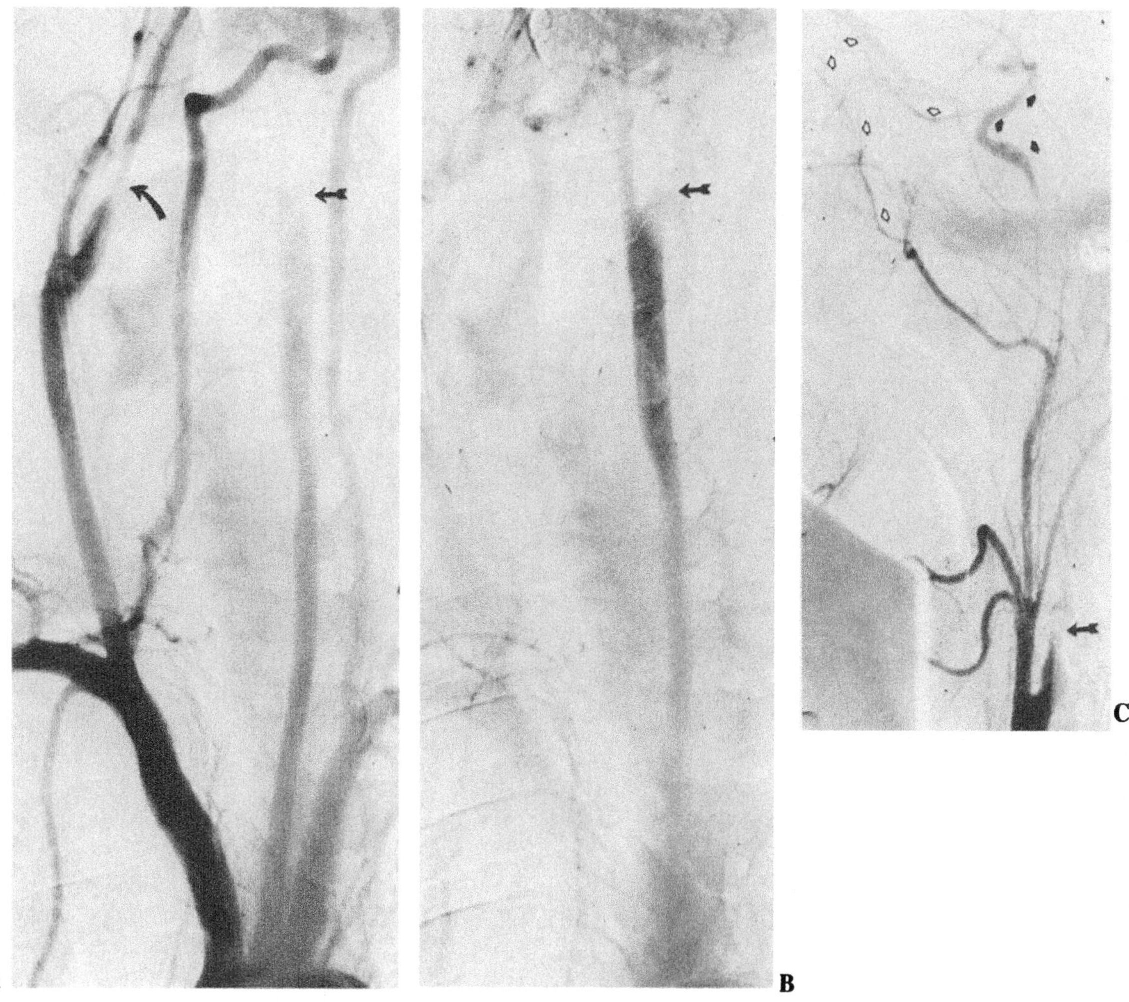

Figure 1.34. Occlusion, proximal internal carotid with delayed emptying of left common carotid artery. Stenosis also present in proximal right internal carotid: Collateral filling of intracranial left internal carotid artery via meningeal supply from the ophthalmic artery. **A.** Examination of the aortic arch in right posterior oblique projection demonstrates a long segment of irregular stenosis of right internal carotid over a distance of 8 mm, beginning 15 mm above bifurcation (*curved arrow*). Complete occlusion of left internal carotid artery is observed at the bifurcation (*arrow*). **B.** Two seconds later, delayed emptying of left common carotid is noted with improved visualization of the site of arterial occlusion (*arrow*). **C.** Examination of the head demonstrates occlusion of left internal carotid artery (*arrow*). External carotid artery is visualized fully with ethmoidal and frontal collaterals to ophthalmic artery (*open arrowheads*) to opacify internal carotid artery (*black arrowheads*).

The identification of patterns of involvement enables one to predict the site or sites of arterial involvement.[62]

In the acute stroke, mass may be identified in up to 25% of cases and is usually present in the first two weeks, but can be identified up to one month after the insult (Fig. 1.37).

Contrast enhancement is most effective from 7 to 11 days[7,65] and is the result of a breakdown in the blood-brain barrier or a loss in cerebral autoregulation. The image of increased density may be seen in isodense or hypodense zones (Figs. 1.38, 1.39, 1.41). In any zone of brain in which a breakdown of blood-brain barrier or loss in autoregulation occurs at some time in the course of resolution, a ring lesion may be visualized[6,67] (Fig. 1.39). Thus, occasionally a ring lesion is observed if sequential studies are ob-

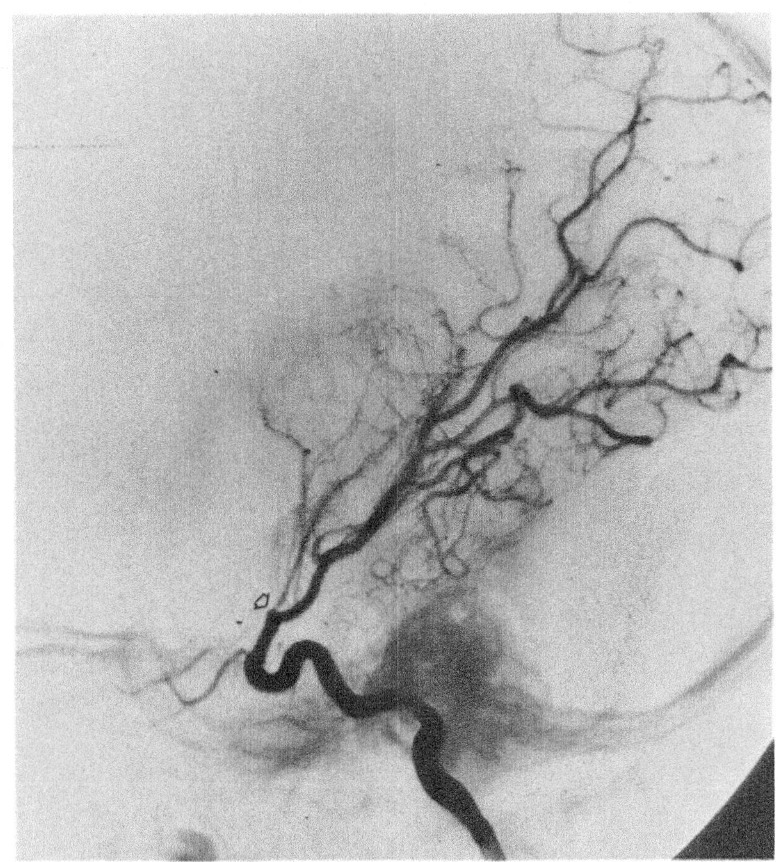
A

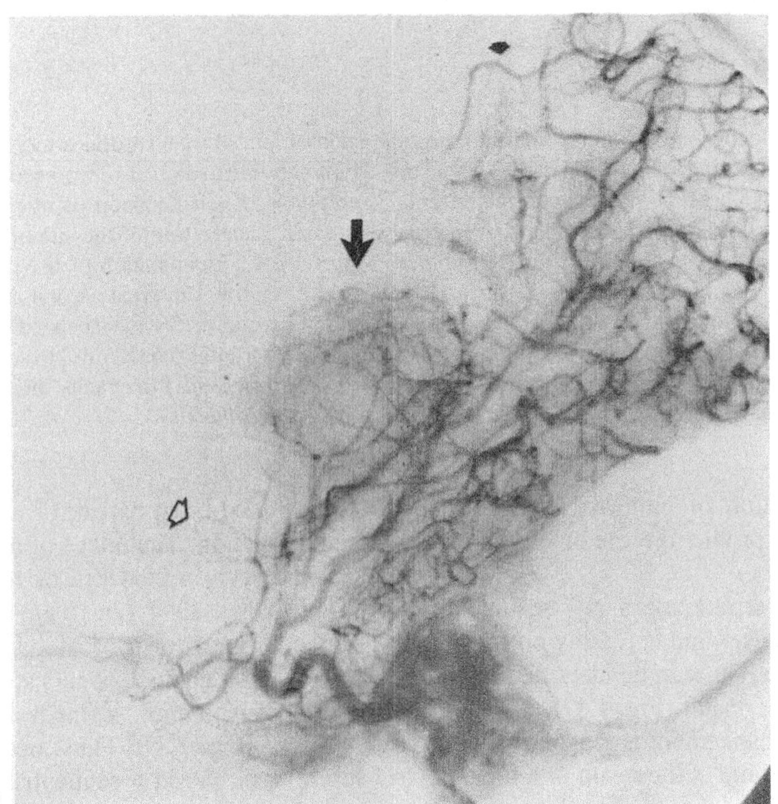
B

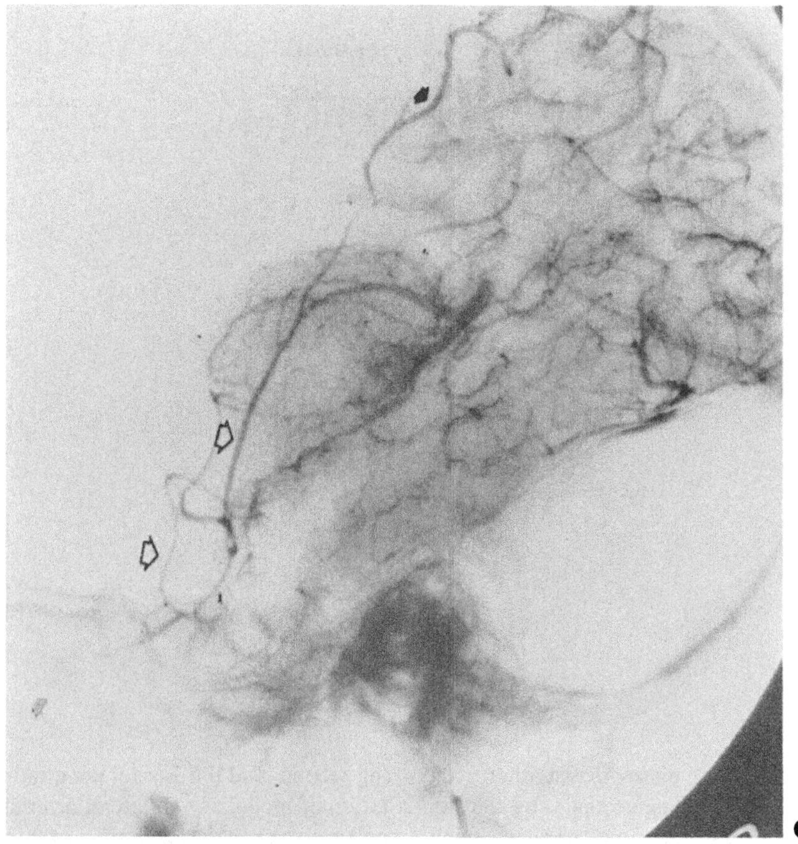

Figure 1.35. 2½-Year-old female developed an acute hemiparesis following viral infection. The computed tomogram demonstrated a cerebral infarct. **A.** Arterial phase, right internal carotid arteriogram in early arterial phase, demonstrates complete occlusion of internal carotid artery (*open arrowhead*) distal to anterior choroidal artery. Marked dilatation of branches of the posterior cerebral artery are present, including penetrating vessels that are serving as collaterals. **B.** One second later, leptomeningeal collaterals are identified arising posteriorly from posterior cerebral artery to middle cerebral artery (*black arrowhead*) and anteriorly from posterior cerebral branches to anterior temporal branches of middle cerebral artery (*open arrowhead*). In addition, diffuse blush in the region of the basal ganglionic and thalamus is seen due to dilatation of penetrating arteries (*arrow*). **C.** One second later in the intermediate phase, veins are being opacified. Leptomeningeal branches from the posterior cerebral artery to the middle cerebral artery are well seen anteriorly (*open arrowheads*) and posteriorly (*black arrowhead*).

tained during evolution of a cerebral infarct.

In the acute infarct, no abnormality may be observed in the first 2 to 3 days, but delayed scans at 7 to 10 days will be positive. However, in some instances the follow-up scan may show significant changes 24 hours after a negative scan (Fig. 1.43). Delayed hemorrhage may also be observed on follow-up scans when little or no hemorrhage is observed on the initial scan. This warrants careful consideration prior to early anticoagulation (Fig. 1.44). The sensitivity of these studies is dependent on the volume of brain affected.[7] An advantage of CT is that serial studies in problem cases may permit the demonstration of evolution of pathophysiologic changes so that one may make an accurate diagnosis and reduce errors in management.

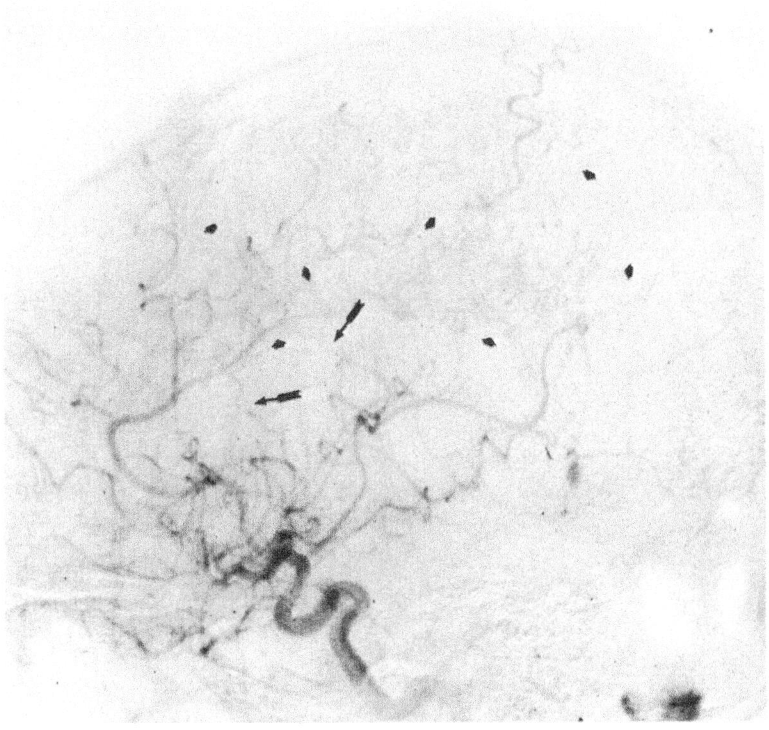

Figure 1.36. Patient with disseminated atherosclerotic vascular disease affecting second- and third-order arteries with telangiectatic collateral channels. Left common carotid arteriogram in the midarterial phase demonstrates disseminated vascular disease affecting branches of anterior and middle cerebral artery, some of which are marked with *arrows*. As a consequence of disseminated vascular disease affecting second- and third-order penetrating arteries, dilatation of medullary collateral arterial channels have occurred (*arrowheads*), giving the appearance of a telangiectatic blush in which distinct vessels cannot be distinguished. (Reprinted with permission from *Neuroradiology;* Burrows and Leeds, 1981, Churchill Livingstone Inc.)

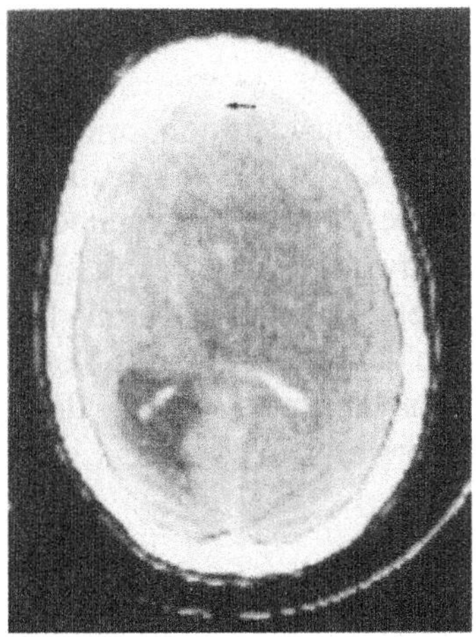

Figure 1.37. Holo-hemispheric cerebral infarct with marked midline shift and transtentorial herniation. Noncontrast CT scan demonstrates decrease in density of right cerebral hemisphere with marked midline shift from right to left. Falx is bowed to the left (*arrow*). Left atrium and occipital horn are dilated, reflecting transtentorial herniation.

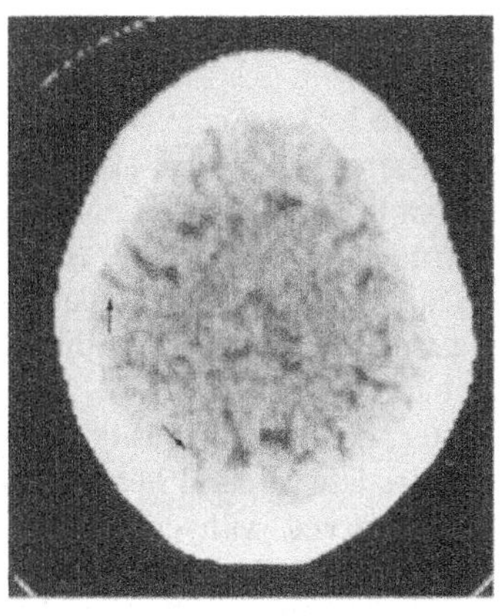

A

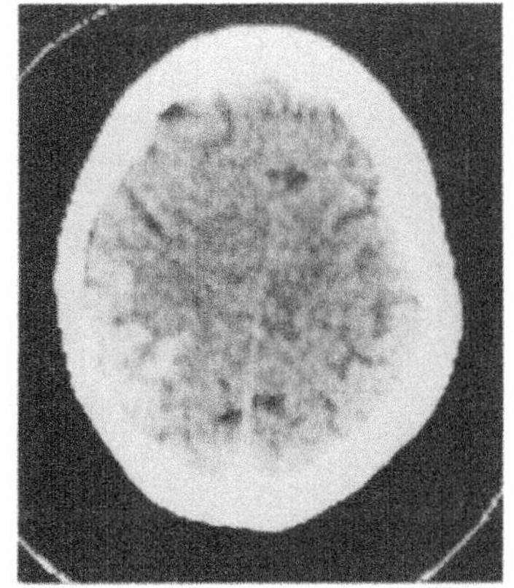

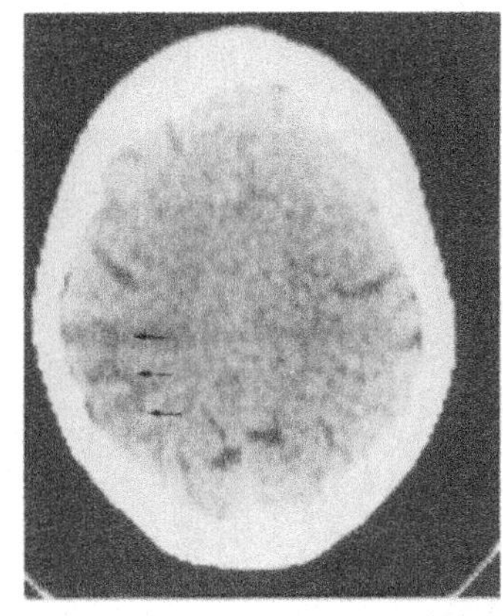

B, C

Figure 1.38. Middle cerebral artery infarct—cortical surface. **A.** Noncontrast CT scan demonstrates only focal absence of cortical sulci on left posterior parietal region (*arrows*) compared with right side. **B.** Post contrast infusion CT scan in same area as **A;** cortical and gyral hyperperfusion is seen. **C.** On noncontrast CT scan, 3 weeks later, dilated cortical sulci are observed in the posterior parietal region (*arrows*).

Figure 1.39. Combination of superficial and deep cortical involvement in middle cerebral artery distribution including lenticulostriate arteries. **A.** On post contrast infusion CT scan, hyperperfusion is noted on cortical surface, island of Reil, lenticular nucleus (*double ring*) (*arrows*), and caudate nucleus. **B.** 16-mm higher, contrast enhancement of gyri on surface and tail of caudate (*open arrowhead*) are seen. ▷

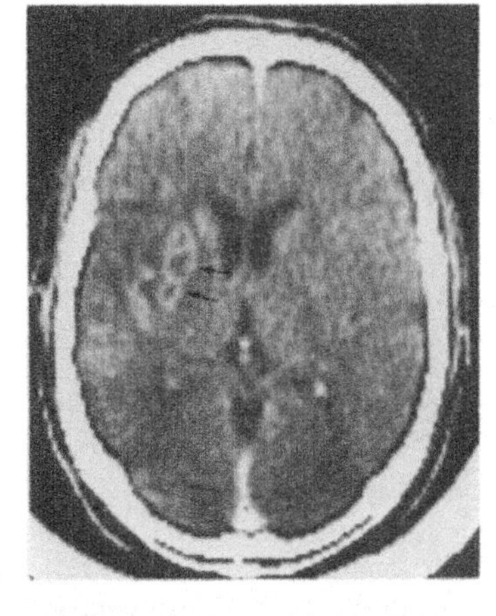

A

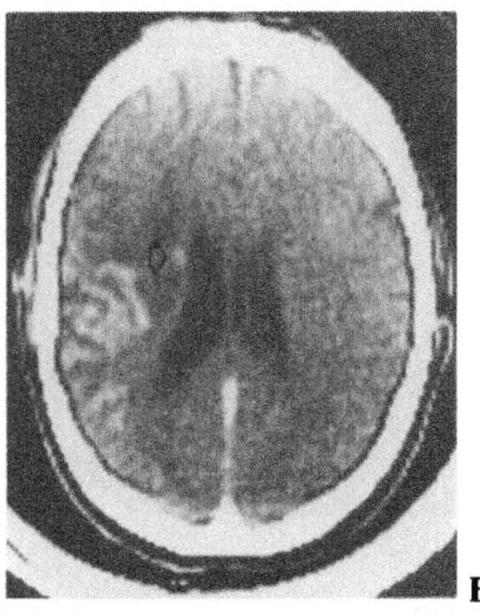

B

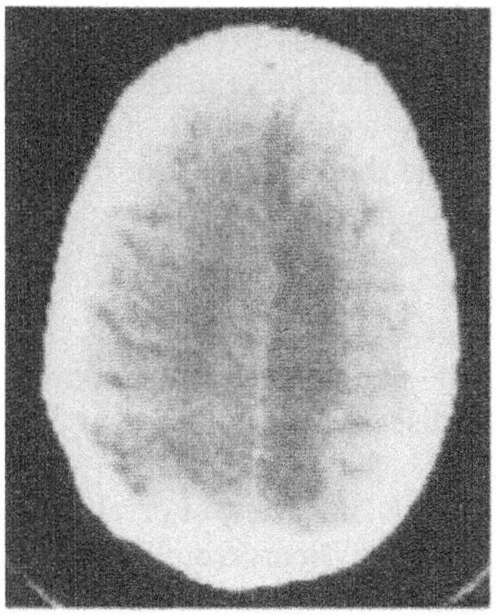

Figure 1.40. Old anterior cerebral artery infarct. On noncontrast CT scan, a well-defined low-density linear band of moderate thickness parallels the interhemispheric fissure on the right.

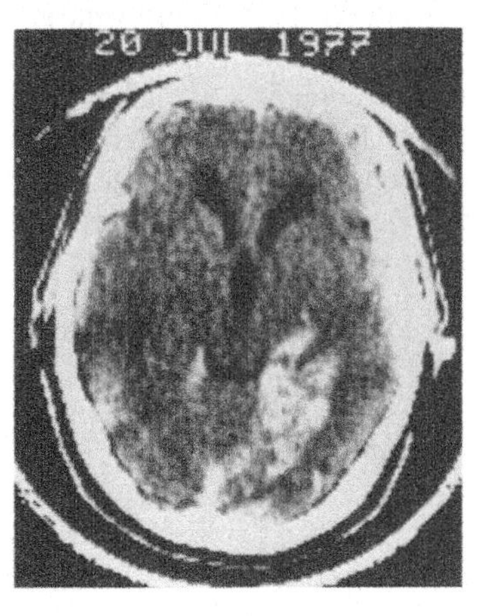

Figure 1.41. Acute infarct confined to posterior cerebral artery distribution. On post infusion CT scan, a well-demarcated zone of contrast enhancement is observed within the posterior medial aspect of right temporal lobe and occipital lobe.

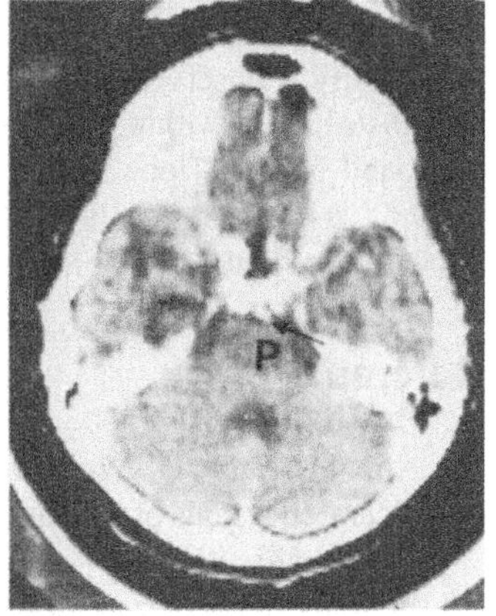

Figure 1.42. Acute infarct confined to pontine branches of basilar artery. On post infusion CT scan, a sharply demarcated oval lesion is observed in the pons (*P*) compressing the prepontine cistern and displacing the basilar artery forward (*arrow*).

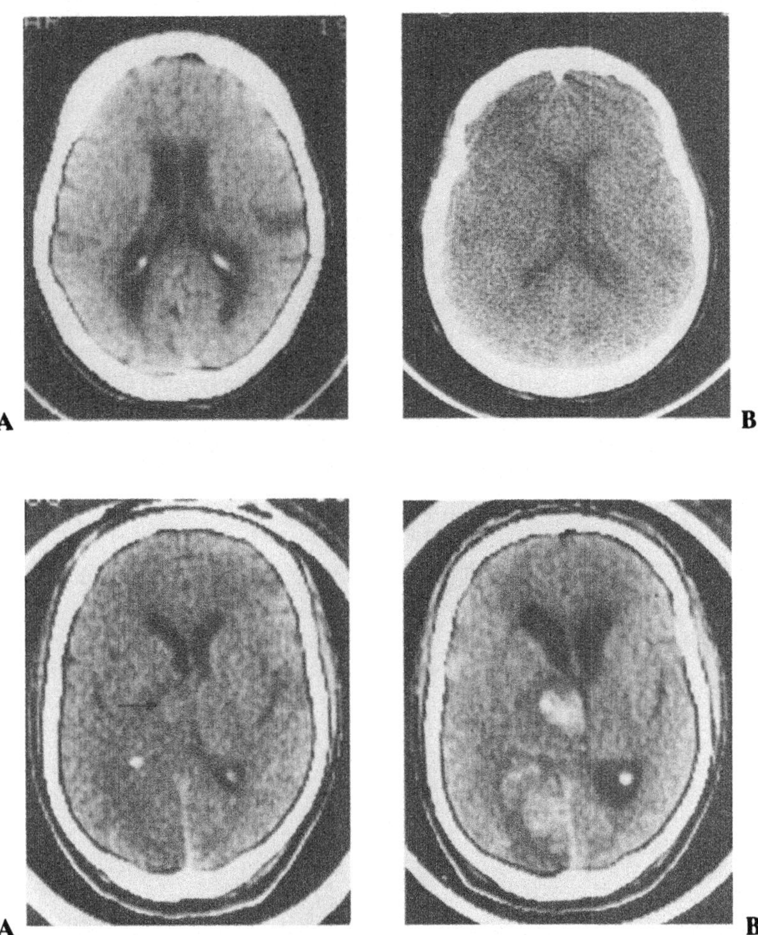

◁ **Figure 1.43.** Acute changes 24 hr after a normal-appearing scan in a patient with an acute stroke. **A.** On noncontrast CT scan, only slight ventricular dilatation is seen with a dilated sulcus on the right. **B.** 24 hr later, diminished density of the entire left cerebral hemisphere is observed with compression of the left lateral ventricle and midline shift to the right owing to the presence of carotid artery occlusion.

Figure 1.44. Posterior cerebral artery infarct with delayed hemorrhage. **A.** On noncontrast CT scan, low density is observed in left posterior cerebral artery distribution within thalamus, medial temporal lobe, and occipital lobe. Focal hemorrhagic infarct (*arrow*) is present in thalamus. Midline shift is present as well as compression of the left lateral and third ventricles. **B.** 72 hr later extensive hemorrhage is seen within the left thalamus occipital lobe and atrial portion of the left lateral ventricle. Midline shift is again noted, but as a consequence of the hemorrhage compressing the third ventricle, obstructive hydrocephalus has developed.

References

1. Atik M, Dein IO, Wolfson NJ: Significance of ulcerated lesions of the carotid arteries. Am Surg 39:681–687, 1973
2. Bergeron RT, Wood EH: Oral contraceptives and cerebrovascular complications. Radiology 92:231–238, 1969
3. Bickerstaff ER: Neurological complication of oral contraceptives. Clarendon Press, Oxford, 1975
4. Broman T, Olsson O: Technique for the pharmacodynamic investigation of contrast medium for cerebral angiography. Acta Radiol 45:96–100, 1956
5. Buell U, Kazner E, Rath M, Steinhoff H, Kleinhans E, Lanksch W: Sensitivity of computed tomography and serial scintigraphy in cerebrovascular disease. Radiology 131:393–398, 1979
6. Burrows EH, Leeds NE: Review of cerebrovascular disease and stroke. Neuroradiology I & II. Churchill Livingstone Inc., New York, 1981
7. Campbell JK, Houser OW, Stevens JC, Wahner HW, Baker HL, Jr., Folger WN: Computed tomography and radionuclide imaging in the evaluation of ischemic stroke. Radiology 126:695–702, 1978
8. Christenson PC, Ovitt TW, Fisher HD III, Frost MM, Nudelman S, Roehrig H: Intravenous angiography using digital video subtraction. Intravenous cervicocerebrovascular angiography. Am J Neuroradiol 1:379–386, 1980

9. Citron BP, Halpern M, MCCarron M, Lundberg GD, McCormick R, Pincus IJ, Totter D, Haverback BJ: Necrotizing angitis associated with drug abuse. New Engl J Med 283:1003–1011, 1970
10. Cole FM, Yates P: Intracerebral microaneurysms and small cerebrovascular lesions. Brain 90:759–768, 1967
11. Crawford ES, Wukasch DW, Debakey ME: Hemodynamic changes associated with carotid artery occlusion: An experimental and clinical study. Cardiovasc Res 1:3–10, 1962
12. Dodge PR, Swartz MN: Bacterial Meningitis—A review of selected aspects. II. Special neurologic problems, post meningitis complications and clinicopathological correlations. New Eng J Med 272:954–960, 1965
13. Edwards JH, Kricheff II, Gorstein F, Riles T, Imparato A: Atherosclerotic subintimal hematoma of the carotid artery. Radiology 133:123–129, 1979
14. Edwards JH, Kricheff II, Riles T, Imparato A: Angiographically undetected ulceration of the carotid bifurcation as a cause of embolic stroke. Radiology 132:369–373, 1979
15. Eisenberg RL, Nemzek WR, Moore WS, Mani RL: Relationship of transient ischemic attacks and angiographically demonstrable lesions of carotid artery. Stroke 8:483–486, 1977
16. Eisenman JI, Jenkin CG, Pribram HF: Evaluation of the cerebral circulation by arch aortography supplemented by subtraction technique. Am J Roentgenol 115:14–16, 1971
17. Faris A, Poser CM, Wilmore DW, Agnew CH: Radiologic visualization of neck vessels in healthy men. Neurology 13:386–396, 1963
18. Ferris EJ, Levine HL: Cerebral arteritis: Classification. Radiology 109:327–341, 1973
19. Fields WS, Lemac NA: Joint study of extracranial arterial occlusion. VII, Subclavian steal—A review of 168 cases. JAMA 222:1139–1143, 1972
20. Gomensoro JB, Maslenikov V, Azambuja N, Field WS, Lemac NA: Joint study of extracranial arterial occlusion. VIII, Clinical-radiographic correlation of carotid bifurcation lesions in 177 patients with transient cerebral ischemic attacks. JAMA 224:985–991, 1973
21. Handa J, Handa H, Nakano Y, Okuno T: Computed tomography in Moya Moya: Analysis of 16 cases. Computed axial tomography, Copyright, University Park Press, 1977, Vol. 1, No. 3, Printed in USA
22. Hass WK, Fields WS, North RR, Kricheff II, Chase NE, Bauer RB: Joint study of extracranial arterial occlusion. JAMA 203:159–166, 1968
23. Hilal SK, Solomon GE, Gold AP, Carter S: Primary cerebral arterial occlusive disease in children; Part I. Acute acquired hemiplegia. Radiology 99:71–86, 1971
24. Hilal SK, Solomon GE, Gold AP, Carter S: Primary cerebral arterial occlusive disease in children. Part II. Neurocutaneous syndromes. Radiology 99:87–94, 1971
25. Houser OW, Baker HL, Jr., Sandok BA, Holley KE: Cephalic arterial fibromuscular dysplasia. Radiology 101:605–611, 1971
26. Houser DW, Sundt TM, Jr., Holman CB, et al: Atheromatous disease of the carotid artery. Correlation of angiographic, clinical and surgical findings. J Neurosurg 4:321–331, 1974
27. Huckman M, Shenk GI, Neems RL, Tinor R: Transfemoral cerebral arteriography versus direct percutaneous carotid and brachial arteriography: Comparison of complication rates. Radiology 132:93–97, 1979
28. Kaufman DM, Leeds NE: Focal abnormalities with subdural empyema. Neuroradiology 11:169–173, 1976
29. Kerber CW, Cromwell LD, Drayer BP, Bank WO: Cerebral ischemia. I. Current angiographic techniques, complications and safety. Am J Roentgenol 130:1097–1103, 1978
30. Kilgore BB, Fields WS: Occlusive disease in adults. In Newton TH and Potts DG (eds.): Radiology of the Skull and Brain. Vol. 2, Book 4. CV Mosby, St. Louis, 1974
31. Kishore PRS, Chase NE, Kricheff II: Carotid stenosis and intracranial emboli. Radiology 100:351–356, 1971
32. Lassen NA: The luxury-perfusion syndrome and its possible relation to acute metabolic acidosis localized within the brain. Lancet 2:1113–1115, 1966
33. Latchaw RE, Gabrielson TO, Seeger JF: Cerebral angiography in meningeal sarcomatosis and carcinomatosis. Neuroradiology 8:131–139, 1974a.
34. Latchaw RE, Seeger JE, Gabrielson TO: Vertebrobasilar arterial occlusions in children. Neuroradiology 8:141–147, 1974b.
35. Launay M, Fredy P, Merland JJ, Bories J: Narrowing and occlusion of arteries by intracranial tumors. Review of literature and report of 25 cases. Neuroradiology 14:117–126, 1977
36. Leeds NE, Abbot KH: Collateral circulation in cerebrovascular disease in childhood via rete mirabile and perforating branches of anterior choroidal and posterior cerebral arteries. Radiology 85:628–634, 1965
37. Leeds NE, Goldberg HI: Lenticulostriate artery abnormalities: Value of direct serial magnification. Radiology 97:377–383, 1970
38. Leeds NE, Goldberg HI: Angiographic manifes-

tations in cerebral inflammatory disease. Radiology 98:595–604, 1971

39. Leeds NE, Goldberg HI: Abnormal vascular patterns in benign intracranial lesions: Pseudo tumors of the brain. Am J Roentgenol 118:576–585, 1973
40. Leeds NE, Rosenblatt R: Arterial wall irregularities in intracranial neoplasms: The shaggy vessel brought into focus. Radiology 103:121–124, 1972
41. Lin JP, Siew FP: Glioblastoma multiforme presenting angiographically as intracranial atherosclerotic vascular disease. Radiology 101:353–354, 1971
42. Maddison FE, Moore WS: Ulcerated atheroma of the carotid artery: Arteriographic appearance. Am J Roentgenol 107:530–534, 1969
43. Mani RL: Computer analysis of factors associated with thrombus formation observed on pull-out angiograms. Invest Radiol 10:378–384, 1975
44. Mani RL, Eisenberg RL: Complications of catheter cerebral arteriography: Analysis of 5000 procedures. II. Relation of complication rates to clinical and arteriographic diagnoses. Am J Roentgenol 131:867–869, 1978
45. Mani RL, Eisenberg R: Complications of catheter cerebral arteriography: Analysis of 5000 procedures. III. Assessment of arteries injected, contrast medium used, duration of procedure and age of patient. Am J Roentgenol 131:871–874, 1978
46. Mani RL, Eisenberg RL, McDonald EJ, Jr., Pollak JA, Mani JR: Complications of catheter cerebral arteriography: Analysis of 5000 procedures. I. Criteria and incidence. Am J Roentgenol 131:861–865, 1978
47. Martin MJ, Whisnant JP, Sayre GP: Occlusive vascular disease in the extracranial cerebral circulation. Arch Neurol 3:530–538, 1960
48. Mori H, Maeda T, Suzuki Y, Hisada K, Kadoya S: Brain scan in cerebrovascular moya-moya disease. Am J Roentgenol 124:583–589, 1975
49. Radu EW, Moseley IF: Carotid artery occlusion and computed tomography. A clinicoradiological study. Neuroradiology 17:7–12, 1978
50. Ridley A, Cavanaugh JB: Lymphocytic infiltration in gliomas: Evidence of possible host resistance. Brain 94:117–124, 1971
51. Riggs HE, Rupp C: Variations in form of circle of willis. Arch Neurology 8:8–14, 1963
52. Roberson GH, Scott WR, Rosenbaum AE: Thrombi at the site of carotid stenosis. Radiology 109:353-356, 1973
53. Ross Russel RW: Observations on intracerebral aneurysms. Brain 86:425–442, 1963
54. Rumbaugh CL, Bergeron RT, Fang HCH, McCormick R: Cerebral angiographic changes in the drug abuse patient. Radiology 101:335–344, 1971
55. Shillito J, Jr.: Carotid arteritis: A cause of hemiplegia in childhood. J Neurosurg 21:540–551, 1964
56. Simmons CR, Tsao E, Smith LL, Hinshaw DB, Thompson JR: Angiographic evaluation in extracranial vascular occlusive disease. Arch Surg 107:785–790, 1973
57. Sole'-Llenas J, Mercader JM, Pons-Tortella E: Morphological aspects of the vessels of the brain tumors. Neuroradiology 13:51–54, 1975
58. Stein BM, McCormick WF, Rodriquez JN, Taveras JM: Postmortem angiography of cerebral vascular system. Arch Neurol 7:545–559, 1962
59. Taveras JM: Multiple progressive intracranial arterial occlusions: A syndrome of children and young adults. Am J Roentgenol 106:235–268, 1969
60. Toole JF, Janeway R, Choi K, Cordell R, Davis C, Johnston F: Transient ischemic attacks due to atherosclerosis. Arch Neurol 32:5–12, 1975
61. Vander Ecken H, Adams RD: The anatomy and functional significance of the meningeal arterial anastomoses of the human brain. J Neuropath Exp Neurol 12:132–157, 1953
62. Weisberg LA: Computerized tomographic enhancement patterns in cerebral infarction. Arch Neurol 37:21–25, 1980
63. Whisnant JP, Martin MJ, Sayre GP: Atherosclerotic stenosis of cervical arteries. Arch Neurol 5:429–432, 1961
64. Wood EH, Correll JW: Atheromatous ulceration in major neck vessels as a cause of cerebral embolism. Acta Radiol [Diagn] (Stockh) 9:520–536, 1969
65. Yock DH and Marshall WH: Recent ischemic brain infarcts at computed tomography: Appearance pre and post contrast infusion. Radiology 117:559–608, 1975
66. Zimmerman RD, Leeds NE, Naidich TP: Carotid cavernous fistula associated with intracranial fibromuscular dysplasia. Radiology 122:725–726, 1977
67. Zimmerman RD, Leeds NE, Naidich TP: Ring blush associated with intracerebral hematoma. Radiology 122:707–711, 1977

2

Digital Subtraction Angiography in the Evaluation of Patients with Cerebrovascular Disease

Robert D. Zimmerman, Norman E. Leeds, and Mark J. Goldman

Introduction

Since its clinical introduction in 1980 digital subtraction angiography (DSA)[2,4,11,20,21] has become an increasingly popular tool used in the workup of patients with cerebrovascular disease. The procedure uses digitized fluoroscopy[13,14,16] to obtain high-quality angiographic images with low intra-arterial iodine concentration (under 5%).[2] Its uncritical usage, however, may lead to erroneous diagnoses and inappropriate therapy. Therefore, a knowledge of the current technique, its intrinsic limitations, and future potential is very important.

Physical Principles[13,10]

DSA represents an early and significant application of what has come to be known as digital radiography. All digital systems share the common feature of having an x-ray image "recorded" directly within a computer rather than on film, as it is in traditional radiography. [Computed tomography (CT) scanning is the first and best-known radiographic system to use digitized data recording.] The x-ray exposure is made on an image intensifier with digital fluoroscopy, and the signal from the intensifier is "read" by a video camera exactly as it is in traditional fluoroscopy. The analogue video signal is digitized, and the acquired data are stored within and manipulated by the computer to yield subtraction images. With routine film subtraction angiography (FSA), an initial film is obtained without contrast (the "mask"). The densities on this mask image are photographically inverted and then superimposed on subsequent films within the series where intravascular contrast is present. Since the mask film contains an exact inversion of all bony- and soft-tissue densities, the superimposition cancels out all densities present except those produced by contrast material within vascular structures. With DSA these operations are all performed electronically. The computer reverses the densities on the initial mask image and superimposes the mask on all subsequent images.

There are several advantages to DSA over FSA. First, good subtraction requires exact superimposition of all structures. Assuming no patient motion, this superimposition (or registration) is easily performed by the computer with its precise spatial encoding of data. Mechanical superimposition of radiographic images can never be this accurate. Second, DSA uses digital density measurements, which are intrinsically more precise than analogue measurements. Subtraction of densities is therefore more accurate than that of the purely analogue film subtraction systems. "Perfect" subtraction with complete elimination of all background (nonvascular) density is routinely obtained with DSA and rarely obtained with FSA. Third, since the background density is "0," computerized enhancement produces increased intravascular density with no increase in background noise, thus allowing for visualization of vessels with low intra-arterial contrast concentration. The contrast enhancement is logarithmic rather than linear (as it is in photographic FSA), and this eliminates subtraction artifacts produced by the superimposition of intravascular contrast on structures of markedly different radiographic density. (The background density in cerebrovascular arteriography ranges from low density of the soft tissue of the neck to the intermediate density of the cranial vault and finally to the very high density of the petrous bones.) The key to obtaining excellent DSA studies lies in the ability to obtain complete subtraction. If the patient moves during the procedure, superimpostion is incomplete and misregistration artifacts are produced. Computerized enhancement increases the density of both vessels and superimposed structures, and image quality suffers greatly. This is a constant problem when studying the extracranial carotid arteries where swallowing may obscure one of the carotid bifurcations superimposed upon adjacent pharyngeal structures. A fourth advantage to DSA over FSA is that the radiation dose for an average DSA study is one tenth the dose from arteriogram, because extensive fluoroscopy necessary for selective angiography is eliminated.[17] Finally, individual examinations are less expensive because of film cost savings. With routine arteriography, up to 100 films are exposed during the procedure at a cost of several hundred dollars. With DSA the study is recorded and stored on magnetic tape and only two to three pieces of film (costing less than $20.00) are used to produce hard copies of the diagnostic images. Subtraction of film angiography is a time-consuming laborious task requiring a high level of technical skill. With DSA the subtraction is performed by the computer and is therefore instantaneous and requires no special skills.

Comparative studies of image quality between DSA and FSA show that digital systems have greater density resolution (because of the superiority of digital versus analogue data recording and computer enhancement techniques), but FSA has much greater spatial resolution. DSA systems[3] generally resolve one to two line pairs per millimeter compared with 10 to 12 line pairs per millimeter with film screen systems commonly used in FSA. Spatial resolution in DSA is dependent on many components. These can be divided into the "imaging train" and computerized components. The imaging train consists of the image intensifier and video camera; at present it is the "weak link" in the digital system. Prior to the advent of DSA there was no clinical need for high resolution fluoroscopic systems. The advent of DSA has created just such a demand. Image intensifier improvements include (1) larger fields of view (14- to 16-inch fields are now available, whereas in the past a 9-inch field was standard); (2) an increase in the number of line pairs per millimeter that can be resolved; and (3) increased sensitivity due to a decrease in filtering of lower energy x-ray beams. Improvements in video systems include (1) an increase in the number of lines on the video monitor from 500 to 1,000; (2) an increase in the signal-to-noise ratio from approximately 500 to 1 to greater than 1,000 to 1; and (3) marked increase in the dynamic range (to allow for better visualization of large differences in densities encountered with DSA). In the computerized portion of DSA systems, spatial resolution is limited by "pixel" size. This term is short for picture element and has the same meaning as with CT. It represents the small area or volume to which the computer assigns a specific density determination. DSA systems have gone from 256 × 256 pixel matrices to 512 × 512 matrices. (1,024 × 1,024 matrices are becoming available.) As the pixel number increases, the pixel size is reduced, improving spatial resolution (at some cost to density resolution). These technologic advances will undoubtedly improve the spatial resolution of digital systems. Whether this will allow DSA to achieve the spatial resolution commonly obtained with FSA is unclear.

Injection Site

DSA equipment provides great flexibility and may be used to perform arteriography in a variety of ways. Contrast may be injected intravenously (digital intravenous angiography, DIVA) or intra-arterially. Arterial injections may be made into the aortic arch (digital arch arteriography, DAA) or into individual vessels following selective catheterization. Each site has its individual advantages and disadvantages.

Digital Intravenous Angiography

DIVA Technique

The most common site of venous puncture is the anticubital vein. Contrast may be injected peripherally or centrally. With peripheral injections a 6- to 8-inch catheter is advanced into the antecubital vein. The contrast is injected following which additional fluid (often saline) is also injected to wash the contrast from its peripheral site of injection. This is the technique initially devised for performing DIVA and is still widely used in many centers.[1,11] The major advantages of this technique are its ease, speed, and safety. Because of the peripheral location of the catheter, the procedure may be done by paramedical staff, saving physician time. Occasionally the short catheter abutts against a peripheral valve. This may lead to extravasation of contrast into the soft tissues and a suboptimal study. Other centers have opted to use a longer catheter with multiple side holes (multipurpose or pigtail catheters) and advance it into the superior vena cava.[4,10] With this central site of injection, the contrast bolus is better maintained, increasing intra-arterial contrast concentration and leading to better arterial opacification, especially intracranially. It is not necessary to flush the contrast bolus from its peripheral location; therefore, additional injections of fluid are not necessary. When a satisfactory antecubital vein cannot be found, the catheter may be inserted into the femoral vein and advanced into the inferior vena cava.

The volume of contrast used per injection ranges from 30 to 50 cc injected at 10 to 25 cc/sec using a power injector (hand injection does not yield an adequate bolus of contrast). A variety of iodinated contrast materials may be employed usually in a concentration of 76 mg% iodine. Depending on patient weight, 150 to 250 cc of contrast is used per study, and therefore a maximum five to six angiographic runs may be obtained.

The patient is positioned under fluoroscopic control in various obliquities to obtain views of specific areas, in particular the carotid bifurcations. When available, C-arm fluoroscopy is preferable, since it allows for positioning of the fluoroscopic tube while the patient remains in a comfortable (and therefore easily maintained) supine position.

Contrast is injected and multiple sequential images are obtained. It takes a finite time for the contrast bolus to reach the right heart, traverse the lungs, return to the left heart, and enter the arterial system. Therefore, a three- to six-second delay is incorporated into the angiographic

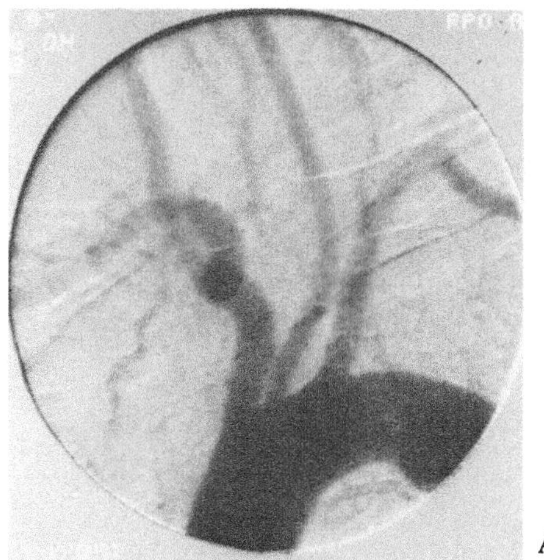
A

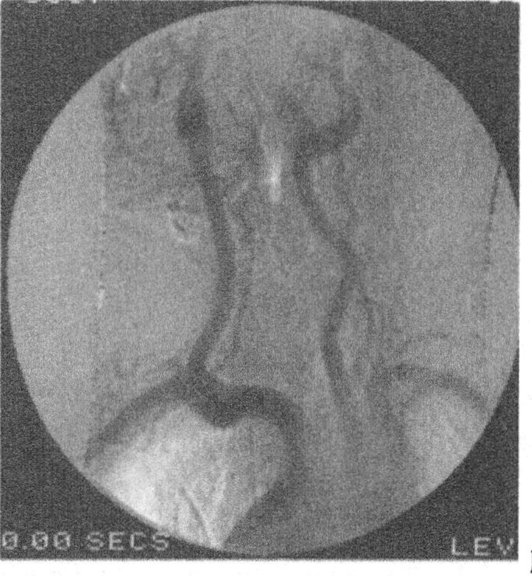

B

Figure 2.1. DIVA of the normal aortic arch. **A.** There is excellent visualization of the aorta and its tributary branches, including the innominate artery, both vertebral arteries, both common carotid arteries, and left subclavian artery. **B.** In another patient, arch study was performed with slightly higher centering to demonstrate excellent visualization of both common carotid arteries and of the origin of the left internal and external carotid arteries.

sequence between obtaining the initial mask image and the performance of the remainder of the angiographic series.

Ideally, this study allows for evaluation of the entire cervical and intracranial vasculature. The area of greatest clinical importance is the region of the carotid artery bifurcations, and therefore right and left posterior oblique views centered on these regions are initially obtained (Fig. 2.1). Additional views of the aortic arch and its proximal branches (Fig. 2.2) and more cephalic intracranial structures (Fig. 2.3) are obtained. If, for any reason, the carotid bifurcation views are suboptimal (Fig. 2.2C), repeat examinations through this area should be obtained in preference to either intracranial or proximal series.

Complications of DIVA

Because of the intravenous route of injection, DIVA is a safe and relatively noninvasive study

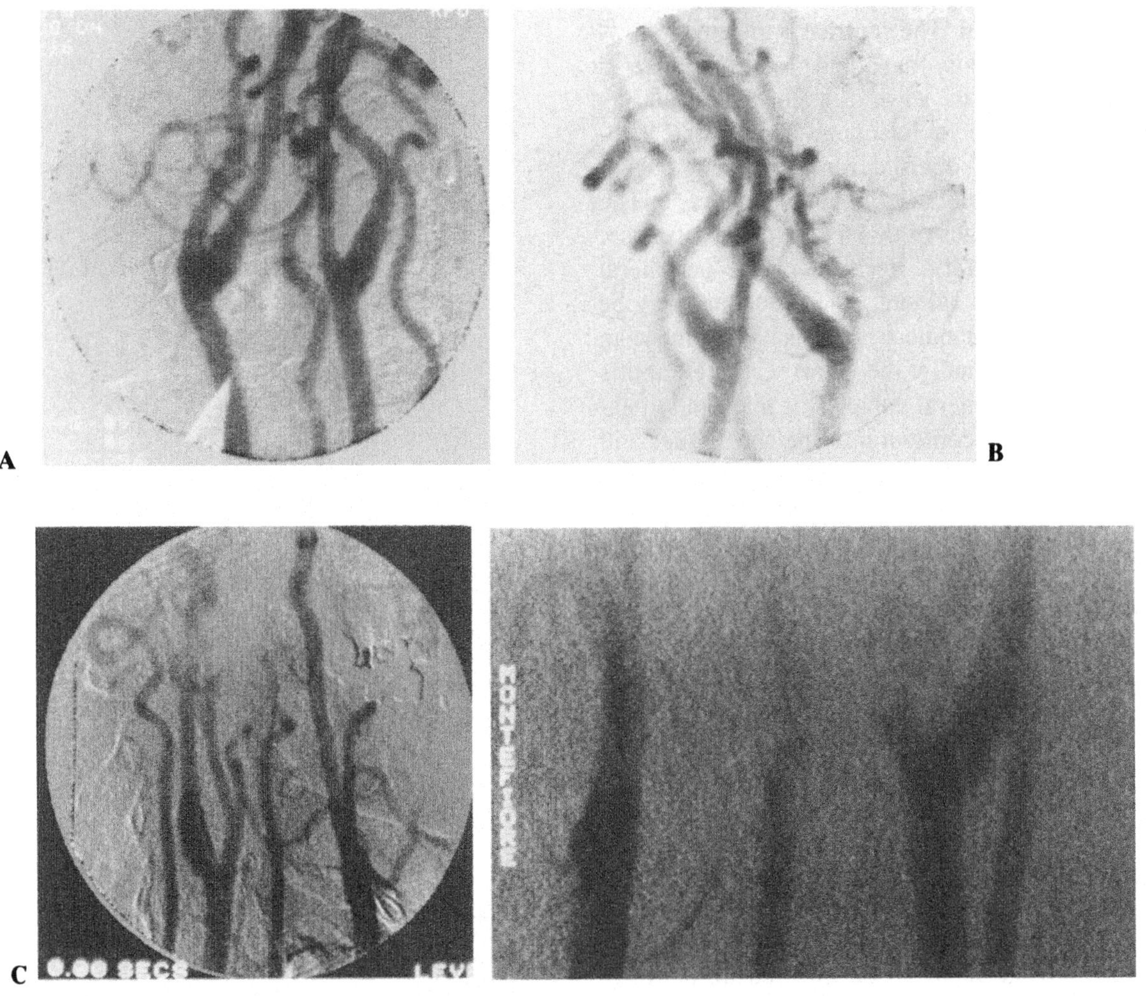

Figure 2.2. The normal carotid artery bifurcations on DIVA. Right posterior oblique (RPO) **(A)** and left posterior oblique (LPO) **(B)** views in the same patient demonstrate excellent visualization of both carotid arteries in two separate projections. The distal common carotid arteries, their bifurcations, and the proximal internal and external carotid arteries are well visualized without vascular overlap. More commonly, carotid artery bifurcations are well seen in only one projection. Thus, in another patient the LPO view **(C)** demonstrates the right common carotid artery bifurcation and the internal and external carotid arteries to great advantage. But the left carotid bifurcation and internal carotid artery origin are overlapped by the external carotid artery. Magnified view of the RPO projection **(D)** shows the left common carotid artery, its bifurcation, and the left internal carotid artery to advantage. On this view the right carotid artery bifurcation and internal carotid artery are overlapped by the external carotid artery.

that can be performed on an outpatient basis. The major arteriographic complications (such as infarction) do not occur. Extravasation of contrast material is uncommon (less than 1%) with both peripheral and central injection. Aside from pain and local swelling, no significant sequellae have been reported with extravasation either into the arm (peripheral injection) or mediastinum (central injection). Rarely, patients with significant compromise of cardiac or renal function showed deterioration after DIVA due to the large amount of contrast necessary to obtain an adequate study. Thus, patients with severe renal or cardiac disease are probably not ideal candidates for outpatient DIVA, since the contrast load must be curtailed (often leading to an inadequate study) if the examination is to be performed safely.

Results of DIVA

Visualization of arterial structures with DIVA is generally excellent. Studies correlating DIVA with selective arteriography demonstrated that DIVA is both accurate and sensitive when the study is of adequate quality.[1,4,10,15,19] The full range of vascular pathology is demonstrable. Ulcerations are clearly seen (Figs. 2.4, 2.8) even when these lesions are small. Vascular occlusions are reliably seen (Figs. 2.5, 2.6, 2.8). Regions of stenosis are identified and accurately quantified (Figs. 2.5–2.8). Evaluation of the intracranial vasculature is somewhat more variable[15,21] (Figs. 2.3, 2.6). Difficulties with imaging in the intracranial vasculature are caused by (1) attenuation of the x-ray beam by the calvarium and dense petrous bones; (2) inadequate intra-arterial contrast concentration due to dilution of the contrast bolus as it progresses cephalad; (3) limitations in spatial resolution which make it difficult (at least at the present time) to visualize small but important intracranial vessels such as lenticulostriate arteries and small middle cerebral artery branches; and (4) nonselective technique produces extensive overlap of different vascular territories, in particular on lateral views, obscuring significant intracranial vascular structures. Despite these limitations, good visualization of the intracranial carotid arteries, basilar artery, and proximal anterior middle and posterior cerebral arteries is often obtained (Fig. 2.3).

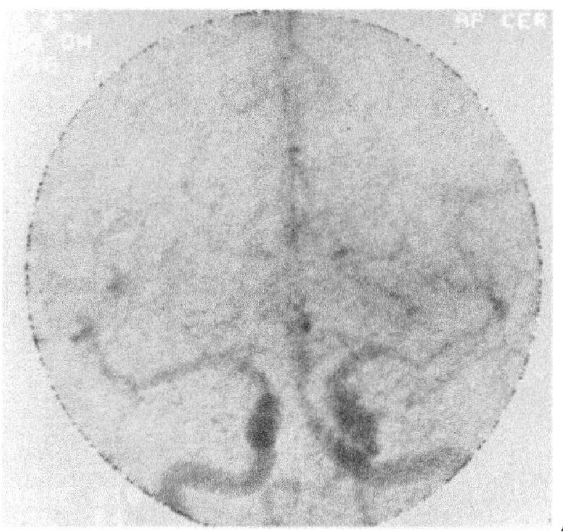

A

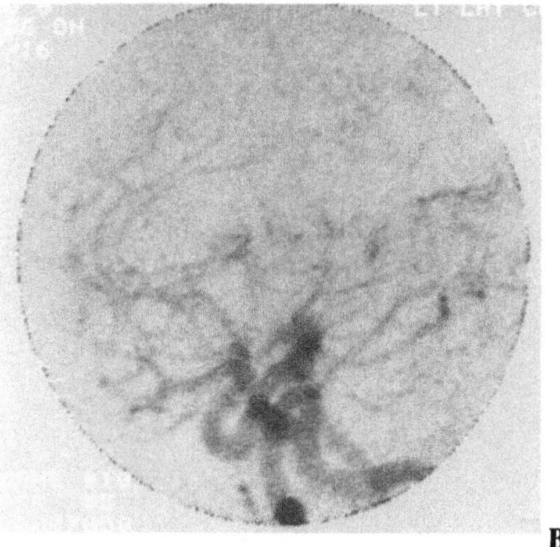

B

Figure 2.3. Normal intracranial circulation on DIVA. On the frontal view **(A)** the internal carotid arteries are visualized bilaterally and are particularly well seen in their petrosal, precavernous, and supraclinoid segments. The cavernous segments are suboptimally seen owing to redundancy of these portions of the vessels. Between the distal internal carotid arteries the basilar artery is visualized after it originates from the two vertebral arteries. The horizontal segments of the anterior and middle cerebral arteries are well seen, and the middle cerebral artery trifurcations are identified. Secondary and tertiary order middle cerebral artery branches and the lenticulostriate artery are not well seen. The steep lateral oblique view **(B)** "unravels" the cavernous carotid arteries. Individual middle and anterior cerebral artery branches are also well seen, but vascular overlap is so severe that overall evaluation is difficult.

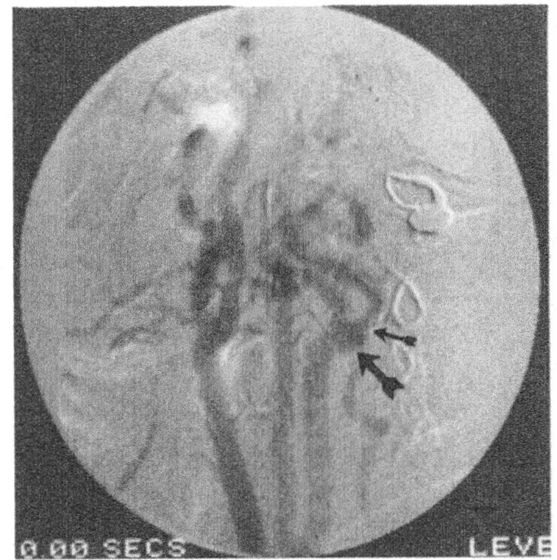

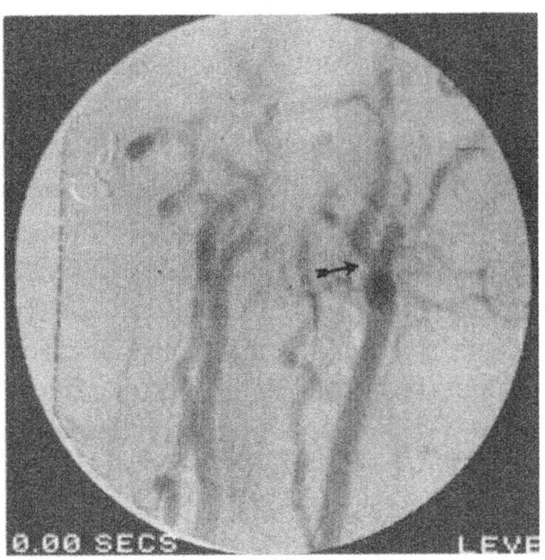

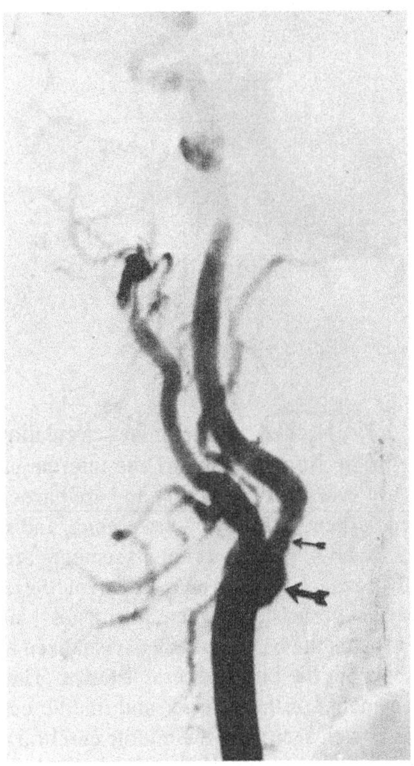

Figure 2.4. Ulcerated plaque visualized on DIVA. The RPO view **(A)** demonstrates an outpouching (ulceration) from the posterior aspect of the common carotid artery bifurcation (*large arrow*). Just distal to the ulceration there is narrowing of the internal carotid artery (*small arrow*), which is better appreciated on the LPO **(B)** view (*small arrow*). The ulceration is not well identified, since it is seen en face. There is excellent correlation between the DIVA study and the lateral carotid angiogram **(C)**, which confirms the presence of the area of ulceration (*large arrow*) and stenosis (*small arrow*).

In a relatively short period of time, DIVA has proved to be a sensitive and specific diagnostic study in a majority of patients. Suboptimal studies do occur, however, owing to a variety of factors. The incidence of suboptimal studies has been reported as low as 5%[19] and at least potentially as high as 60%.[8] Most authors place the incidence of suboptimal studies at between 15% and 30%.[1,4,10,15] Many factors may affect the incidence of suboptimal studies, including the quality of the digital subtraction equipment, the population of patients under study, and the criteria of study adequacy.

A major cause of suboptimal study is patient motion producing misregistration and degradation of DIVA images. The most common type of motion artifact encountered is induced by swallowing (an involuntary response of the contrast agent injected). With the patient in the oblique projection, the ipsilateral carotid artery bifurcation overlies the pharyngeal region and when swallowing occurs, adequate visualization of this portion of the carotid artery may be impossible. To avoid or decrease swallowing, oral local anesthesia may be used (e.g., viscous lidocaine). This does appear to decrease the swallowing response to a certain extent; however, it may create an unwarranted risk of aspiration in ambulatory and, therefore, unmonitored patients. These swallowing-induced artifacts cause suboptimal visualization of 10% of the carotid bifurcations studied in our experience. The problem may be reduced in the future with the introduction of a nonionic contrast agent that appears to cause less involuntary

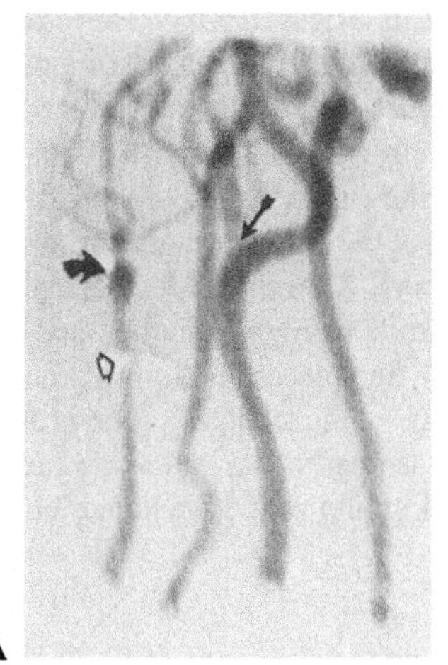
A

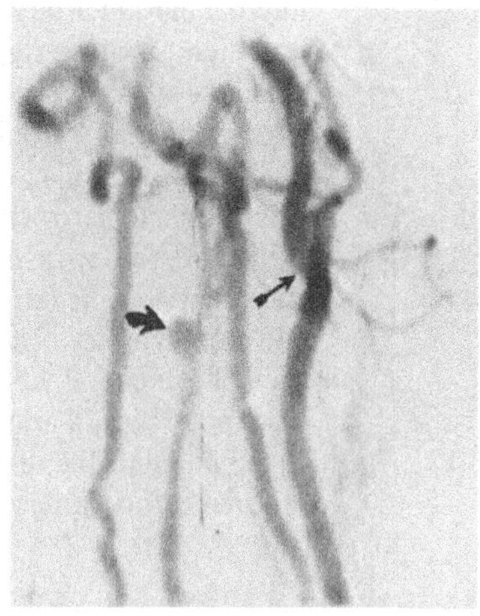
B

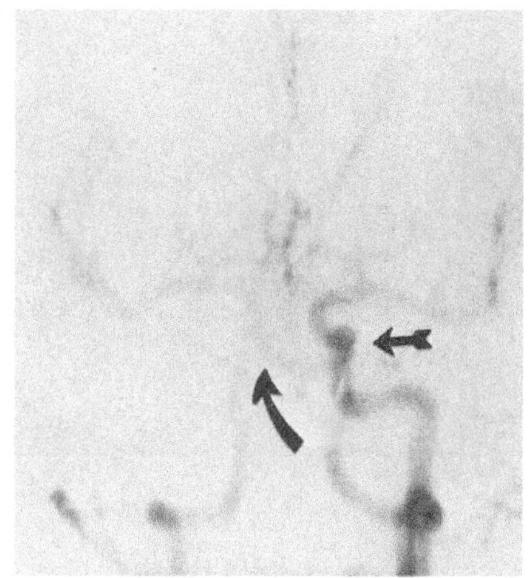
C

Figure 2.5. Severe atherosclerotic disease identified on DIVA in a patient with left cerebral transient ischemic attacks and an asymptomatic right carotid bruit. On the RPO **(A)** view the right common carotid artery is small in caliber owing to decreased flow. There is a severe stenosis of the distal common carotid artery (*open arrowhead*). The internal carotid artery is occluded (*curved arrow*). The left common carotid artery is normal in caliber, but at the origin of the left external artery (*arrow*) a tight stenosis (80%–90%) is identified. On the LPO view (*B*) the small caliber of the right common carotid artery and the occlusion of the right internal carotid artery are clearly identified. The plaque in the common carotid artery is not well seen. The left external carotid artery stenosis is completely obscured because the common carotid artery bifurcation is overlapped by the internal and external carotid artery orifices. On a frontal intracranial series **(C)** there is filling of the left internal carotid artery (*arrow*) and of the vertebral basilar system (*curved arrow*). Both right and left anterior and middle cerebral arteries fill, but there is no filling of the occluded right internal carotid artery.

swallowing. Respiratory motion may also occasionally degrade images, especially toward the end of the angiographic series. The power-injected bolus of contrast produces the sudden onset of heat and burning and may cause involuntary bulk movement as the patient is "jolted" by the contrast material. Quite obviously, therefore, the patient must be highly cooperative for this study to be performed. Patients with decreased mentation or consciousness are not candidates for this procedure.

Another source of suboptimal studies is poor cardiac output (5% of patients in our experience). In these patients slow circulation time causes dilution of the contrast bolus, thereby decreasing the intra-arterial contrast concentration to a point where it is too low for adequate visualization of arterial structures.

One of the most difficult problems to assess is the effect of vascular overlap on the diagnostic adequacy of DIVA studies. These studies are by nature nonselective, with overlap an intrinsic limitation that will not be eliminated with technical improvement in digital subtraction angiography equipment. Prior to the advent of DIVA, selective angiography was deemed necessary, since arch arteriography (essentially the equivalent of DIVA studies) failed to demonstrate many significant lesions.[6] Despite this fact, a series correlating DIVA results with that of selective arteriography has shown a very low incidence of suboptimal studies due to overlap (5%–10%).[19] There is, however, a statistical bias in these studies, since they include normal examinations. The fact that a portion of an artery overlapped by superimposed vascular structures is shown to be normal on subsequent arteriography does not lead to the conclusion that DIVA studies without follow-up arteriography are adequate for evaluation of these regions. It is common for the external carotid artery or vertebral artery to overlap all or a

A 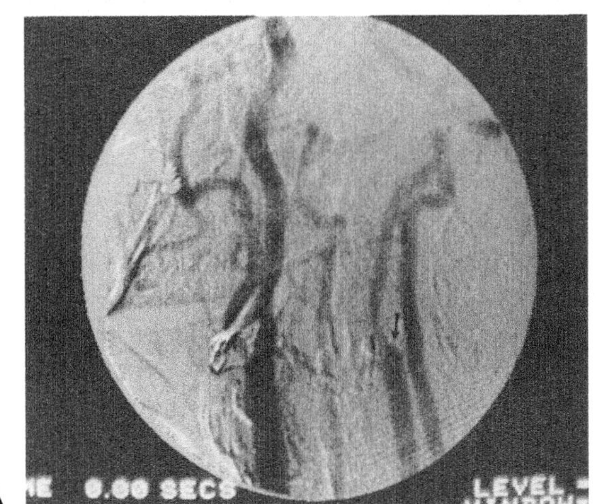

Figure 2.6. Severe atherosclerotic involvement identified on DIVA in a patient with asymptomatic carotid bruits bilaterally. Examination of the RPO view **(A)** demonstrates complete occlusion of the left internal carotid artery at its origin (*arrow*). There is mild stenosis of the right internal crotid artery origin, which is somewhat obscured by artifacts produced by swallowing. A frontal intracranial view **(B)** demonstrates good filling of the right internal carotid artery with mild narrowing of the precavernous portion of this vessel (*open arrow*). The distal left internal carotid artery fills retrograde (*arrow*) from the opposite carotid artery. These findings are better seen on the oblique lateral view **(C)**. The stenosis of the precavernous carotid artery is identified (*open arrow*) as is the filling of the distal stump of the occluded left internal carotid artery.

B 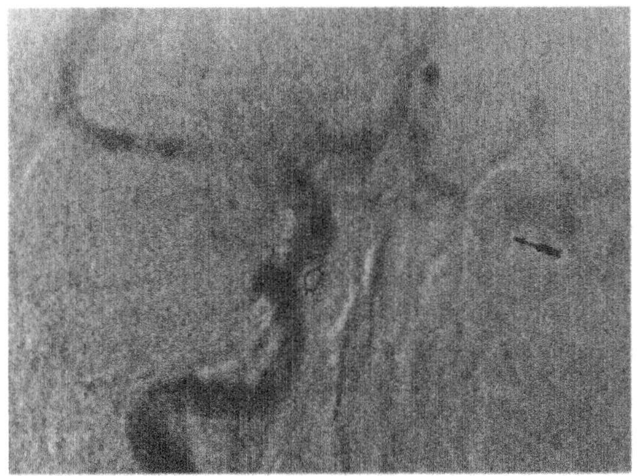

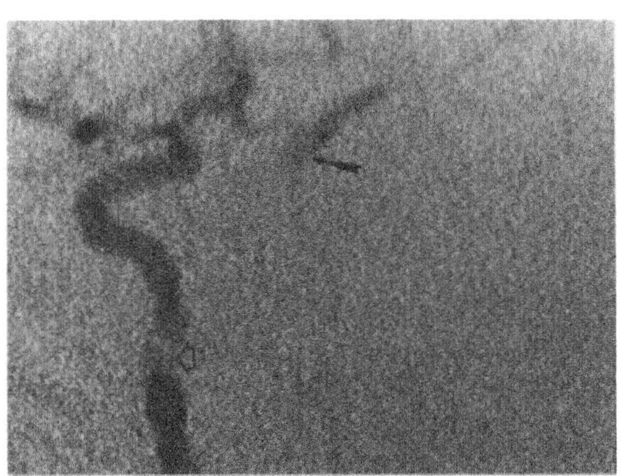 C

A 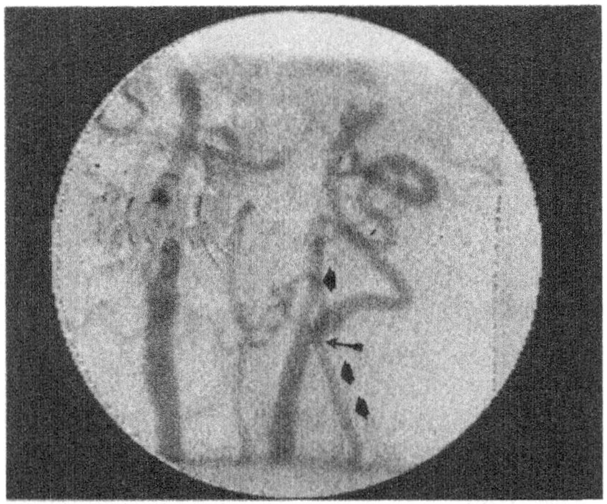

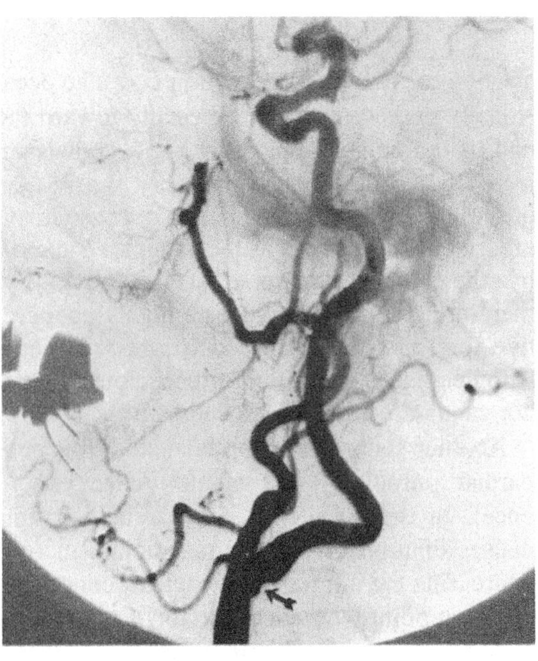 B

Figure 2.7. Limitation of DIVA due to nonselective technique. On an RPO view **(A)** both carotid arteries appear normal. Note that the left internal carotid artery origin is overlapped by a small left vertebral artery (*small arrowheads*). The lateral film from a selective left carotid angiogram **(B)** demonstrates an ulcerated plaque at the origin of the internal carotid artery (*arrow*) that was not visualized on the DIVA study because of the overlap of the plaque by the small vertebral artery and because of the inability to obtain a true lateral projection of this focal area of atherosclerosis.

portion of the common carotid artery bifurcation and proximal internal carotid artery. Since these are common sites of atherosclerotic involvement, care must be taken to determine that these regions are well seen. More recently several investigators studied the adequacy of DIVA by using traditional criteria for adequate arteriography in patients with cerebrovascular disease. The major criteria for adequacy was visualization of significant areas (in particular, the carotid artery bifurcations and cavernous internal carotid arteries) in two projections without vascular overlap. By these criteria only 41% of carotid artery bifurcations were adequately visualized with DIVA and in only 28% of patients was there bilateral adequate carotid artery bifurcation visualization.[7] One of the weaknesses of DIVA (and any other nonselective arteriographic technique) is the inability to obtain a true lateral projection, because the two carotid arteries are superimposed on this view. Unfortunately, this is the most sensitive view for demonstrating atherosclerotic disease on selective angiography, since the majority of atherosclerotic plaques arise along the posterior wall of the common carotid artery bifurcation and extend into the carotid artery origin.[23] In one recent study[9] focal areas of atherosclerosis with ulceration and/or stenosis were identified on the lateral projection only in 37% of patients. Focal, rather than circumferential lesions are more likely to be missed because of the inability to obtain multiple unobstructed views of the carotid artery bifurcations. Small focal areas of ulceration or, less commonly, noncircumferential stenoses or webs are the types of lesions that may be missed on DIVA studies (Figs. 2.7, 2.8). The more common circumferential stenoses and large areas of ulceration will be identified with a high degree of accuracy.

In summary, determination of the adequacy of DIVA studies both in general and in any specific case must be done with great care. To determine if follow-up arteriography is necessary in any single patient, the referring physician and radiologist should be guided by practicality. The question that we must continually ask ourselves is "Will a selective arteriogram (with all its attendant cost and risk) demonstrate findings that might alter therapeutic decisions from those that would be made on the basis of a DIVA study alone?"

Indications for DIVA

Screening Tests in Patients with Asymptomatic Bruits. Many patients over 50 years of age have asymptomatic carotid bruits. In the past it was not feasible to examine these patients en masse. DIVA allows for safe, accurate, and relatively inexpensive evaluation of these patients on an ambulatory basis. Patency of the carotid arteries can be assessed and therapeutic regimens instituted. DIVA has proved to be particularly valuable in patients with bruits who are to undergo surgery (in particular, cardiac surgery), since these patients are at risk for cerebral infarction compared with the normal patient population. The purpose of the study is to identify severe stenoses or occlusions that are asymptomatic so that prophylactic carotid surgery may be performed when indicated. DIVA is clearly the procedure of choice in these patients.

Evaluations of Patients with Ill-Defined Neurologic Abnormalities. Occasionally patients have neurologic symptoms that are difficult to assess clinically. In these patients DIVA is an effective tool in determining the status of the cervicocerebral vasculature. Where significant abnormalities (ulcerations, stenoses, or occlusions) are encountered, ischemia may be invoked as a cause for the patient's clinical abnormalities. If the DIVA study is normal, a major occlusive lesion of the extracranial arteries may be ruled out.

Postoperative Examination. Following endarterectomy, DIVA may be used to assess the effectiveness of surgery. The endarterectomy site may be identified and residual stenoses or ulcerations seen (Fig. 2.10). Since carotid artery atherosclerosis is often bilateral, DIVA may also be used to ascertain the severity and/or progression of disease in the contralateral unoperated carotid artery.[5] DIVA may also be used to evaluate the patency and effectiveness of external to internal carotid artery anastomoses.

Evaluation of Patients with Transient Ischemic Attacks. DIVA may prove to be inadequate in from 20%[10] to 50% (authors experience) of patients with transient ischemic attacks or amaurosis fugax (in whom there is a high index of suspicion of a surgically treatable vascular le-

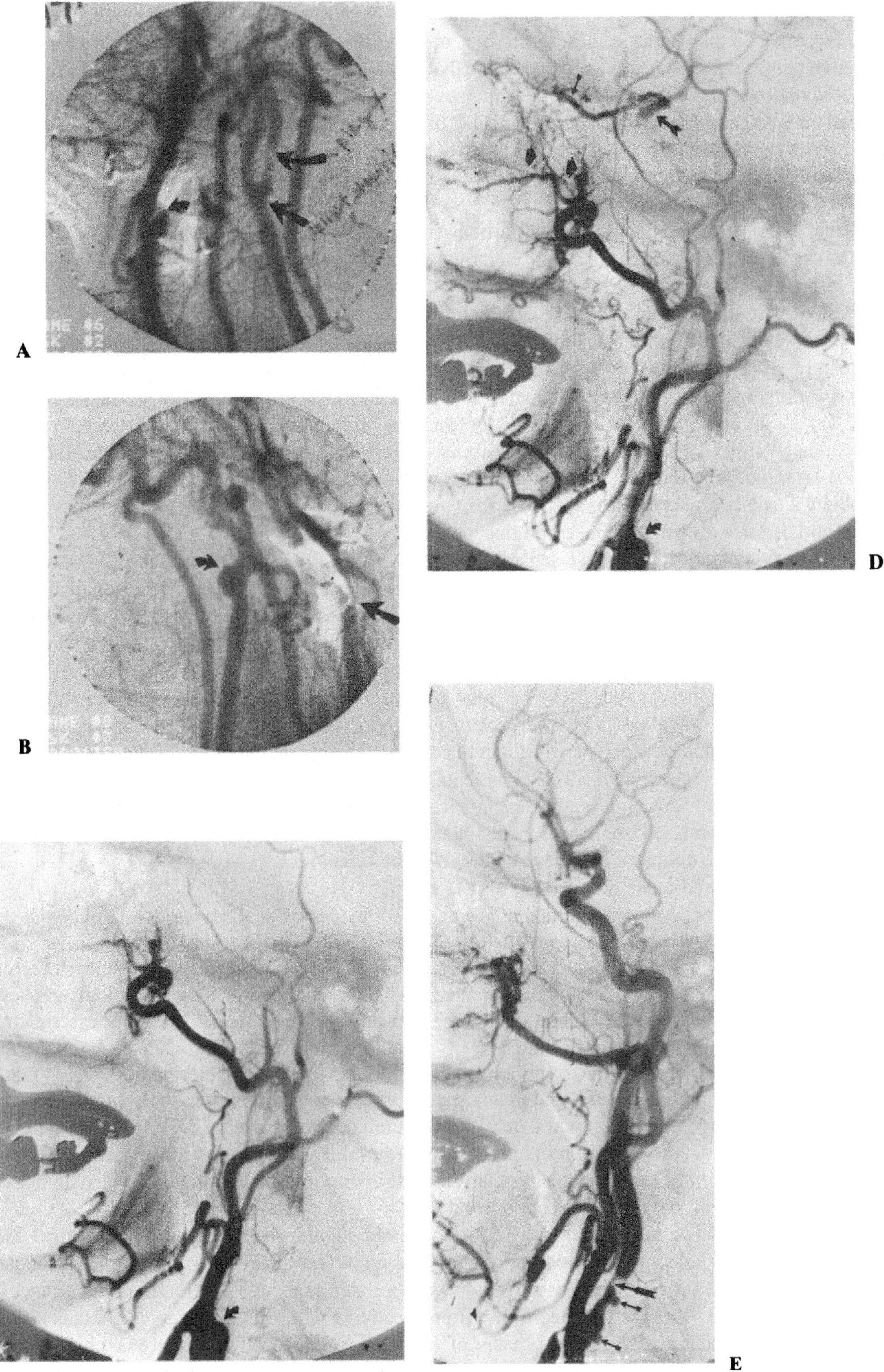
A
B
C
D
E

sion). The frequency of inadequate DIVA examinations is dependent on the amount of information required to make a therapeutic decision, which is, in turn, affected by the referring physician's treatment philosophy. For example, a DIVA study demonstrating complete carotid occlusion may be adequate in some clinical circumstances (Figs. 2.5, 2.6) and inadequate in other circumstances (Fig. 2.7). It will be nondefinitive if the patient is a candidate for extracranial-intracranial bypass, and the superficial temporal artery is poorly visualized because of its small caliber and the nonselective nature of DIVA. The extent of atherosclerosis and the pattern of collateralization is also difficult to assess on DIVA because it is not selective, and yet many surgeons consider this information important in choosing patients for bypass surgery (Fig. 2.7). In our experience, a minimally patent but very narrow internal carotid artery (the "string sign")[12] may be mistaken for an external carotid artery branch; thus a lesion that is potentially treatable by endarterectomy may go undetected.

Arteriography is also occasionally warranted in patients with transient ischemic attacks and normal DIVA, since endarterectomy may be performed to eliminate embolization from shallow nonstenotic plaques (often not visible even on conventional selective arteriography),[6] especially in patients who have failed to respond to medical management. In these patients arteriographic identification of small intracranial lesions not visible on DIVA (Fig. 2.9) may explain the patients' ischemic symptoms and obviate the need for surgical exploration of the carotid bifurcation.

DIVA is definitive when it clearly demonstrates a hemodynamically significant stenosis (greater than 50%)[5] and/or a large area of ulceration in the symptomatic carotid artery. When the remainder of the carotid artery and the proximal and middle cerebral arteries are well visualized and normal (Figs. 2.4–2.6), arteriography will yield little additional significant information. Arteriography may thus be avoided in precisely those patients who are at greatest risk for ischemic complications of selective angiography.

Evaluation of Intracranial Disease. DIVA may be used to evaluate intracranial pathology when high quality arteriography is unnecessary, dangerous, or unlikely to yield clinically significant results.[21] Thus, DIVA has replaced arteriography in the evaluation of intrasellar and suprasellar masses.[15] Giant aneurysms, which may mimic CT appearance of large pituitary adenomas, are easily identified. DIVA also allows for assessment of the position of the carotid arteries and the anterior cerebral artery prior to transphenoidal approach to the pituitary fossa. When a vascular blush is visualized, lesions such as suprasellar meningiomas may be suspected and arteriography performed. When vascular lesions such as giant aneurysms or ar-

◁ **Figure 2.8.** Severe atherosclerosis identified on DIVA: Value of selective arteriography providing additional information in a patient with right cerebral transient ischemic attacks. RPO view **(A)** demonstrates a complete occlusion of the right internal carotid artery just distal to its origin (*curved arrow*). The left carotid artery also shows atherosclerotic involvement with mild narrowing of the common carotid artery bifurcation (*straight arrow*) and more severe narrowing of the internal carotid artery approximately 1 cm distal to the origin of this vessel. The LPO view **(B)** confirms the right carotid occlusion (*curved arrow*), but the left carotid bifurcation and proximal internal carotid artery are not well seen owing to a combination of overlap of vascular structures and to "swallowing" artifacts. Selective right carotid arteriography **(C)** confirms the presence of an occlusion of the internal carotid artery (*curved arrow*). On a later film **(D)** there is visualization of the distal internal carotid artery (*large arrow*), which is reconstituted via collateral circulation from the internal maxillary artery (*arrowheads*) to the ophthalmic artery (*small arrows*). The type and degree of collateral filling of the internal carotid artery cannot be identified on DIVA because of the marked reduction in flow in the carotid artery and the nonselective nature of the study. The selective left carotid angiogram **(E)** demonstrates more severe involvement of the left carotid artery then can be appreciated on the DIVA study. There are multiple areas of ulceration present (*small arrows*) in both common carotid artery bifurcation and internal carotid artery. The stenosis of the internal carotid artery is greater than 90% (*large arrow*).

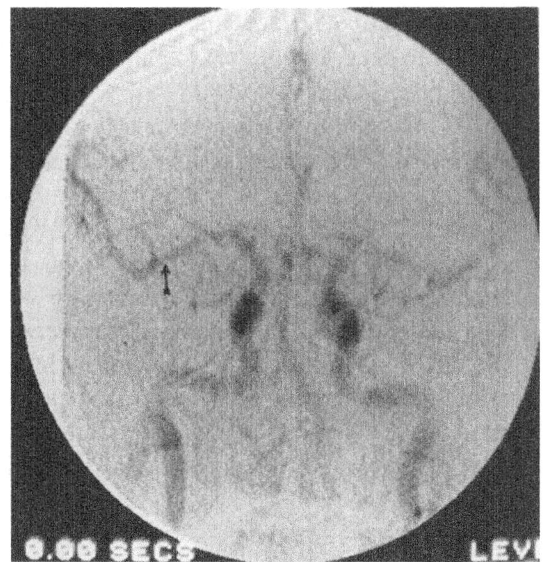

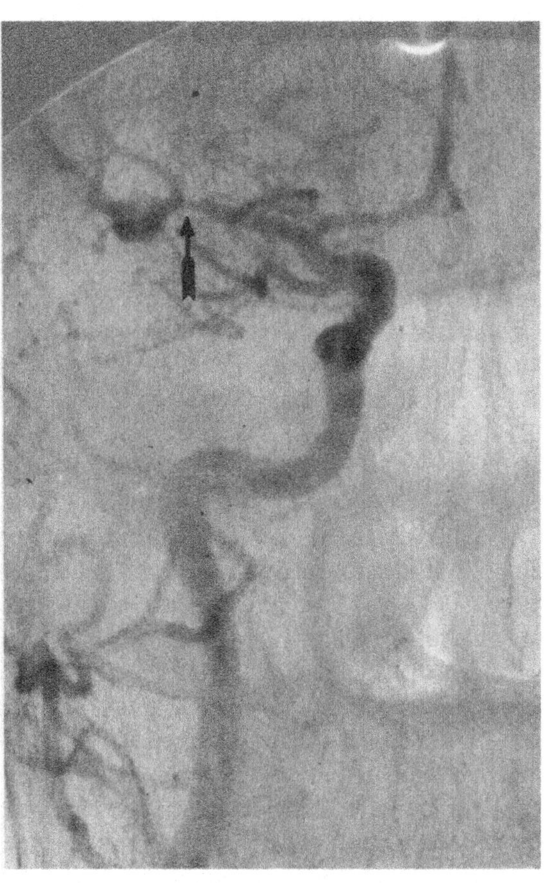

Figure 2.9. Limitation of DIVA in the evaluation of intracranial atherosclerotic disease. In this patient with right cerebral transient ischemic attacks, the DIVA examination is normal. On a frontal intracranial examination **(A)** the middle cerebral artery appears normal. Selective right common carotid arteriography, however, demonstrates a stenosis of the right middle cerebral artery just proximal to its trifurcation **(B)**.

teriovenous malformations are diagnosed or suspected on CT, but surgery is not contemplated, DIVA may be used to confirm the diagnosis and effectively delineate the vascular lesions. In patients with subarachnoid hemorrhage, DIVA serves a complementary role to arteriography. The nonselective nature of DIVA and the limited spatial resolution of digital systems prevent adequate visualization of the aneurysm and its relationship to the surrounding vascular structures; therefore, the definitive study remains an arteriogram. DIVA may be used to assess the extent and progression of arterial spasm.[18] Because DIVA is noninvasive, multiple studies may be performed as often as necessary to follow the development and regression of spasm prior to surgery, obviating the need for multiple arteriographic procedures. DIVA may be used for the preoperative evaluation of some intracranial neoplasms. An overall assessment of tumor vascularity and the major arterial and venous displacements may be obtained. DIVA is actually superior to selective arteriography in demonstrating dural venous sinus thrombosis in patients with meningiomas abutting against the sinus,[15] since with DIVA, the entire vascular system is flooded and failure to opacify a midline dural sinus is more strongly indicative of thrombosis. In general, however, DIVA gives only gross information on the site and nature of intracranial neoplasms, and therefore if angiography is performed for diagnostic purposes (rather than for vascular roadmapping), arteriography remains the procedure of choice.

Digital Arch Arteriography[3,22,24]

Digital equipment may be used to perform aortic arch arteriography. DAA has several advantages when compared with DIVA and traditional film arch angiography (FAA). In the past FAA was used predominantly as an adjunct to selective arteriography in evaluating patients with cerebrovascular disease. The major limitation of FAA lies in the large volumes of contrast necessary to adequately opacify the vascular tree. As much as 65 cc of 76 mg% iodine con-

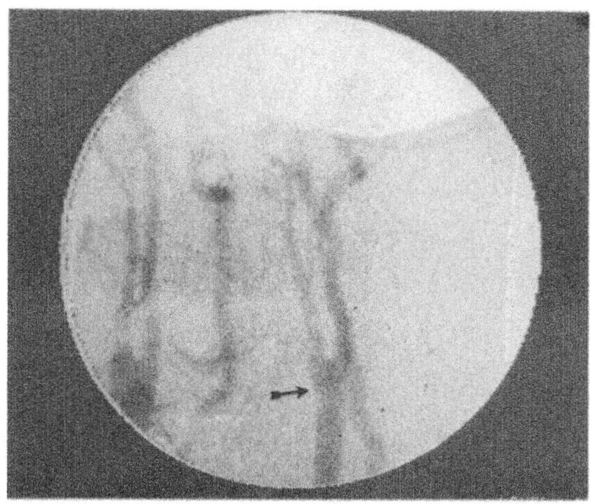
A

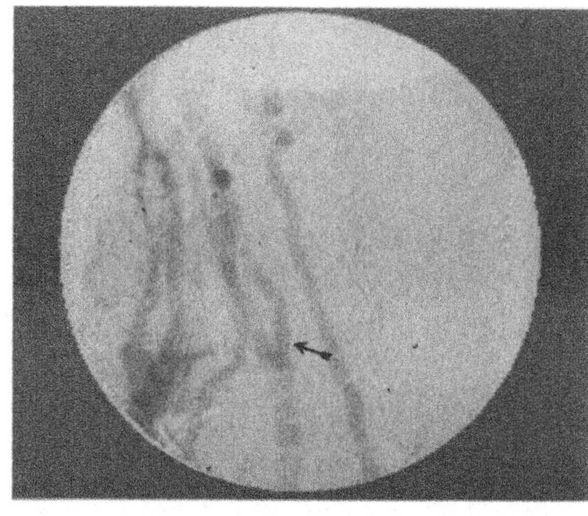
B

Figure 2.10. DIVA in postoperative evaluations. The patient is status post left carotid endarterectomy (initial arteriogram demonstrated 85% stenosis with ulceration of this vessel). DIVA demonstrates a normal distal common carotid artery and a normal carotid bifurcation with a widely patent internal carotid artery demonstrated on both RPO (AM) and steep RPO views. The distal common carotid artery and proximal internal carotid artery are slightly patulous (*arrows*), a finding typically seen after endarterectomy.

centration contrast material must be used, and therefore a maximum of two or, at most three series may be obtained with FAA. Vascular overlap is common, and the study is rarely adequate for full assessment of the cervicocerebral vasculature. The large volume of contrast used may flood the already compromised cerebrovascular system, producing an increase in ischemic symptom. Finally, the large volumes of contrast and rapid injection rates required for adequate arterial opacification necessitate the use of specialized large-bore catheters (7 French) with multiple side holes. Thus, if selective arteriography is to be performed at the same sitting, the catheter and contrast material must be changed during the procedure.

At those institutions where selective studies are performed with small, thin-walled catheters (5 French), arch studies must be performed after selective arteriography, and therefore the FAA cannot serve as a preliminary test or a screening test. In this setting, routine FAA has been shown to be of little diagnostic value.[7] Despite its limitations, FAA does serve a useful function when done as a preliminary test in patients undergoing arteriography for cerebrovascular disease. It may be used as a "road map," delineating the origins and proximal portions of the major branches of the aorta. Although the value of this "road map" has been questioned, since it is not required for subsequent selective catheterization, it is both intuitively obvious and emperically true that a clear visualization of the often tortuous and/or anomolous arterial anatomy around the aortic arch facilitates catheterization of these vessels, particularly when the arch angiogram indicates that standard catheterization techniques are unlikely to yield successful catheterization of the appropriate vessel. Arch arteriography also provides a method for preliminary evaluation of the cerivcocerebral vasculature. Lesions of the proximal common carotid arteries, subclavian arteries (Fig. 2.11) and vertebral artery origins can be identified, and the carotid artery bifurcations may be evaluated. Severely stenotic and/or ulcerated lesions can be identified, and the risk of blindly catheterizing severely diseased vessels avoided. Using digital subtraction angiography equipment, virtually all the disadvantages of FAA can be eliminated, because with digital technique very small amounts of contrast can be used to obtain excellent arterial opacification. The iodine concentration of the contrast material can be varied from as low as 20 mg% to as much as 60 mg%. Depending on the concentration of the contrast used, volumes ranging from 5 to 20 cc injected at rates varying from 5 to 10 cc/sec yield excellent results. Thus, virtually any combination of catheter and contrast

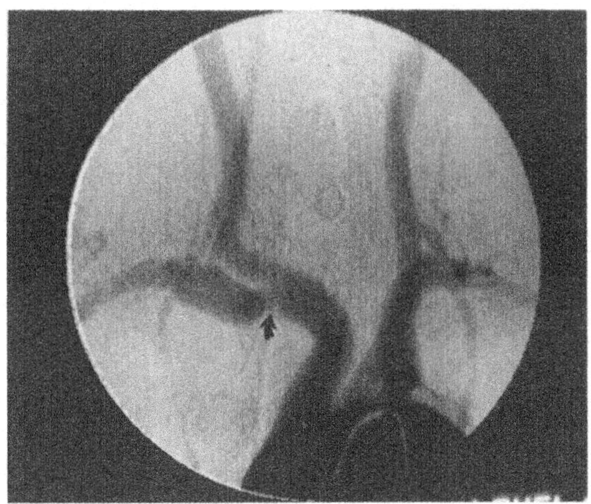

Figure 2.11. DAA of the aortic arch. Catheter is noted in the aorta, and a stenotic lesion is identified in the right subclavian artery (*curved arrow*). To obtain a study of similar technical quality, three to four times the amount of contrast would be necessary using either traditional film arch angiography (FAA) or DIVA.

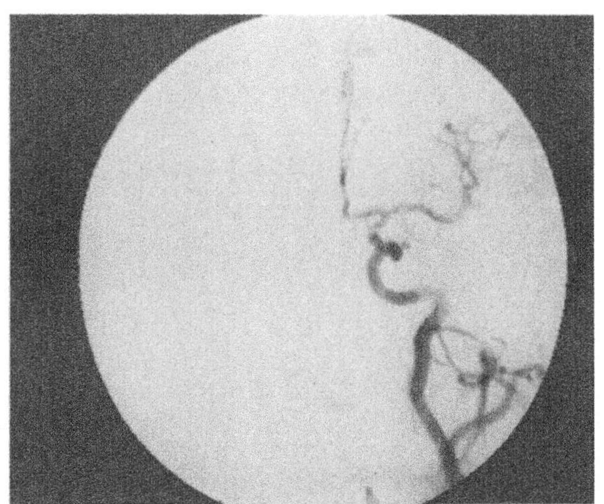

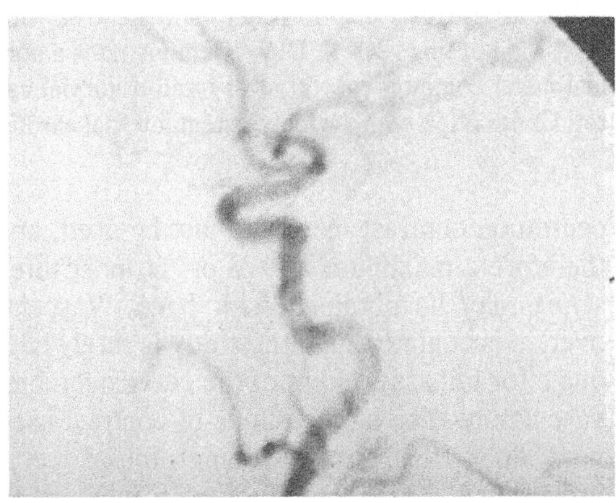

Figure 2.12. Selective digital subtraction arteriography. Lateral **(A)** and frontal **(B)** views of the carotid artery demonstrate excellent extra- and intracranial filling. The internal carotid artery is well visualized as are the anterior and middle cerebral arteries. Because of limitations of spatial resolution, smaller branches such as the lenticulostriate arteries are not well seen, but overall visualization is much better than with nonselective digital techniques (DIVA or DAA).

can be used, depending on physician preference and clinical circumstance. Because the amount of contrast per injection is small (from one tenth to one fifth of the dose used in FAA), there is no flooding of the vascular system and therefore ischemia does not occur. Contrast may be injected through small-bore catheters, and the study performed prior to selective angiography even in those centers preferring 5 French catheters. In fact, it is possible to use the same end-hole selective cerebral catheter (5–7 French) and the same contrast material for both arch and selective studies, thus avoiding time-consuming exchanges during the procedure. There is virtually no limitation to the number of series that may be obtained; therefore suboptimal studies due to motion may be repeated. Suboptimal studies due to vascular overlap may be minimized by obtaining multiple projections.

Because the contrast is injected directly into the aortic arch, DAA also requires a much smaller contrast load (typically 20%–30%) than that used with DIVA, the contrast load per se is not a limiting factor in obtaining an adequate study. With DIVA, a maximum of six series may be obtained so that repeat evaluation of specific areas that were suboptimal because of motion artifact or vascular overlap may require subsequent repeat examination. With DAA, suboptimal studies are less commonly encountered. The contrast produces involuntary swallowing (as it does with DIVA), but opacification of the carotid arteries occurs so rapidly that the "swallowing" artifacts usually occur after adequate visualization of these areas have been obtained. The short lag time between injection and vessel opacification makes suspension of breathing easier in patients with respiratory compromise, and the small bolus of contrast used produces less patient pain and therefore less involuntary head jerking. Deterioration of renal and cardiac function are not observed; therefore the procedure may be used in patients with compromise of these functions. Finally, with DAA the option to perform selective angiography where safe and when indicated is readily and immediately available, thus allowing for greater study flexibility. Thus, DAA is ideal as an initial step in all patients undergoing arteriography for the evaluation of cerebrovascular disease.

Selective Digital Subtraction Arteriography

Selective arteriography may be performed using digital subtraction angiographic equipment. The contrast concentration and/or dose may be decreased somwhat, but the main advantage of performing selective digital subtraction arteriography lies in the ability to obtain instaneous subtraction of the entire angiographic series. The study may be performed rapidly, and film costs are decreased using digital technique. Since the spatial resolution of the digital system does not yet approach that of traditional film screen systems, fine arteriographic detail, expecially of secondary and tertiary branches, is not well seen; therefore, when fine arteriographic detail is required, traditional arteriography is preferred. In those cases where small-vessel arterial detail is not of importance, selective digital subtraction arteriography is preferred.

References

1. Chilcote WA, Modic MT, Pavilcek WA, et al: Digital subtraction angiography of the carotid arteries: A comparative study in 100 patients. Radiology 139:287–295, 1981
2. Christianson BC, Ovitt TW, Fisher HD, Fost MM, Nudelman S, Roehrig H: Intravenous angiography using digital video subtraction: Intravenous cervico-cerebrovascular angiography. AJNR 1:379–386, 1980 and AJR 1980;135:1144–1151
3. Crummy AB, Stieghorst MF, Turski PA et al: Digital subtraction Angiography current status and use of intra-arterial injection. Radiology 145:303–307, 1982
4. Crummy AB, Strother CM, Sackett JF et al: Computerized fluoroscopy: Digital subtraction for intravenous angio-cardiography and arteriography. AJR 135:1131–1140, 1980
5. Durward QJ, Ferguson GG, Barr HW: The natural history of asymptomatic carotid bifurcation plaques. Stroke 13:459–464, 1982
6. Edwards JH, Kricheff II, Riles T, Imparato A. Angiographically undetected ulceration of the carotid bifurcation as a cause of embolic stroke. Radiology 132:369–373, 1979
7. Goldstein SJ, Freid AM, Young B, Tibbs PA: Limited usefulness of aortic arch angiogram in the evaluation of carotid occlusive disease. AJNR 2:559–564, 1981
8. Hoffman MG, Gomes AS, Pais SO: Pitfalls and limitations in the interpretation of intravenous carotid digital subtraction angiography (DSA). Presented at the 68th Annual Meeting of the Radiologic Society of North America. Chicago, Illinois, November 30, 1982
9. Kasef LG: Positional variations of the common carotid artery bifurcation implications for digital subtraction angiography. Radiology 145:3077–3078, 1982
10. McGinnis B, Hesselink JR, Ackerman R, Davis KR, Taveras JM: The use of subtraction angiography in the evaluation of cerebral transient ischemic attacks. Presented at the 68th Annual Meeting of the Radiologic Society of North America, Chicago, Illinois, November 30, 1982
11. Meany TF, Weinstein MA, Buonocore E et al: Digital subtraction angiography of the human cardiovascular system. AJR 135:1153–1160, 1980 and SPIE 223:272–278, 1980
12. Mehegan JT, Olcott C: The carotid "string" sign. The differential diagnosis in management. AJR 140:137–142, 1980
13. Mistreta CA: Development of digital subtraction angiography. In Mistreta CA, Crummy AB, Strother CM, Sackett JF (eds.): Digital Subtraction Angiography: An Application of computerized Fluoroscopy. Publishers Inc., Chicago, Illinois, 1982, pp 7–15
14. Mistretta CA, Crummy AB, Strother CM: Digital angiography: A perspective. Radiology 139:273–276, 1981
15. Modic MT, Weinstein MA, Shilcote WA et al: Digital subtraction angiography of the intracranial vascular system. A Comparative study in 55 patients. AJNR 2:527–534, 1981
16. Ovitt TW, Christianson TC, Fisher HD et al: Intravenous angiography using digital video subtraction: Xray imaging system. AJR 135:1141–1144, 1980
17. Pavlicek W, Weinstein MA, Modic MT, Buonocore E, Ducaesneau MA: Patient doses during digital subtraction angiography of the carotid arteries: Comparison with conventional angiography. Radiology 145:683–685, 1982
18. Pinto RS, Kricheff II, DeFillip G, Lin JP: Cere-

bral vasospasm secondary to acute ruptured intracranial aneurysm: Assessment of vessel calibre and circulation time prior and after medical therapy. Presented at XI Symposium Neuroradiologicum, Washington, D.C., October 1982

19. Smith JRL, Carmody RF, Seeger JF, McIntyre KE: Digital intravenous subtraction angiography in the detection of cervical cerebral atherosclerotic disease. Presented at the 69th Annual Meeting of the Radiological Society of North America, Chicago, Illinois, November 30, 1982
20. Strother CM, Sackett JF, Crummy AB et al: Clinical applications of computerized fluoroscopy. Radiology 136:781–783, 1980
21. Strother CM, Sackett JF, Crummy AB et al: Intravenous video arteriography of the intracranial vasculature: Early experience. AJNR 2:215–218, 1981
22. Strother CM, Steighorst MF, Tursten PA, Sackett JF, Peppler WW: Intraarterial digital subtraction angiography. SPIE 34, 1981 Digital Radiography 235–238
23. Sundberg J: Localization of atheromatosis and calcification in the carotid bifurcation: A post mortem radiographic investigation. Acta Radiol 22:521–528, 1981
24. Zimmerman RD, Goldman MJ, Auster M, Chen C, Leeds NE: Aortic arch digital arteriography—An alternative technique to digital venous angiography and routine arteriography in the evaluation of cerebrovascular insufficiency. Presented XI Symposium Neuroradiologicum, Washington, D.C., October 1982 Accepted for Publication, AJNR, 1983

3

Antithrombotic Therapy in Ischemic Cerebrovascular Disease

Robert Coté, C. W. McCormick, and Henry J. M. Barnett

Introduction

Stroke is well documented as both a major medical and a social problem, having a great economic impact on society.[198] Of equal importance is the loss of independence and human dignity secondary to neurologic dysfunction. The vast majority of strokes are due to cerebral ischemia,[130,157] the most common underlying cause of which is atherosclerosis with its various thromboembolic complications. Ultimately, better and more specific treatment and stroke preventive therapy will emerge from improved understanding of the pathogenetic mechanisms involved. Since brain recovery following established infarction is limited, major therapeutic emphasis must be focused on prevention.

Classification and Definitions

Clinical stroke syndromes may be described in many ways, but a very useful classification is based principally on temporal profile (and to a lesser extent, severity) of the neurologic deficit. A *transient ischemic attack (TIA)* is defined as an episode of temporary focal neurologic dysfunction of vascular origin lasting less than 24 hours. Most commonly these attacks last between 5 and 30 minutes. The risk of subsequent stroke in TIA patients is estimated to be about 35% over five years, or approximately 7% per year, with some suggestion that the highest risk occurs in the first few months after the initial TIA. Similar figures apply to risk of death in TIA patients, chiefly from myocardial infarction. Recent figures from the Canadian Cooperative Stroke Study estimate the combined risk of stroke or death following TIA as 13% during the first year, 22% at two years, and 30% at three years.[17]

Reversible ischemic neurologic deficit (RIND), by definition, is a temporary focal neurologic deficit of vascular origin persisting more than 24 hours, but resolving completely within a few weeks. The prognosis for events of this type is imperfectly known, but the pathogenetic mechanisms and therapeutic implications appear to be similar to TIA.

The *progressing stroke (PS)* or *stroke-in-evolution* is less crisply defined but is generally regarded as a focal neurologic deficit of vascular origin which continues to increase in severity (or further extends its vascular distribution) after the patient's admission to observation. The rapidity of worsening may vary considerably from minutes through hours to days, and the underlying pathogenetic mechanisms may be diverse. In rare instances of so-called "slow stroke," progression may occur over weeks to months, closely mimicking a cerebral tumor. The profile of worsening may be either smooth or stepwise. Recognition of the progressing stroke appears to have very real therapeutic implications.

A *completed stroke (CS)* or *established stroke* is defined as a focal neurologic deficit of vascular origin which has stabilized. In the carotid system, a stroke is considered to be completed if it has remained stable for 18 to 24 hours, whereas this period is extended to 48 to 72 hours for strokes in the vertebrobasilar territory. Depending on the amount and anatomic location of damaged brain tissue, neurologic deficit may vary from minimal to calamitous.

The term *partial nonprogressing stroke (PNS)* describes a minimal to moderate permanent focal neurologic deficit of vascular origin. A PNS can be regarded as the minor end of the spectrum of completed stroke. Many lacunar strokes fall within this group.

Although these clinical categories are obviously overlapping and arbitrary, they permit some correlation between pathophysiology and clinical presentation, suggesting guidelines for rational therapy. For example, TIA, RIND, and progressing stroke indicate ischemia with limited or no tissue necrosis and reflect viability and potential "recoverability" of brain substance. On the other hand, completed strokes represent brain necrosis and imply "nonrecoverability" of some cerebral tissue.

Epidemiology

Data from a variety of studies indicate that brain infarction predominates by about four to one over intracerebral hemorrhage.[119] In the prospective Harvard Stroke Registry,[158] based on 694 patients, 53% had "thrombotic" strokes; 31%, cerebral embolism; 10%, cerebral hematoma; and 6%, subarachnoid hemorrhage from aneurysm or AVM (arteriovenous malformation). Grouping the thrombotic and embolic strokes together into a single category of ischemic stroke yields a total of 84%. The thrombosis group was subdivided into two categories: those involving large arteries (34%) and those with lacunar infarction (19%). The high incidence of emboli in this study is due to the recognition of artery-to-artery emboli in addition to the classical cardiac sources. Lacunar infarction contributes significantly, being responsible for about one stroke in five.

Risk Factors

Several risk factors predispose to increased risk of stroke. Arterial *hypertension* is the major contributory factor in the development of both ischemic and hemorrhagic stroke.[120,123,132,175,198] Framingham Study data[120] indicate that atherothrombotic brain infarction (ABI) occurs seven times more often in hypertensive patients as compared with normotensives, the risk being proportional to the level of blood pressure.

There is a strong relationship between *cardiac disease* and stroke, particularly ischemic stroke. The Framingham Study[119] showed a threefold increase in risk of cerebral infarction (after adjustment for hypertension) in patients with cardiac left ventricular hypertrophy or prior history of coronary heart disease. Other types of heart disease are known to be associated with increased risk of cardioembolic stroke, including rheumatic valvular disease, acute myocardial infarction, prosthetic heart valves, subacute bacterial endocarditis, and certain cardiac arrhythmias, especially atrial fibrillation.[235] Heart disease can be viewed as a factor that increases the risk of stroke. An alternative view is that both diseases are linked through common precursors, namely, atherosclerosis and hypertension.

Age is a powerful variable associated with increased stroke incidence. As both atherosclerosis and hypertension increase with age and are themselves strong stroke precursors, they may account for the increased risk with age.

Diabetes mellitus has been regarded frequently as a risk factor for ischemic stroke.[198,119,132,113] Framingham Study data[119] indicate increased risk of cerebral infarction for diabetic patients. The mechanism is not clear, but might be explained by the contribution of diabetes to atherogenesis in cervicocranial vessels.[88]

The status of *hyperlipidemia* as a risk factor for stroke is controversial. In one study[121] an association between lipid values and cerebral infarction was found only in patients under 50 years of age; in this group, risk of stroke appears to be directly related to lipid levels.

Cigarette smoking is a contributory risk factor for cerebral infarction especially in men.[198,119] Lastly, certain studies[122,212] have reported an increased incidence of ischemic stroke with higher *hematocrit* values. Other possible risk factors have been suggested, but the association is not clear for obesity, lack of physical activity, and stress.

Recently, a significant decline in the incidence of stroke was reported[84,85]; the decline is greatest for ischemic stroke, less for intraparenchymatous hemorrhage, and not at all for subarachnoid hemorrhage. The overall reduction in one of these studies approached 50% over a 25-year period. Reasons for the decline have not been clearly identified, although it is tempting to link it, in part, to improved recognition and treatment of hypertension, the principal risk factor for cerebral infarction.

Pathogenesis of Ischemic Cerebrovascular Disease

The pathogenesis of cerebral ischemia is complex and diverse, involving the interplay of various factors which differ widely in significance among individual patients.

Atherosclerosis

Atherosclerosis is a disease of arteries which has long been recognized as the leading cause of death in the western world, principally through myocardial and cerebral infarction.

Three stages of atherosclerosis have been described pathologically. The *fatty streak* commonly found in young persons consists of a focal accumulation of intimal smooth muscle cells with both intracellular and extracellular lipid, mostly cholesterol and cholesterol esters. Grossly, this is a flattened yellowish lesion that causes no symptoms. The *fibrous plaque* is a more advanced stage of atherosclerosis; it has a whitish appearance and protrudes into the arterial lumen. Microscopically it consists of lipid-containing smooth-muscle cells, surrounded by more lipids, collagen, and proteoglycans. The relationship between the fatty streak and the fibrous plaque is a matter of controversy.[238] The third stage is the *complicated plaque*, a fibrous plaque altered by ulceration, calcification, hemorrhage, or mural thrombosis. Such lesions may become symptomatic by diminishing cerebral perfusion or from embolism. Four fundamental phenomena are involved in atherogenesis—migration and proliferation of smooth-muscle cells in the intima, deposition of intracellular and extracellular lipid, accumulation of connective tissue and proteoglycans, and superimposition of mural thrombosis.[164,239]

Various hypotheses of atherogenesis have been advanced.[128,147,164,179,238] The most widely accepted at this time is the "response-to-injury" hypothesis, considerably refined and advanced since Virchow's time. The main premise of this theory is that processes initiated in response to intimal injury or disruption of the vascular endothelium ultimately lead to formation of the atherosclerotic plaque. Certain factors such as hypertension, smoking, hyperlipidemia, etc., may lead via various mechanisms to endothelial damage, exposing the underlying connective tissue to circulating blood elements, especially platelets. Adhesion of platelets to subendothelial collagen is followed by further platelet aggregation, leading to release from platelet granules of a variety of substances, including a mitogenic factor.[179,238] This factor stimulates smooth-muscle cell migration to the intima. Concurrently, elaboration of large amounts of connective tissue, particularly collagen and elastin, contributes to the growth of the plaque. Deposition of lipids is also enhanced by disruption of the endothelial barrier. Critical in symptom production is the final stage of mural thrombosis,[163,164,239] which results in further arterial stenosis or thromboembolism. Thus, platelets play an important role not only in initial atherogenesis, but also in the thromboembolic complications of established plaques.

Atherosclerosis is a diffuse process with a predilection for certain arterial sites. Atherosclerotic involvement of arteries seems to proceed temporally in a definite sequence.[202] In the carotid system, fatty streaks first appear during infancy, but not in the vertebrobasilar or intracranial arteries until puberty. Solberg and Eggen[196] studied the distribution of the various stages of atherosclerotic lesions in the cervicocranial arteries. All types of lesions were most prevalent near the bifurcation of the common carotid and in the distal internal carotid. Lesions in the vertebrobasilar system were much more uniformly distributed.

Thrombogenesis

Thrombosis and hemostasis both involve complex interactions among related factors and systems,[15,86,159,187,194] including integrity of the arterial wall, platelet function, coagulation system, fibrinolytic system, and blood flow dynamics.

The intact arterial endothelium prevents thrombosis and hemostasis by two mechanisms. First, it forms a physical barrier between circulating platelets and subendothelial collagen. Second, intact endothelial cells elaborate a prostaglandin known as prostacyclin (PGI_2), which acts as both a potent inhibitor of platelet aggregation and as a vasodilator.[194]

If platelet adherence and aggregation occur secondary to endothelial disruption, then the so-called "release reaction" occurs. Among the factors released is a phospholipid designated as platelet factor 3, essential to the coagulation mechanism. At least three of the known release factors—serotonin, epinephrine, and thromboxane A_2, cause vasoconstriction. The last is also a potent platelet aggregant. A "biological balance" is maintained between the mutually antagonistic actions of prostacyclin on the one hand and thromboxane A_2 on the other.

Exposed subendothelium can also activate the extrinsic arm of the coagulation cascade via release of tissue thromboplastin. The end product of this process is the production of thrombin, an enzyme that converts fibrinogen to fibrin and thus stabilizes the platelet aggregate, resulting in the formation of a mature thrombus. Adsorption of factor XII on a foreign surface such as exposed subendothelial collagen initiates the second pathway of the coagulation cascade, the intrinsic system.

The fibrinolytic system plays an important role in the maintenance of fluidity in the blood. Plasminogen, a pro-enzyme in plasma, is converted into the activated enzyme plasmin, a protease that degrades fibrin into soluble fragments. The activator that converts plasminogen to plasmin is present in most body tissues, including endothelium.

Normal plasma contains several protease inhibitors that can neutralize activated clotting factors; the most important of these inhibitors is antithrombin III, which plays a major role in maintaining hemofluidity.

Hemodynamics play an important role in thrombogenesis. Stasis and local disruption of laminar flow both contribute to thrombus formation.

Extracranial vs. Intracranial Lesions

A number of studies have emphasized the importance of atherosclerotic lesions in the extracranial cervicocerebral circulation.[72,108,139] Martin and co-workers[139] studied the distribution of atherosclerosis in the extracranial and intracranial circulation in patients over 50 and found that extracranial involvement predominated over intracranial lesions in 93% of cases. Fisher et al[72] devised an "atherosclerotic index" for evaluating the pattern of atherosclerotic involvement in the entire carotid and vertebrobasilar system (both extra- and intracranially) in patients over 40. In general, the index was highest in the aorta, followed, in order, by the coronary, carotid, cerebral, and vertebral arteries (the last two being about equal). Their data clearly showed a predominance of atherosclerotic involvement in the larger arteries of the neck over that in the intracranial vessels. Angiographic data from the Joint Study of Extracranial Arterial Occlusion[95,96] emphasizes the importance of the extracranial as compared with the intracranial circulation.

Thrombotic Occlusions

Extracranial atheroma plays a major role in cerebral infarction. In a landmark study, Fisher[74] reported a series of cases of symptomatic occlusion of one or both carotid arteries, the most frequent manifestation being contralateral hemiplegia. Occlusion of extracranial arteries may be silent clinically; this has been documented by both pathologic studies[74,139] and angiographic data.[56] The presence or absence of neurologic dysfunction (and the degree of cerebral necrosis, if any) under these circumstances is determined by several factors: status of collateral flow, variations in vascular anatomy, blood pressure, blood oxygenation, viscosity of blood, and presence of other obliterative vascular lesions.

Apart from simple occlusion or tight stenosis of the vascular lumen, the thrombotic process may bring about ischemic damage by anterograde extension of thrombus ("stagnation thrombus") or secondary embolism to distal intracranial branches. Castaigne et al[35] have suggested that more than 80% of cerebral infarctions occurring in the setting of internal carotid artery occlusion are due to these mechanisms, either singly or in combination.

Intra-Arterial Emboli

Intra-arterial emboli arise in complicated atherosclerotic lesions in proximal vessels (usually extracranial) and pass distally to lodge in small-caliber cerebral arteries. These emboli may be of two types: platelet-fibrin emboli and so-called atheromatous-debris emboli.

Moore et al[161] report that ulcerated nonstenotic lesions at the carotid bifurcation have a serious prognosis: a stroke incidence of 12.5% per year in patients with definite ulceration of the carotid artery on angiography, the presumed mechanism being distal embolization. Pessin and colleagues[173] studied angiographically a group of patients with carotid stenosis or occlusion in the setting of acute stroke. Two thirds had evidence of embolism distal to the extracranial carotid lesion. This mechanism has also been reinforced by pathologic data from Lhermitte et al,[134] who found a high incidence of emboli as opposed to thrombosis in situ in their study of middle cerebral artery occlusions. Edwards and collaborators[50] stressed the limitations of angiography to detect ulcerative lesions at the carotid bifurcation, reporting that 40% of ulcers found at surgery were not diagnosed preoperatively by angiography.

Platelet-Fibrin Emboli

In 1959 Fisher[61] provided the first suggestion that cerebral microemboli might be of platelet origin while observing whitish material coursing through the retinal arteries of a patient during an attack of amaurosis fugax. A few years later Ross-Russell[180] made similar observations in two patients. Clinico-pathologic correlation of this mechanism was provided by McBrien et al.[141]

A further contribution was made by Gunning et al[90] who studied a series of patients with carotid atheroma. Examination of endarterectomy specimens showed fresh platelet-fibrin thrombus on the luminal surface of plaques in patients who had their most recent clinical event within the previous seven weeks. In patients with more remote events, no such thrombus was found. It is tempting to speculate that atherosclerotic lesions may go through certain phases where the risk of clinical embolic events is increased. In this regard, Whisnant[230] has stated that the risk of stroke is highest during the initial three-month period after the first TIA. Rarely brain surgery has provided an opportunity for direct visualization of embolic material in cortical vessels.[16]

In an experimental study, Honour and Ross-Russell[102] produced platelet embolism secondary to vascular injury and found that successive platelet emboli (arising from the same injured segment of cerebral artery) followed identical paths, lodging in small terminal branches. A subtle and thoughtful discussion of this mechanism is contained in a recent review by Schmidley and Caronna.[185]

Atheromatous Debris Emboli

The concept of emboli arising from ulcerated atheromatous plaques was mentioned by a few early writers.[76,169] Recognition of their occurrence in cerebral vessels was noted by Meyer[151] and Winter.[234] In the latter instance, two cases are reported of cerebral infarction clearly related to cholesterol emboli in small cerebral vessels. Hollenhorst[101] described "bright plaques" in the retinal arteries of patients with occlusive carotid system disease and suggested that these were actually cholesterol emboli arising from proximal ipsilateral carotid or aortic lesions. This suggestion was confirmed pathologically by David et al.[44] Symptoms associated with atheromatous retinal emboli may range from nothing at all through amaurosis fugax to frank retinal infarction.

In a review of atheromatous emboli in the central nervous system, Soloway and collaborators[197] noted that such emboli were generally of small size, tending to lodge in vessels with diameters less than 100 μm. Experimental studies in animals[227] have shown that atheromatous cerebral embolism is followed by initiation of a thrombotic process with participation of platelets and other blood elements. On occasion, scanning electron microscopic studies have shown cholesterol crystals being disgorged from the depths of human atheromatous lesions.[14] More recent data[23] has also linked cholesterol emboli to hemispheric TIAs and cerebral infarction.

The relative roles of the two types of artery-to-artery emboli in the pathogenesis of clinical cerebral ischemic symptoms are not known. It seems well established that microembolism of both varieties can produce transient ischemic events, but the contribution of these mechanisms to the development of completed cerebral infarction is less well understood.

Hemodynamic Factors

In an earlier era, the concept of focal vasospasm was thought to account for much of the symptomatology of ischemic cerebrovascular disease. In the 1950s Denny-Brown[46] formulated the concept of the "hemodynamic crisis," referring to focal cerebral ischemic attacks resulting from transient falls in systemic blood pressure, with subsequent decreased blood flow to specific regions of the brain perfused by stenotic arteries.

Other studies[17,184,150] had shown reduced blood flow and EEG abnormalities with postural changes, but correlation with symptoms of focal ischemia was very poor. In 1964 Brice[27] showed, in an important study, that the luminal cross-sectional area must be less than 2 mm^2 before producing any appreciable change in blood flow or pressure gradient. Clinical observation of TIA patients during attacks has not shown any change in systemic blood pressure,[153] and deliberate reduction of systemic blood pressure by means of drugs and postural changes in a group of TIA patients failed to produce focal events, but rather symptoms of diffuse cerebral hypoperfusion, chiefly syncope.[126] Autopsies of patients surviving a few days or weeks after cardiac arrest have not shown a correlation between the site of recent cerebral infarcts and the location or degree of cervicocranial atherosclerotic lesions, although the correlation was good for old infarcts. The authors concluded that the superimposition of severe systemic hypotension on cervicocranial atherosclerosis is not a major cause of brain infarction.[215]

Orthostatic TIAs have been described at times in patients with severe and diffuse occlusive disease of major extracranial vessels in both carotid and/or vertebrobasilar systems.[104,204,205] This syndrome of "primary orthostatic cerebral ischemia" usually implies generalized, nonfocal cerebral ischemic symptoms related to erect posture, but without a simultaneous significant drop in systemic blood pressure. Clinically, such patients usually experience postural light-headedness or syncope, blurring of vision, unsteadiness, gait difficulties, and changes in mentation and/or memory. Less commonly such patients have discrete focal events, and this mechanism is a very uncommon cause of focal cerebral ischemia. Several possible explanations for this phenomenon have been advanced, most of them emphasizing the possibility of focal cerebral dysautoregulation. Arrhythmias generally produce symptoms of diffuse cerebral ischemia as opposed to focal manifestations,[146,176,226] except of course where arrhythmias predispose to an increased likelihood of cerebral embolism.

In the pathogenesis of cerebral ischemia, vasospasm plays a significant role only in certain specific instances: subarachnoid hemorrhage, hypertensive encephalopathy, and the aura phase of migraine. Fisher[69] described a series of patients over 40 with focal cerebral ischemic symptoms in whom angiograms were negative and other causes of cerebral ischemia excluded. Visual phenomena are prominent and headache absent in about half the patients. These he designated as "transient migrainous accompaniments" (TMAs).

A rare hemodynamic cause of focal posterior circulation ischemia is the subclavian steal syndrome.[171] Symptoms may follow vigorous arm exercise ipsilateral to a subclavian artery that is the site of occlusion or very tight stenosis proximal to the origin of the vertebral artery on the same side. This results in "stealing" of blood from the vertebrobasilar circulation owing to reversal of flow in the vertebral. The phenomenon is a common angiographic finding, but the clinical picture with vertebrobasilar ischemic symptoms is rare, and probably never develops without advanced obliterative disease in several of the other major cerebral arteries.

Hematologic Factors

A variety of disorders and drugs may be accompanied by hypercoagulability, which may infrequently give rise to focal cerebral ischemic events. A state of altered coagulability may be seen in pregnancy, in the puerperium, postoperative status, with oral contraceptive therapy, with known or occult cancer, inflammatory bowel disease, and in such hematological disorders as sickle cell anemia and paroxysmal nocturnal hemoglobinuria.[15]

Risk of stroke is increased in women taking oral contraceptives.[37,223] Recent studies[110,111] have focused attention on vessel wall changes, especially intimal hyperplasia, with or without associated thrombosis. Many reports[149,165,174,225] have linked "the oral contraceptive pill" with coagulation abnormalities, including decreased antithrombin-3 levels, decreased fibrinolytic activity, and possibly enhanced platelet aggregation.

Schneiderman et al[186] have called attention to a hypercoagulable state predisposing to stroke in patients with inflammatory bowel disease. The patients in their study had none of the conventional risk factors for stroke, but coagulation studies showed thrombocytosis, decreased partial thromboplastin time, and elevation of fibrinogen and blood clotting factor VIII levels. These values returned to normal after therapeutic control of intestinal inflammation.

The exact role of primary platelet abnormalities in cerebral ischemia remains to be accurately defined. A significant problem exists in determining whether platelet abnormalities are the cause of or merely secondary to cerebral ischemic events. Thrombocytosis appears to be associated with TIA and stroke in a fairly predictable way.[133,193] Wu et al[240] found a close association between platelet hyperaggregability and ischemic attacks in patients with thrombocythemia.

Reports[47,118,207,241] of increased numbers of circulating platelet aggregates in stroke patients have attracted great interest. Al-Mefty and colleagues[6] suggest from their work that a group of patients exists with none of the conventional explanations for cerebral ischemia, the sole cause of whose symptoms is increased platelet adhesiveness and/or aggregation. Dougherty et al[47] studied patients with acute cerebral ischemia and found increased platelet aggregation during the acute phase, with a return to normal within 10 days to 6 weeks after the initial event. They concluded that platelet dysfunction does not play a primary role in initiating cerebral ischemia, but suggested that as a secondary phenomenon it might contribute to a worsening of the initial ischemic insult.

Hyperviscosity associated with certain hematologic disorders such as polycythemia, sickle cell anemia, Waldenstrom's macroglobulinemia, and other paraproteinemias may lead to diffuse or focal cerebral ischemia.[136,155,192,236] The pathogenesis of cerebral ischemia in so-called "hyperviscosity syndromes" may be due to relative stasis of blood in the cerebral microcirculation, delayed clearance of clotting factors, or an increased number of platelets. In patients with polycythemia, Thomas[208] reported a significant decrease in cerebral blood flow, with improvement after reduction of hematocrit by venesection. Other studies[209] have shown a similar inverse relationship between cerebral blood flow and hematocrit. Two recent studies[122,212] have reported an increased incidence of cerebral infarction in patients with high hematocrit values, suggesting the possible importance of blood rheology in association with other factors in the pathogenesis of cerebral ischemia.

In sickle cell anemia, hyperviscosity secondary to changes in red cell morphology seems to play a prominent role in occlusion of small vessels and in the occurrence of stroke, mainly in children. Large vessel involvement is also found in this condition.[201]

Heart Disease and Cerebral Emboli

Focal cerebral ischemia may be caused by a variety of cardiac conditions. The common mechanism is thrombosis with emboli passing from heart to brain.

Myocardial infarction with mural thrombosis is a regular source of cardioembolic stroke.[98] The risk of stroke has been found to rise with increasing myocardial infarction size.[210] The incidence of ischemic stroke after myocardial infarction increases with higher serum creatine phosphokinase (CPK) levels. The mechanisms include increased risk of mural thrombosis with extensive endocardial damage or coagulation disturbance known to occur with myocardial infarction. The risk of cerebral embolism is highest within the first two months after myocardial infarction, but damage to myocardium will produce akinetic segments or aneurysms, a potential embolic source for years afterwards.[14]

Cardiac valvular disease, particularly rheumatic mitral stenosis (with or without atrial fibrillation), is a common cause of cerebral emboli[41,107]: Thrombus forms within the atrium (or its appendage) or on the valvular surface with subsequent embolization. Other cardiac disorders known to be associated with cerebral emboli include rheumatic involvement of other heart valves, marantic endocarditis[127] (nonbacterial thrombotic endocarditis or NBTE), infective endocarditis,[87,190] prosthetic heart valves,[79] right-to-left shunts, atrial myxoma,[242] mitral valve prolapse,[19,20] possibly mitral annulus calcification,[45] and cardiomyopathy.[144]

In patients with mitral valve prolapse, thrombus formation is known to occur on the abnormal myxomatous heart valve with subsequent liberation into the systemic circulation. Pathologic evidence is increasing in support of this association,[18,38] and in younger patients with cerebral and retinal ischemia this possibility must always be considered.[19]

Atrial myxoma is a rare but eminently treatable condition. Neurologic manifestations include TIAs, stroke, or syncope.[242] Of patients with such cardiac tumors, 50% experience cerebral emboli consisting of either myxomatous material itself or pieces of thrombus originating from the surface of the tumor.

Cardiac arrhythmia is an uncommon cause of focal cerebral ischemic events. In a series of patients who received cardiac pacemakers for bradyarrhythmias, only 2 out of 290 patients experienced focal neurologic symptoms that could be related to an episode of arrhythmia.[176] Most patients experience symptoms of global cerebral ischemia, particularly syncope, rather than focal cerebral ischemic symptoms.[140,226]

Certain types of arrhythmia, especially atrial fibrillation[100] and the bradycardia-tachycardia syndrome,[22,55] increase the risk of cerebral embolism. Thrombus formation in the atrium, with subsequent embolization, is the underlying mechanism.

Lacunes

Lacunes (or lacunar infarcts) are small cavities resulting from ischemic infarction in the territory of small, deep, penetrating cerebral arteries.[64] They may vary from 0.5 mm up to 15 mm in diameter. They are the most common pathologic cerebrovascular lesion at autopsy, found in about 10% of necropsied brains.[66] The most common sites of occurrence are the lenticular nuclei, basis pontis, caudate nucleus, thalamus, internal capsule, and subcortical white matter of the hemispheres. There is a very strong correlation between the presence of lacunes and hypertension.

Lacunes present with five well-recognized syndromes: pure motor hemiparesis,[71] pure sensory stroke,[63] dysarthria-clumsy-hand syndrome,[65] ataxic hemiparesis syndrome,[70] (formerly known as homolateral ataxia-crural paresis), and the full-blown lacunar state (état lacunaire). The clinical outcome for individual small lacunar strokes may be very good, but the cumulative effects of multiple lacunes can result in a lacunar state with pseudobulbar palsy. In some cases lacunar stroke may be preceded by TIAs, as, for example, 23% of the time in the Harvard Cooperative Stroke Registry.[158] Many lacunes are found at postmortem, which because of small size or particular location, have been asymptomatic.

Fisher described occlusion of small penetrating arteries by a process he designated as "segmental arterial disorganization" or lipohyalinosis.[66] Pathologic changes in these vessels include derangement of normal arterial architecture, foam cells in the arterial wall, deposits of fibrinoid material, extravasation of blood, and focal enlargement of the arterioles in some instances.

Angiographic and CT scan investigation of patients with lacunar strokes is very often negative. When associated with cervicocranial atheroma, the interrelationship among causative factors in a given case can be perplexing.

Nonatherosclerotic Vasculopathy

Under this general heading are included a variety of uncommon and even rare causes of cerebral ischemia. These entities should be considered when the cause of cerebral ischemic symptoms is obscure and particularly in younger patients. These vasculopathies may be divided for convenience into two general groups:

1. Inflammatory cerebral vasculopathies (vasculitis). These include systemic lupus erythematosus,[115] polyarteritis nodosa,[78] scleroderma,[53] granulomatous angiitis,[29] giant-cell arteritis (temporal or cranial arteritis),[233] Behçet's syndrome,[114] Takayasu's disease,[112] and syphilitic angiopathy.[222]
2. Noninflammatory cerebral vasculopathies. Included in this category are diverse conditions such as spontaneous dissection of cervicocranial arteries,[73] fibromuscular dysplasia,[103,195] Moya-Moya disease,[166] and homocystinuria.[91] Distal embolization may occur from thrombus in a cerebral aneurysm.[36]

Physical Damage to Arteries

Occasionally extravascular structures may impinge on extracranial arteries. Compression of a vertebral artery in patients with cervical spondylosis, especially when the head is rotated or hyperextended, is a very rare cause of ischemia.[188] Congenital or rheumatoid atlantoaxial subluxation may produce vertebral compression with secondary brainstem infarction.[116] Thrombosis and thromboembolism may occur as secondary developments following trauma,[25] chiropractic manipulation,[189] work activities, and spontaneous head turning.[167,189] The mechanism in the vertebrobasilar cases is stretching and compression of the vertebral arteries at the atlantoaxial level, causing intimal damage and triggering the thrombotic process. More direct trauma will injure the carotid artery in the neck.

Venous Thrombosis

Aseptic intracranial venous thrombosis is a well-known, but relatively uncommon entity occurring in certain specific clinical situations including pregnancy, puerperium, oral contraceptive therapy,[52] malignant cachexia, dehydration, and congestive heart failure (especially in the elderly,[216]) in postoperative patients, polycythemia, and closed-head injuries. The septic variety of cerebral thrombosis (cerebral thrombophlebitis) has become uncommon, but occurs with chronic ear and mastoid infections, intracranial infections, overwhelming systemic sepsis, and in postoperative neurosurgical patients. Anticoagulant therapy for these conditions is hazardous since venous infarction of brain is commonly hemorrhagic.

Mimics

A wide variety of conditions may simulate or mimic cerebral ischemia. Perhaps the most important are tumors,[43] subdural hematoma,[177] focal seizures,[67] and primary labyrinthine disorders.

Antithrombotic Therapy—General Considerations

The antithrombotic treatment of ischemic cerebrovascular disease remains one of the most controversial subjects in all of medicine. A pessimistic view is that the outlook for TIA patients is altered very little from the natural history of the disease, regardless of what therapy is chosen.[214] A very extensive literature has accumulated in this area, and a few hopeful trends have begun to emerge.

Anticoagulants and the Coagulation System

Anticoagulation is the most venerable form of medical therapy for cerebral ischemia. Despite more than 25 years of usage[170] and numerous clinical trials, the exact role of these drugs remains to be accurately defined. As with all forms of treatment including surgery and antiplatelet drugs, the rationale for the usage of anticoagulants is prophylactic. They have no role to play in the reversal of established ischemic deficits.

There are two major groups of anticoagulant agents—heparin, a rapidly acting anticoagulant that must be given parenterally and the coumarin derivatives, slower acting but administered orally.

The pharmacologic action of heparin is complex, interfering with the coagulation process at

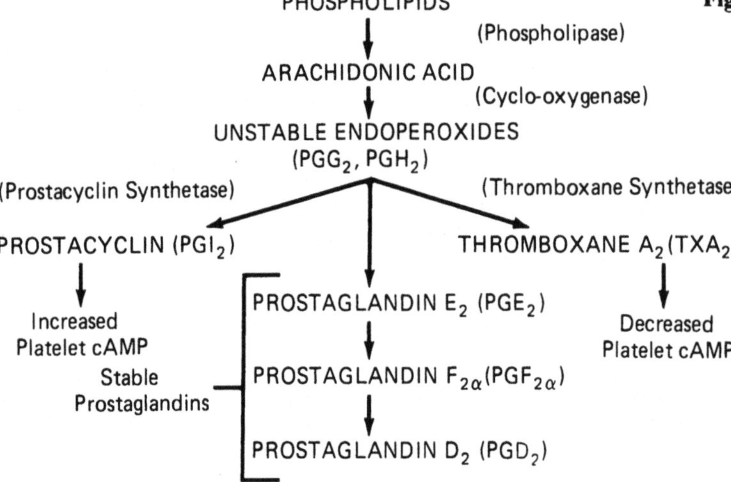

Figure 3.1. Arachidonic Acid Pathway.

several points. The oral anticoagulants produce a deficiency of clotting factors by antagonizing vitamin K action in the liver and thereby inhibiting formation of clotting factors II, VII, IX, and X. The action of heparin may be quickly reversed by administering of protamine sulphate, whereas the coumarin derivatives are blocked by vitamin K.

The major side effect of both classes of anticoagulants is hemorrhage, which may originate from various body sites. The most tragic complication of anticoagulant therapy is the occurrence of cerebral hemorrhage. There is some suggestion that the risk of cerebral hemorrhage increases after the first year of anticoagulant therapy.[229]

Thrombi that develop in vivo are considerably different in composition than blood clots formed in vitro, the latter being a mixture of all blood elements. Thrombi, according to the hemodynamic circumstances in which they form, are composed of a variable mixture of red (predominantly red cells and fibrin) and white (mostly platelet aggregates) components. The former predominates in thrombi formed in conditions of slow flow and vascular stasis, whereas platelet aggregates occur more frequently at sites of rapid flow. It is probably simplistic, yet not unreasonable, to suggest that anticoagulants might, therefore, be more effective in situations of vascular stasis, whereas antiplatelet effectiveness might predominate in higher velocity arterial diseases. The situation is almost certainly not so simple.[86]

Antiplatelet Drugs and the Arachidonic Acid Cascade

A great deal of attention has been focused on the potential role of antiplatelet drugs in the management of cerebrovascular disease and other vascular disorders. These agents act through diverse effects on the platelet arachidonic acid cascade.

The unstable endoperoxides are capable of elaborating either prostacyclin (PGI_2) via the enzyme prostacyclin synthetase, or thromboxane A_2 (TXA_2) via the enzyme thromboxane synthetase (Fig. 3.1). These substances have diametrically opposite biologic effects. PGI_2 is formed primarily from arachidonic acid in endothelial cells and acts as a vasodilator and natural platelet antiaggregant, whereas TXA_2 is elaborated principally in circulating platelets and functions as a vasoconstrictor and stimulates platelet aggregation. It is thought that these mutually antagonistic activities form a basic biologic homeostatic mechanism to prevent the adherence and aggregation of platelets to intact endothelium under normal circumstances, yet favor hemostasis and thrombogenesis in pathologic situations.

Excellent comprehensive reviews of these mechanisms have been provided by Moncada and Vane,[160] Fuster and Chesebro,[81] and Harlan and Harker.[92] The antiplatelet drugs that have thus far been most thoroughly tested in ischemic cerebrovascular disease are acetylsalicylic acid (aspirin or ASA), dipyridamole (Persantine), and sulfinpyrazone (Anturane). Many other drugs have been shown to have antiplatelet activity, but have not been used in the treatment of cerebrovascular disease.[82,83]

ASA exerts its antiplatelet effect by means of irreversible acetylation of the cyclooxygenase enzyme in the arachidonic acid pathway.[7,181] Cyclooxygenase in circulating platelets is much more sensitive to the effect of ASA than is that in the endothelial cells, thereby favoring the suppression of TXA_2 production over that of PGI_2, the end result being enhanced platelet antiaggregation.

Dipyridamole exerts its platelet antiaggregant effect as a phosphodiesterase inhibitor,[156,224] interfering with the breakdown of platelet cyclic adenosine monophosphate (AMP). The fact that ASA and dipyridamole exert their individual effects at completely different sites has led to speculation that the two agents together might prove more effective in the management of ischemic cerebrovascular disease than either agent given alone.

Sulfinpyrazone probably exerts its major antiplatelet effect via reversible inhibition of cyclooxygenase.[4,143,200]

Several new approaches to antiplatelet therapy would seem theoretically attractive.[160] These include selective inhibition of thromboxane synthetase (or TXA_2 itself), direct administration of PGI_2, and suppression of platelet aggregation by means of dietary eicosapentaenoic acid.

Antithrombotic Therapy—Specific Indications

Asymptomatic Patients

Risk factors for ischemic stroke have been discussed in a previous section. There is now conclusive evidence to show that adequate treatment of hypertension reduces the risk of ischemic stroke[109,219,220] and, furthermore, that treatment of hypertension following an initial stroke reduces the incidence of subsequent cerebral infarction.[24] It is not known at this time what impact, if any, the treatment of diabetes and hyperlipidemia has on stroke incidence, nor is it known if stopping smoking will in any way affect the recurrence rate of cerebral ischemia.

The issue of prophylactic antiplatelet therapy for patients theoretically at risk of stroke due to the presence of risk factors has not as yet been tested in clinical trials. ASA therapy is a reasonable recommendation for male patients with asymptomatic carotid bruits.[158]

TIA, RIND, and Minor Stroke

The data presented in this section are almost entirely drawn from studies of patients with TIAs, as specific trials of patients with RIND and minor stroke have not as yet been undertaken. Most workers in the field presume the pathogenetic mechanism of RIND and minor stroke to be much the same as for TIA and extrapolate this thinking to embrace similar therapeutic implications.

An exception to this of course is lacunar infarction, where a different pathologic vascular process is operative. It is generally agreed that control of systemic hypertension is the keystone of management for lacunes and that anticoagulant therapy may be hazardous because of coexistent hypertension. Since platelet deposition might play a role in the further complication of lipohyalinosis in small vessels, antiplatelet drugs might have a theoretically beneficial role. This has never been tested in any clinical trial.

Anticoagulants

Existing data bearing on this issue have been interpreted differently by various authorities. An exhaustive review of available data relating to anticoagulant efficacy in TIA patients was compiled in 1977.[86] The eight studies in the literature, four randomized[11–13,172] and four nonrandomized,[60,80,191,230] were analyzed. The conclusion was that

> . . . the evidence is unconvincing that anticoagulants are of benefit to patients with TIA in terms of increased survival and reduced incidence of stroke. Further, the evidence that anticoagulants are of benefit in reducing the number of TIA recurrences remains equivocal. Even if there were some reduction in the frequency of TIA, one must ask if this is really a benefit when the four randomized trials showed that 16 persons in the treatment group died, compared with only 10 in the control group, and correspondingly there were 13 major bleeding problems in the treatment group, compared with only 4 in the control group.

In a more recent interpretation of the same data, plus two additional nonrandomized studies,[57,213] Byer and Easton[30] commented that

> These data have been discussed in detail and interpreted quite differently by different writers. Much of the difference of opinion centres on whether one attributes meaning to trends or only to statistically significant data, and whether one attributes meaning to nonrandomized studies or only randomized and controlled ones. Most of the studies have involved too few patients, the follow-up periods have been too short, and the controls have been inadequate to determine the definitive role of anticoagulation in the treatment of transient ischemic attacks. On balance, however, when properly used, anticoagulation may reduce the risk of further transient ischemic attacks and subsequent cerebral infarction.

Despite these uncertainties, some authorities recommend continued use of anticoagulants as the initial treatment for TIA,[146,183] believing the risk of stroke to be highest within the first two to three months.[231]

There remains a need to mount still another study utilizing modern methodology. This would require a large, randomized, prospective trial with a sufficient number of patients and a follow-up period long enough to provide a definitive answer to this vexing question. Whether this will ever be done in an era when other forms of stroke-preventive therapy are emerging is a moot point.[21,142]

Antiplatelet Therapy

Interest in antiplatelet therapy for ischemic cerebrovascular disease began in the early 1970s with two anecdotal reports by Harrison et al[94] and Mundall et al[162] of successful therapy of amaurosis fugax with ASA. This was soon followed by a retrospective study by Dyken et al[48] showing a reduction of TIA incidence in patients treated with aspirin.

These early leads culminated in two large studies[31,59] designed to evaluate the effectiveness of ASA in a prospective, randomized fashion. The American Aspirin in TIA (AITIA) Study showed a reduced TIA incidence for ASA-treated patients, but it did not show a significant reduction in the endpoints of stroke and death. The larger Canadian Cooperative ASA-Anturane Trial, in which TIA and minor stroke were the criteria for entry, indicated that ASA therapy reduced stroke incidence over the length of the trial by 50% in men, with no benefit for women. Sulfinpyrazone was of no value in either sex, despite earlier promising observations,[26,54] Sex difference in response to antiplatelet agents has been demonstrated in other clinical and experimental situations as well,[93,117,125,135,218] although the underlying mechanisms are far from clear. The data from the Canadian Cooperative Study suggest an increased benefit from the combination of ASA and sulfinpyrazone as compared with ASA alone.[31,131] Benefit from the combination was not significant, and nothing short of a major trial would prove this hypothesis.

Dipyridamole has theoretical attractiveness. In 1971 Sullivan et al[203] showed that the combination of oral anticoagulants and dipyridamole reduced the incidence of embolism in patients with prosthetic heart valves. In 1969 Acheson et al[2] reported no definite benefit to a group of patients with ischemic cerebrovascular disease treated with this drug. Olsson et al compared a group of TIA and RIND patients treated with anticoagulants to a group treated with combination (ASA-dipyridamole) antiplatelet therapy.[168] The anticoagulant-treated patients showed slightly fewer subsequent cerebral ischemic events than did the antiplatelet therapy group, but both groups were said to benefit, and antiplatelet therapy was safer in regard to hemorrhagic complications. The problem with this study was the absence of a simultaneous control group.

Two additional randomized prospective trials of antiplatelet therapy in ischemic cerebrovascular disease are currently underway.[58,217] A multicenter trial in England has been mounted to further evaluate the efficacy of ASA therapy in stroke-threatened patients, utilizing two different dosage regimens to answer the question about optimal dosage. Another multicenter trial in the United States and Canada is underway to evaluate the effectiveness of combination antiplatelet therapy with ASA and dipyridamole as opposed to ASA alone.

Progressing Stroke

Anticoagulants in Progressing Stroke

Byer and Easton[30] recently analyzed three randomized[12,33,62] and three nonrandomized studies[60,152,228] examining this issue and concluded that anticoagulants probably benefit patients with progressing stroke. The available data do not conclusively prove efficacy in this situation, but suggest it.[86,154]

In circumstances where it is reasonable to assume that deterioration is on the basis of extending thrombus or repeated artery-to-artery emboli, and when hemorrhage has been ruled out, immediate anticoagulation with heparin is to be considered, followed by early conversion to oral anticoagulants. Neurologic deterioration may occur due to other causes including hemorrhage, cerebral edema, and general medical conditions; accurate diagnosis is mandatory before instituting anticoagulation. Diagnostic accuracy in progressing stroke has been much improved by the advent of CT scanning.[182]

Antiplatelet Drugs in Progressing Stroke

There are no available data regarding the effect of antiplatelet drugs such as ASA, dipyridamole, and sulfinpyrazone upon the clinical course or outcome of stroke-in-evolution. There would be concern that a process of active thrombogenesis, with the coagulation cascade already stimulated, might be less likely to benefit from platelet antiaggregants than from anticoagulants.

Completed Stroke

Anticoagulant Therapy in Completed Stroke

In a review[86] of seven randomized* and two nonrandomized studies[106,211] of completed stroke it was concluded that ". . . the findings are consistent and clear that no therapeutic benefit from anticoagulants derives to patients with completed stroke." In fact, such therapy may even be hazardous in certain instances.[30]

Antiplatelet Drugs in Completed Stroke

There are no data to evaluate the efficacy of antiplatelet agents in preventing subsequent cerebral infarction in completed stroke patients. It seems reasonable to expect that ASA therapy might reduce the incidence of subsequent cerebral ischemia in male patients who have suffered initial stroke. Presumably the pathogenetic mechanisms of recurrent atherothrombotic stroke are the same as for an initial event. The Canadian Cooperative Study showed that ASA did not have a beneficial effect in patients with advanced arterial disease. Those with both carotid and vertebrobasilar symptoms or those with angiographic evidence of extensive involvement of a large number of cerebral arteries had no reduction in vascular endpoints.[16]

Cerebral Emboli of Cardiac Origin

Anticoagulants in Cardiogenic Cerebral Emboli

In patients with rheumatic heart disease (particularly mitral stenosis) and recent myocardial infarction, anticoagulants reduce the incidence of both initial and subsequent embolic stroke.† More controversial are the issues of when to initiate therapy and how long to maintain it.[232] The tendency over the years has been to earlier therapy following initial embolic stroke, recognizing nonetheless that a small risk may exist in converting an ischemic (or slightly hemorrhagic) stroke into a hemorrhagic one. The Study Group on Antithrombotic Therapy[86] recommended initiation of treatment with *oral anticoagulants* at the time the patient is seen following an embolic event. Therapeutic anticoagulation will be achieved several days later.

Easton and Sherman[49] have advocated that patients with probable cerebral embolism from any cardiac source should be anticoagulated immediately, provided that bacterial endocarditis and intracranial hemorrhage have been excluded, since there is a high probability of a second embolus occurring within the first one to three weeks. Anticoagulation should be maintained for about three months in myocardial infarction, after which time the risk of recurrent embolism decreases abruptly, but continued indefinitely in the following situations where the embolic source cannot be eliminated: all patients with rheumatic heart disease, those with prosthetic mitral valves, nonvalvular atrial fibrillation, and persistent cardiomyopathy.

* References 11, 12, 51, 99, 105, 138, 145.

† References 1, 3, 10, 32, 34, 39–41, 75, 169, 178, 206, 221, 237.

The use of prophylactic anticoagulant therapy in patients with cardiac disease who have not experienced prior embolic events is less clear. Recently some predictive factors for embolization following myocardial infarction have emerged,[9,210] and it is now probably reasonable to suggest that patients with large anterior infarcts, congestive heart failure, ventricular aneurysms, or mural thrombi (on echocardiogram) should be anticoagulated for at least three months. Regarding patients with rheumatic valve disease, it is suggested that patients with "prominent" rheumatic heart disease should be anticoagulated indefinitely.[49] This would include patients with obvious mitral stenosis, large left atrium, congestive heart failure, atrial fibrillation, and atrial thrombi demonstrated by echocardiography. For lesser degrees of rheumatic heart disease it is not clear if the benefits of long-term anticoagulation outweigh the risks.

Controversy concerns the patient with nonvalvular atrial fibrillation who has never had an embolus. There is strong evidence of increased risk of stroke in this situation,[68,100,235] but prophylactic anticoagulant therapy has not been universally agreed upon for this group of patients.

Three studies[89,124,203] in patients with mechanical prosthetic heart valves have shown benefit from combination therapy with anticoagulants and dipyridamole, and two other trials[8,42] have demonstrated similar results with anticoagulants and ASA. The latter combination may be hazardous in terms of excessive gastrointestinal bleeding. A reasonable recommendation might be to administer anticoagulants after inserting biologic prosthetic valves for three months in uncomplicated situations and indefinitely in those who have artificial valves and manifest thromboembolism, left atrial enlargement, or fibrillation.

Anticoagulants are contraindicated in bacterial endocarditis complicated by cerebral embolism.[77,190]

Antiplatelet Drugs in Cardiogenic Cerebral Emboli

One study suggests that sulfinpyrazone decreases thromboembolism in patients with mitral stenosis.[199] Antiplatelet therapy may be reasonable for patients with embolic events secondary to mitral valve prolapse, but insufficient data are available to justify conclusive statements in this regard.[18]

Summary of Therapeutic Recommendations

In recent years several authors have attempted to collate all the data regarding the treatment of various forms of ischemic cerebrovascular disease into comprehensive plans of patient management. Very thorough and useful reviews have been published regarding the management of TIA,[30,146,157,183] progressing stroke,[154] completed stroke,[28] and cerebral embolism.[49]

It must be recognized that in a disorder of diverse etiology and complex pathogenesis such as ischemic cerebrovascular disease, no single management approach is either possible or desirable, and each case must be considered on an individual basis. The following general recommendations are based on an interpretation of the data in the literature and from personal experience:

1. Angiography should be reserved for those patients with threatened stroke presenting with carotid artery symptoms, and in whom surgery would be indicated should an accessible lesion be found. Angiography is not indicated in most patients with posterior circulation TIAs.
2. Carotid endarterectomy is recommended for patients with carotid system TIAs, RIND, or minor stroke ipsilateral to a surgically accessible stenotic and/or ulcerated proximal internal carotid artery atheromatous lesion.[129] The combined morbidity and mortality risk for angiography and surgery in the particular institution should be known and must be at or below 3%. No patient should be submitted to endarterectomy without a careful assessment by a physician or surgeon expert in the interpretation of the signs and symptoms of neurologic disease.
3. Aspirin therapy, at the time of writing, is the first line of antithrombotic treatment to be administered for threatened stroke in male patients. It will be the definitive treatment for patients with carotid symptoms in whom surgical procedures are not contemplated for any reason; as a prelude to and a

Table 3.1. The place of anticoagulants in preventing calamitous stroke.

Presentation	Indication	Confidence in recommendation	Type of anticoagulant	Duration of treatment	Subsequent treatment
TIA	Failure to stop TIAs with antiplatelet therapy.	++	Coumadin	3 months	Platelet antiaggregants
	Progression to PNS.	++			
PNS	As above, despite antiplatelet treatment.	++	Coumadin	3 months	Platelet antiaggregants
	Primary presentation and within few days of occurrence.	+			
Progressing stroke (Short of complete)	Stepwise progression over days to weeks.	+++	Heparin followed by coumadin	3 days	Platelet antiaggregants
	Slow progression over hours to days.	+++		3 months	
Completed stroke	Nil	++++	—	—	—
Myocardial infarction	Major infarction; transmural; septal; with congestive heart failure.	+++	Coumadin	3 months	—
	Evidence for emboli.	++++	Coumadin	3 months	—
	Subsequent akinetic segment containing thrombi or producing emboli.	+++	Coumadin	3 months	Platelet antiaggregants
Rheumatic heart disease	Atrial fibrillation and mitral stenosis.	+	Coumadin	Until surgery	—
	Same, with systemic emboli. Thrombi visualized in atrium.	++++	Coumadin	Until surgery	—
Prosthetic heart valve	Valve insertion.	++++	Coumadin	Indefinitely. (?) Stop at 3 months	Combined with persantine
Atrial fibrillation with myocardial infarction or rheumatic heart disease	Without emboli.	?	?	?	?
	With emboli.	++	Coumadin	Indefinitely (?) 3 months	(?) Platelet antiaggregants
Prolapsing mitral valve	With emboli, despite antiplatelet treatment.	+++	Coumadin	3 months	Platelet antiaggregants

sequel to carotid endarterectomy if this is carried out; and for patients with vertebrobasilar TIA.

4. In male patients, failure to eliminate TIA with aspirin is not uncommon, and the next step recommended is the addition of dipyridamole.
5. The optimum dosage of platelet antiaggregants has become a debated subject. Based on clinical trials, the recommended dose of aspirin is 325 mg by mouth every six hours. An enteric-coated form is advised where plain ASA cannot be tolerated.[5] Alternatively, cimetidine may be given concurrently.[97] Some would recommend a lower dosage of ASA,[137] but this is hypothetical and based on animal experimental work. The issue remains unresolved. The recommended dosage of dipyridamole, on empirical grounds, is 50 mg four times daily.
6. Platelet antiaggregant treatment in female patients presents a greater dilemma.[16] The recommended approach is to start empirically with a combination of ASA and dipyridamole.
7. Anticoagulant therapy in stroke prevention has its enthusiasts, its cautious users, and a large number of clinicians who deny it any place. The problem is one of uncertain scientific data coupled with the hazards of its use. Table 3.1 presents an algorithm based on an attempt to balance conflicting evidence and is not to be construed as an alternative to the judicious use of a surgical approach to carotid-territory symptoms.
8. Risk factor management in all likelihood is as important in stroke prevention as any other measure currently available. Hypertension control is mandatory, and despite the difficulties that may be encountered in dose-adjustment and compliance, blood pressure must be maintained at or below 160/90 mm Hg in all ages and in both sexes. Cigarette smoking should be abandoned; hemoglobin levels above 16 should be treated by intermittent phlebotomy; diabetes should be detected and regulated; cardiac irregularities should be given strict attention; and reasonable dietary intake of fat should be recommended. The role of other risk factors is less certain and the benefit or their management less certain.
9. The asymptomatic bruit is recognized as a risk factor, and its presence demands that attention be paid to associated conditions, particularly hypertension. Prophylactic platelet antiaggregants are recommended if the bruit is recognized as coming from the cerebral arteries and is not transmitted from the heart.
10. Antispasmodic and so-called vasoactive drugs have no credible status in stroke prevention.

References

1. Abernathy WS, Willis PW: Thromboembolic complications of rheumatic heart disease. Cardiovas Clin 5, 2:131–175, 1973
2. Acheson J, Danta G, Hutchinson EC: Controlled trials of dipyridamole in cerebral vascular disease. Br Med J 1:614–615, 1969
3. Adams GF, Merrett JD, Hutchinson WM, Pollok AM: Cerebral embolism and mitral stenosis: survival with and without anticoagulants. J Neurol Neurosurg Psychiatry 37:378–383, 1974
4. Ali M, McDonald JWD: Reversible and irreversible inhibition of platelet cyclooxygenase and serotonin release by nonsterioidal antiinflammatory drugs. Thromb Res 13:1057–1065, 1978
5. Ali M, McDonald JWD, Thiessen JJ, Coates PE: Plasma acetylasalicylate and salicylate and platelet cylcooxygenase activity following plain and enteric-coated aspirin. Stroke 11:9–13, 1980
6. Al-Mefty O, Marano G, Rajaraman S, Nugent GR, Rodman N: Transient ischemic attacks due to increased platelet aggregation and adhesiveness. Ultrastructural and functional correlation. J. Neurosurg 50:449–453, 1979
7. Al-Mondhiry H, Marcus AJ, Spaet TH: On the mechanism of platelet function inhibition by acetysalicylic acid. Proc Soc Exp Biol Med 133:632–636, 1970
8. Altman R, Boullon F, Rouvier J, Raca R, de la Fuente L, Favalavo R: Aspirin and prophylaxis of thromboembolic complications in patients with substitute heart valves. J. Thorac Cardiovasc Surg 72:127–129, 1976
9. Asinger RW, Mikell FL, Elsperger J, Hodges M: Incidence of left-ventricular thrombosis after acute transmural myocardial infarction. N Engl J Med 305:297–302, 1981
10. Askey JM, Cherry CB: Thromboembolism associated with auricular fibrillation. JAMA 144:97–100, 1950

11. Baker RN: An evaluation of anticoagulant therapy in the treatment of cerebrovascular disease: Report of the Veterans Administration cooperative study of atherosclerosis. Neurology 11:4. 2:132–138 1961
12. Baker RN, Broward JA, Fang HC, Fisher CM, Groch SN, Heyman A, Karp HR, McDevitt E, Scheinberg P, Schwartz W, Toole JF: Anticoagulant therapy in cerebral infarction. Report on cooperative study. Neurology 12:823–835, 1962
13. Baker RN, Schwartz WS, Rose AS: Transient ischemic strokes. A report of a study of anticoagulant therapy. Neurology 16:841–847, 1966
14. Barnett HJM: Pathogenesis of transient ischemic attacks. In P Scheinberg (ed.): Cerebrovascular Diseases. Raven Press, New York, 1976, pp 1–21
15. Barnett HJM: Platelet and coagulation function in relation to thromboembolic stroke. Adv Neurol 16:45–70, 1977
16. Barnett HJM: The pathophysiology of transient cerebral ischemic attacks: Therapy with platelet antiaggregants. In Medical Clinics of North America 63:649–679, 1979
17. Barnett HJM: Progress towards stroke prevention. Robert Wartenberg Lecture. Neurology 30:1212–1225, 1980
18. Barnett HJM: Embolism in mitral valve prolapse. Annu Rev Med 33:489–507, 1982
19. Barnett HJM, Boughner DR, Taylor DW, Cooper PE, Kostuk WJ, Nichol P: Further evidence relating mitral valve prolapse to cerebral ischemic events. N Engl J Med 302:139–144, 1980
20. Barnett HJM, Jones MW, Boughner DR, Kostuk WJ: Cerebral ischemic events associated with prolapsing mitral valve. Arch Neurol 33:777–782, 1976
21. Barnett HJM, Peerless SJ, McCormick CW: In answer to the question "As compared to what?". A progress report on the EC/IC Bypass Study. Stroke 11:137–140, 1980
22. Bathen J, Sparr S, Rokseth R: Embolism in sinoatrial disease. Acta Med Scand 203:7–11, 1978
23. Beal MF, Williams RS Richardson EP Jr, Fisher CM: Cholesterol embolism as a cause of transient ischemic attacks and cerebral infarction. Neurology 31:860–865, 1981
24. Beevers DG, Fairman M, Hamilton M, Harpur JE: Antihypertensive treatment and the course of established cerebral vascular disease. Lancet i:1407–1409, 1973
25. Bell HS: Basilar artery insufficiency due to atlanto-occipital instability. Am Surg 35:695–700, 1969
26. Blakely JA, Gent M: Platelets, drugs and longevity in a geriatric population. In J Hirsh, JF Cade, AS Gallus, E Schonbaun (eds.): Platelets, Drugs and Thrombosis, Karger, Basel, 1975, pp 284–291
27. Brice JG, Dowsett DJ, Lowe RD: Haemodynamic effects of carotid artery stenosis. Br Med J 2:1363–1366, 1964
28. Buonanno F, Toole JF: Management of patients with established ("completed") cerebral infarction. Stroke 12:7–16, 1981
29. Burger PC, Burch JG, Vogel FS: Granulomatous angiitis. An unusual etiology of stroke. Stroke 8:29–35, 1977
30. Byer JA, Easton JD: Therapy of ischemic cerebrovascular disease. Ann Intern Med 93:742–756, 1980
31. Canadian Cooperative Study Group (Barnett, HJM et al): A randomized trail of aspirin and sulfinpyrazone in threatened stroke. N Engl J Med 299:53–59, 1978
32. Carter AB: The immediate treatment of cerebral embolism. Q J Med 26:335–348, 1957
33. Carter AB: Anticoagulant treatment in progressing stroke. Br Med J 2:70–73, 1961
34. Carter AB: Prognosis of cerebral embolism. Lancet 2:514–519, 1965
35. Castaigne P, Lhermitte F, Gautier J-C, Escourolle R, Derouesne C: Internal carotid artery occlusion. A study of 61 instances in 50 patients with postmortem data. Brain 93:231–258, 1970
36. Cohen MM, Hemalatha CP, D'Addario RT, Goldman HW: Embolization from a fusiform middle cerebral artery aneurysm. Stroke 11:158–161, 1980
37. Collaborative Group for the Study of Stroke in Young Women: Oral contraception and increased risk of cerebral ischemia or thrombosis. N Engl J Med 288:871–878, 1973
38. Cook AW, Bird TD, Spence AM, Pagon RA, Wallace JF: Myotonic dystrophy, mitral-valve prolapse and stroke. Lancet 1:335–336, 1978
39. Cosgriff SW: Prophylaxis of recurrent embolism of intracardiac origin. JAMA 143:870–872, 1950
40. Cosgriff SW: Chronic anticoagulant therapy in recurrent embolism of cardiac origin. Ann Intern Med 38:278–287, 1953
41. Coulshed N, Epstein EJ, McKendrick CS, Galloway RW, Walker E: Systemic embolism in mitralvalve disease. Br Heart J 32:26–34, 1970
42. Dale J, Myhre E, Storstein O, Stormorken H, Efskind L: Prevention of arterial thromboembolism with acetylsalicylic acid: a controlled clinical trial in patients with aortic ball valves. Am Heart J 94:101–111, 1977

43. Daly DD, Svien HJ, Yoss RE: Intermittent cerebral symptoms with meningiomas. Arch Neurol 5:287–293, 1961
44. David NJ, Klintworth GK, Friedberg SJ, Dillon M: Fatal atheromatous cerebral embolism associated with bright plaques in the retinal arterioles. Report of one case. Neurology 13:708–713, 1963
45. DeBono DP, Warlow CP: Mitral annulus calcification and cerebral or retinal ischaemia. Lancet 2:383–386, 1979
46. Denny-Brown D: Recurrent cerebrovascular episodes. AMA Arch Neurol 2:94–110, 1960
47. Dougherty JH Jr, Levy De, Weksler BB: Platelet activation in acute cerebral ischemia. Lancet 1:821–824, 1977
48. Dyken ML, Kolar OJ, Jones FH: Differences in the occurrence of carotid transient ischemic attacks associated with antiplatelet aggregation therapy. Stroke 4:732–736, 1973
49. Easton JD, Sherman DG: Management of cerebral embolism of cardiac origin. Stroke 11:433–442, 1980
50. Edwards JH, Kricheff II, Riles T, Imparato A: Angiographically undetected ulceration of the carotid bifurcation as a cause of embolic stroke. Radiology 132:369–373, 1979
51. Enger E, Boyensen S: Long-term anticoagulant therapy in patients with cerebral infarction. A controlled clinical study. Acta Med Scand 178 (Suppl) 438:1–61, 1965
52. Estanol B, Rodriguez A, Conte G, Aleman JM, Loyo M, Pozzuto J: Intracranial venous thrombosis in young women. Stroke 10:680–684, 1979
53. Estey E, Liberman A, Pinto R, Meltzer M, Ransohoff J: Cerebral arteritis in scleroderma. Stroke 10:595–597, 1979
54. Evans G: Effect of platelet suppressive agents on the incidence of amaurosis fugax and transient cerebral ischemia. In FH McDowell, RW Brennan, (eds.): Cerebral Vascular Diseases, Eighth Conference. Grune and Stratton Inc, New York, 1973, pp 297–299
55. Fairfax AJ, Lambert CD, Leatham A: Systemic embolism in chronic sinoatrial disorder. N Engl J Med 295:190–192, 1976
56. Faris AA, Poser CM, Wilmore DW, Agnew CH: Radiologic visualization of neck vessels in healthy men. Neurology 13:386–396, 1963
57. Fazekas JF, Alman RW, Sullivan JF: Vertebral-basilar insufficiency: management of patients with vertebral-basilar insufficiency. Arch Neurol 8:215–220, 1963
58. Fields WS, Lemak NA, et al: The ASA-dipyridamole study. Manual of instructions to investigators. Unpublished, 1978
59. Fields WS, Lemak NA, Frankowski RF, Hardy RJ: Controlled trial of aspirin in cerebral ischemia. Stroke 8:301–316, 1977
60. Fisher CM: The use of anticoagulants in cerebral thrombosis. Neurology 8:311–332, 1958
61. Fisher CM: Observations of the fundus oculi in transient monocular blindness. Neurology 9:333–347, 1959
62. Fisher CM: Anticoagulant therapy in cerebral thrombosis and cerebral embolism: a national cooperative study, interim report. Neurology 11:4 119–131, 1961
63. Fisher CM: Pure sensory stroke invloving face, arm and leg. Neurology 15:76–80,1965
64. Fisher CM: Lacunes: Small, deep cerebral infarcts. Neurology 15:774–784, 1965
65. Fisher CM: A lacunar stroke: The dysarthria—clumpsy hand syndrome. Neurology 17:614–617, 1967
66. Fisher CM: The arterial lesions underlying lacunes. Acta neuropath (Berl) 12:1–15, 1969
67. Fisher CM: Transient paralytic attacks of obscure nature: The question of non-convulsive seizure paralysis. Can J Neurol Sci 5:267–273, 1978
68. Fisher CM: Reducing risks of cerebral embolism. Geriatrics 34:57–66, 1979
69. Fisher CM: Late-life migraine accompaniments as a cause of unexplained transient ischemic attacks. Can J Neurol Sci 7:9–17, 1980
70. Fisher CM, Cole M: Homolateral ataxia and crural paresis: a vascular syndrome. J Neurol Neurosurg Psychiatry 28:48–55, 1965
71. Fisher CM, Curry HB: Pure motor hemiplegia of vascular origin. Arch Neurol 13:30–44, 1965
72. Fisher CM, Gore I, Okabe N, White PD: Atherosclerosis of the carotid and vertebral arteries—extracranial and intracranial. J Neuropathol Exp Neurol 24:455–476, 1965
73. Fisher CM, Ojemann RG, Roberson GH: Spontaneous dissection of cervico-cerebral arteries. Can J Neurol Sci 5:9–19, 1978
74. Fisher M: Occlusion of the carotid arteries. Arch Neurol Psychiatry 65:346–377, 1951
75. Fleming HA, Bailey SM: Mitral valve disease, systemic embolism and anticoagulants. Postgrad Med J 47:599–604, 1971
76. Flory CM: Arterial occlusions produced by emboli from eroded aortic atheromatous plaques. Am J Pathol 21:549–565, 1945
77. Foote RA, Reagan TJ, Sandok BA: Effects of anticoagulants in an animal model of septic cerebral embolization. Stroke 9:573–579, 1978
78. Ford RG, Siekert RG: Central nervous system manifestations of periarteritis nodosa. Neurology 15:114–122, 1965
79. Friedli B, Aerichide N, Grondin P, Campeau L:

Thromboembolic complications of heart valve prostheses. Am Heart J 81:702–708, 1971
80. Friedman GD, Wilson WS, Mosier JM, Colandrea MA, Nichaman MZ: Transient ischemic attacks in a community. JAMA 210:1428–1434, 1969
81. Fuster V, Chesebro JH: Antithrombotic therapy: Role of platelet-inhibitor drugs. I. Current concepts of thrombogenesis: role of platelets. Mayo Clin Proc 56:102–112, 1981
82. Fuster V, Chesebro JH: Antithrombotic therapy. Role of platelet inhibitor drugs. II. Pharmacologic effects of platelet-inhibitor drugs. Mayo Clin Proc 56:185–195, 1981
83. Fuster V, Chesebro JH: Antithrombotic therapy. Role of platelet-inhibitor drugs. III. Management of arterial thromboembolic and atherosclerotic disease. Mayo Clin Proc 56:265–273, 1981
84. Garraway WM, Whisnant JP, Furlan AJ, Phillips LH II, Kurland LT, O'Fallon WM: The declining incidence of stroke. N Engl J Med 300:449–452, 1979
85. Garraway WM, Whisnant JP, Kurland LT, O'Fallon WM: Changing pattern of cerebral infarction: 1945-1974. Stroke 10:657–663, 1979
86. Genton E, Barnett HJM, Fields WS, Gent M, Hoak JC: Cerebral ischemia: the role of thrombosis and of antithrombotic therapy. Study group on antithrombotic therapy. Stroke 8:150–175, 1977
87. Greenlee JE, Mandell GL: Neurological manifestations of infective endocarditis: a review. Stroke 4:958–963, 1973
88. Grunnet ML: Cerebrovascular disease: diabetes and cerebral atherosclerosis. Neurology 13:486–491, 1963
89. Groupe de recherche PACTE: Prevention des accidents thromboemboliques systemiques chez les porteurs de protheses valvulaires artificielles: essai cooperatif controle du dipyridamole. Coeur 9:915–969, 1978
90. Gunning AJ, Pickering GW, Robb-Smith AHT, Ross Russell R: Mural thrombosis of the internal carotid artery and subsequent embolism. Q J Med New Series XXXIII: 129:155–195, 1964
91. Harker LA, Slichter SJ, Scott CR, Ross R: Homocystinemia. Vascular injury and arterial thrombosis. N Engl J Med 291:537–543, 1974
92. Harlan JM, Harker LA: Hemostasis, thrombosis, and thromboembolic disorders. The role of arachidonic acid metabolites in platelet vessel wall interactions. Med Clin North Am 65:855–880, 1981
93. Harris WH, Salzman EW, Athanasoulis CA, Waltman AC, DeSanctis RW: Aspirin prophylaxis of venous thromboembolism after total hip replacement. N Engl J Med 297:1246–1249, 1977
94. Harrison MJG, Marshall J., Meadows JC, Ross Russell RW: Effect of aspirin in amaurosis fugax. Lancet 2:743–744, 1971
95. Hass WK: Occlusive cerebrovascular disease. Med Clin North Am 56:1281–1297, 1972
96. Hass WK, Fields WS, North RR, Kricheff II, Chase NE, Bauer RB: Joint study of extracranial arterial occlusion. II. Arteriography, techniques, sites and complications. JAMA 203:961–968, 1968
97. Hass WK, Hazzi C: Cimetidine protection against gastric side effects of long term aspirin therapy in transient ischemic attacks. In JS Meyer, H Lechner, M Reivich, EO Ott and A Araniba (eds.): Cerebral Vascular Diseases II. (The Proceedings of the International Salzburg Conference, Sept. 28–30, 1978) Excerpta Medica, Amsterdam, 1981, pp 207–210
98. Hellerstein HK, Martin JW: Incidence of thromboembolic lesions accompanying myocardial infarction. Am Heart J 33:443–452, 1947
99. Hill AB, Marshall J, Shaw DA: Cerebrovascular disease: trail of longterm anticoagulant therapy. Br Med J 2:1003–1006, 1962
100. Hinton RC, Kistler JP, Fallon JT, Friedlich AL, Fisher CM: Influence of etiology of atrial fibrillation on incidence of systemic embolism. Am J Cardiol 40:509–513, 1977
101. Hollenhorst RW: Significance of bright plaques in the retianl arterioles. JAMA 178:23–29, 1961
102. Honour AJ, Ross-Russell RW: Experimental platelet embolism. Br J Exp Pathol 43:350–362, 1962
103. Houser OW, Baker HL Jr, Sandok BA, Holley KE: Fibromuscular dysplasia of the cephalic arterial system. Handbook Clin Neurol 11:366–385, 1972
104. Houser OW, Sundt, TM Jr, Holman CB, Sandok BA, Burton RC: Atheromatous disease of the carotid artery. Correlation of angiographic, clinical and surgical findings. J Neurosur 41:321–331, 1974
105. Howard FA, Cohen P, Hickler RB, Locke J, Newcomb T, Tyler HR: Survival following stroke. JAMA 183:921–925, 1963
106. Howell DA, Tatlow WFT, Feldman S: Observations on anticoagulant therapy in thromboembolic disease of the brain. Can Med Assoc J 90:611–614, 1964
107. Hutchinson EC, Stock JPP: Paroxysmal cerebral ischaemia in rheumatic heart disease. Lancet 2:653–656, 1963
108. Hutchinson EC, Yates PO: Carotico vertebral stenosis. Lancet 1:2–8, 1957

109. Hypertension Detection and Follow-up Program Cooperative Group: Five-year findings of the hypertension detection and follow-up program. 1. Reduction in mortality of persons with high blood pressure, including mild hypertension. JAMA 242:2562–2571, 1979
110. Irey NS, Manion WC, Taylor HB: Vascular lesions in women taking oral contraceptives. Arch Pathol 89:1–8, 1970
111. Irey NS, McAllister HA, Henry JM: Oral contraceptives and stroke in young women: A clinicopathologic correlation. Neurology 28:1216–1219, 1978
112. Ishikawa, K: Natural history and classification of occlusive thromboaortapathy (Takayasu's Disease). Circulation 57:27–35, 1978
113. Jakobson T: Glucose tolerance and serum lipid levels in patients with cerebrovascular disease. Acta Med Scand 182:233–243, 1967
114. James DG: Behcet's Syndrome. N Engl J Med 301:431–432, 1979
115. Johnson RT, Richardson EP: The neurological manifestations of systemic lupus erythematosus. Medicine 47:337–369, 1968
116. Jones MW, Kaufmann JCE: Vertebrobasilar artery insufficiency in rheumatoid atlanto-axial subluxation. J Neurol Neurosurg Psychiatry 39:122–128, 1976
117. Kaegi A, Pineo CF, Shimizu A, Trivedi H, Hirsh J, Gent M; Arteriovenous-shunt thrombosis—prevention of sulfinpyrazone. N Engl J Med 290:304–306, 1974
118. Kalendovsky Z, Austin J, Steele P: Increased platelet aggregability in young patients with stroke. Diagnosis and therapy. Arch Neurol 32:13–20, 1975
119. Kannel WB: Current status of the epidemiology of brain infarction associated with occlusive arterial disease. Stroke 2:295–318, 1971
120. Kannel WB, Dawber TR, Sorlie P, Wolf PA: Components of blood pressure and risk of atherothrombotic brain infarction. The Framingham Study. Stroke 7:327–331, 1976
121. Kannel WB, Gordon T, Dawber TR: Role of lipids in the development of brain infarction. The Framingham Study. Stroke 5:679–685, 1974
122. Kannel WB, Gordon T, Wolf PA, McNamara P: Hemoglobin and the risk of cerebral infarction. The Framingham Study. Stroke 3:409–420, 1972
123. Kannel WB, Wolf PA, Verter J, McNamara PM: Epidemiological assessment of the role of blood pressure in stroke. The Framingham Study. JAMA 214:301–310, 1970
124. Karahara T: Clinical effect of dipyridamole ingestion after prosthetic heart valve replacement—especially on the blood coagulation system. Nippon Kyobu Geka Gakkai Zasshi 25:1007–1021, 1977
125. Kelton JG, Hirsh J, Carter CJ, Buchanan MR: Sex differences in the antithrombotic effects of aspirin. Blood 52:1073–1076, 1978
126. Kendell RE, Marshall J: Role of hypotension in the genesis of transient focal cerebral ischemic attacks. Br Med J 2:344–348, 1963
127. Kooiker JC, MacLean JM, Sumi SM: Cerebral embolism, marantic endocarditis, and cancer. Arch Neurol 33:260–264, 1976
128. Kottke BA, Ravi Subbiah, MT: Pathogenesis of atherosclerosis. Concepts based on animals models. Mayo Clin Proc 53:35–48, 1978
129. Kurtzke J: Formal discussion. In JP Whisnant and BA Sandok (ed.): Cerebral Vascular Diseases, Grune and Stratton Inc, New York, 1974, pp 190–194
130. Kurtzke J (ed.): Epidemiology of cerebrovascular disease. Springer Verlag, Berlin 1969
131. Kurtzke JF: A critique of the Canadian TIA study. Ann Neurol 5:597–599, 1979
132. Lavy S: Medical risk factors in stroke. Adv Neurol 25:127–133 1979
133. Levine J, Swanson PD: Idiopathic thrombocytosis. A treatable cause of transient ischemic attacks. Neurology 18:711–713, 1968
134. Lhermitte F, Gautier JC, Derouesne C: Nature of occlusions of the middle cerebral artery. Neurology 20:82–88, 1970
135. Linos A, Worthington JW, O'Fallon W, Fuster V, Whisnant JP, Kurland LT: Effect of aspirin on prevention of coronary and cerebrovascular disease in patients with rheumatoid arthritis. A long-term follow up study. Mayo Clin Proc 53:581–586, 1978
136. Logothetis J, Silverstein P, Coe J: Neurologic aspects of Waldenstrom's macroglobulinemia. Arch Neurol 3:564–573
137. Marcus AJ: Aspirin and thromboembolism—a possible dilemma. N Engl J Med 297:1284–1285, 1977
138. Marshall J, Shaw DA: Anticoagulant therapy in acute cerebrovascular accidents. A controlled trial. Lancet 1:995–998, 1960
139. Martin MJ, Whisnant JP, Sayre GP: Occlusive vascular disease in the extracranial cerebral circulation. Arch Neurol 3:530–538, 1960
140. McAllen PM, Marshall J: Cardiac dysrhythmia and transient cerebral ischaemic attacks. Lancet 1:1212–1214, 1973
141. McBrien DJ, Bradley RD, Ashton N: The nature of retinal emboli in stenosis of the internal carotid artery. Lancet 1:697–699, 1963

142. McCormick CW: The cooperative study of extracranial-intracranial arterial anastomosis—clinical aspects. In G. Tognoni, S. Garattini (eds.): Drug Treatment and Prevention in Cerebrovascular Disorders, Elsevier/North-Holland Biomedical Press, Amsterdam, 1979, pp 395–403
143. McDonald JWD, Ali M, Nagai GR, Barnett WH, Barnett HJM: Inhibition of platelet prostaglandin synthetase and platelet release reaction by sulfinpyrazone (abstract). Blood 46:1033, 1975
144. McDonald CD, Burch GE, Walsh JJ: Prolonged bed rest in the treatment of idiopathic cardiomyopathy. Am J Med 52:41–50, 1972
145. McDowell F, McDevitt E: Treatment of the completed stroke with long-term anticoagulant: Six and one-half years experience. In RG Siekert and JP Whisnant (eds.): Cerebral Vascular Diseases, Fourth Princeton Conference. Grune and Stratton Inc., New York, 1965, 185–199
146. McDowell FH, Millikan CH, Goldstein M: Treatment of impending stroke. Stroke 11:1–2, 1980
147. McMillan GC: Atherogenesis: The process from normal to lesion. Adv Exp Med Biol 104:3–10, 1977
148. Melamed E, Lavy S, Reches A, Sahar A: Chronic subdural hematoma simulating transient cerebral ischemic attacks. Case report. J Neurosurg 42:101–103, 1975
149. Menon IS, Peberdy M, Rannie GH, Weightman D, Dewar HA: A comparative study of blood fibrinolytic activity in normal women, pregnant women and women on oral contraceptives. J Obstet Gynecol Br Commonwealth 77:752–756, 1970
150. Meyer JS, Leiderman H, Denny-Brown D: Electroencephalographic study of insufficiency of the basilar and carotid arteries in man. Neurology 6:455–477, 1956
151. Meyer WW: Cholesterinkristallembolie Kleine Organarterien und ihre Folgen. Virchow Arch [Pathol Anat] 314:616, 1947
152. Millikan CH: Anticoagulant therapy in cerebrovascular disease. In CH Millikan, RG Siekert, JP Whisnant (eds.): Cerebral Vascular Diseases Third Princeton Conference. Grune and Stratton Inc, New York, 1961, pp 183–185
153. Millikan CH: The pathogenesis of transient focal cerebral ischemia. Circulation 32:438, 1965
154. Millikan CH, McDowell FH: Treatment of progressing stroke. Prog Cardiovasc Dis 22:397–414, 1980
155. Millikan CH, Siekert RG, Whisnant JP: Intermittent carotid and vertebral-basilar insufficiency associated with polycythemia. Neurology 10:188–196, 1960
156. Mills DCB, Smith JB: The influence on platelet aggregation of drugs that affect the accumulation of adenosine 3′:5′—cyclic monophosphate in platelets. Biochem J 121:185–196, 1971
157. Mohr JP: Transient ischemic attacks and the prevention of strokes. N Engl J Med 299:93–95, 1978
158. Mohr JP, Caplan LR, Melski JW, Goldstein RJ, Duncan GW, Kistler JP, Pessin MS, Bleich HL: The Harvard cooperative stroke registry. Neurology 28:754–762, 1978
159. Moncada S, Amezcua JL: Prostacyclin, thromboxane A_2 interactions in haemostasis and thrombosis. Haemostasis 8:252–265, 1979
160. Moncada S, Vane JR: Arachidonic acid metabolites and the interactions between platelets and blood-vessel walls. N Engl J Med 300:1142–1147, 1979
161. Moore WS, Malone JM, Boren C, Roon AJ Goldstone J: Asymptomatic ulcerative lesions of the carotid artery—natural history and effect of surgical therapy compared. Stroke 10:96, 1979
162. Mundall J, Quintero P, von Kaulla KN, Harmon R, Austin J: Transient monocular blindness and increased platelet aggregability treated with aspirin: A case report. Neurology 22:280–285, 1972
163. Mustard JF, Packham MA, Kinlough-Rathbone R: Platelets, thrombosis and atherosclerosis. Adv Exp Med Biol 104:127–144, 1977
164. Mustard JF, Packham MA, Kinlough-Rathbone RL: Platelets and thrombosis in the development of atherosclerosis and its complications. Adv Exp Med Biol 102:7–30, 1978
165. Nilsson IM, Astedt B, Isacson S: The effect of hormones on coagulation and fibrinolysis. Proceedings of the International Society for Thrombosis and Hemostasis, 2nd Congress, 1971, p 86
166. Nishimoto A, Takeuchi S: MoyaMoya disease. Handbook Clin Neurol 12:352–383, 1972
167. Okawara S, Nibbelink D: Vertebral artery occlusion following hyperextension and rotation of the head. Stroke 5:640–642, 1974
168. Olsson J-E, Brechter C, Bäcklund H, Krook H. Muller R, Nitelius E, Olsson O, Tornberg A: Anticoagulant vs. antiplatelet therapy as prophylactic against cerebral infarction in transient ischemic attacks. Stroke 11:4–9, 1980
169. Otken LB: Experimental production of atheromatous embolization. Arch Pathol 68:685–689, 1959

170. Owren PA: The results of anticoagulant therapy in Norway. Arch Intern Med 111:240–247, 1963
171. Patel A, Toole JF: Subclavian steal syndrome: Reversal of cephalic blood flow. Medicine 44:289–303, 1965
172. Pearce JMS, Gubbay SS, Walton JN: Long-term anticoagulant therapy in transient cerebral ischaemic attacks. Lancet 1:6–9, 1965
173. Pessin, MS, Hinton RC, Davis KR, Duncan GW, Roberson GH, Ackerman RH, Mohr JP: Mechanisms of acute carotid stroke. Ann Neurol 6:245–252, 1979
174. Poller L, Thomson J.M.: Clotting factors during oral contraception: Further report. Br Med J 2:23–25, 1966
175. Prineas J, Marshall J: Hypertension and cerebral infarction. Br Med J 1:14–17, 1966
176. Reed RL, Siekert RG, Merideth J: Rarity of transient focal cerebral ischemia in cardiac dysrhythmia. JAMA 223:893–895, 1973
177. Robin JJ, Maxwell JA, Pitkethly DT: Chronic subdural hematoma simulating transient ischemic attacks. Ann Neurol 4:154, 1978
178. Rogers PH, Sherry S: Current status of antithrombotic therapy in cardiovascular disease. Progress Cardiovas Dis 19:235–253, 1976
179. Ross R, Glomset JA: The pathogenesis of atherosclerosis. N Engl J Med 295:369–377 and 420–425, 1976
180. Ross-Russell RW: Observations on the retinal blood-vessels in monocular blindness. Lancet 2:1422–1428, 1961
181. Roth GJ, Stanford N, Majerus PW: Acetylation of prostaglandin synthase by aspirin. Proc Nat Acad Sci USA 72:3073–3076, 1975
182. Ruff RL, Dougherty JH Jr: Evaluation of acute cerebral ischemia for anticoagulant therapy: Computed tomography or lumbar puncture. Neurology 31:736–740, 1981
183. Sandok BA, Furlan AJ, Whisnant JP, Sundt TM Jr: Guidelines for the management of transient ischemic attacks. Mayo Clin Proc 53:665–674, 1978
184. Scheinberg P, Stead EA Jr: The cerebral blood flow in male subjects as measured by the nitrous oxide technique. J Clin Invest 28:1163–1171, 1949
185. Schmidley JW, Caronna JJ: Transient cerebral ischemia: Pathophysiology. Prog Cardiovasc Dis 22:325–342, 1980
186. Schneiderman JH, Sharpe JA, Sutton DMC: Cerebral and retinal vascular complications of inflammatory bowel disease. Ann Neurol 5:331–337, 1979
187. Schwartz CJ, Chandler AB, Gerrity RG, Naito HK: Clinical and pathological aspects of arterioal thrombosis and thromboembolism. Adv Exp Med Biol 104:111–126, 1977
188. Sheehan S, Bauer RB, Meyer JS: Vertebral artery compression in cervical spondylosis. Neurology 10:968–986, 1960
189. Sherman DG, Hart RG, Easton JD: Abrupt change in head position and cerebral infarction. Stroke 12:2–6, 1981
190. Siekert RG, Jones HR Jr: Transient cerebral ischemic attacks associated with subacute bacterial endocarditis. Stroke 1:178–183, 1970
191. Siekert RG, Whisnant JP, Millikan CH: Surgical and anticoagulant therapy of occlusive cerebrovascular disease. Ann Intern Med 58:637–641, 1963
192. Silverstein A, Doniger DE: Neurologic complications of myelomatosis. Arch Neurol 9:534–544, 1963
193. Singer G: Migrating emboli of retinal arteries in thrombocythaemia. Br J Ophthalmol 53:279–281, 1969
194. Smith JB: The prostanoids in hemostasis and thrombosis. A review. Am J Pathol 99:743–804, 1980
195. So EL, Toole JF, Moody DM, Challa VR: Cerebral embolism from septal fibromuscular dysplasia of the common carotid artery. Ann Neurol 6:75–78, 1979
196. Solberg LA, Eggen DA: Localization and sequence of development of atherosclerotic lesions in the carotid and vertebral arteries. Circulation 43:711–724, 1971
197. Soloway HB, Aronson SM: Atheromatous emboli to central nervous system. Arch Neurol 11:657–667, 1964
198. Stallones RA, Dyken ML, Fang HCH, Heyman A, Seltser R, Stamler J (Epidemiology Study Group): Report of the Joint Committee for Stroke Facilities. I. Epidemiology for stroke facilites planning. Stroke 3:360–371, 1972
199. Steele P, Rainwater J: Favourable effect of sulfinpyrazone on thromboembolism in patients with rheumatic heart disease. Circulation 62:462–465, 1980
200. Steele PP, Weily HS, Genton E: Platelet survival and adhesiveness in recurrent venous thrombosis. N Engl J Med 288:1148–1152, 1973
201. Stockman JA, Nigro MA, Mishkin MM, Oski FA: Occlusion of large cerebral vessels in sickle-cell anemia. N Engl J Med 287:846–849, 1972
202. Strong JP, Eggen DA, Tracy RE: The geographic pathology and topography of atherosclerosis and risk factors for atherosclerotic lesions. Adv Exp Med Biol 104:11-31, 1977
203. Sullivan JM, Harken DE, Gorlin R: Pharmaco-

logic control of thromboembolic complications of cardiac-valve replacement. N Engl J Med 284:1391–1394, 1971
204. Sundt TM Jr, Siekert RG, Piepgras DG, Sharbrough FW, Houser OW: Bypass surgery for vascular disease of the carotid system. Mayo Clin Proc 51:677–692, 1976
205. Sundt TM Jr, Whisnant JP, Piepgras DG, Campbell JK, Holman CB: Intracranial bypass grafts for vertebral-basilar ischemia. Mayo Clin Proc 53:12–18, 1978
206. Szekely P: Systemic embolism and anticoagulant prophylaxis in rheumatic heart disease. Br Med J 1:1209–1212, 1964
207. Ten Cate JW, Vos J, Oosterhuis H, Prenger D, Jenkins CSP: Spontaneous platelet aggregation in cerebrovascular disease. Thromb Haemost 39:223–229, 1978
208. Thomas DJ: The influence of blood viscosity on cerebral blood flow and symptoms. In Greenhalgh RM, Rose FC (eds.): Progress in Stroke Research, Pitman Medical, England, 1979, pp 47–55
209. Thomas DJ, Duboulay GH, Marshall J, Pearson TC, Ross Russell RW, Symon L, Wetherley-Mein G, Zilkha E: Effect of hematocrit on cerebral blood-flow in man. Lancet 2:941–943, 1977
210. Thompson PL, Robinson JS: Stroke after acute myocardial infarction. Relation to infarct size. Br Med J 2:457–459, 1978
211. Thygesen P, Christensen E, Dyrbye M, Eiken M, Frantzen E, Gormsen J, Lademann A, Lennox-Buchthal M, Ronnov-Jessen V, Therkelsen J: Cerebral apoplexy. A clinical, radiological, electroencephalographic, and pathological study with special reference to the prognosis of cerebral infarction and the result of long-term anticoagulation therapy. Dan Med Bull 11:233–257, 1964
212. Tohgi H, Yamanouchi H, Murakami M, Kameyama M: Importance of the hematocrit as a risk factor in cerebral infarction. Stroke 9:369–374, 1978
213. Toole JF, Janeway R, Choi K, Cordell R, Davis C, Johnston F, Miller HS: Transient ischemic attacks due to atherosclerosis. Arch Neurol 32:5–12, 1975
214. Toole JF, Yuson CP, Janeway R, Johnston F, Davis C, Cordell R, Howard G: Transient ischemic attacks: A prospective study of 225 patients. Neurology 28:746–753, 1978
215. Torvik A, Skullerud K: How often are brain infarcts caused by hypotensive episodes? Stroke 7:255–257, 1976
216. Towbin A: The syndrome of latent cerebral venous thrombosis: Its frequency and relation to age and congestive heart failure. Stroke 4:419–430, 1973
217. UK-TIA Study Group: design and protocol of the UK-TIA aspirin study in drug treatment and prevention in cerebrovascular disorders (ed.) Tognoni G and Garattini S. Amsterdam: Elsevier, 1979
218. Uzunova AD, Ramey ER, Ramwell PW: Gonadal hormones and pathogenesis of occlusive arterial thrombosis. Am J Physiol 234:H454–H459, 1978
219. Veterans Administration Cooperative Study Group on Antihypertensive Agents: Effects of treatment on morbidity in hypertension. I. Results in patients with diastolic blood pressures averaging 115 through 129 mm Hg.
220. Veterans Administration Cooperative Study Group on Antihypertensive Agents: Effects of treatment on morbidity in hypertension. II. Results in patients with diastolic blood pressure averaging 90 through 114 mm Hg.
221. Veterans Administration Hospital Investigators: see ref #50
222. Vatz KA, Scheibel RL, Keiffer SA, Ansari KA: Neurosyphilis and diffuse cerebral angiopathy. A case report. Neurology 24:472-476, 1974
223. Vessey MP, Doll R: Investigation of relation between use of oral contraceptives and thromboembolic disease. A further report. Br Med J 2:651–657, 1969
224. Vigdahl RL, Mongin J Jr, Marquis NR: Platelet aggregation. IV. Platelet phosphodiesterase and its inhibition by vasodilators. Biochem Biophys Res Commun 42:1088–1094, 1971
225. Von Kaulla E, Droegemueller W, Aoki N, Von Kaulla KN: Antithrombin III depression and thrombin generation acceleration in women taking oral contraceptives. Am J Obstet Gynecol 109:868–873, 1971
226. Walter PF, Reid SD Jr, Wenger NK: Transient cerebral ischemia due to arrhythmia. Ann Intern Med 72:471–474, 1970
227. Warren BA, Vales O: Electron microscopy of the sequence of events in the atheroembolic occlusion of cerebral arteries in the animal model. Br J Exp Pathol 56:205–215, 1975
228. Whisnant JP: Discussion of "Progressing stroke: anticoagulant therapy." In: Millikan CH, Siekert RG, Whisnant JP, (eds.): Cerebral Vascular Diseases, Third Princeton Conference, Grune and Stratton Inc, New York, 1961, pp 156–157
229. Whisnant JP, Cartlidge NEF, Elveback LR: Carotid and vertebral basilar transient ischemic attacks: effect of anticoagulants, hypertension, and cardiac disorders on survival and stroke

occurrence—A population study. Ann Neurol 3:107–115, 1978

230. Whisnant JP, Matsumoto N, Elveback LR: Transient cerebral ischemic attacks in a community. Rochester, Minnesota, 1955 through 1969. Mayo Clin Proc 48:194–198, 1973
231. Whisnant JP, Matsumoto N, Elveback LR: The effect of anticoagulant therapy on the prognosis of patients with transient cerebral ischemic attacks in a community. Rochester, Minnesota, 1955 through 1969. Mayo Clin Proc 48:844–848, 1973
232. Whisnant JP, Millikan CH, Sayre GP Wakim KG: Effect of anticoagulants on experimental cerebral infarction. Clinical implications. Circulation 20:56–65, 1959
233. Wilkinson IMS, Russell RWR: Arteries of the head and neck in giant cell arteritis. Arch Neurol 27:378–391, 1972
234. Winter WJ Jr: Atheromatous emboli: A cause of cerebral infraction. Arch Pathol 64:137–142, 1957
235. Wolf PA, Dawber TR, Thomas HE Jr, Kannel WB: Epidemiologic assessment of chronic atrial fibrillation and risk of stroke: The Framingham Study. Neurology 28:973–977, 1978
236. Wood, DH: Cerebrovascular complications of sickle cell anemia. Stroke 9:73–75, 1978
237. Wood P: An appreciation of mitral stenosis I. Clinical Features and II. Investigation and Results. Br Med J 1:1051–1063 and 1113–1124, 1954
238. Woolf N: The origins of atherosclerosis. Postgrad Med J 54:156–161, 1978
239. Woolf N: Thrombosis and atherosclerosis. Br Med Bull 34:2, 137–142, 1978
240. Wu Kun-Yu K: Platelet hyperaggregability and thrombosis in patients with thrombocythemia. Ann Intern Med 88:7–11, 1978
241. Wu KK, Hoak JC: Increased platelet aggregates in patients with transient ischemic attacks. Stroke 6:521–524, 1975
242. Yufe R, Karpati G, Carpenter S: Cardiac Myxoma: a diagnostic challenge for the neurologist. Neurology 26:1060–1065, 1976

4

Principles of Vascular Surgery

Charles G. Rob

We do not know when vascular surgery began, but it developed slowly during many centuries.[35,80] The pace gradually increased from about 1900 to 1945 and then accelerated dramatically for the next 39 years from the end of World War II to the present day. But when these developments are reviewed, one is made aware that only two genuinely new ideas have been introduced into vascular surgery since 1945, and in each case the idea was produced by a resident and not by a chairman, a professor, or an established surgeon.[85] Most of the ideas that led to the advances of this present golden era of vascular surgery were conceived in the experimental laboratory or clinical practice during the years preceding World War I. It is of interest to report that a concept such as the use of vein grafts to restore arterial flow was introduced into clinical practice by Goyanes[41] of Madrid in 1906, developed further by Lexer[65] and Pringle,[82] and then only used occasionally until Kunlin[60] introduced the operation of long femoral to popliteal bypass grafting using the saphenous vein and Julian et al[58] published their paper in 1952, "The Direct Surgery of Atherosclerosis."

The symptom of intermittent claudication was first described in 1831 by Bouley,[10] a young French veterinary student who correctly determined that the cause was thrombosis of the femoral artery. His patients were horses who could only limp or walk slowly when the muscle pain began, hence the word claudication, which is derived from the Latin word "claudicare," to limp.

Blood vessels were possibly sutured by Hallowell as reported by Lambert[61] in 1762 and others, but the first proven and successful procedures were reported by Eck[34] in 1877. He anastomosed the portal vein to the inferior vena cava in Pavlov's laboratory in Leningrad. The modern technique of vascular anastomosis was developed by Dorfler[30] and improved by Carrel.[13] In 1912 Carrel was awarded the Nobel prize for his work on the transplantation of organs and blood vessels. In 1897 Murphy[77] of Chicago introduced the invagination technique of end-to-end arterial and venous anastomosis but this is rarely used today.

These early vascular reconstruction operations were soon followed by the development of the associated reconstruction operations of thrombectomy, embolectomy, thromboendarterectomy, and aneurysmorrhaphy. Delbet[25] in 1906 discussed the operations of arterial and venous thrombectomy but the results were disappointing. It was dos Santos[31] 41 years later who realized that the correct operation for an established arterial thrombosis was not thrombectomy but thromboendarterectomy, the difference being the establishment by the surgeon of a plane of cleavage in the media. The throm-

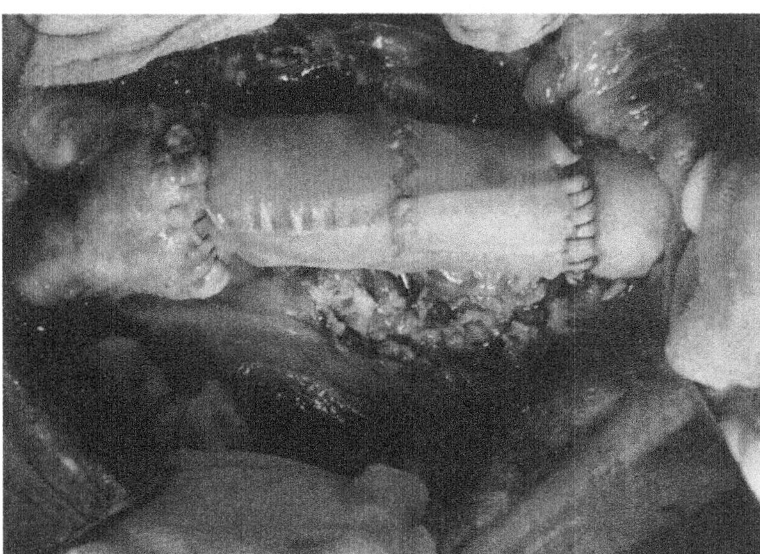

Figure 4.1. Dacron prosthesis. In 1954 this prosthesis of Dacron cloth was inserted into the abdominal aorta. The patient had an aneurysm caused by tuberculous adenitis. Prosthesis was made from a Dacron shirt and fashioned into a tube with Dacron thread. The piece of Dacron placed into this patient functioned long after the original batch of shirts were worn out.

bus, intima, any atheromatous plaques, the internal elastic lamina, and the inner layers of the media were removed. After this operation the arterial wall consists of the adventitia, the external elastic lamina, and the outer layers of the media, which is rapidly covered by a layer of psuedointima consisting of cells deposited from the bloodstream. In 1888 Matas[68,69] of New Orleans reported the operation of aneurysmorrhaphy, and by 1903 he had performed a number of these operations. The procedure, which is an arterial repair using the wall of the sac of the aneurysm, is still used today in certain special situations such as saccular aneurysms of the arch of the aorta. The treatment of an intracranial aneurysm by occluding the neck with a clip or suture is a similar procedure.

The word embolus is derived from a similar Greek word meaning a plug or stopper. The operation of arterial embolectomy was attempted by Sabaneyev,[88] and reported by Mosny and Dumont[75] in 1911. In 1913 Bauer[3] reported the succesful removal of an embolus lodged at the bifurcation of the abdominal aorta. After this, many reports of the surgical removal of emboli from the arterial system were published, but the results were less satisfactory than had been hoped,[44] and some were frankly disappointing. This all changed when Fogarty[37] and his colleagues introduced the balloon catheter for embolectomy. Many consider this to be one of the two truly original concepts introduced into vascular surgery between the end of World War II and today. The results of arterial embolectomy are now good, and many limbs, organs, and lives have been saved.

The use of substitutes or grafts to restore the flow through the arterial and venous systems goes back to the end of the last century. Carrel and Guthrie[14,15] working in Chicago used antogenous homologous, and heterologous grafts to replace both arteries and veins. They also used solid tubes of a variety of relatively inert materials. The first clinical procedure was the use of an autogenous vein graft by Goyanes[41] in 1906, and today autogenous veins are the most widely used and best substitutes for small- and medium-sized arteries.[84]

Because of the occasional need for an arterial substitute when a coarctation of the aorta could not be repaired by direct anastomosis, Gross[43] and his colleagues introduced into clinical practice the concept of arterial banking based on earlier work by Carrel[13] and others. For a few years from 1951 to about 1953 arterial homografts were widely used. But in 1952 a major advance occurred. Voorhees et al[99] introduced the entirely new concept of replacing a segment of the arterial system with a tube of partially porous and pliable plastic cloth. At first they used Vinyon-N cloth, but they soon abandoned this material in favor of Dacron (Fig. 4.1). This advance has changed arterial surgery in a most significant way and, in our opinion, constitutes a great step forward; it was totally different from previous procedures where tubes of steel, glass, aluminum, and other materials were used.[14] Today these tubes are crimped, and they are the best substitute for the aorta and iliac arteries. They are also satisfactory for arteries down to the size of the superficial femoral artery, provided that the prosthesis does not cross a joint.

A variety of other arterial substitutes have been used. New materials arousing the greatest interest today are made of collagen or expanded polytetrafluoroethylene.[12] Grafts of collagen may be divided into two main categories: those made of human collagen and those using collagen of another species, and those that have been reinforced with a mesh of Dacron fibers. The bovine arterial heterograft was introduced in 1958,[87] the carotid artery of a steer having been digested with ficin and tanned with glutaraldehyde. The Sparks Mandril[95] is a graft with great theoretical appeal. It consists of the patient's own collagen reinforced with a mesh of Dacron. The problems with the Sparks Mandril include the need to leave the mandril in position for at least six weeks to give time for the collagen to form and the fact that the resulting tube has no stretch and is therefore difficult to sew into position. It is probable that the collagen tube that will be most useful in clinical practice is the reinforced umbilical vein graft tanned with glutaraldehyde and reinforced with a Dacron mesh.[24] In this connection it is of interest that umbilical vein grafts were first used in 1951 in the research laboratories at Tufts Medical School in Boston,[1] but these were fresh umbilical veins and they all failed.

Grafts of expanded polytetrafluoroethylene have been used by many surgeons,[12] and early results have been good. This product is a useful arterial substitute for patients who do not have a suitable long saphenous vein.

Alternatives When the Saphenous Vein Is Not Available

The saphenous vein is the best substitute for arteries of the limbs and for coronary arteries, but sometimes it is diseased, anatomically unsuitable, or has been stripped. In these patients an alternative is required, and the best alternatives to use in a number of situations have caused considerable debate. Our view of this subject is as follows. For small arteries when donor vessels such as the radial artery are available and when only a short length is required, an autogenous arterial graft is best. For large arteries such as the abdominal aorta or iliac arteries a prosthesis of Dacron is preferred. For all other situations the autogenous saphenous vein is preferred. When it is not available and the site for the graft does not cross a joint such as the knee, a tube of Dacron with an external valor gives good results. For situations where the graft crosses the knee joint or involves arteries such as the tibial or peroneal, an autogenous vein graft from another site is best. If this is not available, a collagen tube reinforced with a Dacron mesh can be used. The Dardik-type umbilical vein graft is an example of this[24]; an alternate being a graft of polytetrafluoroethylene.[12]

An important principle of arterial surgery is that the continued patency of an arterial reconstruction operation depends to a great extent on the efficiency of the arterial inflow and the adequacy of the arterial outflow. This is well illustrated in the reconstruction of the arteries of the lower limb. Many patients have aortoiliac stenosis, thrombosis of the superficial femoral artery, and occlusion of the distal arteries in the foot and leg. The first essential is to restore a normal blood flow at a normal blood pressure to the common femoral artery. This may be achieved by reconstruction of the aortoiliac segment or in poor risk patients by an extraanatomical bypass graft such as the axillary femoral[8,99a] or femoro-femoral bypass graft.[70] With blood flow restored improvement may be so good that further surgery may be unnecessary. If it is necessary, the success of a femoropopliteal or femorotibial bypass graft depends to a great extent on the patency of the distal vascular bed and especially on the patency of the plantar arterial arch. The profunda femoral artery is also of great importance, and a good flow through this artery is often sufficient to ensure the viability of the limb. The relatively minor operation profundaplasty[62] is a very useful procedure.

Reconstruction of the carotid circulation in the neck illustrates the development of a particular procedure.[86] Thrombosis of the internal carotid artery was described by Penzoldt[81] in 1881. In the 1881 edition of *Manual of Diseases of the Nervous System* Gowers[40] discussed the clinical picture of thrombosis of the internal carotid and vertebral arteries in the neck. In 1905 Chiari[19] and in 1914 Hunt[50] stressed the importance of investigating the state of the carotid arteries in all patients with an apoplectic stroke.

Hunt was first to recognize the importance of occlusion of the extracranial as opposed to the intracranial cerebral arteries as a cause of cerebral vascular insufficiency. He began his paper with the following statement:

> The object of the present study is to emphasize the importance of obstructive lesions of the main arteries of the neck, in the causation of softening of the brain and more especially to urge the routine examination of these vessels in all patients who have cerebral symptoms of vascular origin. In other words the author would advocate the same attitude towards this group of cases as towards intermittent claudication, gangrene and other vascular symptoms of the extremities, and never omit a detailed examination of the main arterial stem.

In general, clinicians continued to believe that arterial thrombosis occurred with few exceptions in the intracranial arteries such as the middle cerebral. One reason was that at that time a definitive diagnosis of carotid or vertebral arterial thrombosis was only possible at autopsy or with a surgical exploration, and the cervical portions of these arteries were rarely examined in the postmortem room.

Moniz[73] introduced cerebral angiography in 1927, but it was not until 1936 that Sjoquist[92] demonstrated a thrombosis of the internal carotid artery by arteriography. Improved efficiency in the technique of arteriography led to a better understanding of the importance and frequency of these lesions. In 1951 Johnson and Walker[57] reviewed the literature from 1936 to 1950 and found that 101 instances of thrombosis of the internal carotid artery had been demonstrated by arteriography and reported six from their own series of 500 carotid arteriograms. This work, combined with the studies of Hultquist[49] who found a carotid artery thrombosis in 4.4% of 1,300 routine autopsy examinations and Fisher[36] who demonstrated a thrombosis of one or of both internal carotid arteries in 6.5% of 432 unselected postmortem examinations, led to the suggestion that extracranial cerebral arterial occulsion was more frequent than had been suspected.

The definitive work that demonstrated the real incidence of occlusive disease of the extracranial cerebral arteries was performed by Hutchinson and Yates.[51,52] They made a careful clinical and pathologic study of 83 patients who had died as a result of a lesion considered on clinical ground to be a cerebrovascular abnormality. In each patient the whole length of the carotid and vertebral arteries from their origin at the base of the neck to the smaller branches were carefully studied. Forty patients or 48.2% showed significant disease of the cervical portions of the carotid or vertebral arteries.

A review of the literature in 1954 showed that the following surgical procedures had been tried in the management of thrombosis of the internal carotid artery and found to be ineffective: arterectomy,[16] sympathectomy or sympathetic nerve block,[64,93] formation of an arteriovenous anastomosis between the common carotid artery and internal jugular vein,[4,94] revascularization of the brain by a graft of temporal muscle[45] ligature of the external carotid artery, and the formation of an anastomosis between the external and internal carotid arteries.[21] The first thromboendarterectomy of the internal carotid artery was performed by Strully, Hurwitt, and Blankenbery,[96] but they operated on a patient with a complete carotid thrombosis and the artery rapidly rethrombosed. The first report of a successful reconstruction of the internal carotid artery was in 1954 when a carotid stenosis was successfully corrected in a patient suffering from transient cerebral ischaemic attacks.[33] Subsequently in 1955, Carrea et al.[12a] reported that they had performed such an operation in 1951 and DeBakey[24a] reported in 1975 that he had performed a successful carotid thromboendarterectomy in 1953.

Reconstruction of the subclavian veretebral circulation has been practiced for almost as long as carotid reconstruction, but the indications are still unclear in many patients. A variety of surgical procedures have been described and well reviewed by Crawford et al,[22a] Mozersky et al,[75a] and Edwards and Mulheriu.[34a]

Technique of Vascular Anastomosis

The technique of vascular anastomosis differs between normal and diseased arteries. An artherosclerotic artery is often thickened, calcified, and the intima severely ulcerated at the site of suture; this may so change the technique of arterial anastomosis that it hardly resembles the suture of an injured normal artery.

The Suture or Anastomosis of a Normal Artery

This may be required because of an injury to a young person's artery or because a diseased process in an individual without gross arterial disease necessitates an arterial resection or bypass. The first step is to decide which form of arterial repair is required. The types of repair include lateral suture, end-to-end anastomosis, a patch graft angioplasty, and reconstruction with a blood vessel graft. In general, lateral suture should be avoided unless the injury to the arterial way is transverse and there has been only minimal damage to the arterial wall. It is better to repair such an injury with a patch graft angioplasty or to divide the vessel completely and perform an end-to-end anastomosis. The reasons are first that a lateral repair may constrict the lumen and second that the damage to the arterial wall may be much more extensive than is expected. Figures 4.2 and 4.3 illustrate this point.

The surgeon first strips back the loose outer layers of the sheath of the artery. This usually should leave the adventitia nearly intact. Any damaged arterial wall is then removed and the vessels or graft examined to see that they are not twisted. At this point an assistant approximates the ends to be sutured. The surgeon then passes the needle of the arterial suture through the vessel wall into the lumen and brings the same needle out of the opposite side of the

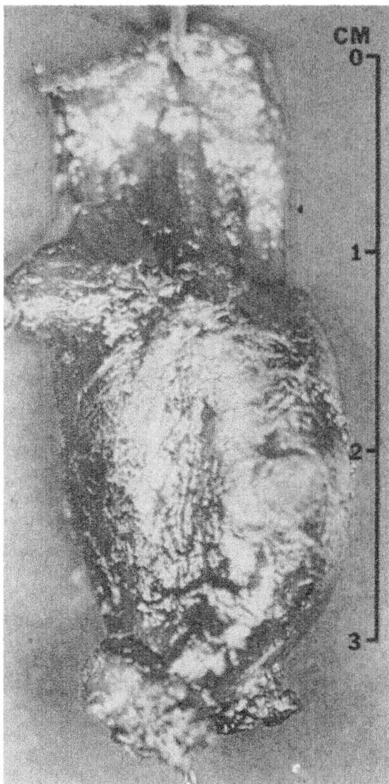

Figure 4.2. Outer wall of common carotid artery from patient who became hemiplegic about 30 min after a heavy rope compressed his neck in an industrial accident. Note bruising and discoloration of adventitia.

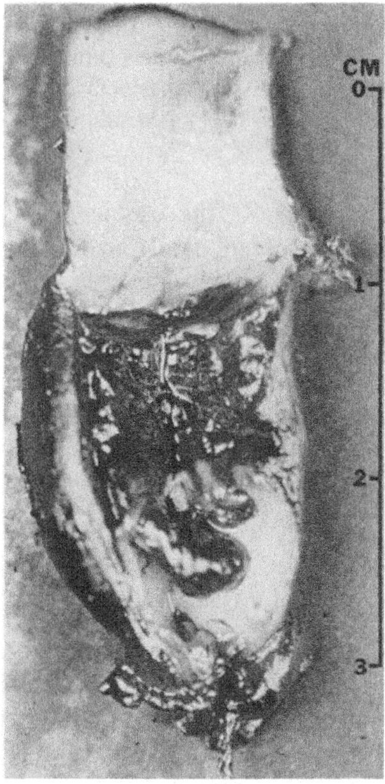

Figure 4.3. Lumen of carotid artery shown in Fig. 4.2. Note complete disruption of intima and thrombus on surface. After damaged segment had been resected, continuity was restored with autogenous vein graft. During the operation, carotid flow was maintained with an indwelling shunt. Hemiplegia cleared within four hours.

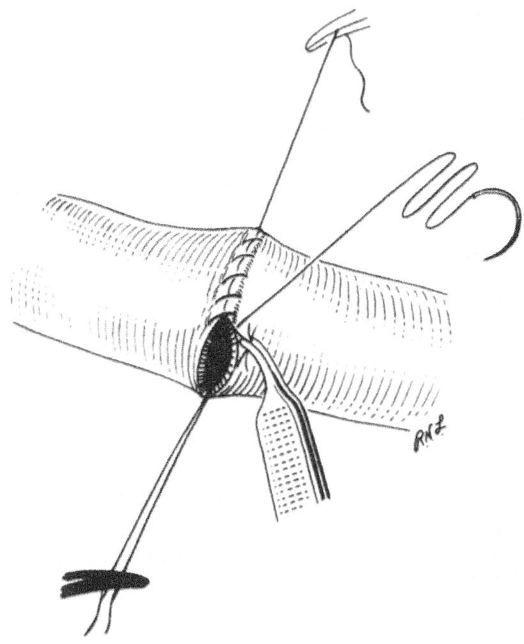

Figure 4.4. Classic method of arterial anastomosis. Procedure was introduced by Dorfler and Carrel in 1899 and 1908. Two or three stay sutures are inserted to steady blood vessels, anastomosis is completed with continuous or interrupted sutures.

vascular repair. In the classic technique developed by Dorfler[30] and Carrel,[13] three such sutures are passed and the suture line is then triangulated. In actual practice surgeons vary considerably from this, depending on the situation in an individual patient. The suture line is then completed usually with a continuous suture but in young patients and those in whom a stenosis may develop a series of interrupted sutures are used (Fig. 4.4).

Anastomosis of a Diseased Artery

Today most vascular operations are performed on patients with atherosclerosis. The first step is to remove from the vessel wall any calcified plaques that may interfere with passing the needle. These can be removed and the outer layers of the wall of the artery left in positioin for the surgeon to use for the anastomosis. The intima of the distal artery must be carefully cut or sutured down so that intimal dissection will not occur. The lumen of the vessel must be irrigated so that all loose fragments of atheroma or thrombus are removed. The suture line is then inserted with the surgeon taking large bites of the vessel wall. Again, continuous or interrupted sutures may be used depending on the requirements of the individual patient.

Microsurgery is the ultimate test of a vascular suture and needle.[53,54] Most manufacturers restrict the term microsuture to those incorporating an 8-0 or smaller suture. The majority of microsutures are made of monofilament nylon. In microsurgery there is great variation among specialties as to the type of needle used. Ophthalmologists, the principal pioneers in the field, prefer spatulated needles with a sharp point and trapezoid configuration. Its cutting edges permit penetration of the cornea, and the lower rounded edges decrease the risk of deep penetration. Microvascular and microneural surgeons prefer a taper needle whose sharp tip ensures atraumatic penetration and minimizes trauma to delicate blood vessels and nerves. Needle diameter has decreased progressively from 130 to 50μm, and nylon suture size has decreased from 21μm (10-0) to 18μm (11-0). Today very sharp atraumatic needles are available from half circle to one-eight circle in shape as well as simple straight needles. Ocular aides include loupes in the form of achromatic double-operating telescopes with a magnification of 2.5 to 6.0 × and a working distance of 10 to 21 inches, zoom microscopes with fast controlled focusing and magnification, a variety of beam-splitting devices that permit the participation of an active surgical assistant, and brilliant fiberoptic light sources. The microinstruments are characterized by precision tips, light weight, balanced proportions, graded pinch closure, and nonreflective surfaces. Because divided blood vessels contract, atraumatic clamp approximators are used.

It is possible to achieve a patency rate of 90% in vessels of 1 mm in diameter. The key to success is not anticoagulants or antiplatelet agents but rather impeccable technique.[23]

Lymph Vessel Anastomosis

Although it is technically possible to perform end-to-end anastomosis of lymph vessels, clinical applications are limited owing to segmental destruction rather than localized interruption. *Lymphnodo-capsularvenous shunts* were introduced in 1968 by Nielubowicz and Olszewski.[78,79] Their experience included 31 clinical procedures with good results in secondary lymphedema. In 1974 Clodius and Wirth[20] introduced a modification in which the fibrosed pulp of the lymph nodes is removed, thus producing a lymphnodo-capsularvenous shunt.

Bench Surgery

The idea of the removal of an organ such as the kidney from the body and the reconstruction of the smaller blood vessels on a bench, followed by the reimplantation of the kidney back into the body was introduced by Mori et al[74] in 1967. In 1974 Belzer[5] and his group from San Francisco reported the added requirement of extracorporeal hypothermic continuous perfusion and the microvascular repair of lesions of the smaller branches of the renal arteries. They perfused the kidney with a pulsatile flow of hypothermia type-specific homologous cryoprecipitated plasma. The technique has extended the time available for repair of the kidney to up to 70 hours. Bench surgery of this type has been of particular value in patients with fibromuscular-hyperplasia involving the secondary and tertiary branches of the renal arteries, in some patients with renal injuries or tumors, and in patients with aneurysms arriving from the smaller branches of the renal arteries.

Technique of Thromboendarterectomy

The operation of thromboendarterectomy is frequently used for reconstruction of the internal carotid artery. The vessels are clamped and a longitudinal incision made over the zone of arterial disease. The surgeon then establishes a plane of cleavage in the media and separates the intima, the plaques of atheroma, any thrombus, the inner layers of the media, and the internal elastic lumina from the rest of the artery. In the case of the carotid bifurcation the inner core is divided at the proximal end, the core is then removed from the external carotid artery, and the dissection carefully continued up the internal carotid artery to the top of the plaque of atheroma. The whole inner core is now removed. It is very important to remove completely the distal end of the plaque of atheroma. Atheroma may be left proximally in the common carotid artery or distally in the external carotid artery, but the outflow must be into a segment of the internal carotid artery which has a normal wall. If this is done it is not necessary to tack down the distal intima.

An indwelling shunt continues and usually improves the circulation to the distal artery during the period of arterial clamping. Some surgeons use such a shunt in every case[98] and others shunt selected patients. All are agreed that every patient who is operated on for an acute stroke should have a shunt. Likewise, every patient who has a poor retrograde flow from the internal carotid artery, patients who develop symptoms with preoperative compression of the cervical carotid arteries, and patients who have arteriographic evidence of an inadequate circle of Willis should also be shunted.

After the thromboendarterectomy has been completed the surgeon inspects the lumen and flushes it with heparinized saline to make certain that all loose fragments have been removed. The arterial incision is then closed either directly or with a patch graft angioplasty. After the suture line is dry the wound is sutured in layers (Fig. 4.5).

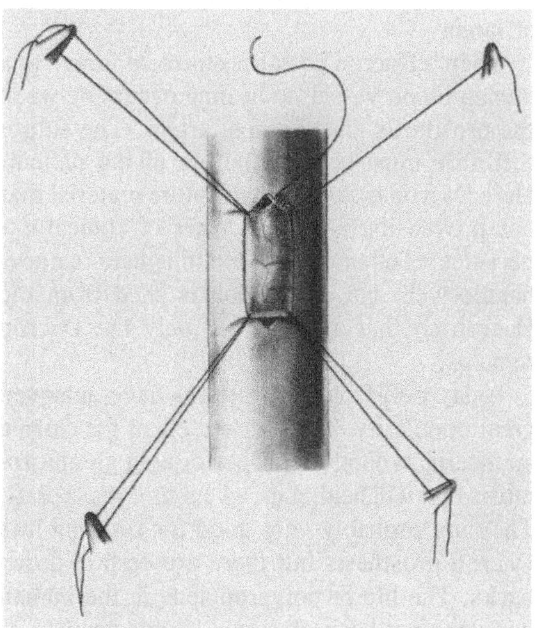

Figure 4.5. Patch graft angioplasty. Technique may be used to close arterial defect or incision. Four stay sutures are placed and the graft—usually of autogenous vein—is sutured into position with continuous suture. As objective is to enlarge lumen, the patch must be under no tension.

Vascular Sutures

The technical aspects of blood vessel suture and anastomosis were established before World War II and reviewed by Horsley in 1921.[47] Today minor variations have been made but the methods of vascular suture, either continuous or interrupted, everting or end-to-end, have essentially followed the techniques originally described. Stapling devices have not achieved general acceptance in vascular surgery and the nonsuture techniques over a variety of tubes are not used routinely in clinical practice today.

For vascular closure two major types of suture are required: first, a suture for use when healing will occur at the suture line and, second, a suture for use when no healing occurs as is the case when a Dacron or other plastic prosthesis is inserted. Silk, which has been used in vascular surgery for more than 80 years, slowly absorbs and therefore should not be used for the anastomosis of a plastic prosthesis. Silk is not available in such fine threads as nylon or polypropylene but it is satisfactory as a 4-0 or 5-0 suture for the closure of a thromboendarterectomy incision or for the direct anastomosis of vessels of the size of the internal carotid artery or larger.

When a Dacron prosthesis is to be joined to a human blood vessel no healing occurs between the prosthesis and the host artery. The suture therefore must last for the life of the patient. Here Dacron is an excellent suture material that has proved itself with 30 years of clinical experience. Teflon-coated multifilament sutures handle well, but the Teflon is shed from the Dacron so that after a year only the Dacron remains.

Today polypropylene sutures have achieved great popularity. They are excellent for closing an arterial wound or for performing an anastomosis that will heal, e.g., a venous bypass graft. They are probably very good for suturing in a Dacron prosthesis but there are certain drawbacks. The life of polypropylene in the human body has not been observed for longer than 15 years. Dacron is known to survive more than 30 years. Polypropylene knots may slip if improperly tied and very occasionally these sutures break. Polypropylene sutures, do, however, provide an excellent dry closure and we use them extensively.

Continuous or Interrupted Sutures

Continuous sutures are widely used, but if there is a tendency to a purse-string action, interrupted sutures are preferred. This also applies to a vascular suture line in a child whose growth is incomplete. In many patients having bypass grafts or small-vessel anastomosis it is best to use interrupted sutures.

Hemostatic Agents

Bleeding from arteries and veins usually presents no problem. But proper hemostasis is essential to any operation. Occasionally a vascular suture line may bleed, particularly if a Dacron prosthesis is sutured to a markedly diseased artery. Usually all that is required is two to five minutes of compression followed occasionally by an additional suture or sutures. During this period of compression it is advantageous to wrap the suture line with a hemostatic gauze such as Surgicel,[56] an absorbable gauze made of oxidized regenerated cellulose. Other such agents include alginates, fibrin foam, and gelatin sponge. The advantages of Surgicel is that it can be used to wrap the suture line and be left in the body if necessary.

Blood Vessel Clamps

The development of microsurgery has focused attention upon instrumentation. It has been known for a long time that certain blood vessel clamps inflict more damage on the vessel wall than others. In 1956 Henson and Rob[46] reported that rubber-covered bulldog clamps, the tape tourniquet, and Crile vascular clamps were the least traumatic to the vessel wall whereas the Blalock, Craaford, and Potts clamps produced considerable damage. Since then the Fogarty series of rubber-covered clamps have been introduced and these cause little damage.

Anticoagulant Drugs and Fibrinolysins

In 1916 McLean[72] discovered that an impure extract of liver inhibited the coagulation of blood. In 1933 Charles and Scott[17] purified this substance so that it could be used clinically. Howell and Holt[48] gave it the name heparin, and Murray[76] of Toronto was the man who popularized its use in vascular surgery. Today heparin is used systemically in vascular surgery during the actual period of vascular clamping, it being neutralized with an equivalent dose of protamine sulphate at the time the clamps are removed. It is also used as a dilute solution for flushing the lumen of open vessels, and it is instilled into the lumen distal to clamps. The use of long-term anticoagulation with coumadin has not been popular because of the risk of wound hematoma if it is used in the immediate postoperative period. Many surgeons believe that a good vascular repair does not need postoperative anticoagulation and that anticoagulation does not prevent thrombosis if the repair is technically unsatisfactory.

Heparin is a good fibrinolysin, but streptokinase is even better and is being used with increasing frequency to treat patients with all forms of recent venous or arterial occlusions, including acute coronary artery thrombosis.[72a]

Microemboli (Aspirin, Dipyridamole, Ibuprofen and Sulfinpyrazone)

The development of platelet aggregations on plaques of atheroma may result in microemboli which cause problems such as transient attacks of cerebral ischemia or ischemia of a finger or toe. The use of drugs such as aspirin, dipyridamole (Persantine) ibuprofen or sulfinpyrazone (Anturane) may prevent this problem by inhibiting the platelet aggregation. It is known that platelet aggregation increases with age, particularly after 60 years. A Canadian cooperative study of transient ischemic attacks showed that of men treated with 10 grains of aspirin twice a day, 48% had fewer attacks or strokes. Sulfinpyrazone was no different from a placebo, and females treated with either aspirin or sulfinpyrazone received no benefit.

Dextran and Blood

Blood should be available for transfusion in every patient who has direct vascular surgery. It is often not required but it may be needed and therefore should be available. A normal hematocrit is important whenever any part of the body is ischemic and this, in addition to blood loss, may be the indication for a blood transfusion. Dextran, either of the clinical or the low-molecular type, is a plasma expander and increases the blood volume, thus reducing post-operative thrombosis, especially of small-blood vessels. Dextran must be used with caution in the immediate postoperative period because of the increased risk of hematoma formation. With dextran there is also the risk of cardiac failure, particularly in older patients, because the increased blood volume increases the work of the heart.

Extraanatomical Blood Vessel Grafts[99]

The procedure of femoro-femoral bypass grafting was introduced in 1960[71] and was soon followed by the axillary-femoral graft[8] and the splenic to femoral grafts.[66] Since then a number of other arterial lesions have been treated in this way. Of special interest are those designed to restore arterial flow to the brain. These include axillary to axillary,[75a] subclavian to carotid, and carotid to carotid bypass grafts in the neck, reconstruction of a stenosed external carotid artery in patients with a symptomatic internal carotid occlusion,[88a] and in particular the various extranial to intracranial bypass grafts. In 1967 Yasargil[100] reported such a bypass anastomosing the superficial temporal artery to a cortical branch of the middle cerebral artery. Since then occipital to cerebellar artery, superficial temporal to superior cerebellar artery, and other extracranial to intracranial bypass grafts have been used.[2a] In addition, the radial artery and the saphenous vein have been used to bypass occluded vessels in this region[2,18] (Figs. 4.6-4.8). Although the indications for these operations on the intracranial cerebral circulation are subject to change, they may be summarized as follows: transient ischemic attacks due to stenosis of the middle cerebral artery, symptomatic patients with thrombosis of one internal carotid artery, severe distal stenosis of the internal carotid artery, and some patients with cerebral ischemia associated with stenosis or thrombosis of multiple cerebral arteries.

Arterial Embolectomy, Arterial and Venous Thrombectomy

In the past the results of arterial embolectomy were little better than that of conservative care.[44] This all changed in 1963 when the Fogarty[37] balloon catheter was introduced. Today

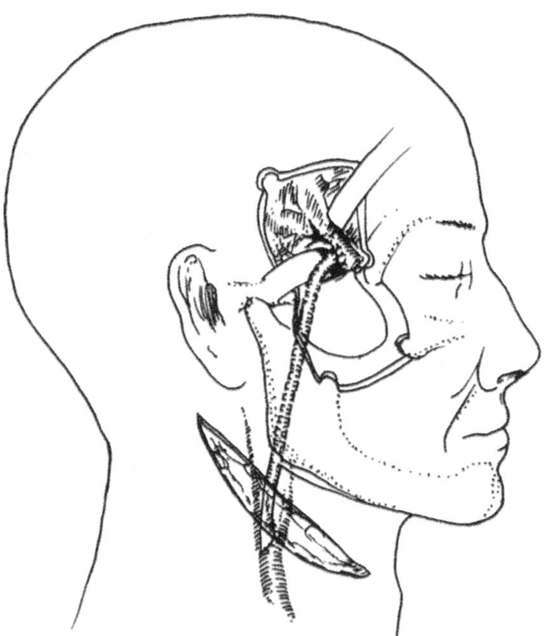

Figure 4.6. One form of extraanatomic bypass graft. An autogenous vein graft is anastomosed to side of common carotid artery proximally and to middle cerebral artery distally.

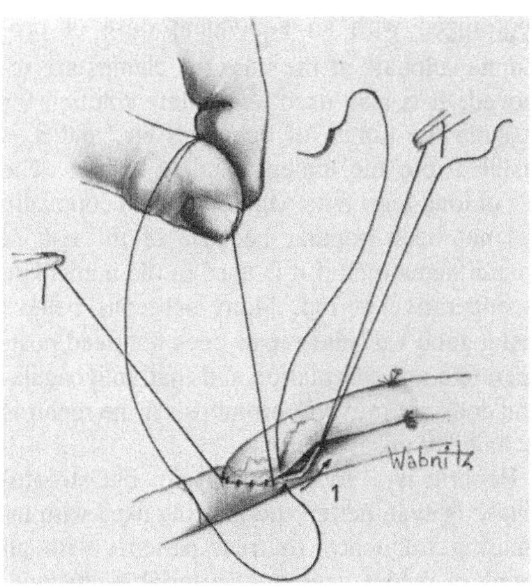

Figure 4.8. Anastomosis of vein graft to the artery is then completed with either continuous or interrupted sutures.

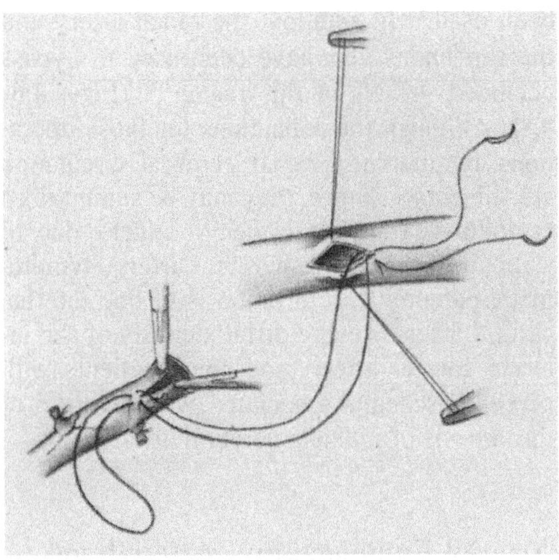

Figure 4.7. Technique of inserting saphenous vein bypass graft. Vein graft is removed, prepared, and reversed. Distal end of vein is then anastomosed to proximal artery. End of vein is enlarged as shown and anchored into position over arterial incision.

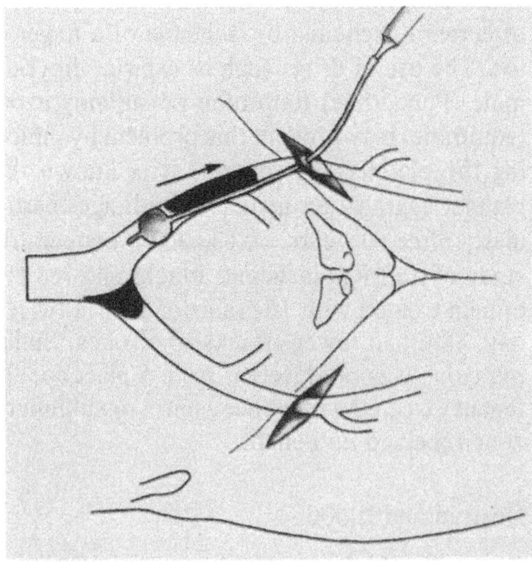

Figure 4.9. Fogarty embolectomy balloon catheter. Great advantage of this type of catheter is that emboli can be extracted from accessible site in the arterial tree. In this figure an aortic bifurcation embolus is being extracted. Under local anesthesia, incisions are made over each common femoral artery. Transverse arteriotomy incisions are made and Fogarty catheters passed up into the abdominal aorta; embolus is extracted first on one side and then on the other.

arterial embolectomy is the standard treatment for this problem[42] (Fig. 4.9).

After an arterial injury or in a variety of other situations, thrombi form in the arterial system and spread distally. These can be removed with a Fogarty catheter at the time of arterial repair. The same applies to venous thrombi. After an arterial injury the presence of a good retrograde arterial flow does not guarantee that the distal arterial tree is patent. In these patients it is wise to pass a Fogarty catheter in every case before closing the artery.

Although useful when an acute injury is repaired, venous thrombectomy gives less satisfactory results when the reason for operating is thrombophlebitis.[26] It may be that the establishment of an arteriovenous fistula between the saphenous vein and superficial femoral artery may so increase the rate of blood flow that fewer of these patients suffer a postoperative recurrence of the venous thrombosis in the iliofemoral venous system.

Infected Blood Vessel Grafts

This is a most serious but fortunately uncommon complication of vascular surgery. In a series of 664 operations on the abdominal aorta and iliac arteries at the University of Rochester, 2.3% of the patients developed an infection involving the Dacron graft.[55] Most of these patients received prophylactic antibiotics in the form of cephalothin and kanamycin from the night before surgery for three to five days. Once a graft has become infected, the only certain way to cure the patient is to remove the infected graft, ligature the arteries, and restore the circulation with an extraanatomical bypass graft.[67] But if there is no evidence that the suture lines of the graft are infected (hemorrhage) or that the neointima is infected (thrombosis, septicemia), there is a place for conservative and local treatment.[89,97] But, in general, an aggressive approach with removal of the infected graft is best and should not be delayed for long.

The Vascular Laboratory

The main purpose of a vascular diagnostic laboratory is to detect, diagnose, and document vascular disease in a variety of locations, including the extracranial circulation and the peripheral arterial and venous trees. Such studies are also capable of estimating the functional significance of a problem in contrast to angiography, which outlines the anatomic lesion alone.[6,38]

The basic measurements in a noninvasive vascular diagnostic laboratory include the study of blood velocity, blood vessel size and shape, blood pressure, and limb volume. Blood velocity is measured by the continuous wave Doppler ultrasonic device; some units are directionally sensitive and may be used for semiquantitative analysis.[38] The shape and size of a blood vessel are best studied by ultrasonic echography using both the A and B mode and the B-scan techniques.[7] This is of special value in the diagnosis of abdominal aortic aneurysms.[63] Extremity blood pressure measurements use blood pressure cuffs and a Doppler velocity detector as a recording device. The Doppler may also be used to study the flow in the external carotid arteries. The oculoplethysmograph measures the internal carotid or ophthalmic artery pressures.[39,59] Limb or digit volume measurement known as plethysmography is today measured by either the pulse volume recorder[83] or the phleborheograph.[22]

In the case of cerebrovascular disease, current techniques available to the clinician are limited to the measurement of hemodynamically significant lesions. These, combined with a study of cervical bruits, have proved to be very useful. But the picture is changing rapidly as imaging techniques using either the echo B-scan or Doppler develop satisfactorily and it becomes possible to diagnose noninvasively shallow ulcerated plaques.[6]

Therapeutic Techniques in Diagnostic Radiology

Boijsen and Anders[9] recently reviewed this relatively new field. Of special interest to vascular surgeons are the intravascular therapeutic techniques. In 1964 Dotter and Judkins[32] introduced the technique of mechanical dilatation of stenosed arteries. With major modifications by Grunzig,[43a,b] this technique has been used in the circulation to the limbs, kidneys, and coronary arteries. It has not yet been used for stenosis of the carotid arteries because of the theoretical risk of embolization but has worked well for stenotic lesions of the subclavian innominate and occasionally the vertebral arteries. Angiomatous lesions of the brain and spinal[29,28] cord have been treated by embolization via a Seldinger catheter. This method has been of special value in the management of congenital arteriovenous malformations of the head and neck, which can be very difficult to treat by other means. In some of these patients, embolization may so reduce the blood flow through the lesion that excision becomes possible. Various methods of treatment of carotid-cavernous sinus arteriovenous fistulas have been reported since the first attempt by Brooks[11] in 1930. The most well known is the detachable balloon technique of Serbinenko.[90]

General Management

The general management of a patient with atherosclerosis is important at all times, before, during and after an operation. It is a sobering thought that many vascular surgeons do not treat their patients primary disease—atherosclerosis. In my opinion a most important concept is that the surgeon who performs an arterial reconstruction operation must accept the responsibility for the care and efficient follow-up of each patient for the remainder of that patient's life. The surgeon must either do this himself or he must make certain that it is done by the patient's internist or family doctor. In 1960 Singer and Rob[91] published a three-year follow-up of 339 patients who had complained of intermittent claudication and who, for a variety of reasons, were not operated on. During this period of three years, 74 or 20.6% of these patients died, usually from a myocardial infarction. Then in 1977 DeWeese and Rob[27] published a complete follow-up of 103 consecutive patients who had a femoral to popliteal artery bypass using the long saphenous vein. Here the mortality was 74 patients or 71.8% at 10 years. Again, the main cause of death was myocardial infarction.

Perhaps the answer may be a greater use of coronary bypass operations in these patients who have generalized atherosclerosis. But there are many nonsurgical procedures that may be used to help these patients including:

Stopping tobacco smoking
Treatment of diabetes mellitus
Treatment of arterial hypertension
Treatment of anemia
Reduction of body weight
Correction of cardiac arrhythmia (including pacemakers)
Eating less, particularly cholesterol and sugar
Regular exercise
Care of ischemic extremities
Vasodilator drugs
Anticoagulants and fibrinolysins
Aspirin, persantine, sulfinpyrazone, ibuprofen

Although many operations on arteries, veins, or lymphatics are performed for injuries, congenital abnormalities, inflammatory diseases, as part of the resection of a malignant tumor, or for one of the more unusual forms of occlusive arterial disease such as arteritis, thromboangiitis obliterans, or polyarteritis nodosa, the vast majority of such operations are performed for atherosclerosis. Surgeons should never forget that atherosclerosis, although usually segmental in distribution, is a general disease and the surgical operation can only have a local effect, whether it be on the blood vessels of the heart, brain, limbs, kidneys, or other organs.

References

1. Anzula B, Palmer TH, Welch CS: Long femoral and iliofemoral grafts. Surg Forum 243–244, 1951
2. Ausman, JI: Cerebral Revascularization: Extracranial-Intracranial Bypass Procedures for Cerebrovascular Disease. Vascular Surgery Symposia Specialists. Miami 343–357, 1978

2a. Barrett HJM, Peerless SJ: The collaborative EC/IC bypass study. Cerebrovascular Diseases. Proceedings of 12th Princeton Conference. Raven Press, New York, 1981, pp 271–288

3. Bauer, F: Fall von Embolus Aortae Abdominalis operation heilung. Cbl Chir 2:1945–1956, 1913
4. Beck CS, McKhann CF, Belnap WD: Revascularization of the brain through establishment of a cervical arteriovenous fistula. J Pediatr 35: 317–322, 1949
5. Belzer FFO, Salvatierra O, Perloff D, Grausz H: Surgical correction of advanced fibromuscu-

lar dysplasia of the renal arteries. Surgery 75:31–37, 1974

6. Bernstein EF: The Noninvasive Vascular Diagnostic Laboratory. Vascular Surgery. Najarian JS, Delaney JB, Symposia Specialists. Miami 33–46, 1978
7. Bernstein EF, Shea MA, Murphy AE, Housman LB: Experimental and clinical experience with transcutaneous Doppler ultrasonic flowmeters. Arch Surg 101:21–25, 1970
8. Blaisdell FW, Hall AD: Axillary femoral artery bypass for lower extremity ischaemia. Surgery 54 : 563–572, 1962
9. Boijsen E, Anders L: Therapeutic Techniques in Diagnostic Radiology. Advances in Surgery Yearbook Publishers. Chicago 1978
10. Bouley J: Claudication intermittente des membres posterieurs determinee par l'obliteration des arteres femoralis. Rec de Med Veter 8:517–527, 1831
11. Brooks B: The treatment of traumatic arteriovenous fistula. South Med J 23:100–111, 1930
12. Campbell CD, Brooks DH, Webster NW, Bahnson HT: The use of expanded microporous polytetrafluoroethylene for limb salvage: A preliminary report. Surgery 79:485–493, 1976

12a. Carrea R, Molnis M, Murphy G: Surgical treatment of spontaneous thrombosis of the internal carotid artery in the neck. Acta Neurol Latinoamer 1:71–77, 1955

13. Carrel A: Results of the transplantation of blood vessels, organs and limbs. JAMA 51: 1662–1667, 1908
14. Carrell A: Permanent intubation of the thoracic aorta. J Exp Med 16:17–24, 1912
15. Carrel A, Guthrie CC: Uniterminal and biterminal venous transplantation. Surg Gynecol Obstet 2:226–286, 1906
16. Chao WH, Kwan ST, Lyman RS, Loucks WW: Thrombosis of the left internal carotid artery. Arch Surg 37:100–107, 1938
17. Charles AF, Scott DA: Studies on Heparin: (3) The purification of Heparin. J Biol Chem 102: 437–448, 1933
18. Chater N, Popp J: Microsurgical vascular bypass for occlusive cerebrovascular disease: Review of 100 cases. Surg Neurol 6:115–118, 1976
19. Chiari H: Über das Verhalten des Teilungswinkels der Carotis Communis bei der Endarteriitis Chronica Deformans. Verh Dtsch Ges Pathol 9:326–342, 1905
20. Clodius L, Wirth R: A new model for chronic lymphedema of the extremities. Plastica 2:115–122, 1974
21. Conley JJ, Pack GT: Surgical procedure for lessening the hazards of carotid bulb excision. Surgery 31:834–849, 1952
22. Cranley JJ, Canos AJ, Sull WJ, Gross AM: Phleborheographic technique for diagnosing deep venous thrombosis of the lower extremities. Surg Gynecol Obstet 141:331–338, 1975

22a. Crawford ES, DeBakey ME, Morris GC, Howell JF: Surgical treatment of occlusion of the innominate, common carotid and subclavian arteries: a 10 year experience. Surgery 65:17–31, 1969

23. Daniel RK, Swartz WM: Advances in Microsurgery. Advances in Surgery Yearbook Publishers. Chicago 11:285–339, 1977
24. Dardik H, Dardik II: Successful arterial substitution with modified human umbilical vein. Ann Surg 183:252–261, 1976

24a. DeBakey ME: Successful carotid endarterectomy for cerebrovascular insufficiency—nineteen year follow up. JAMA 233:1083–1085, 1975

25. Delbet P: Chirurgie Arterielle et Veineuse: Les Modernes Acquisitions. JB Bailliere et Fils, Paris, 1906
26. DeWeese JA: Thrombectomy for acute iliofemoral venous thrombosis. J Cardiovasc Surg 5:703–705, 1964
27. DeWeese JA, Rob CG: Autogenous venous grafts ten years later. Surgery 82:775–786, 1977
28. Djindjian R, Cophignon J, Theron J: Embolisation by supraselective arteriography from the femoral route in neurology: review of 60 cases. Neuroradiology 6:20–33, 1973
29. Doppman JL, DiChiro G, Gmmaya A: Obliteration of spinal cord arterio-venous malformation by percutaneous embolisation. Lancet 1:477–485, 1968
30. Dorfler J: Uber arteriennaht. Beitr Klin Chir 25:781–783, 1899
31. dos Santos JC: Sur la desobstruction des thromboses arterielles anciennes. Mem Acad Chir 73:409–416, 1947
32. Dotter CT, Judkins MP: Transluminal treatment of arteriosclerotic obstruction. Description of a technique and a preliminary report of its application. Circulation 30:654–667, 1964
33. Eastcott HHG, Pickering GW, Rob CG: Reconstruction of internal carotid artery. Lancet 2:994–996, 1954
34. Eck NY: Ligature of the portal vein. Voen Med J 1:120, 1877

34a. Edwards WH, Mulheri, JL: The surgical approach to significant stenosis of vertebral and subclavian arteries. Surgery 87:20–28, 1980

35. Erichsen JE: Observations on aneurism. London Sydenham Soc, 1844
36. Fisher M: Occlusion of the carotid arteries. AMA Arch Neurol Psychiatry 72:187–193, 1954

37. Fogarty TJ, et al: A method for extraction of arterial emboli and thrombi. Surg Gynecol Obstet 116:241–245, 1963
38. Fronek A, Johansen K, Dilley RB, Bernstein EF: Noninvasive physiological tests in the diagnosis and characterization of peripheral arterial occlusive disease. Am J Surg 126:205–210, 1973
39. Gee W, Mehigan JT, Wylie EJ: Measurement of collateral cerebral hemispheric blood pressure by ocular pneumoplethysmography. Am J Surg 130:122–129, 1975
40. Gowers WR: Manual of Diseases of the Nervous System, Churchill, London, 2:403, 1888
41. Goyanes J: Nuevos trabajos de cirugia vascular, substiticion plastica de las venas o arterioplastia venosa, aplicada como nuevo metodo al tratamiento de los aneurismios. Siglo Med 53:546–561, 1906
42. Green RM, DeWeese JA, Rob CG: Arterial embolectomy before and after the Fogarty Catheter. Surgery 77:24–32, 1975
43. Gross RE, Hurwitt ES, Bill AH Jr, Peirce EC II: Methods for Preservation and Transplantation of Arterial Grafts. Surg Gynecol Obstet 88:689–701, 1949
43a. Gruntzig A, Hopff H: Perkutane Rekanalisation chronischer arterielle Verschlusse mit liuen nerem Dilatationskatheter. Dtsche med Wsch 99:2502–2506, 1974
43b. Gruntzig A, Kunke DA: Technique of percutaneous transluminal angioplasty with Gruntzig balloon catheter. Am J Radiol 132:547–522, 1979
44. Haimovici H: A study of 330 unselected cases of embolism of the extremities. Angiology 1:20–45, 1950
45. Henschen C: Operative Revaskularisation des zirkulatorisch geschädigten Gehirns durch Auflage gestielter Muskellappen. Arch Klin Chir 264:392, 1950
46. Henson GF, Rob CG: A comparative study of the effects of different arterial clamps on the vessel wall. Br J Surg 43:561–564, 1956
47. Horsley JS: Suturing Blood Vessels. JAMA 77:117–121, 1921
48. Howell WH, Holt E: Two New Factors in Blood Coagulation Heparin and Pro-Antithrombin. Am J Physiol 47:338–341, 1918
49. Hultquist GT: Uber Thrombose and Embolie der Arteria Carotis, Gustav Fischer, Jena, 52 and 399
50. Hunt JR: The role of the carotid arteries in the causation of vascular lesion of the brain with remarks as certain features of symptomatology. Am J Med Sci 147:704–712, 1914
51. Hutchinson EC, Yates PO: The cervical portion of the vertebral artery: A clinico-pathological study. Brain 79:319–327, 1956
52. Hutchinson EC, Yates PO: Carotico-verebral stenosis. Lancet 1:2–5, 1957
53. Jacobson JH: Microsurgical Technique in repair of the traumatized extremity. Clin Orthop 29:132–139, 1963
54. Jacobson JH, Suarez EL: Microsurgery in the anastomosis of small blood vessels. Surg Forum 11:243–244, 1960
55. Jamieson GG, DeWeese JA, Rob CG: Infected arterial grafts. Ann Surg 181:850–852, 1975
56. Jantet GH, Rob CG: An experimental and clinical investigation of a new hemostatic absorbable gauze. Br J Surg 48:270–271, 1960
57. Johnson HC, Walker AE: The angiographic diagnosis of spontaneous thrombosis of internal and common carotid arteries. J Neurosurg 8: 631–644, 1951
58. Julian OC, et al: Direct surgery of arteriosclerosis. Ann Surg 136:459–474, 1952
59. Kartchner MM, Rae LP, Morrison FD: Noninvasive detection and evaluation of carotid occlusive disease. Arch Surg 106:528–539, 1973
60. Kunlin J: Le traitement de l'ischemic arteritique par la greffe veineuse longue. Rev Chir Paris 70:206–236, 1951
61. Lambert M: Wound of an artery treated by pin suture: Extract of a letter read by W. Hunter. Med Obs 2:360–364, 1762
62. Leeds FH, Gilfillan RS: Revascularization of the lower limb: Importance of profunda femoris artery. Arch Surg 82:25–31, 1961
63. Leopold, GR, Goldberger LE, Bernstein EF: Ultrasonic detection and evaluation of abdominal aortic aneurysms. Surgery 72:936–945, 1972
64. Leriche R, Fontaine R: L'Anesthesie Isolee du Ganglion Etiole. Pr Med 42:849–854, 1934
65. Lexer E: Die ideale Operation des Arteriellen und des Arteriovenosen Aneurysma. Arch Klin Chir 83:459–477, 1907
66. Louw JH: Spenecto-femoral and axillary to femoral bypass grafts in diffuse atherosclerotic occlusive disease. Lancet 1:1401–1404, 1963
67. Mannick JA, Williams LE, Nabseth DC: The Late Results of Axillo-Femoral Grafts. Surgery 68:1038–1043, 1970
68. Matas R: Traumatic aneurysm of the left brachial artery: Incision and partial excision of the sac recovery. Med News NY 53:462–466, 1888
69. Matas R: An operation for the radical cure of aneurysm based upon arteriorrhaphy. Ann Surg 37:161–196, 1903
70. McCaughan JJ, Kahn SF: Cross over graft for unilateral occlusive disease of the ilio-femoral arteries. Ann Surg 151:26–31, 1960
71. McCaughan JJ, Kahn SF: Cross over graft for

unilateral occlusive disease of the ilio-femoral arteries. Ann Surg 151:26–32, 1960
72. McLean Jr: The Thromboplastic Action of Cephalin. Am J Physiol 41:250–257, 1916
72a. Merx W, Doerr R, Rentrop P, Blanke H, Karsch KR, Mathey DG: Evaluation of the effectiveness of intracoronary streptokinase infusion in acute myocardial infarction: postprocedure management and hospital course in 204 patients. Am Heart J 1181–1187, 1981
73. Moniz E: L'Encephalographie arterille, son importance dans la localizarion des tumeurs Cerebralis. Rev Neurol 2:72–81, 1927
74. Mori S, Awane Y, Geno A: Ex situ repair of renal artery for renovascular hypertension. Arch Surg 94:370–377, 1967
75. Mosney M, Dumont MJ: Embolie femorala au cours d'un retrecissement mitral pur arterotomie. Bull Acad Med 51:73–76, 1911
75a. Mozersky DJ, Sumner DS, Barnes RW, Strandness DE: Subclavian revascularisation by means of a subcutaneous axillary-axillary graft. Arch Surg 106:20–23, 1973
76. Murray G: Heparin in Surgical Treatment of Blood Vessels. AMA Arch Surg 40:307–325, 1940
77. Murphy JB: Resection of arteries and veins in continuity: End to end suture, experimental and clinical research. Med Rec 51:73–88, 1897
78. Nielubowicz J, Olszewski W: Experimental lymphovenous anastomosis. Br J Surg 55:449–453, 1968
79. Nielubowicz J, Olszewski W: Surgical lymphaticovenous shunts in patients with secondary lymphoedema. Br J Surg 55:440–448, 1968
80. Osler W: Remarks on arteriovenous aneurysm. Lancet 1:949–955, 1915
81. Penzoldt F: Über Thrombose der Carotis. Dtsch Arch Klin Med 28:80–85, 1881
82. Pringle JH: Two cases of vein grafting for the maintenance of a direct arterial circulation. Lancet 1:1795–1796, 1913
83. Raines JK, Darling RC, Buth J, Brewster DC, Austen WG: Vascular laboratory criteria for the management of peripheral vascular disease of the lower extremities. Surgery 79:21–29, 1976
84. Rob CG: Graft Materials in Vascular Surgery Symposium. Symposia Specialists Miami
85. Rob CG: A History of Arterial Surgery. Arch Surg 105:821–823, 1972
86. Rob CG: The origin and development of surgery for occlusive disease of the carotid arteries. Rev Surg 29:1–6, 1972
87. Rosenburg N, Gaughran ERL, Henderson L, Lord GH, Douglas JF: Use of enzyme digested heterografts as segmented arterial substitutes. Arch Surg 76:275–287, 1958
88. Sabaneyev IF: The problem of vascular suture. Russk Chir Arch 2:132–140, 1895
88a. Schuler JJ, Flanigan P, DeBord JR, Ryan TJ, Castronuovo JJ, Lim LT: The treatment of cerebral ischemia by external carotid artery revascularisation. Arch Surg 118:567–572, 1983
89. Scott WH, Barker WF, Cannon JA et al: Management of Arterial Occlusive Disease. Dale, WA Year Book Publishers 1971
90. Serbinenko FA: Balloon catheterization and occlusion of major cerebral vessels. J Neurosurg 41:125–134, 1974
91. Singer A, Rob CG: The fate of the claudicator. Br Med J 2:633–636, 1960
92. Sjoquist O: Über intrakranielle Aneurysmen der Arteria Carotis und deren Beziehung zur Ophthalmophegischen Migräne. Nervenarzt 9: 233–241, 1936
93. Sousa Pereira A de: La Chirurgie Sympathique dans La Traitement des Embolies et Thrombosis Cerebrales XII Congres Soc. Ins Chir, London 375–378, 1947
94. Sousa Pereira A de: Surgical Treatment of Internal Carotid Thrombosis. Ann Surg 141:218–224, 1955
95. Sparks CH: Silicone mandril method for growing reinforced autogenous femoropopliteal artery grafts in situ. Ann Surg 177:293–304, 1973
96. Strully KJ, Hurwitt ES, Blankenberg HW: Thromboendarterectomy for thrombosis of the internal carotid artery in the neck. J Neurosurg 10:474–481, 1953
97. Szilagyi ED, Smith RG, Elliott JP, Virandecid MP: Infection in Arterial Reconstruction with Synthetic Grafts. Ann Surg 176:321-327, 1972
98. Thompson JE: Surgery for Cerebrovascular Insufficiency (Stroke). Charles C Thomas, Springfield, Ill., 1968
99. Voorhees AB, Jaretzki A, Blakemore AW: The use of tubes constructed from Vinyon "N" cloth in bridging arterial defects. Ann Surg 135:332–336, 1952
99a. Ward RE, Holcroft JW, Conti S, Blaisdell FW: New concepts in the use of axillo-femoral-bypass grafts. Arch Surg 118:573–576, 1983
100. Yasargil MF: Microsurgery Applied to Neurosurgery. Academic Press, New York, 1969

5

Carotid Endarterectomy

Jack M. Fein

Introduction

The common carotid bifurcation is the most frequent site for atherosclerotic lesions which produce cerebral ischemia. In the last 15 years the etiologic relationship of such lesions to cerebral symptoms has been clarified. Diagnostic methods have been refined to assist in the identification of patients with carotid lesions and in the selection of those suitable for surgery. Carotid endarterectomy has now become the procedure of choice for many patients at risk of stroke. Intraoperative monitoring of brain function and improved surgical techniques have lowered the morbidity and mortality of endarterectomy. This chapter describes the current surgical management of patients with atherothrombotic lesions of the extracranial carotid artery.

Pathophysiology of Carotid Occlusive Disease

The majority of ischemic strokes are associated with atherosclerotic lesions of the extracranial arteries. This was demonstrated in 75% of 3,788 patients with cerebrovascular insufficiency subjected to four-vessel angiography.[80] In a Mayo Clinic study reported by Houser and Baker[91] in 1968, only 28 of 5,000 patients with ischemic symptoms had lesions due to causes other than atherosclerosis. These included problems such as fibromuscular hyperplasia, blood dyscrasias, arteritis, and collagen vascular disease.

Atheroslerosis in the carotid arteries originates as a subintimal collection of fatty cells that are recognized grossly as a fatty streak.[93] A response from the connective tissue layer to the fatty streak often results in fibrous proliferation in the subendothelial layer. Alternatively, several streaks may coalesce into a larger lipid plaque. Atheroma forming on the posterior wall of the common carotid artery usually originates from lipid plaque. As the plaque develops, it extends into the external carotid artery and for approximately 1 to 2 cm into the internal carotid artery (Fig. 5.1). The lesion is hemodynamically more threatening in the smaller diameter internal carotid artery than in the larger common carotid artery. In contrast to the fibrous type of atheroma, which affects the vertebral arteries, lipid atheroma tends to ulcerate, due either to rupture of lipid-laden phagocytes into the lumen or from hemorrhage into the plaque from the lumen.[95] In 75 consecutive plaques removed at endarterectomy, we found that 40 had some degree of superimposed thrombus.[55] This was usually concentrated proximal to the point of maximal stenosis. These findings make it likely that symptoms are related either to hemo-

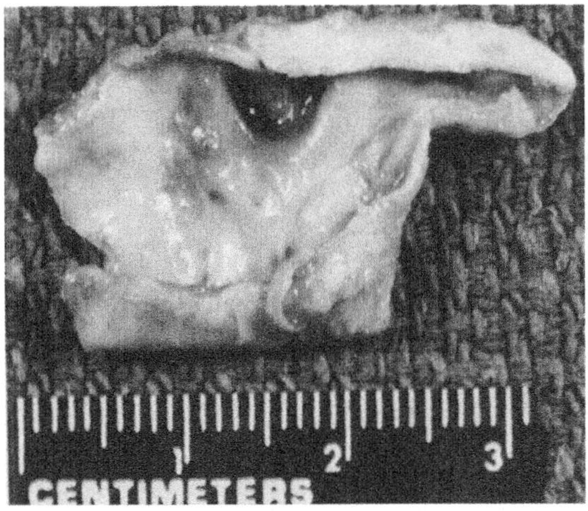

Figure 5.1. Atherosclerotic plaque removed from right carotid bifurcation in 58-year-old man with transient monocular blindness and transient hemispheric ischemic attacks. Plaque extends for 1.5 cm into internal carotid artery. Deep ulcer containing platelet thrombus is seen.

dynamically significant stenosis or to emboli released from the ulcerated plaque.

Denny-Brown[39,40] first proposed that atherosclerotic lesions of the carotid arteries produced hemodynamic insufficiency. Foerster and Guttman[68] described a patient in whom attacks of blindness recurred in the right eye. One attack occurred under ophthalmoscopic examination, and the vessels running to the upper part of the retina became bloodless as vision was lost in the lower visual field. In earlier reports by Leob and Meyer[105] and Crawford et al,[35] lesions near the carotid bifurcation appeared to be hemodynamically significant when they compromised the lumen by more than 30%. Intraoperative measurement, however, demonstrated that pressure gradients did not develop until the lumen was compromised by 47% or more. Brice et al[22] concluded that significant stenosis occurred when the cross-sectional area was reduced to 5 mm^2 or less. Removal of the stenotic plaque in another group of patients[14] eliminated the intravascular pressure gradient which averaged 80 mm Hg. Average carotid blood flow then increased from 24 mL/min to 208 mL/min. The progressive development of stenotic lesions at the carotid bifurcation was described by Javid et al.[97] With serial angiography they studied 92 patients harboring atheromas for one to nine years. A significant increase in the degree of stenosis was noted in 62% of patients. In 35% the lumen was further compromised by more than 25% of its diameter in one year. None of the lesions regressed. Consecutive examination of specimens removed at surgery in 65 patients[55] indicated that in those specimens where the lumen was compromised by more than 50%, the incidence of intraplaque hemorrhage was 90%, whereas hemorrhage was found in only 20% of smaller lesions. This was confirmed by Lusby et al,[110] who also noted that plaques recently distended by hemorrhage had a greater susceptibility to form platelet aggregates on the intimal surface.

Many patients with transient ischemic attacks (TIAs) have carotid lesions that do not compromise the lumen significantly but harbor ulcers[126] that release emboli to the distal circulation (Fig. 5.2). Emboli to systemic arteries

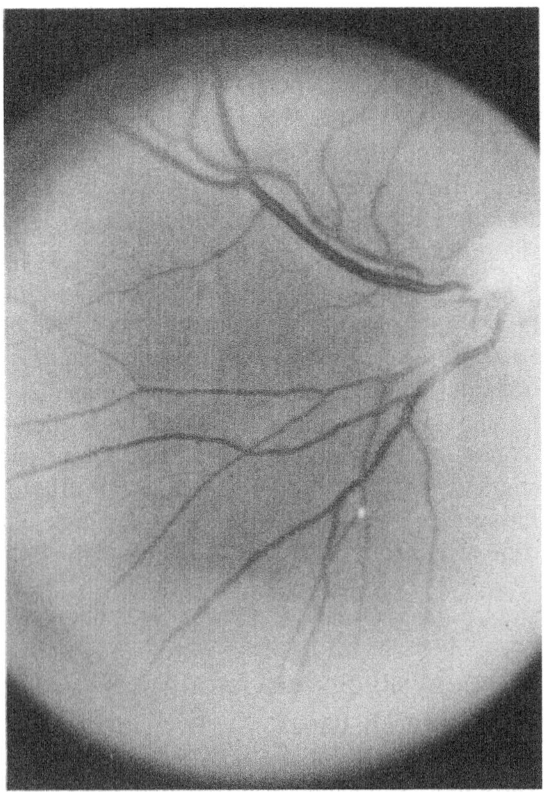

Figure 5.2. Fundus photograph of the right eye in the patient described in Fig. 5.1. Fundus photograph was taken during an episode of transient monocular blindness. Small white embolus at junction of inferior temporal artery branches is seen

were described in 1926 by Benson[13] and similar events were described in the cerebral circulation by Winter.[171] Millikan[118] proposed that emboli were primarily responsible for the symptoms of cerebral ischemia. Emboli were identified in the retina by Witmer and Schmid[172] and described as "bright plaques" by Hollenhorst.[89] Fisher[64] described a patient in whom emboli were observed during the course of an attack of amaurosis fugax. Two types of emboli are of clinical significance. White particles represent platelet-fibrin emboli, whereas shiny yellowish masses represent cholesterol fragments.[92] Most patients with amaurosis fugax were found to have an ulcerative lesion of the carotid bifurcation responsible for their symptoms. Kallorits et al[100] studied 45 patients with transient visual disturbances and found a source of emboli near the common carotid bifurcation in 43 (96%). The prognosis of patients with ulcerative lesions may depend on the size of the ulcer crater. Moore et al[121] followed 67 patients with 72 asymptomatic nonstenotic ulcerative lesions found at angiography. The annual stroke rate over seven years was 0.4% for patients with minimal ulcers, but was as high as 12.5% per year for those with large or compound ulcers.

Diagnosis

Diagnostic evaluation of patients with carotid artery occlusive disease is designed to exclude other causes of symptoms and to identify a remediable lesion if possible.[57,79,86] Significant lesions may be found in asymptomatic patients whereas ischemic symptoms may be found in the absence of a lesion. Selection of patients for surgery is generally reserved for symptomatic patients with an appropriate lesion.

A careful history of the onset, duration, and resolution of ischemic symptoms characterize the clinical syndrome and its probable site of origin. Aside from the general neurologic examination, a neurovascular examination is performed. This should include a careful funduscopic examination. Retinal artery pressure measurements are performed and any asymmetry is noted.[102] The presence of an audible bruit over the orbits or at the anterior cervical triangle has a high correlation with internal carotid artery stenosis. A variety of noninvasive testing techniques were developed to facilitate identification of extracranial carotid artery lesions. Patients with TIA, reversible ischemic neurologic deficit (RIND), progressive stroke (PS), or nondebilitating completed stroke will require angiography whether or not the screening tests are revealing. These tests, however, are of value in patients with atypical complaints who may be harboring silent but threatening lesions. The discovery of a very high-grade stenosis, a large ulcer crater, or fragment of thrombus projecting into the lumen usually requires surgery irrespective of the clinical history.

Arteriography

Digital subtraction angiography (DSA) is now routinely employed in patients with cerebrovascular symptoms. The limited resolution of current DSA techniques, however, requires that arterial angiography be performed prior to carotid endarterectomy. Three-vessel selective angiography is required in patients with symptoms referable to the carotid artery distribution. This provides information regarding the presence of intracranial small-vessel disease and the pattern of collateral circulatory filling.

In the Joint Stroke Study[80] 41.2% of the patients examined by four vessel angiography had accessible lesions only, 33% had both accessible and inaccessible lesions, and 25% had either no lesions (10.4%) or inaccessible lesions only (6.1%). Multiple lesions were present in surgically accessible sites in 67.3% of patients. More specifically, one-third of the patients were found to have lesions involving the common carotid bifurcation. Stenotic lesions of the right carotid bifurcation were as frequent as those in the left carotid bifurcation (34%). Occlusions at these locations were also equally distributed (8.5%).

The angiographic diagnosis of atherosclerotic lesions is usually straightforward for hemodynamically significant stenosis (Figs. 5.3 and 5.4). Ulcerative lesions may be more difficult to identify (Figs. 5.5, 5.6). Of 75 consecutive endarterectomy specimens, 47% were reported by Newton[127] to show ulceration, and all but 6% were demonstrated on preoperative angiography. However, Edwards et al.[49] found a signifi-

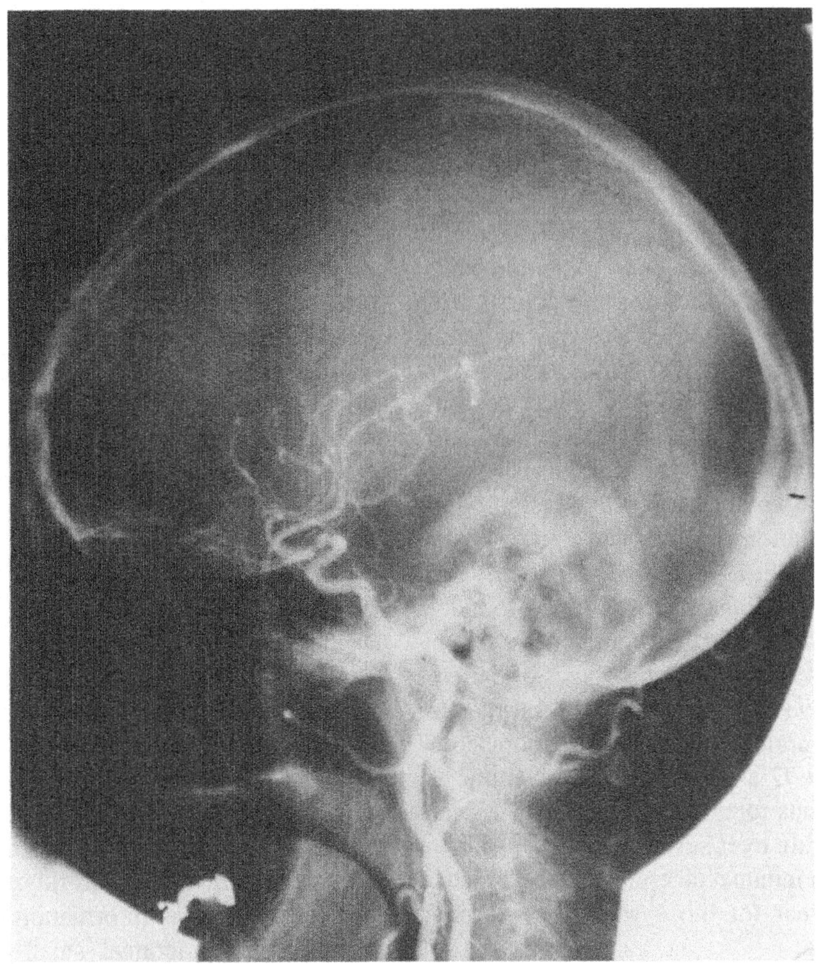

Figure 5.3. Left lateral angiogram of patient with transient hemispheric ischemic attacks. There is a high-grade stenoic lesion originating on posterior wall of internal carotid artery and compromising the lumen by about 90% of its diameter.

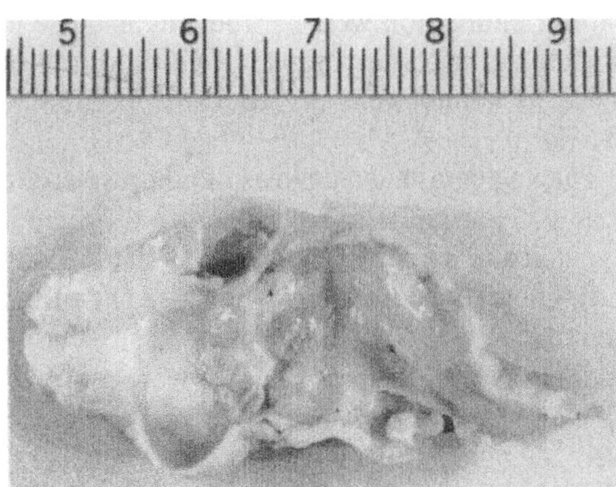

Figure 5.4. Specimen removed from patient described in Fig. 5.3. There is a high-grade stenotic lesion at posterior wall of internal carotid artery as well as a small ulceration just proximal to it, which was not visualized on the arteriogram.

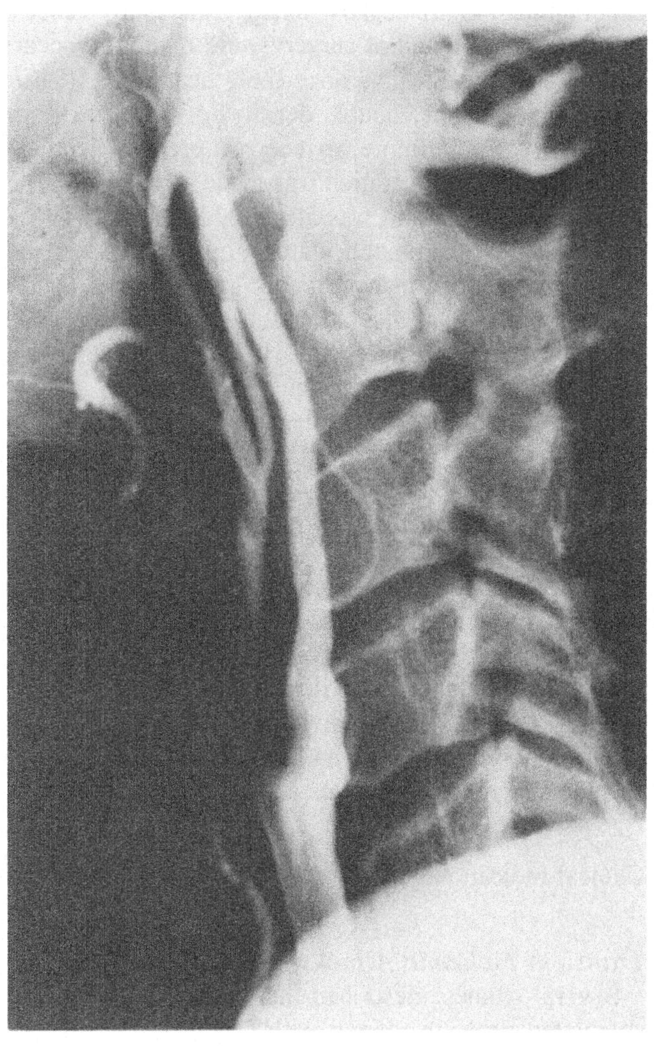

Figure 5.5. Left lateral carotid angiogram in 41-year-old female with recurrent transient hemispheric ischemic attack. There are multiple ulcerative defects in the posterior wall near the origin of the internal carotid artery.

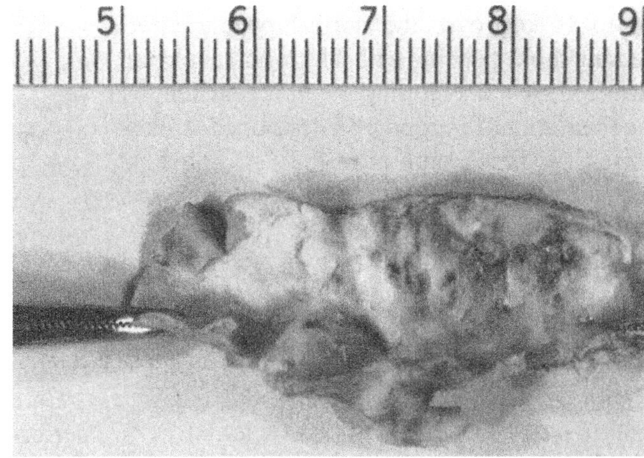

Figure 5.6. Specimen removed from patinet described in Fig. 5.5. There are two larger ulcers in the posterior wall of the internal carotid artery as well as numerous smaller ulcerations that were not visualized on the arteriogram. All of the ulcer craters contained platelet thrombi.

cant number of false negative angiograms. Only 12 of 20 ulcers found at surgery were demonstrated angiographically, since the other 8 did not exhibit a niche, double density, or mural irregularity. Furthermore, an incorrect preoperative diagnosis of ulceration was made in 17 of 50 carotid arteries and was attributable to the presence of a subintimal hematoma in the arterial wall. Although many patients have angiographic evidence of ulceration and stenosis in the same lesion, Moore and Hall[122] demonstrated that the presence of ulcers within plaques was unrelated to the degree of stenosis.

Selection of Patients for Surgery

A variety of indications for carotid endarterectomy have been proposed and in the last 15 years considerable experience has accumulated to support or refute these positions. It is worthwhile to consider these individually, since the risk-benefit ratio of surgery in the clinical-radiographic subgroups of patients are different.

Clinical Indications

Transient Ischemic Attacks

Several studies* described the frequency of completed stroke in patients with TIA. The difference in frequency of stroke in these studies may have been related to differences in the frequency of associated disease and other risk factors in the populations studied. In concert, however, these studies indicated that 25% to 40% of patients with TIA suffered completed stroke within five years. The risk of completed stroke in such patients was therefore increased up to 16-fold over the normal population.[169] Among those patients with TIA who developed stroke, 51% did so during the first year following their initial TIA, and 21% developed strokes during the first month after the first attack.[169] Although the relationship of TIA to stroke was variable, it was related to the length of follow-up.[116] It was difficult, however, to predict which individuals with TIA would develop a stroke. There was little correlation between sex,[77,113,169] age,[113,169] number of attacks,[1,8,169] or the presence of diabetes mellitus[163] and the subsequent occurrence of stroke. The presence of hypertension in patients with TIA increased the risk of stroke in some series[8,113,163] but not in others.[73,77]

The medical management of patients with TIA using anticoagulants was described in both retrospective and prospective randomized studies. While several retrospective studies favored the use of warfarin sodium (Coumadin),[63,131] prospective randomized studies[9,133] were unable to show a significant benefit when the complications of anticoagulants were also considered. The role of aspirin was evaluated in several studies.[17,25,60,148] Fields et al[60] found a reduction in the rate of TIAs but not in the rate of stroke over a six-month follow-up. In the Canadian Study[25] a reduction in the risk of stroke was found in male patients. The number of ischemic events was small, however, and the significance of these differences was questioned.[103,116] In other studies aspirin appeared to have a beneficial effect,[35] but Sorensen et al[148] were unable to confirm the benefits of aspirin therapy. In each of the foregoing studies it should be recognized that the arterial lesions responsible for TIA were not defined by arteriography so that inferences regarding efficacy for specific lesions are difficult to draw. The results of carotid endarterectomy in 316 patients with TIA and specific carotid lesions were compared with the results of medical management in the Joint Study.[58] Further TIA occurred in 38% of the surgically treated group and in 54.5% of the medically managed patients. In the surgical group these episodes usually occurred contralateral to the operated artery. Occurrence of new stroke in the follow-up period was 4% in the surgical group and 12.4% in the nonsurgical group. These differences favored surgical treatment for patients with TIA. In larger series[42,153,160,161,177] the surgical morbidity and mortality rates were lowest in patients with TIAs compared with other cerebrovascular syndromes. The presence of cerebral hemisphere TIA associated with an appropriate carotid lesion is considered a strong indication for carotid endarterectomy.

Acute Stroke

Carotid endarterectomy should ideally be performed in patients who are neurologically

* References 2,6,8,9,63,73,77,113,133,144,169,181.

stable, with minimal or no neurologic deficit. On occasion, surgery may also be appropriate in a more acute setting. A distinction should be made, however, between patients who present with an acute and completed stroke and patients with an acute progressing stroke.

After onset of an acute ischemic insult, a series of pathophysiologic changes conspire to make surgical intervention undesirable. Neuronal injury may be irreversible. Restoration of blood flow under such circumstances may not improve cellular metabolism and function. Additionally, injury to the vasculature may result in the "no reflow" phenomenon with inability to perfuse the microcirculation.[3] If reflow is successful, breakdown of the blood-brain barrier may occur and will predispose the brain to hemorrhagic infarction.[24,178]

Clinical studies of patients[12,14,37,48,139,176] who have undergone surgery for acute stroke have borne out these anticipated results. Wylie reported on 14 operations performed within two days of the onset of symptoms.[176,179] Ten patients were worse after surgery and nine of the ten died. Autopsies obtained in eight of these patients showed massive hemorrhagic infarction in each. In a comparable group of 14 patients treated nonsurgically, however, only two patients died. Julian[99] operated on 26 patients urgently. Twenty had immediate relief of their signs and symptoms, but 5 of the 26 continued to have symptoms or became worse, and one died. Blaisdell et al[14,15] found that there was a mortality of 42% in 50 patients operated on within two weeks following an acute stroke, whereas the mortality was only 20% for nonsurgical patients, and only 5% for those operated with neurologic deficits of more than two weeks' duration. Similarly, in a study by Bauer et al[12] a mortality rate of 38% was found in patients undergoing endarterectomy within two weeks of the onset of a stroke. This was considerably higher than the 23% mortality rate in a comparable group of nonsurgical patients. Ojemann[130] reported on a small group of nine patients with sudden severe deficit who underwent urgent carotid endarterectomy. There was improvement in four, no change in one, and four deaths. They concluded that patients with sudden total deficits, especially those who were drowsy, should not be operated on. Several other series confirmed the poor results obtained in patients with acute deficits[94,160,178] and form a consensus that such patients should be managed primarily by nonsurgical means.

Progressive Stroke

The prognosis of patients with untreated progressive stroke is poor. In Millikan's series[119] of 204 cases, 69% became hemiparetic, 5% monoparetic, 14% died, and only 12% returned to normal by 14 days after onset. There are five[6,27,63,65,119] studies with appropriate control subjects which indicate that patients treated with anticoagulation have a lower frequency of infarction than patients not treated. We currently treat such patients with a continuous infusion of heparin at a rate of 800 to 1,200 units/h to achieve an activated partial thromboplastin time (APTT) which is twice the control value. This regimen is maintained for three weeks after progression has been arrested. In the presence of a nondebilitating residual deficit and a correctable lesion, surgery is then undertaken. In some patients there is further progression of the neurologic deficit despite therapeutic levels of anticoagulation, and angiography and emergency carotid endarterectomy may be indicated.[43,66,78] In Fisher's series[66] emergency carotid endarterectomy was undertaken within 12 hours of onset of symptoms in 55 patients, 26 with stenosis and 29 with occlusion. The outcome was closely related to the preoperative condition, with good to excellent results in more than 80% of patients with crescendo TIA or mild to moderate progressive stroke. Patients with completed and extensive stroke, however, did poorly, with a combined morbidity-mortality rate of 32% related to either hypertensive hemorrhage or hypotension. Of 18 patients with progressive stroke operated on by Goldstone,[78] 10 exhibited a slowly progressive pattern preoperatively, and 8 showed a waxing and waning or stuttering pattern. Each made a dramatic and complete recovery with no morbidity after emergency carotid endarterectomy.

Chronic Completed Stroke

Although the operative mortality rate for patients with deficits greater than two weeks' duration was only 5%,[114] it is generally agreed that the long-term outlook for patients with extensive and stable deficits is not improved by carotid endarterectomy.[173,184] Bauer et al[11] found that in patients with a dense hemiparesis or hemiplegia, the cumulative survival rate at 42 months for surgical patients was 58% compared with 72% for nonsurgical patients. In patients who have a minimal deficit and who are functionally independent, the risk of another completed stroke is similar to that in patients with TIA. Such patients may be good candidates for endarterectomy.

Atypical or Nonhemispheric TIAs

Some authors have suggested that in the presence of carotid stenosis, carotid endarterectomy may be indicated[5,33,69,177] in patients with atypical or nonhemispheric TIAs. McNamara et al[115] found, however, that over a three-year period following endarterectomy, 8 of 18 patients (44%) with nonhemispheric TIAs continued to have ischemic episodes postoperatively. By contrast, recurrent ischemic attacks developed in only 8 of 52 patients (15%) with hemispheric transient ischemia who had carotid endarterectomy on the appropriate side. According to Fields et al,[61] 24 patients with unilateral carotid stenosis had carotid endarterectomy for vertebrobasilar transient ischemia. Ten patients (42%) continued to have recurrent ischemic episodes during follow-up. Eight of 20 patients (40%) treated nonsurgically also experienced recurrent transient ischemia. In a small number of patients with vertebrobasilar insufficiency,[117] the carotid arteries may contribute prominently to the posterior circulation. This may be related to enlarged posterior communicating arteries or to large vestigial trigeminal, acoustic or hypoglossal arteries. We would generally advocate a conservative approach to patients with vertebrobasilar symptoms and carotid stenosis unless dependence of the posterior circulation on carotid flow can be demonstrated.

Angiographic Indications

Patients with TIA, progressive stroke, or mild stroke may be candidates for carotid endarterectomy if an appropriate lesion that is hemodynamically significant or the source of emboli is found near the carotid bifurcation. Many patients have multiple lesions, which influence the risk-benefit ratio for surgery. Subgroups of patients have been identified based on a combination of these lesions.

Unilateral Carotid Stenosis

In patients with a single stenotic lesion ipsilateral to the symptomatic hemisphere, the results of surgery were related to the degree of residual neurologic deficit. In 218 patients with TIA,[11] those treated nonsurgically had a 42-month survival rate of 64%, whereas the surgically treated patients had a survival rate of 81%. The quality of this survival was analyzed[61] in 94 patients, 45 of whom were operated on and 49 of whom were treated medically. Of the operated patients, 6% developed cerebral infarction during follow-up study. In the presence of a persistent partial deficit, the difference in survival rates of 49 surgical (82%) compared with 44 nonsurgical (54%) patients also favored surgery.[11] In 74 patients with completed strokes, however, 34 nonsurgical patients had a cumulative survival rate of 76%, whereas 40 surgical patients had a survival rate of only 47%. Endarterectomy, therefore, appears to be of benefit in patients with TIA or partially resolved stroke who have stenosis of a single carotid artery.[109,111,125]

Ulcerative Plaque

Many patients have lesions that are not hemodynamically significant, but contain ulcer craters that are a source of emboli. It is of interest to note, however, that Hertzer et al[84] found a 9.9% risk of intraoperative deficit and 4.5% risk of intraoperative stroke in patients with ulcerated atheroma. Comparable risks in nonulcerated atheroma were 0.7% and 0%, respectively.

Bilateral Carotid Stenosis

Most surgeons advocate endarterectomy for the symptomatic patient with bilateral carotid stenosis although not all agree that the asymptomatic side should be treated. According to Bauer,[11] surgery on the symptomatic side did not increase survival rates at 42 months in patients with bilateral carotid stenosis. In Field's report,[61] however, the quality of survival was better in surgically treated patients. Of 94 surgical patients, 45% remained asymptomatic throughout the period of follow-up, whereas only 26% of the 73 nonsurgical patients remained asymptomatic. There are few studies of the natural history of bilateral carotid stenosis. In most cases stenosis of a contralateral carotid artery is discovered incidental to the symptomatic carotid artery. Levin[106] followed 60 patients with bilateral stenosis who had unilateral reconstruction. Two patients became symptomatic within two years and were subsequently operated on. Ojemann[130] and others,[162] however, recommend that surgery be performed on the symptomatic side first and the opposite side within two to four weeks. In our experience, the higher grade lesion is more often on the symptomatic side whereas the contralateral side usually provides cross flow through the circle of Willis.

Carotid Stenosis and Contralateral Carotid Occlusion

This is the most common combination of multiple lesions in this author's practice. In the Joint Stroke Study,[59] nearly two-thirds of the patients with internal carotid occlusion had significant contralateral stenosis. Of the 557 patients who had this combination of lesions, 55% had symptoms related to the occlusion, 16% had symptoms related to both carotid systems, and 10% had symptoms related to the stenosis only. Twenty percent of the patients were asymptomatic or had symptoms related to the vertebrobasilar territory. In other series[4] the deficit was referable to the side of occlusion in 92% and to the side of stenosis in 8%. Earlier studies showed a significantly higher surgical morbidity in this group compared with patients operated on for a unilateral carotid stenosis only. At the end of a 66-month follow-up,[62] 63% of medically treated patients were alive, whereas only 34% of surgically treated patients were still living. This difference was related to the initial surgical mortality of 28%. Perioperative strokes were related to carotid clamping, shunt insertion, or shunt removal. Postoperative strokes involved the contralateral occluded side in 33% of cases.[4] In a similar group, however, Patterson[132] described no morbidity after endarterectomy in 23 patients, and Heilbrun[83] described similar results in his series.

Our approach differs. The side of symptoms, the patency of the circle of Willis, and the size of the superficial temporal artery are considered. Patients with symptoms related to the stenotic side only undergo endarterectomy. Those patients with symptoms referable to the occluded side or to both sides and who have a large (~1.2 mm diameter) superficial temporal artery undergo extracranial/intracranial (EC-IC) bypass first, followed by endarterectomy. This sequence is chosen since on the occluded side the degree of middle cerebral filling seen after a bypass may be significantly greater than that seen after contralateral endarterectomy. Bypass does not require a period of major vessel clamping and probably provides additional cerebral protection during subsequent endarterectomy. The requirements for an intraoperative shunt decreased in 45 patients who had a previous contralateral EC/IC bypass.[54]

Internal Carotid Occlusion

Sixteen percent of the patients in the Joint Study[59] had complete occlusion of the internal carotid artery. Several studies described a high morbidity and mortality from the presenting ischemic event,* but of greater interest is the future risk in patients who have survived the initial event with minimal deficits. In 95 patients with no deficit, who were managed conservatively, the mortality rate was 43% and the new stroke rate was 25%. Of 135 patients followed by Furlan,[74,75] however, the incidence of new stroke ipsilateral to the occlusion was 2% per year. This is greater than expected for the normal population, but less than in patients with TIA.[34] A prospective study of 47 patients revealed a 5% annual ipsilateral stroke rate during a mean follow-up of 2.9 years.[35]

Carotid endarterectomy is generally contraindicated in the clinical setting of an acute deficit or with angiographic evidence of an occlusion that extends intracranially. There may, however, be a role for acute surgical intervention in the rare patient with a progressive deficit due to fresh thrombosis. It may also be worthwhile to attempt endarterectomy in chronic occlusions that are confined to the extracranial internal carotid artery. Shucart et al[143] were able to restore flow in four patients where there was some retrograde filling of the intracranial internal carotid

* References 67, 38, 44, 47, 140, 166, 81.

artery down to the level of the carotid canal via collateral channels. Ojemann performed 16 operations for completed carotid occlusion more than 24 hours after the occlusion was demonstrated.[130] Flow could be reestablished in only four patients. In these, the occlusion probably did not extend intracranially. In most patients with internal carotid occlusion, flow cannot be reestablished and EC/IC bypass surgery may be a practical alternative if the patient is at risk for future stroke.

Asymptomatic Lesions

Significant controversy surrounds the proper management of patients with asymptomatic lesions. The advent of DSA has made it easy to verify the presence of significant lesions of the carotid bifurcation with little risk. Most of the information used to assess the future risk of asymptomatic lesions, however, was obtained before DSA studies were available. Several series described the prognosis of patients with carotid bruit in whom, however, the presence of significant internal carotid lesions was not verified angiographically. Thompson[157–159] followed a group of 92 patients with asymptomatic carotid bruits. During a 10-year follow-up period, 45% of the patients developed either TIA (26%) or completed strokes (19%). In Trieman's series,[164] however, no strokes occurred in 40 patients with carotid bruits operated on for abdominal aortic disease, but two strokes occurred in 156 patients without bruits. In two series of patients undergoing abdominal aortic surgery,[26,52] there were no perioperative strokes among a total of 127 patients with asymptomatic bruits. Kartchner[101] found an increased risk of stroke in patients who had positive noninvasive tests (oculoplethysmography) prior to coronary revascularization. Spray-Gunderson,[149] however, found no postoperative strokes in 18 patients with positive Doppler examinations prior to a variety of general surgical procedures. Ojemann[130] operated on 19 patients with asymptomatic carotid stenosis with no surgical complications. There was one mild cardiopulmonary complication. In 14 cases the lesion was found during angiography for contralateral symptoms. Nunn[129] performed 28 operations in asymptomatic patients. Transient neurologic deficits occurred in two patients after surgery, but all patients were normal when assessed at 48 months. Twenty four operations were performed in patients who had previously undergone endarterectomy on the opposite side. Two operations preceded major surgical procedures and two were done in patients evaluated for carotid bruit alone. The prognosis for patients with asymptomatic bruits is generally good if untreated; however, the morbidity of prophylactic procedures in these patients is also very low. In the hands of a surgeon whose combined morbidity mortality is less than 2%, we recommend endarterectomy for hemodynamically significant or deeply ulcerative lesions.

Physiologic and Anesthetic Consideration

Anesthetic Agent

Regional anesthesia induced by cervical block[88,138] allows the surgeon to utilize the patient's mental status as an indication of cerebral function during endarterectomy. In the anxious patient, however, surgical exposure may be limited and may lead to significant technical errors. Rainer et al[137] utilized regional block in 257 consecutive cases, with an operative mortality rate of only 0.8%. The authors attributed this to awareness of the patient's intraoperative neurologic status. In patients who were intolerant to carotid clamping, Hobson et al[87,88] terminated the surgical procedure and resorted to general anesthesia and a shunt at a second operation.

Regional anesthesia does not enjoy the same popularity it did several years ago.[104] Endotracheal intubation and general anesthesia allow better airway control and the ability to maintain optimal blood gas concentrations.[155] The author has used general anesthesia in 405 carotid endarterectomies with an anesthetic combined morbidity and mortality rate of only 0.2%. Since cerebrovascular disease has a profound effect on cerebral hemodynamics, the choice of an agent is related to its effect on metabolism and flow.[154,174] Other considerations are the ease of administration and the rapidity of recovery at the termination of the surgical procedure.

Barbiturates produce primary suppression of electrophysiologic activity and thereby reduce the cerebral metabolic rate for oxygen

($CMRO_2$).[100,135,147,156] Increasing doses of barbiturates will progressively depress the $CMRO_2$ until the point at which the electroencephalogram becomes isoelectric, but thereafter, do not further depress the $CMRO_2$. Since careful neurologic observation is critical in the immediate postoperative period, we have restricted barbiturate use to induction of anesthesia.

In the last 300 carotid endarterectomies we have used the halogenated inhalational agents halothane and isoflurane. When blood pressure is maintained at normal levels, halothane produces a slight increase in cerebral blood flow (CBF)[30,114,173] and a reduction of $CMRO_2$.[146,154] At halothane concentrations of less than 0.5%, however, CBF will gradually return to normal.[114]

Arterial Blood Gas Levels

Any system of closed ventilation can maintain arterial Po_2 values above 100 mm Hg.[90] Serial measurements of forced inspiratory oxygen (FIo_2) and arterial Po_2 levels will quantitate the degree of pulmonary shunting in the presence of pulmonary disease. Jennett et al[98] reported excellent results using hyperbaric oxygenation during endarterectomy in 14 patients. Heyman,[85] however, reported that ischemic infarction occurred despite jugular venous oxygen tension of 180 mm Hg in a patient who underwent surgery in the hyperbaric chamber. We aim to keep arterial oxygen levels between 120 and 140 mm Hg throughout surgery, raising it between 140 and 160 mm Hg during the period of carotid clamping.

The optimal CO_2 for patients undergoing carotid endarterectomy has been the subject of considerable study. The linear relationship of CO_2 to CBF found in the normal brain is often disturbed with loss of CO_2 reactivity in areas of ischemic infarction.[167] An intracerebral steal effect may be produced by the normal vasodilatation produced by CO_2 in normal areas. Earlier studies by Clark[31] and White[170] demonstrated an increase in jugular venous oxygen saturation during clamping of the internal carotid artery when hypercapnia was induced. Hypercapnia during endarterectomy was then introduced by Wells[168] to increase cerebral perfusion during carotid clamping. Smith et al[145] utilized routine hypercarbia ($Paco_2$ 50–70 mm Hg) in 55 carotid endarterectomies. Hypercarbia may be produced by removing the CO_2 absorber, adding CO_2 or using acetazolamide (Diamox). Several authors have since reported on their experience with hypercarbia,[18,23,51] which is less enthusiastic. Ehrenfeld et al[51] studied the effects of CO_2 on downstream cerrebral arterial pressure and the CBF equivalent during carotid endarterectomy in nine patients. Relative hypocarbia resulted in increased internal carotid stump pressure, and on this basis Ehrenfeld thought that hypocarbia produced preferential flow into ischemic areas. However, hypercarbia may induce arrhythmia, particularly when halothane is used.[32] Experimental data from Mitchenfelder[120] indicate, however, that levels of adenosine triphosphate (ATP) were lower and lactic acid was higher in regions of focal ischemia when monkeys were subjected to hypocapnia during middle cerebral artery occlusion. Most surgeons, therefore, try to maintain a high normal Pco_2 during surgery and prefer to use other methods of cerebral protection during carotid clamping.

Systemic Blood Pressure

Patients on an antihypertensive regimen are maintained on their drugs to avoid wide swings in blood pressure intraoperatively.[28] Many of the hypotensive episodes reported during induction of anesthesia are probably related to hypovolemia. Adequate hydration preoperatively is essential and it is useful to ensure a daily intake of 2,500 cc of fluid over three to four days preoperatively. Supportive stockings are used during surgery to prevent pooling of blood in the lower extremities and thereby maintain systemic blood pressure. Ehrenfeld[51] and Fourcade[70] determined that norepinephrine-induced hypertension produced a proportional increase in the internal carotid artery (ICA) stump pressure with a mean ratio between systemic and ICA stump pressure of 2 to 1 in their patients. Boysen[19] noted that angiotension induced increases of systemic blood pressure also produced the same increase in ICA stump pressure in patients with good collateral circulation. In the ischemic brain with a decreased ability to autoregulate, supporting cerebral perfusion by such agents is generally very effective.

Surgical Technique

Expeditious and precise technique is important in performing carotid endarterectomy since either prolonged periods of clamping or rough handling of the plaque significantly increase the risk of ischemia. Our technique now includes use of the operating microscope, microinstruments, and microsuture material. The Zeiss OPMI operating microscope is fitted with a 250-mm objective, a pair of inclined binocular tubes, and 12.5× ocular lenses. The illumination and detailed visualization have made selection of the plane for endarterectomy more precise, the plaque is excised more completely, and the arteriotomy incision can be repaired more accurately. The necessity for a vein patch graft has been relegated to occasional secondary operations for postoperative stenosis.

The patient is placed in the supine position and a brief electroencephalographic recording is made with the patient awake. Endotracheal intubation is carried out, and the patient is anesthetized. The head is supported on a small doughnut ring and is turned about 30° away from the side of operation. A thyroid bag is inflated under the shoulders and the operating table is flexed. The position of the carotid bifurcation in relation to the cervical spine is verified on the angiogram. In 80% of the author's cases, the bifurcation was found in relation to the C4 body or the C3-4, C4-5 interspace (Table 5.1). A more difficult dissection should be anticipated when the bifurcation is displaced above the C3-4 interspace. The origin of the external occipital artery from the external carotid artery is also noted. The medial segment of the hypoglossal nerve is often fixed in position by the artery, and its origin often will provide a clue to the location of the hypoglossal nerve in relation to the carotid bifurcation.

Table 5.1. Relationship of carotid bifurcation to cervical spine level in 403 patients.

Level	Percent
C2-3 Interspace	3
C3 Body	10
C3-4 Interspace	35
C4 Body	30
C4-5 Interspace	15
C5 Body	7

The skin is infiltrated with xylocaine containing epinephrine (1/200,000). An oblique skin incision is made along the anterior border of the sternomastoid muscle and is curved posteriorly to avoid the parotid gland, the lower branches of the facial nerve, and the greater auricular nerve. The incision enters one of the transverse skin folds inferiorly (Fig. 5.7) and is carried down to the platysma layer. The platysma is then opened separately using sharp dissection and the Malis bipolar cautery (Fig. 5.8). The fascial plane between the sternomastoid muscle and the midline structures is entered and separated sharply (Fig. 5.9). By leaving the sternomastoid fascia intact, postoperative swelling of the muscle is minimized. The carotid pulse is then palpated gently and leads directly to the carotid sheath (Fig. 5.10). The internal jugular vein is usually identified first and dissection is carried out along its medial border. The facial vein is usually the largest of several venous branches that enter the internal jugular vein (Fig. 5.11). If a patch graft is anticipated, the vein is then doubly ligated, and a 2-cm segment between the ligatures can be harvested. The vein is opened longitudinally with a Potts scissor and the intima is irrigated with saline. 4-0 silk stay sutures secure the corners of the vein graft to a wet tongue blade that is temporarily stored in a Petri dish with a solution containing 1,000 units of heparin in 20-cc of saline. The descending hypoglossal nerve is medial to the internal jugular vein. The carotid sheath between the vein and the nerve is exposed and grasped with a Gerald's forceps. The sheath is opened sharply here and the artery is separated from the jugular vein using a sharp dissecting technique (Fig. 5.12). The common carotid artery is then isolated from its surrounding fascia, and an umbilical tape ligature is placed around it to help mobilize the artery from the sheath. The tape is passed through a length of a No. 8 French rubber catheter and will later form an occluding tourniquet (Fig 5.13). A Wheatlander retractor is positioned with the teeth of the retractor laterally against the sternomastoid muscle and medially against the subcutaneous tissue. Sharp dissection is carried out on the lateral side of the common carotid artery up to the carotid bifurcation. The external carotid ar-

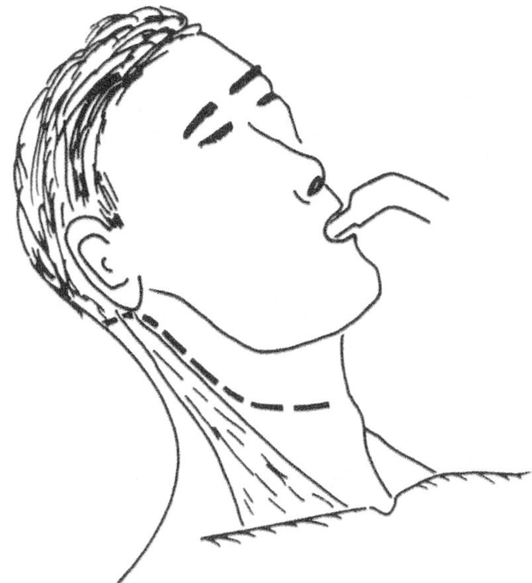

Figure 5.7. Incision for carotid endarterectomy is sigmoid-shaped with a posterior extension below the ear to avoid injury to the inferior auricular nerve. The incision follows the anterior border of the sternomastoid muscle down to about the level of the thyroid cartilage where it is then medially directed.

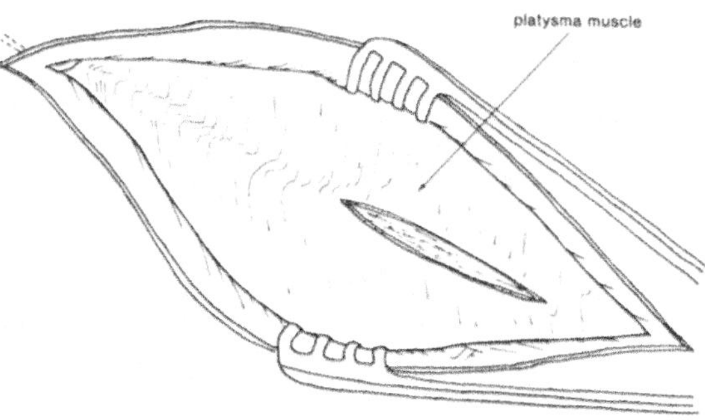

Figure 5.8. After incision in skin and subcutaneous tisseus, edges of the wound are retracted. Sternomastoid muscle may be palpated below the platysma. An oblique incision is made in the platysma muscle.

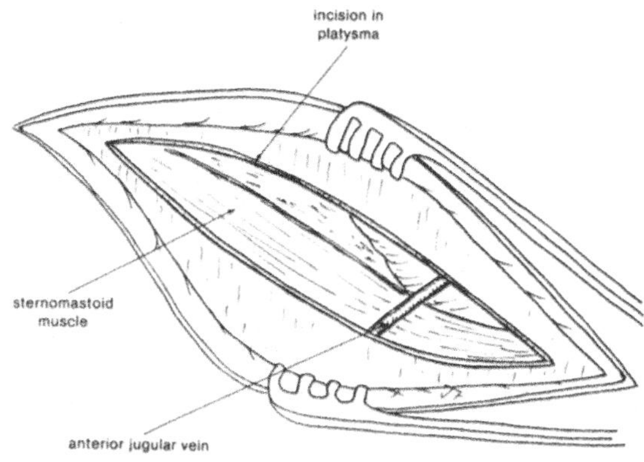

Figure 5.9. The incision through the platysma exposes the belly and fascia of the sternomastoid muscle. Care is taken not to injure the anterior jugular vein.

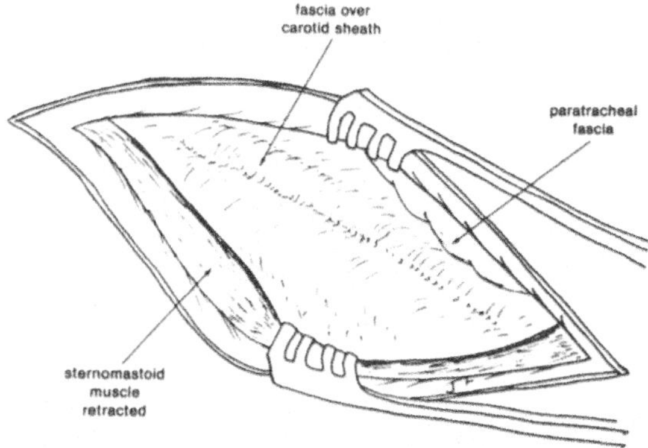

Figure 5.10. The fascia between the sternomastoid muscle laterally and the paratracheal fascia medially is opened, and underlying carotid sheath containing the internal jugular vein laterally and the carotid artery more medially is palpated.

tery and superior thyroid artery are exposed and isolated with an umbilical tape tourniquet (Fig. 5.14). After dissecting the internal carotid artery free from its fascial surroundings, it is isolated in a tourniquet (Fig. 5.15). It is usually necessary to mobilize the hypoglossal nerve before the distal portion of the internal carotid artery can be dissected free of its fascia. The hypoglossal nerve usually crosses the carotid bifurcation just below the digastric muscle, and a small branch artery and vein are within its

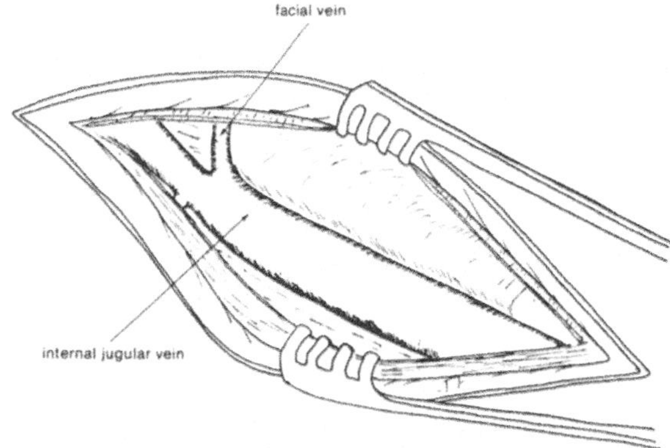

Figure 5.11. The internal jugular vein is usually encountered first and exposed so that it can be preserved. The facial vein crossing the mandible enters the internal jugular vein and may be divided if necessary.

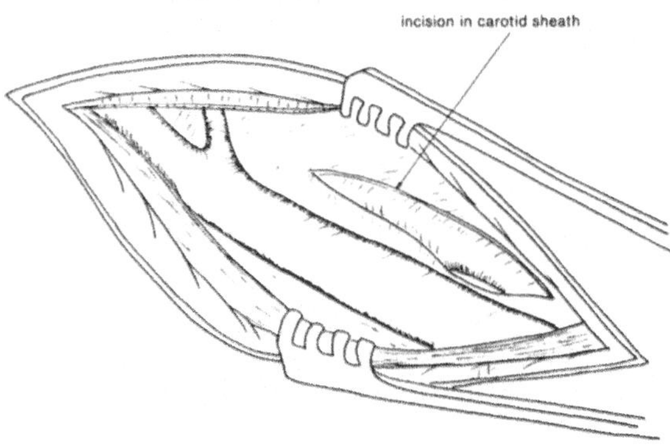

Figure 5.12. Carotid sheath around the common carotid artery is incised sharply and the artery is exposed.

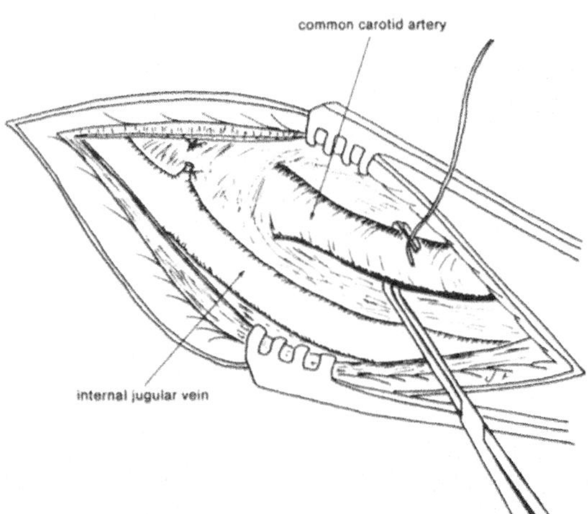

Figure 5.13. Carotid sheath is sharply dissected from the ventral surface of the common carotid artery and care is taken not to injure the underlying vagus nerve. The carotid artery is dessected free of the carotid sheath the vagus nerve and a right angle clamp is passed around the common carotid artery. An umbilical tape ligature is then passed with the clamp around the artery. The facial vein has been ligated and divided.

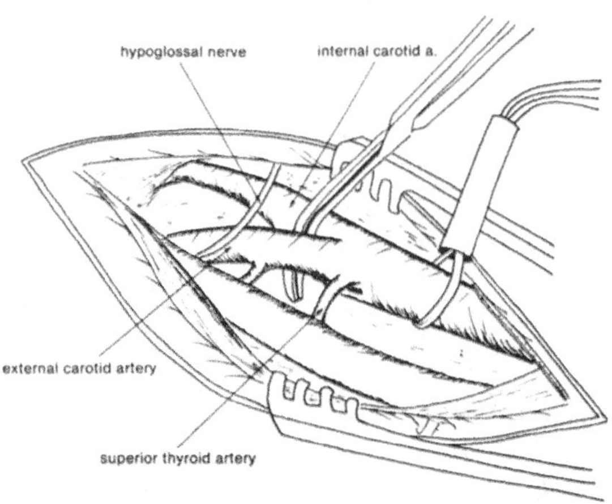

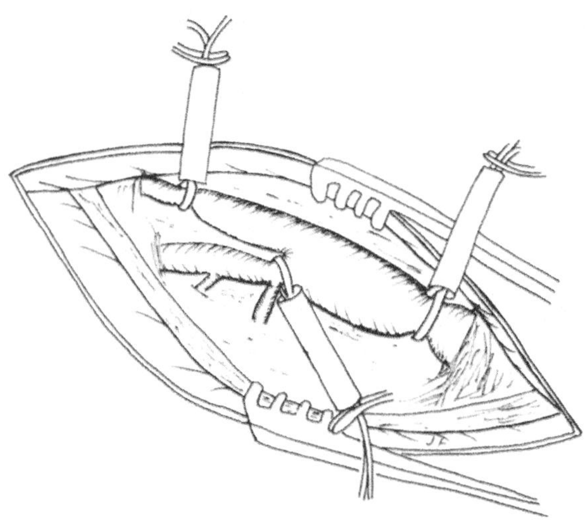

Figure 5.15. Umbilical tape ligatures have ben placed around the external carotid artery, including the superior thyroid artery in the ligature. Ligatures have also been placed around the common carotid and internal carotid arteries. If is often necessary to dissect and mobilize the hypoglossal nerve to obtain distal exposure of the internal carotid artery.

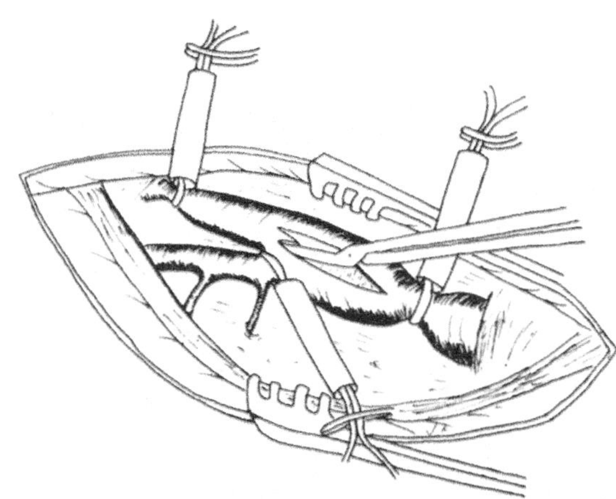

Figure 5.16. After stump pressure measurements have been made, the umbilical tape ligatures are closed. Arteriotomy is started with a no. 11 scalpel blade and continued with a Potts scissors. This author prefers to open both the artery and the plaque to expose the lumen of the plaque.

◁ **Figure 5.14.** The umbilical tape ligature tourniquet has been positioned around the common carotid artery. Dissection is then carried up the carotid sheath to the carotid bifurcation, usually identifiable by the superior thyroid artery branch. The external carotid artery and the superior thyroid artery are then isolated from the bifurcation.

neurovascular bundle. After the external carotid artery, internal carotid artery, and hypoglossal nerve are fully mobilized, the patient is given 5,000 units of heparin intravenously. The pressure in the common carotid artery is then measured through a No. 21 butterfly needle. Ligatures around the common and external carotid arteries are then closed and a repeat measurement is made which represents the ICA stump pressure.

At this point changes in the EEG associated with clamping are noted and a decision is made regarding the use of a shunt. It should be noted that there have been three schools of thought on the use of a shunt. Some advocate the routine use of a shunt,[96,161] others contend that a shunt should never be used.[21,56,180] A third school holds that shunts be used in selected cases[76,150–152] where preoperative assessment and intraoperative monitoring suggest that the patient may be at especially high risk for cerebral ischemia with clamping. This author agrees that the last approach is the most rational. Therefore, if the stump pressure is maintained above 50 mm Hg and there are no immediate changes in the EEG, a shunt is not used.

An arteriotomy incision is started on the common carotid artery with a No. 11 scalpel blade and the lumen is exposed. The incision is extended with a Potts scissor from a point 3 cm proximal to the common carotid artery bifurcation to a point 3 cm distal to the bifurcation on the internal carotid artery (Fig. 5.16). This incision should extend well beyond the distal end of the plaque (Fig. 5.17). In high-risk patients an intraluminal shunt is placed. The tapered shunt currently in use has a flange at either end and an irrigating channel at the center which is used to verify flow and to inject drugs. The distal end of the shunt is first passed up the internal carotid artery through the tourniquet, while the proximal end is closed with a rubber shod clamp. The proximal end is then threaded down the common carotid artery and secured with the tourniquet. Patency of each limb of the shunt is verified separately by noting back flow through the irrigating limb. Tension of the tourniquets may need to be readjusted accordingly.

The operating microscope is introduced and focused on the surface of the carotid artery. Endarterectomy is started with a microdissector (Fig. 5.18) in the cleavage plane between the plaque and the outer media.[29] The plane should be selected so that the stenosis is relieved and all ulcer craters are removed. A uniform plane is developed by passing a blunt microdissector around the vessel circumference (Fig. 5.19). The plane should be maintained throughout the length of the arteriotomy exposure. If a smooth plane is achieved, it is unnecessary to remove the outermost layer of plaque. If too much plaque is removed, the pink color of the adventitia becomes visible and should forewarn that perforation of the wall may occur. The plaque is then amputated proximally with a curved flat microscissor (Fig. 5.20). After the proximal plaque has been separated from the wall of the common carotid artery, it is dissected away from the orifice of the external carotid artery. It is useful to insert a blunt nerve hook between the plaque and the wall of the external carotid artery to separate the plaque cleanly from the orifice of the artery (Fig. 5.21). The plaque is cut sharply and dissected from the wall of the internal carotid artery. The plaque usually extends along the posterior wall for 3 to 5 mm beyond its termination on the anterior wall (Fig. 5.22). Thorough endarterectomy is required distally. The residual wall is inspected at 10× to 16× magnification to ensure that free debris or intimal tags do not remain. If a tag of plaque remains distally in the internal carotid artery, 7-0 prolene tacking sutures are placed vertically to secure it against the intima.[175] The same sequence is followed if an internal shunt is used (Figs. 5.23–5.25). The arteriotomy is then closed with a continuous 6-0 prolene suture (Fig. 5.26). Prior to completing the suture repair, the shunt is removed (Fig. 5.27), and the internal carotid artery tourniquet is loosened temporarily to allow back flow of air and debris through the arteriotomy opening. The arteriotomy is closed completely, and the common and external carotid tourniquets are opened to allow debris to pass into the external carotid artery. Finally, the internal carotid artery tourniquet is opened. Residual bleeding from the arteriotomy line can usually be managed with Gelfoam, cottonoids, and gentle pressure. Once hemostasis is achieved, a Jackson-Pratt drain is placed in the operative bed, and the muscle and subcutaneous layers are closed over the drain with Vicryl suture. The skin is closed with nylon suture.

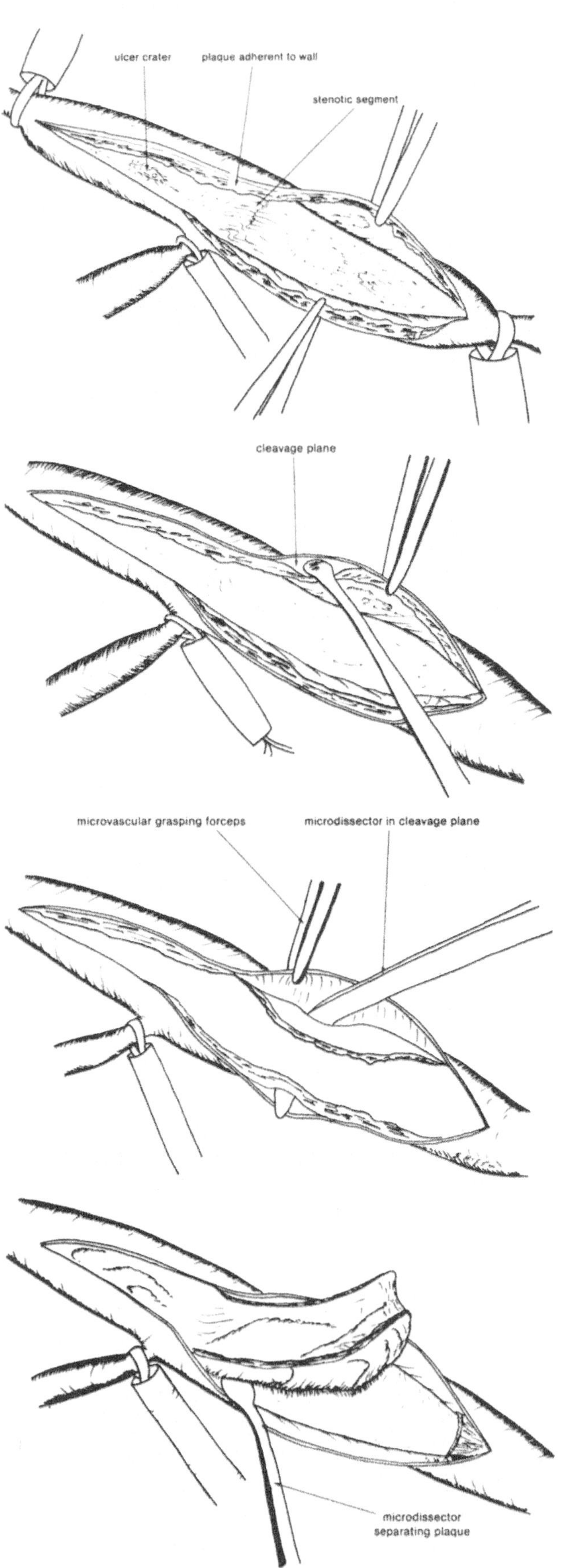

Figure 5.17. Arteriotomy has been completed. Atherosclerotic plaque extends from the common carotid artery through approximately 2 cm of the internal carotid artery. Both stenotic and ulcerative lesions are seen. Care is taken to use microvascular nontraumatic forceps to manipulate the arterial wall.

Figure 5.18. Dissection is started here without the use of an internal shunt. A microdissector is used with the microscope at 6–10 times magnification to develop a cleavage plane to be developed throughout the exposure.

Figure 5.19. Once this cleavage plane has been developed it is made continuous around the circumference of the carotid artery with a curved microdissector. This allows the same plane to be developed throughout the exposure.

Figure 5.20. The proximal portion of plaque in the common carotid artery has ben mobilized and amputated. The plaque is then mobilized as a single specimen from the common carotid artery toward the orifice of the external carotid artery.

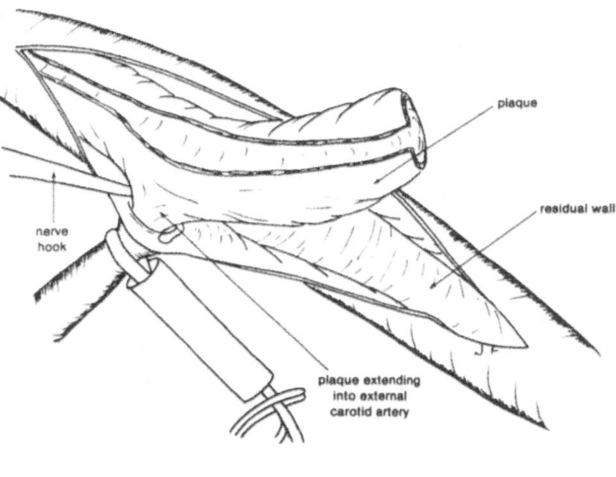

Figure 5.21. The plaque extending into the external carotid artery is mobilized completely and separated from the residual arterial wall. This can then be amputated so that residual fragments of plaque do not extend into the lumen of the common carotid artery.

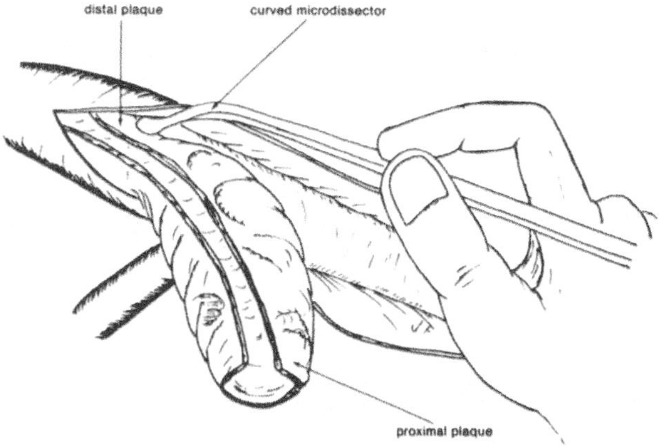

Figure 5.22. The plaque is then mobilized distally in the internal carotid artery maintaining the same cleavage plane between plaque and arterial wall.

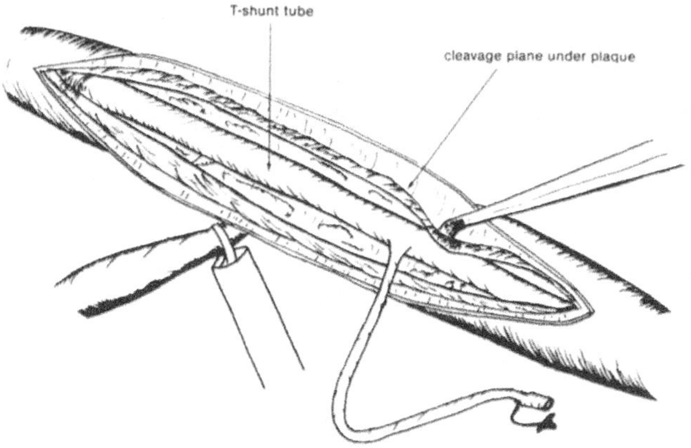

Figure 5.23. Use of an internal shunt is illustrated. Cleavage plane between plaque and arterial wall has been developed, and plaque will be mobilized underneath the shunt.

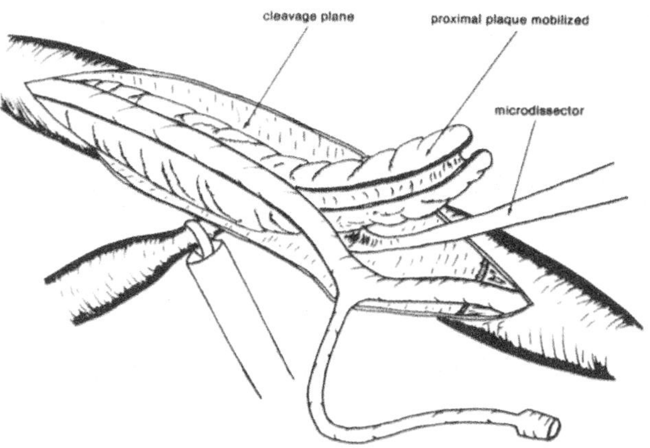

Figure 5.24. Proximal portion of plaque has been amputated, and the plaque is mobilized from the cleavage plane and to one side of the shunt.

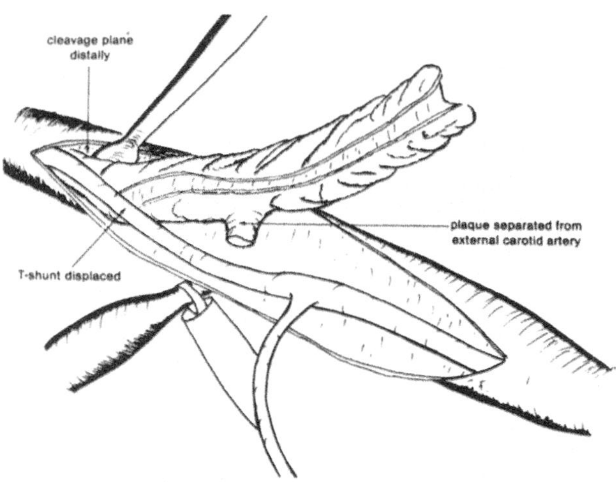

Figure 5.25. Distal portion of plaque is being mobilized. Proximal portion has been delivered out of the arteriotomy.

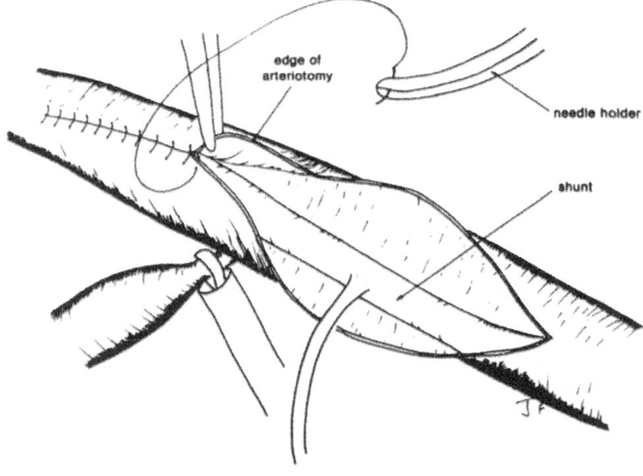

Figure 5.26. Once the plaque is completely mobilized and the surgeon is sure that there are no distal tags of plaque, the arteriotomy is closed with a continuous suture using 6-0 prolene. Suturing begins at the distal end and the shunt tube is oversewn.

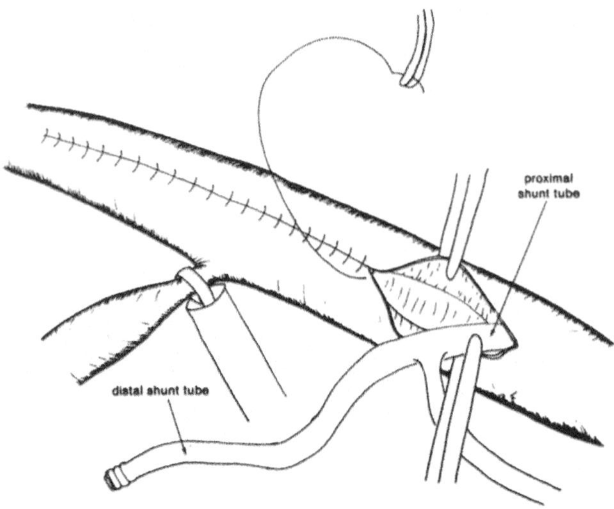

Figure 5.27. When most of the arteriotomy has been sutured, the distal end of the shunt is removed and the proximal portion of the shunt is removed. Tourniquets are reapplied and the arteriotomy is completely closed.

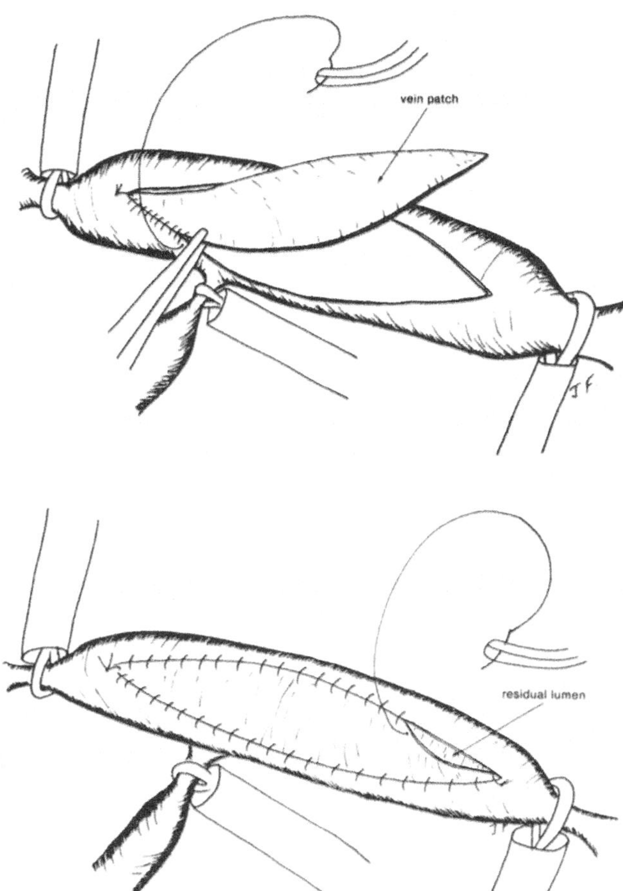

Figure 5.28. In a small number of cases a vein patch graft may be used to reduce the chances of postoperative stenosis. This has become significantly less frequent with use of the operating microscope. When a vein patch graft is utilized, the leading edge of the patch is sewn first on one side with a continuous suture technique using 7-0 prolene.

Figure 5.29. The second side of the graft is sutured. Before complete closure, back flow from the internal carotid artery is permitted to wash out air and debris. The internal carotid artery is reclampled. The common carotid and external carotid tourniquets are then opened to allow debris to wash into the external circulation. Finally, the internal carotid ligature is opened and reflow is established.

When the internal carotid artery is congenitally narrow or in cases of reoperation for postoperative stenosis, primary closure of the arteriotomy may further compromise the lumen.[108] A vein patch graft has been used to repair the carotid artery in 34 cases. The patch is positioned by placing one corner of the vein graft in the apex of the arteriotomy (Figs. 5.28,5.29). A double armed 6-0 prolene suture is used. If a shunt is used to maintain flow, it is removed before completing the second suture line.

Intraoperative Monitoring

A number of manuevers during surgery can induce ischemia or aggravate preexisting ischemic states. Manipulation of the artery, before or after the arteriotomy is made, or insertion or removal of a shunt can result in distal embolization. Alterations in blood pressure or temporary carotid clamping may also precipitate ischemic changes. Various monitoring techniques have been devised to detect the early changes of cerebral ischemia so that corrective action can be undertaken.

Electroencephalography

Electroencephalography is routinely used by the author to detect the presence of cerebral ischemia during surgery. A baseline EEG is performed prior to intubation with the patient fully awake. The EEG is then monitored continually thereafter. Symmetric leads were placed in frontal, central, occipital, and temporal areas. Recordings were bipolar to an electrode over the vertex at a paper speed of 30 mm/s. A symmetrical pattern dominated by 8 to 12 Hz rhythms with amplitudes ranging between 25 to 100 μV was found. Deeper levels of anesthesia produced symmetrically slower activity of 2 to 6 Hz with amplitudes ranging between 50 to 150 μV. In 40 patients with neurologic deficits before surgery, focal asymmetries were found on the awake EEG. These were further accentuated during anesthesia in 30 patients. There was a reduction of normal background activity associated with variable amounts of irregular slowing.

In 34 patients new EEG findings appeared during surgery (Table 5.2). Focal slowing (theta or delta wave activity) appeared after carotid clamping in 20 patients and a shunt was promptly placed. Normal background activity returned in 15 patients within two minutes and in 4 patients within five minutes. In one patient the shunt was not functional immediately because the proximal ligature on the common carotid artery was too tight. This problem was corrected five minutes later when the EEG pattern showed prompt improvement. In two patients bilateral slowing to theta frequencies was associated with relative hypotension and was corrected with an increase in blood pressure. Focal delta wave activity appeared during dissection and manipulation of the carotid artery in a 62-year-old patient who had an ulcerative plaque. An internal shunt was placed; however, the abnormal pattern persisted. He woke up with a new deficit, probably related to thromboembolism resulting from the manipulation. In one patient with ipsilateral stenosis and a contralateral occlusion, a contralateral delta focus and ipsilateral theta activity appeared during clamping and persisted despite placement of a shunt. He awoke with a new deficit referable to the contralateral hemisphere. In 10 patients EEG changes developed unrelated to the period of clamping or manipulation. In five of these patients the changes resolved spontaneously and in three the changes resolved with less anesthesia. In two patients the changes persisted, and both patients awoke with deficits that resolved within 24 hours in one and persisted in the other.

Table 5.2. EEG changes in 265 carotid endarterectomies.

	Number
I. Baseline EEG	
1. Normal before anesthesia	225
2. Abnormal before anesthesia	40
II. Anesthetic-induced changes	30
III. Intraoperative changes	34
1. Related to clamping	21
Reversed with shunt	19
Delayed reversal with shunt	1
Not reversed despite shunt	1
2. Related to hypotension	2
3. Related to manipulating carotid	1
4. Unknown causes	10
Reversed spontaneously	5
Reversed with decreased anesthesia	3
Not reversed	2

In Sharborough et al[142] 17 patients had major focal EEG changes within three minutes of carotid clamping. In all 17 patients an intraluminal shunt was used and this produced resolution of the focal changes within two to seven minutes after shunting. In eight patients there were major transient slowings not associated with carotid clamping. The authors rely on EEG changes to predict the presence of a postoperative neurologic deficit. Baker[7] utilized EEG in 213 elective carotid endarterectomies. Twenty-four patients developed EEG abnormalities after cross clamping of the common carotid artery. Seven patients developed alterations associated with episodes of bradycardia or hypotension. EEG abnormalities developed in four operations, despite stump pressures of 70 to 100 mm Hg. These abnormalities disappeared after insertion of a shunt.

Stump Pressure Measurements

Wright and Sweet[175] noted an increased incidence of ischemic symptoms after carotid ligation when distal intracarotid pressure was less than 50 mm Hg. Moore and Hall[123] first utilized stump pressure measurements during endarterectomy. Forty-eight endarterectomies were conducted under local anesthesia, during which stump pressure correlated with tolerance to clamping. Intolerant patients had stump pressures less than 25 mm Hg. Hobson et al[87] confirmed that stump pressures less than 25 mm Hg were consistently associated with intolerance.

On the other hand, pressures in excess of 25 or even 50 mm Hg did not necessarily protect patients from postoperative complications. Three patients with pressures above 50 mm Hg were unable to tolerate clamping of the carotid artery. Hays et al[82] studied a group of patients under general anesthesia and noticed a decrease in postoperative neurologic deficits when ICA back pressure exceeded 50 mm Hg. Between 41 and 50 mm Hg they felt that vasopressor agents alone would improve perfusion and increase tolerance to clamping.

Stump pressure measurements have been used to help decide whether a shunt should be used. This information is available as soon as the arteries are clamped whereas EEG changes may take several minutes to evolve. In normotensive individuals a shunt was used if stump pressure was less than 50 mm Hg or if focal EEG slowing was recognized. In hypertensive individuals a shunt was used if the stump pressure was less than 50% of resting mean blood pressure or if focal EEG slowing occurred. Internal carotid artery stump pressure was less than 50 mm Hg in 15% of normotensive patients and was reduced by more than 50% in 10% of hypertensive patients. We did not encounter any shunt-related complications.

Other methods to assess the adequacy of the cerebral circulation include measurement of jugular venous oxygen saturation,[112] direct measurement of internal carotid artery blood flow,[90] and regional cerebral blood flow.[18,152]

Regional Cerebral Blood Flow

Sundt[150–152] used intraoperative measurements of CBF as a guide for the placement of a shunt. The minimal CBF required to maintain a normal EEG under halothane anesthesia was 18 ml/100 g/min. Temporary shunts were used when a lower CBF was found. Boysen[18] studies the effects of CO_2 on the CBF level after carotid clamping. The average CBF reduction was only 17% during hypocapnia, but 27% and 47% during normocapnia and hypercapnia, respectively. This was probably related to the vasodilatation prior to the clamping and compromised autoregulation ability. By a combination of monitoring techniques, Trojaborg and Boysen[165] found characteristic EEG, stump pressure, and CBF changes in three groups of patients. In the first group CBF was 16 to 36 ml/100 g/min, and the average ICA pressure fell from 96 to 36 mm Hg. Significant EEG changes occurred in 14 patients. In 10 of these patients with EEG flattening, CBF averaged 14 ml/100 g/min, and the washout curve showed a plateau with clamping. In those with EEG slowing only, CBF averaged 18 ml/100 g/min. The EEG was unaffected in three patients with average CBF values of 20 ml/100 g/min. The second group consisted of 16 patients in whom CBF was diminished to 35 to 49 cc/100 g/min, and ICA stump pressures fell from 98 to 47 mm Hg. In six of these patients the EEG remained unchanged despite a reduction in CBF by more than 30%. In the third group of 30 patients CBF was unchanged after test occlusion, ICA pressure fell from 99 to 78 mm Hg, and the mean EEG frequency was unchanged.

Postoperative Considerations

Immediately after extubation, hypertension is exacerbated in most patients with chronic hypertension. This will generally persist and become more severe unless treated and can lead to increased bleeding in the operative bed or from the suture line. Propranolol HCl (Inderal) or methyldopa (Aldomet) is used to lower blood pressure gradually. Postoperative management is then carried out in an intensive care unit for one or two days. Vital signs, serial neurologic observation, and fluid intake and output are recorded on an hourly basis. The ECG is continually monitored. Careful attention should be paid to the patient's mental status and to evidence of restlessness. Local cervical complications may be heralded by irritability, swelling under the dressing, hoarseness, dysphonia, difficulty in swallowing, secretions, or wheezing. If the larynx is displaced by focal mass or swelling, it may be difficult to visualize the vocal cords for endotracheal reintubation. A tracheostomy set should therefore be kept by the bedside and used immediately if reintubation is not successful. The Jackson-Pratt drain is generally removed within 24 hours of surgery. Oral liquids are given on the first postoperative day and advanced to a solid diet on the second postoperative day.

Healing After Carotid Endarterectomy

The histologic changes occurring after endarterectomy[72] explain the tendency for early thrombosis. The adventitia is usually exposed to the lumen after endarterectomy. The luminal surface becomes covered with platelets and fibrin immediately after flow is reestablished. Thrombus formation is then active for 48 hours, but is markedly reduced by intraoperative heparin.[134] After 48 hours inflammatory changes are routinely observed, particularly when the residual media is very thin. These changes further predispose to thrombus formation. After approximately one week reendothelialization may be extensive and is often complete within three months after surgery. The new endothelium originates from adjacent endothelium, and the long axis of the endothelial cells are aligned parallel to the long axis of the vessel. There is less thrombus formation on the surface of vein patch grafts with an intact endothelium than on the adjacent endarterectomized arterial surface.[45]

Complications

The morbidity and mortality of carotid endarterectomy are related to systemic, local, and neurovascular complications.[46,71]

Systemic Complications

Cardiac complications developed in patients who had preoperative evidence of either atherosclerotic or hypertensive cardiac disease. Both major and minor complications developed in 14% of the patients in this series. Atrial arrhythmias were the most common problems followed in frequency by electrocardiographic evidence of endocardial infarction. Two patients had an acute myocardial infarction on the first postoperative day and died. Other systemic complications in order of frequency included urinary tract infections, pneumonia, and transient liver parenchymal enzyme changes.

Local Complications

The early signs of wound hematoma include neck swelling, hoarseness, and difficulty with secretions. This should be distinguished from swelling of the sternomastoid muscle, which is usually less severe and does not compromise the airway. Wound hematoma occurred in two patients within 24 hours of surgery and was evacuated promptly with no sequelae.

Infection of the operative site has been described,[141,142] but has not occurred in the author's series. Infection may spread to the region of the arteriotomy so that aggressive treatment of such a complication is warranted. A cellulitis of the skin edges may be treated with intravenous antibiotics; however, if there is any suspicion that an abscess is present, the wound should be drained.

The hypoglossal nerve may sustain a traction injury during its mobilization, or may be injured when the cautery is used to coagulate small branches of the facial vein prior to its mobilization. Hypoglossal paralysis was one of the more common complications in our series, occurring in six patients. In four patients it resolved within six months of surgery, but in two patients the weakness persisted for one and three years, respectively.

The vagus nerve or recurrent laryngeal nerve may be injured and result in hoarseness. Indirect laryngoscopy will confirm the presence of vocal cord paralysis. This complication occurred in three patients, but resolved spontaneously in two of these individuals. One patient is still hoarse two years after surgery.

Injury to the lower branches of the facial nerve occurs when the dissection is carried up to the parotid gland. This occurred in one case, but is avoidable if the superior aspect of the incision is directed posteriorly (Fig. 5.7)

A vertical skin incision will interrupt cutaneous cervical nerves and result in hypalglesia of the skin in the anterior cervical triangle. This tends to resolve in six months to a year. This complication can be minimized by the oblique incision.

Neurovascular Complications

A series of neurovascular complications may occur in the perioperative period and are usually related to intraoperative technical errors. These are the most serious problems associated with carotid endarterectomy and demand expeditious action. When a patient experiences a TIA postoperatively, a carotid angiogram should be performed. This will invariably show some degree of irregularity of the vessel lumen. Experience in the interpretation of these findings is required to differentiate normal postoperative changes from significant technical errors. Acute carotid thrombosis, however, may be suspected when rapid deterioration occurs in the first 24 hours postoperatively. Other considerations include intracerebral hematoma or cerebral infarction due to emboli. If a CT scan is unrevealing, immediate reexploration of the wound is indicated. Flow may be reestablished with reversal of the deficit if prompt thrombectomy is accomplished. The endarterectomy site is carefully inspected with the microscope to determine if there are specific reasons for thrombus formation such as fragments of plaque, poor arteriotomy suturing technique, stenosis of the suture line or intimal flaps. Each of these problems should be corrected. Postoperative thrombisis developed in three patients. A mild deficit was found in one patient with good collateral circulation, and a profound hemiplegia and aphasia developed in two patients with bilateral carotid disease.

Intraoperative manipulations of the carotid artery may release emboli. Hoyt observed numerous instances of microemboli in the retinal arteries of patients within a few hours following routine endarterectomy.[92] Serial opthalmoscopic examinations are performed postoperatively. In one patient an intravenous heparin infusion was started in a patient who had repeated retinal emboli on the third postoperative day.

Disruption of the suture line may be caused by errors in suturing, such as taking an inadequate bite of tissue. Uneven tension along a continuous suture alone may lead to postoperative bleeding. This has not occurred in the author's series, but has been reported by others.[20,145]

The use of a Fogarty catheter for removing thrombus from the distal portion of the internal carotid artery was described by Davie and Richardson.[36] In several reported cases[10,50,106,124,128] a carotid cavernous fistula was produced by this manuever. This has not occurred in any of the five patients in our series in which the technique was used to remove fresh thrombus. In one patient, however, a dissecting aneurysm of the internal carotid artery was produced by this technique.

It is worth reiterating that carotid endarterectomy is of demonstrated value in properly selected cases. Patient selection has been facilitated by newly developed noninvasive diagnostic techniques and modernized angiographic methods.[53] Microsurgical instrumentation has improved the precision of endarterectomy and monitoring techniques have helped reduce the intraoperative risks inherent in patients with a poor collateral circulation.

References

1. Acheson J, Hutchison EC: Observatioins on the natural history of transient cerebral ischemia. Lancet 2:871–874, 1964
2. Acheson J, Hutchison EC: The natural history of focal cerebral vascular disease. O J Med, 40: 15–23, 1971
3. Ames A III, Wright RL, Kawada M, Thurston JM, Majano G: Cerebral ischemia. II. The No-reflow phenomenon. Am J Pathol 52:437–453, 1968
4. Anderson CA, Rich NM, Collins GJ, McDonald PT: Unilateral internal carotid occlusion: Special considerations. Stroke 8:669–671, 1977
5. Baker WH: Diagnosis and Treatment of Carotid Artery Disease. Futura Publishing Co, Mt Kisco, New York, 1979, p 128
6. Baker RN, Broward JA, Fang HC et al: Anticoagulant therapy in cerebral infarction. Neurology 12:823–835, 1962
7. Baker JD, Gluecklich B, Watson CW, Marcus E, Kamat V, Callow A: An evaluation of electroencephalographic monitoring for carotid study. Surgery 78:787–794, 1975
8. Baker RN, Ramseyer JC, Schwartz W: Prognosis in patients with transient cerebral ischemic attacks. Neurology 18:1157–1165, 1968
9. Baker RN, Schwartz W, Rose AS: Transient ischemic attacks—a report of a study of anticoagulant treatment. Neurology 16:841–847, 1966
10. Barker WF, Stein WE, Kragenbuhl H et al: Carotid endarterectomy complicated by carotid cavernous sinus fistula. Ann Surg 167:568–572, 1968
11. Bauer RB, Meyer TS, Fields WS, Remington R, MacDonald MC, Collen P: Joint study of extracranial arterial occlusion. III. Progress report of controlled study of long term survival in patients with and without operation. JAMA 208:509–518, 1969
12. Bauer RB, Meyer JS, Gotham JE, Gilroy J: A controlled study of surgical treatment of cerebrovascular disease—42 months experience with 183 cases. In Millikan C, Sickert R, Whis-

nant JP (eds.): Cerebral Vascular Disease. Grune & Stratton, New York, 1966
13. Benson RL: Prestent status of coronary arterial disease. Arch Pathol 2:786–916, 1926
14. Blaisdell FW, Clauss RH, Galbraith JG, et al: Joint study of extracranial arterial occlusion. IV A review of surgical considerations. JAMA 209:1889–1895, 1969
15. Blaisdell FW, Hall AD, Thomas AN: Surgical treatment of chronic internal carotid artery occlusion by saline endarterectomy. Ann Surg, 163:103–111, 1966
16. Blaisdell FW, Lim R, Hall AD: Technical results of carotid endarterectomy: Arteriographic assessment. Am J Surg 114:239, 1967
17. Bousser MG, Eschwege E, Haguenau M, Lefaucconnier JM, Thibult N, Touboul D, Touboul PJ: "AICLA" Controlled trial of aspirin and Dipyridamole in the secondary prevention of athero-thrombotic cerebral ischemia. Stroke 14:5–14, 1983
18. Boysen G: Cerebral hemodynamics in carotid surgery. Acta Neurol Scand (Suppl) 52,V.49:1–84, 1973
19. Boysen G, Engell HC, Henriksen H: Effect of uninduced hypertension on internal carotid artery pressure and regional cerebral blood flow during temporary carotid clamping for endarterectomy. Neurology 22:1133–1144, 1972
20. Bland JE, Chapman RD, Wylie EJ: Neurological complications of carotid artery surgery. Ann Surg 171:459–464, 1970
21. Bloodwell RD, Hallman GL, Keats AS, Cooley DA: Carotid endarterectomy without a shunt. Results using hypercarbic general anesthesia to prevent cerebral ischemia. Arch Surg 96:644–651, 1968
22. Brice JE, Dowsett DJ, Lowe RD: Haemodynamic effects of carotid artery stenosis. Br Med J 2:1363–1366, 1964
23. Browly BW: The pathophysiology of intracerebral steal following carbon dioxide inhalation, an experimental study. Scand J Clin Lab Invest (Suppl) 102, XIII:B, 1968
24. Bruteman ME, Fields WS, Crawford ES, DeBakey ME: Cerebral hemorrhage in carotid artery surgery. Arch Neurol 9:458, 1969
25. Canadian Cooperative Study Group: A randomized trial of aspirin and sulfinpyrozone in threatened stroke. N Engl J Med 299:53–59, 1978
26. Carney NI, Stewart WB, DePinto DJ et al: Carotid bruit at a risk factor in aortorilliae reconstruction. Surgery 81:567, 1977
27. Carter AB: Anticoagulant treatment in progressive stroke. Br Med J 2:70–73, 1961
28. Cassidy J: Management of risk factors and other diseases in candidates for microneurosurgical anastomosis in cerebral ischemia. In Fein J, Reichman OH: Microvascular Anastomosis for Cerebral Ischemia. Springer Verlag, New York, 1978
29. Chochinov H, VanWijhe M: The plane of dissection in endarterectomy. Can J Surg 8:10–14, 1965
30. Christensen MS, Holdt-Rosmussen K, Lassen NA: Cerebral vasodilatation by halothane anesthesia in man and its potentiation by hypotension and hypercapnia. Br J Anesth 39:927–934, 1967
31. Clark L: A-V oxygen differences in the protection of cerebral fissures during decreased cerebral blood flow. In Cerebral Vascular Diseases. Fifth Princeton Conference. Grune & Stratton, New York, 1966, pp 210–217
32. Cormally JE: Discussion in Ehrenfeld WK, Hamilton FN, Larson CP, Hickey RF, Severinghaus JW: Effect of CO_2 and systemic hypertension on downstream cerebral arterial pressure during carotid endarterectomy. Surgery 67:87–96, 1970
33. Correl JW, Stern J, Zyroff J, Whelan M: Vertebrobasilar insufficiency relieved by carotid surgery. In Marguth F, Brock M, Kazner E, Klinger M, Schmiedek P (eds.): Advances in Neurosurgery V7, Neurovascular Surgery—Specialized Neurosurgical Techniques. Springer Verlag, Berlin, 1979
34. Craig DR, Meguro K, Watridge C, Robertson JT, Barnett HJ, Fox AJ: Intracranial internal cartoid artery stenosis. Stroke 13:825–828, 1982
35. Crawford ES, DeBakey ME, Garrett HE, Howell J: Surgical treatment of occlusive cerebrovascular disease. Surg Clin North Am 46:873–884, 1966
36. Davie JE, Richardson R: Distal internal carotid thrombo-embolectomy using a Fogarty catheter in total occlusion. J Neurosurg 27:171–177, 1967
37. DeBakey ME, Crawford ES, Cooley DA, Morris CC Jr, Garrett HE, Fields WS: Cerebral arterial insufficiency: one to 11-year results following arterial reconstructive operation. Ann Surg 161:921–945, 1965
38. DeBakey ME, Crawford ES, Morris GC Jr, Cooley DA: Surgical considerations of occlusive disease of the inominate, carotid, subclavian and vertebral arteries. Ann Surg 154:698–725, 1961
39. Denny-Brown D: Treatment of recurrent cerebrovascular symptoms and the question of "vasospasm". Med Clin North Am 35:1457–1474, 1951

40. Denny-Brown D, Meyer JS: The cerebral collateral circulation. 2. Production of cerebral infarction by ischemic anoxia and its reversibility in early stages. Neurology 7:567–579
41. Denton IC, Gutman L: Surgical treatment of symptomatic carotid stenosis and asymptomatic ipsilateral intravascular aneurysm. Case report. J Neurosurg 38:662–665, 1973
42. DeWeese JA, Robb CG, Satran R, Marsh DO, Joynet RJ, Summers D, Nichols C: Results of carotid endarterectomies for transient ischemic attacks—five years later. Ann Surg 178:258–264, 1973
43. Diaz F, Hussman JE, de los Reyes RA, Dujovny M: Successful application of acute cerebral revascularization to stroke in evolution. Presented at annual meeting. Am Heart Assoc, Dallas, Texas, Nov, 1982
44. Dinman FR, Ehni G, Duty WS: Insidious thrombotic occlusion of cervical carotid arteries, treated by arterial graft. A case report. Surgery 38:569–577, 1955
45. Dirrenberger RA, Sundt TM Jr: Carotid endarterectomy: Temporal profile of the healing process and effects of anticoagulation therapy. J Neurosurg 48:201–219, 1978
46. Dunsker SB: Complications of carotid endarterectomy. Clin Neurosurg 23:336–34, 1975
47. Dyken ML, Klutte E, Kolar OJ, Spurgeon C: Complete occlusion of common or internal carotid arteries. Arch Neurol 30:343–346, 1974
48. Easton JD, Sherman DG: Stroke and mortality rate in carotid endarterectomy: 228 consecutive operations. Stroke 8:565–568, 1977
49. Edwards JH, Kricheff II, Riles TS, Imparato AH: Angiographically undetected ulceration of the carotid bifurcation as a cause of embolic stroke. Radiology 132:369–373, 1979
50. Eggers F, Lukin R, Chambers A, Tomsick T, Sawaya R: Iatrogenic carotid-cavernous fistula following Fogarty catheter thrombendarterectomy. J Neurosurg 51:543–545, 1979
51. Ehrenfeld WK, Hamilton FN, Larson CP, Hickery RF, Severinghaus JW: Effect of CO_2 and systemic hypertension on downstream cerebral arterial pressure during carotid endarterectomy. Surgery 67:87–96, 1970
52. Evans WE, Cooperman M: The significance of asymptomatic carotid bruits in pre-operative patients. Presented at the Midwestern Vascular Surgical Society, Chicago, Illinois, Sept, 1977
53. Fein J: A history of surgery of cerebrovascular disease. In Smith R (ed.): Strokes and the Extracranial Arteries. Raven Press, New York, 1984
54. Fein J, Lantos G: Surgical management of patients with carotid occlusions and contralateral stenosis. Neurosurgery (In Press)
55. Fein JM, Waldemar Y: Pathology of specimens removed during carotid endarterectomy. Neurosurgery (In Press)
56. Ferguson GG: Intraoperative monitoring and internal shunts: Are they necessary in carotid endarterectomy? Stroke 13:287–289, 1982
57. Fields WS, Lemak NA: Joint Study of Extracranial Arterial Occlusion VII. Subclavian Steal—A Review of 168 Cases. JAMA 222:1139–1143, 1972
58. Fields WS, Lemak NA: Joint study of extracranial arterial occlusion IX. Transient ischemic attacks in the carotid territory. JAMA 235:2608–2610, 1976
59. Fields WS, Lemak NA: Joint study of extracranial arterial occlusion. X. Internal carotid artery occlusion. JAMA 235:2734–2738, 1976
60. Fields WS, Lemak NA, Frankowski RF et al: Controlled trial of aspirin in cerebral ischemia. Stroke 8:301–316, 1977
61. Fields WS, Maslenikov V, Meyer JS, Hass WK, Remington RP, MacDonald M: Joint study of extracranial arterial occlusion. V. Progress report of prognosis following surgery or nonsurgical treatment for transient cerebral ischemic attacks and cervical carotid artery lesions. JAMA 211:1993–2003, 1970
62. Fields WS, North RR, Hass WK, Galbraith TG, Wylie EJ, Ratenar G, Burns MH, MacDonald MC, Meyer JS: Joint study of extracranial arterial occlusion as a cause of stroke. I. Organization of study and survey of patient population. JAMA 203:153–158, 1968
63. Fisher CM: Use of anticoagulants in cerebral thrombosis. Neurology 8:311–332, 1958
64. Fisher CM: Observations of the fundus oculi in transient monocular blindness. Neurology 9:333–347, 1959
65. Fisher CM: Anticoagulant therapy in cerebral thrombosis and cerebral embolism. A national cooperative study, interim report. Neurology 11:119–131, 1961
66. Fisher CM: Discussion in McDowell FH, Brennan RW (eds.): Cerebral Vascular Diseases. Eighth Princeton Conference, Grune and Stratton, New York, 1973, pp 216
67. Fisher M: Occlusion of the internal carotid artery. Arch Neurol Psychiatry 65:346–377, 1951
68. Foerster O, Guttman L: Cerebral komplikationen bei thrombangiitis obliterans. Arch Psychiat 100:506, 1933
69. Ford J, Baker WH, Ehrenhoft JL: Carotid endarterectomy for nonhemispheric transient ischemic attack. Arch Surg 110:1314–1317, 1975

70. Fourcade HE, Larson CP, Ehrenfeld WH, Heshy RF, Newton TH: The effects of CO_2 and systemic hypertension on cerebral perfusion pressure during carotid endarterectomy. Anesthesiology 33:383–390, 1970
71. Fraser RAR, Corell J, Fein J: Complications of carotid endarterectomy Panel Discussion. Neurosurgery New York City, New York, Nov 1982
72. French BN, Rescastle NB: Sequential morphological changes at the site of carotid endarterectomy. J Neurosurg 41:745–754, 1974
73. Friedman GR, Wilson S, Mosier JM, Colandrea MA, Nickamon HZ: Transient ischemic attacks in a community. JAMA 210:1428–1431, 1969
74. Furlan AJ, Whisnant JP: Long term prognosis following carotid artery occlusion. Stroke 10:105, 1979
75. Furlan AJ, Whisnant JP, Baker HL Jr: Long term prognosis after carotid artery occlusion. Neurology 30:986–988, 1980
76. Galbraith JG: Safeguards in carotid surgery. Surgery 63:1019–1023, 1968
77. Goldner JC, Whisnant JP, Taylor MF: Long-term prognosis of transient cerebral ischemic attacks. Stroke 2:160–167, 1971
78. Goldstone J, Moore WS: Emergency carotid artery surgery in neurologically unstable patients. Arch Surg 111:1284–1291, 1976
79. Gomensoro JB, Maslenikov V, Azambuja N, Fields WS, Lemak NA: Joint study of extracranial arterial occlusion. JAMA 224:985–991, 1973
80. Hass WK, Fields WS, North RR, Kricheff II, Chase NE, Bauer RB: Joint study of extracranial arterial occlusion. II. Arteriography, techniques, sites and complications. JAMA 203:159–166, 1968
81. Hardy WG, Lindner DW, Thomas LM, Gurdjian ES: Anticipated clinical course in carotid artery occlusion. Arch Neurol 6:64–76, 1962
82. Hays RJ, Levinson SA, Wylie EJ: Intraoperative measurement of carotid back pressure as a guide to operative management for carotid endarterectomy. Surgery 72:953–960, 1972
83. Heilbrun P: Overall management of vascular lesions considered treatable with EC-IC bypass—Part I. Neurosurgery 11:239–245, 1982
84. Hertzer NR, Beven EG, Greenstreet RL, Humphries AW: Internal carotid back pressure, intraoperative shunting, ulcerated atheromata, and the incidence of stroke during carotid endarterectomy. Surgery 83:306–312, 1978
85. Heyman A: Discussion in Clark L: A-V oxygen differences in the protection of cerebral tissues during decreased cerebral blood flow. In Millikan C, Siekert R, Whisnant J: Cerebral Vascular Diseases, Fifth Conference, Grune & Stratton, New York, 1966, p 219
86. Heyman A, Felch WS, Kentery RD: Joint study of extracranial arterial occlusion. VI. Racial differences in hospitalized patients with ischemic stroke. JAMA 222:285–289, 1972
87. Hobson RW, Rich NM, Wright C, Fedde N: Operative assessment of carotid endarterectomy: internal carotid arterial back pressure, carotid arterial blood flow, and carotid arteriography. Am Surg 41:603–610, 1975
88. Hobson RW, Wright CB, Sublett JW, Fedde CW, Rich NM: Carotid artery back pressure and endarterectomy under regional anesthesia. Arch Surg 109:682–687, 1974
89. Hollenhorst RW: Significance of bright plaques in the retinal arteries. JAMA 178:23–29, 1961
90. Homi J, Humphries AW, Young JR, Beven EG, Smart JF: Hyperbaric anesthesia in cerebrovascular surgery. Surgery 59:57–65, 1966
91. Houser OW, Baker HL: Fibromuscular dysplasia and other uncommon diseases of the cervical carotid artery: angiographic aspects. Am J Roentgenol 104:201–212, 1968
92. Hoyt WF: Ocular symptoms and signs. Wylie EJ, Ehrenfeld WK (eds.): Extracranial Cerebrovascular Disease: Diagnosis and Management. WB Saunders Co, Philadelphia, 1970
93. Hunt JR: The role of the carotid arteries in the causation of vascular lesions of the brain, with remarks on certain special features of the symptomatology. Am J Med Sci 147:704–713, 1914
94. Hunter JA, Julian OC, Aye WS, Javid H: Emergency operation for acute cerebral ischemia due to carotid artery obstruction: Review of 26 cases. Ann Surg 162:901–904, 1965
95. Hutchinson EC, Yates PO: Carotico-vertebral stenosis. Lancet, 1:2, 1957
96. Javid H, Julian OC, Nye WS et al: Seventeen year experience with routine shunting in carotid artery surgery. World J Surg 3:167–177, 1979
97. Javid H, Ostermiller WE, Hengesh JW, Dye WS, Hunter JA, Najafi H, Julian OC: Natural history of carotid bifurcation atheroma. Surgery 67:80–86, 1970
98. Jennet WB, Ledinghan I McA, Harper AM, Smelbe GD, Miller JD: The effect of hyperbaric oxygen during carotid surgery. In Brock M, Fieschi C, Ingvar D, Lassen NA, Schurmann K (eds.): Cerebral Blood Flow. Springer Verlag, Berlin, 1969, pp 159–160
99. Julian OC, Javid H: Surgical management of cerebral arterial insufficiency. Curr Probl Surg 1971
100. Kallorits CR, Lubow M, Hissong SL: Retinal strokes. I. Incidence of carotid artheroma. JAMA 222:1273–1275, 1972

101. Kartchner MM: Oculoplethysmography in detection of carotid artery disease. Presented at Non-invasive Diagnostic Technique in Vascular Disease. San Diego, California, March, 1977
102. Kobayashi S, Hollenhorst RW, Sundt TM Jr: Retinal artery pressure before and after surgery for carotid artery stenosis. Stroke 2:569–575, 1971
103. Kurtzke JF: Controversy in neurology. The Canadian study of TIA and aspirin, a critique of the Canadian TIA study. Ann Neurol 5:597–599, 1979
104. Lee LF, Johnson ER, Perry MO, Strong MJ: Anesthetic problems in carotid endarterectomy. In Jenkens MT (ed.): Clinical Anesthesiology. Davis Co, Philadelphia, 1968, pp 248–261
105. Leob C, Meyer JS: Strokes Due to Vertebro Basilar Disease. Charles C Thomas, Springfield, 1965
106. Levin SM, Sondheimer FK: Stenosis of the contralateral asymptomatic carotid artery—to operate or not? Vasc Surg 7:3–13, 1973
107. Levine HL, Ferris EJ, Spatz EL: Carotid-cavernous fistula—iatrogenic carotid cavernous fistula due to thrombectomy with a Fogarty catheter. Rev Interam Radiol 1:105–106, 1978
108. Lin PM, Javid H, Doyle EJ: Partial internal carotid artery occlusion treated by primary resection and vein graft. J Neurosurg 13:650–655, 1956
109. Lippman HH, Sundt TM Jr, Holman CB: The post stenotic carotid slim sign, spurious internal carotid hypoplasia. Mayo Clin Proc 45:762–767, 1970
110. Lusby RJ, Ferrell LD, Ehrenfeld WK, Stoney RJ, Wylie EJ: Carotid plaque hemorrhage. Arch Surg 117:1479–1488, 1982
111. Lyons C, Galbraith G: Surgical treatment of atherosclerotic occlusion of the internal carotid artery. Ann Surg 146:487–496, 1957
112. Lyons SE, Clark LC, McDowell H, McArther K: Cerebral venous oxygen content during carotid thrombintinectomy. Ann Surg 160:561–566, 1964
113. Marshall J: The natural history of transient ischemic cerebrovascular attacks. QJ Med 33:309–324, 1964
114. McDowall DG: The effects of clinical concentration of halothane on the blood flow and oxygen uptake of the cerebral cortex. Br J Anesth 39:186–196, 1967
115. McNamara JO, Heyman A, Silver D, Mandel HE: The value of carotid endarterectomy in treating transient cerebral ischemia of the posterior circulation. Neurology 27:682–684, 1977
116. Millikan CH: Treatment of Occlusive Cerebrovascular Disease. In Seidert RG (ed.): Cerebrovascular Surgery Report. Joint Council Subcommittee on Cerebrovascular Disease NINCDS, Bethesda, Md, pp 244–289
117. Millikan CH, Siekert RG: Studies in cerebrovascular disease. I. The syndrome of intermittent insufficiency of the basilar arterial system. Proc Stroke Meet Mayo Clin 30:61–68, 1955
118. Millikan CH, Siekert RG, Shick RM: Studies in cerebrovascular disease. V. The use of anticoagulant drugs in the treatment of intermittent insufficiency of the internal carotid arterial system. Proc Stroke Meet Mayo Clin 30:578–586, 1955
119. Millikan CH, Siekert RG, Whisnant JP (eds.): Cerebral Vascular Disease. Fourth Princeton Conference, Grune & Stratton, New York, 1965, p 183
120. Mitchenfelder JD, Sundt TM Jr: The effect of $PaCO_2$ on the metabolism of ischemic brain in squirrel monkeys. Anesthesiology 38:445–453, 1973
121. Moore WS, Boren C, Malone JM, Roon AJ, Eisenberg R, Goldstone J, Mani R: Natural history of nonstenotic asymptomatic ulcerative lesions of the carotid artery. Arch Surg 113:1352–1359, 1978
122. Moore WS, Hall AD: Ulcerated atheroma of the carotid artery. A cause of transient cerebral ischemia. Am J Surg 116:237–242, 1968
123. Moore WS, Hall AD: Carotid artery back pressures. A test of cerebral tolerance to temporary carotid occlusion. Arch Surg 99:702–709, 1969
124. Motarjeme A, Keifer JW: Carotid cavernous sinus fistula as a complication of carotid endarterectomy. A case report. Radiology 108:83–84, 1973
125. Murphy F, Maccubin DA: Carotid endarterectomy—a long-term follow up study. J Neurosurg 23:156–168, 1965
126. Myer WW: Cholesterinkristallembolie Kleine Organarterien und ihre Folgen. Virchows Arch (Path Anat) 314–616, 1947
127. Newton TH: Radiologic diagnosis of ulcerated atherosclerotic plaque. In McDowell FH, Brenan RW (eds.): Cerebrovascular Diseases. Eighth Conference. Grune & Stratton, New York, 1973, pp 257–259
128. Newton TH, Troost BT: Arteriovenous malformations and fistulae. In Newton TH, Potts DG (eds.): Radiology of the Skull and Brain, Vol. 2, Book 4, CV Mosby, St Louis, 1974, pp 2490–2565
129. Nunn DB: Carotid endarterectomy. Analysis of 234 operative cases. Ann Surg 182:733–738, 1975
130. Ojemann RG, Crowell RM, Roberson GH,

Fisher CM: Surgical treatment of extracranial carotid occlusive disease. Clin Neurosurg 22:214–263, 1974
131. Ollson JE, Muller R, Berneli S: Long term anticoagulant therapy for TIA's and minor stroke with minimum residuum. Stroke 7:444–451, 1976
132. Patterson RH: Risk of carotid surgery with occlusion of the contralateral carotid artery. Arch Neurol 30:188–189, 1974
133. Pearce JMS, Gubbay SS, Walton JM: Long-term anticoagulant therapy in TIA. Lancet 1:6–9, 1965
134. Piepgras DG, Sundt TM, Didisheim P: Effect of anticoagulants and inhibition of platelet aggregation or thrombotic occlusion of endarterectomized cat carotid arteries. Stroke 7:248–254, 1976
135. Pierce EC, Lambertsen CJ, Deutsch S, Chase PE, Linde HW, Phipps RD, Price HL: Cerebral circulation and metabolism during thiopental anesthesia and hyperventilation in man. J Chir Invest 41:1664–1671, 1962
136. Portnoy HD, Avellanosa A: Carotid aneurysm and contralateral carotid stenosis with successful surgical treatment of both lesions. J. Neurosurg 32:476–482, 1970
137. Rainer WG, Gullen T, Bloomquist DC, McCrory CD: Carotid artery surgery, morbidity and mortality in 257 operations. Am J Surg 116:678–681, 1968
138. Rich NM, Hobson RW: Carotid endarterectomy under regional anesthesia. Am Surg 41:253, 1975
139. Robb CG: Operations for acute completed stroke due to thrombosis of the internal carotid artery. Surgery 65:862–865, 1969
140. Robinson RW, Cohen WD, Higano et al: Life table analysis of survival after cerebral thrombosis—ten years experience. JAMA 169:1149–1152, 1959
141. Rosenthal TT, Gaspar MR, Mobesis HJ: Intraoperative arteriography in carotid thromboendarterectomy. Arch Surg 106:806, 1973
142. Sharbrough FW, Messick JM, Sundt TM: Correlation of continuous electroencephalogram with cerebral blood flow measurements during carotid endarterectomy. Stroke 4:674–683, 1973
143. Shucart WA, Garrido E: Reopening some occluded carotid arteries. Report of four cases. J Neurosurg 45:442–446, 1976
144. Siekert RG, Whisnant JP, Millikan CH: Surgical and anticoagulant therapy of occlusive cerebral vascular disease. Ann Intern Med 48:637–641, 1963
145. Smith AL, Neigh JL, Hoffman TC, Wollman H: Effects of general anesthesia on autoregulation of cerebral blood flow in man. J Appl Physiol 29:665–669, 1970
146. Smith AL, Wollman H: Cerebral blood flow and metabolism: Effects of anesthetic drugs and techniques. Anesthesiology 36:378–400, 1972
147. Sokoloff L: The action of drugs on the cerebral circulation. Pharmacol Rev 11:1–85, 1959
148. Sorensen PS, Pedersen H, Marquardsen J, Petersson H, Heltberg A, Simonsen N, Munck O, Andersen LA: Acetylsallicilic acid in the prevention of stroke in patients with reversible cerebral ischemic attacks. A Danish Cooperative Study. Stroke 14:15–22, 1983
149. Stray-Gunderson, : Discussion of Evan WE, Cooperman M: The significance of asymptomatic carotid bruits in pre-operative patients. Presented at the Midwestern Vascular Surgical Society, Chicago, Ill, Sept. 1977
150. Sundt TM, Sharbrough FW, Anderson RE, Michenfelder JD: Cerebral blood flow measurements and electroencephalogram during carotid endarterectomy. J Neurosurg 41:310–320, 1974
151. Sundt TM, Sharbrough FW, Piepgras DG: Correlation of cerebral blood flow and electroencephalographic changes during carotid endarterectomy. Mayo Clin Proc 56:533–543, 1981
152. Sundt TM, Sharbrough FW, Trautman J, Gronert GA: Monitoring techniques for carotid endarterectomy. Clin Neurosurg 22:199–213, 1975
153. Sundt TM Jr, Sandox RA, Whisnant JP: Carotid endarterectomy complications and preoperative assessment of risk. Mayo Clin Proc 50:301–306, 1975
154. Theye RA, Michenfelder JD: The effects of halothane on canine cerebral metabolism. Anesthesiology 29:1113–1118, 1968
155. Theye RA, Michenfelder JD: The effects of nixtrous oxide on canine cerebral metabolism. Anesthesiology 29:1119–1124, 1968
156. Theye RA, Michenfelder JD: Cerebral protection with barbiturates: relations to anesthetic effect. Stroke 9:140–142, 1978
157. Thompson JE: Surgery for Cerebrovascular Insufficiency (Stroke). Charles C Thomas, Springfield, Ill, 1968
158. Thompson JE: In Discussion DeWeese et al, 1973
159. Thompson JE, Austin DJ, Patman RD: Endarterectomy for the totally occluded carotid artery for stroke. Arch Surg 95:791–801, 1967
160. Thompson JE, Austin DJ, Patman RD: Carotid endarterectomy for cerebrovascular insuffi-

ciency. Long-term results in 592 patients followed up to 13 years. Ann Surg 172:663–679, 1970

161. Thompson JE, Talkington CM: Carotid endarterectomy. Ann Surg 184:1, 1976
162. Toole JF: Diagnostic techniques in the medical evaluation and treatment of transient ischemic attacks. Clin Neurosurg 22:148–162, 1975
163. Toole JF, Janeway R, Choi K, Cordell R, Davis C, Johnston F, Miller HS: Transient ischemic attacks due to atherosclerosis: A prospective study of 160 patients. Arch Neurol 32:5–12, 1975
164. Trieman RL, Foran RF, Shore EH, Levin PM: Carotid bruit, significance in patients undergoing an abdominal aortic operation. Arch Surg 106:803, 1973
165. Trojaborg W, Boysen G: Relation between EEG regional cerebral blood flow and internal carotid artery pressure during carotid endarterectomy. Electroencephalogr Clin Neurophysiol 34:61–69, 1973
166. Waltimo O, Kosti M, Fogdholm R: Prognosis of patients with unilateral extracranial occlusion of the internal carotid artery. Stroke, 7:480–482, 1976
167. Waltz AG, Sundt TM, Mitchenfelder JD: Cerebral blood flow, jugular venous PO_2 and lactate concentration and arterial-venous oxygen content during carotid endarterectomy. Eur Neurol 6:346–349, 1971
168. Wells BA, Keats AS, Cooley DA: Increased tolerance to cerebral ischemia by general anesthesia during temporary carotid occlusion. Surgery 54:216–222, 1963
169. Whisnant JP, Matsumoto N, Elveback LR: Transient cerebral ischemic attacks in the community. Rochester, Minn, 1955 through 1969. Mayo Clin Proc 48:194–198, 1973
170. White CW, Allarde RR, McDowall HA: Anesthetic management for carotid surgery. JAMA 202:1023–1027, 1967
171. Winter WJ Jr: Atheromatous emboli: A cause of cerebral infarction. Arch Pathol 64:137–142, 1957
172. Witmer R, Schmid A: Cholesterinkristall als retinaler arterieller embolus. Ophthalmologica 135:432, 1958
173. Wollman H, Alexander SC, Cohen PJ, Chase PE, Melman E, Bekin MG: Cerebral circulation of man during Halothane anesthesia. Effects of hypocarbia and d-tubocuranine. Anesthesiology 25:180–184, 1964
174. Wollman H, Alexander SC, Cohen PJ, Smith TC, Chase PE, Van der Molen RA: Cerebral circulation during general anesthesia and hyperventilation in man. Thiopental induction to niturous oxide and d-tubocuranine. Anesthesiology 26:329–334, 1965
175. Wright RL, Sweet WH: Carotid or vertebral occlusion in the treatment of intracranial aneurysm: Value of early and late reading of carotid and retinal pressures. Clin Neurosurg 9:163–192, 1963
176. Wylie EJ In discussion, Baver RB, Meyer JS, Gotham JE, Gilroy J: A controlled study of surgical treatment of cerebrovascular disease—42 months experience with 183 cases. In Millikan C, Siekert R, Whisnant JP (eds.): Cerebral Vascular Disease. Grune & Stratton, New York, 1966
177. Wylie EJ, Ehrenfeld WK: Extracranial occlusive cerebral vascular disease—diagnosis and management. WB Saunders Co, Philadelphia, 1970, pp 220–221
178. Wylie EJ, Hein MF, Adams JE: Intracranial hemorrhage following revascularization for tretment of acute stroke. J Neurosurg 21:212–215, 1964
179. Wylie EJ, Hun MF, Adams JE: Intracranial hemorrhage following surgical revascularization for treatment of acute strokes. J Neurosurg 21:212–215, 1964
180. Young JR, Humphries AW, Beven EG, deWolfe VG: Carotid endarterectomy without a shunt. Experiences using hyperbaric general anesthesia. Arch Surg, 99:293–297, 1969
181. Ziegler DK, Hassanein R: Prognosis in patients with transient ischemic attacks. Stroke 4:666–673, 1973

6

Occlusive Disease of the Aortic Arch and the Innominate, Carotid, Subclavian, and Vertebral Arteries

Michael E. DeBakey and George P. Noon

Occlusive disease of the great vessels arising from the aortic arch and producing manifestations of cerebrovascular insufficiency and intermittent claudication of the arms is now a well-recognized clinical entity. Among the earliest descriptions of this disease were those by Savory[19] in 1856, Broadbent[1] in 1875, and Penzoldt[16] in 1881. In 1908, Takayasu,[22] a Japanese ophthalmologist, reported retinal vascular changes associated with occlusive disease of the aortic arch, after which the condition was sometimes referred to as Takayasu's disease. Because of the early reports from Japan, the disease, which was found mostly in young women, was considered predominately of Japanese origin. In a report by Shimizu and Sano,[20] the term "pulseless disease" was used to describe the condition. Subsequent reports, however, suggested more widespread geographic distribution, and a number of cases in the male sex were reported.[5,14,15,18] With the more widespread use of angiography in the study of patients with arterial insufficiency, the disease has been recognized with increasing frequency, and the concept has evolved that this form of occlusive disease may be well localized with relatively normal proximal and distal arterial segments. This concept led to the development of surgical techniques that had proved successful in the treatment of similar occlusive disease in other arterial beds of the body.[14]

Etiology and Incidence

The most common cause of extracranial cerebrovascular insufficiency is atherosclerosis. The highest incidence is in the sixth and seventh decades of life. Men are more commonly affected than women. Arteritis involving the aortic arch and the innominate, carotid, and subclavian arteries occurs most often in young women, usually in the fourth decade of life. The disease is rarely of congenital origin.

Extracranial cerebrovascular insufficiency tends to assume certain characteristic patterns according to the site of involvement and anatomic distribution.[7] In one pattern, for example, the disease affects the proximal segments of the major cerebral arteries as they arise from the aortic arch; it may produce complete or incomplete occlusion, and in about one-half of the patients, more than one of these arteries is affected. In almost all patients with this pattern, the occlusive process is well localized, with a relatively normal distal arterial bed, and is therefore amenable to surgical treatment. In a second pattern the occlusive lesion, which is also usually well localized, tends to occur at the bifurcation of the common carotid arteries and the origin of the internal carotid arteries, and at the origin of the vertebral arteries. Although in most of these patterns the atherosclerotic occlusive process tends to produce stenosis of the

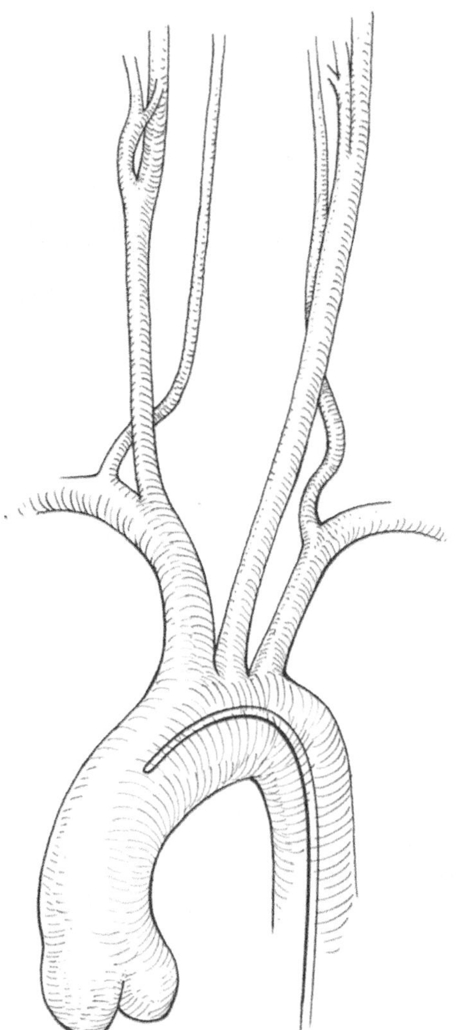

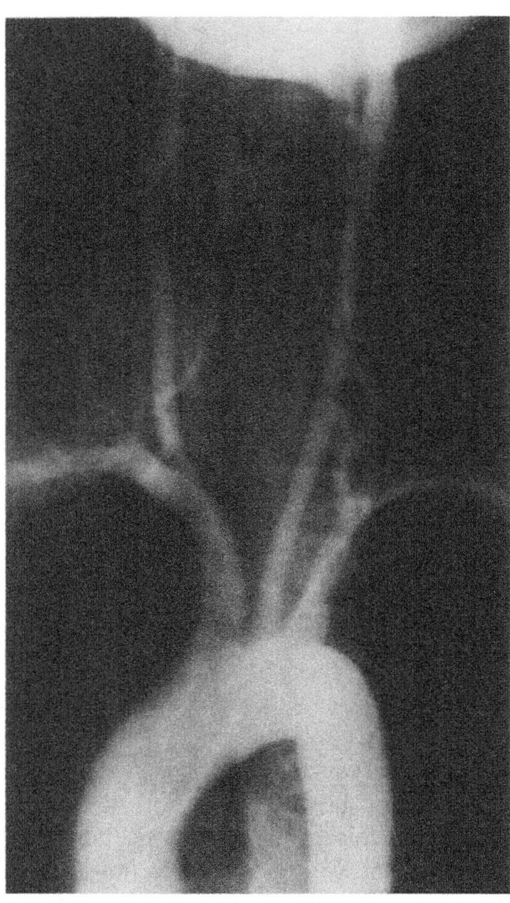

Figure 6.1. Arteriography performed according to intra-arterial catheter techniques. An aortogram is made to visualize aortic arch and brachiocephalic vessels. Selective catheterization of these vessels is performed when indicated. Serial roentgenograms are made to show flow of contrast material through arteries, collateral circulation, and "steal."

lumen, in some patients the lesion is ulcerative, with little or no stenosis. Portions of the fibrin and thrombi that develop on the surface of such lesions may break off, be swept up by the bloodstream, and produce emboli that may cause repeated episodes of transient ischemic attacks.

Clinical Manifestations

The clinical manifestations of occlusive disease of the aortic arch and of the innominate, carotid, subclavian, and vertebral arteries are varied. Neurologic deficits, ophthalmologic manifestations, and ischemic symptoms in the arms may appear alone or in combination. Neurologic symptoms are varied, occurring as transient ischemic attacks or as prolonged, progressive, or permanent neurologic deficits. They may be localized to the carotid or vertebrobasilar distribution, or they may be systemic (lightheadedness, syncope, seizures, confusion, dementia, or drowsiness). The "steal" syndrome usually results from subclavian arterial occlusive disease. Exercise of the arms results in retrograde blood flow through the vertebral artery of the affected subclavian artery, which

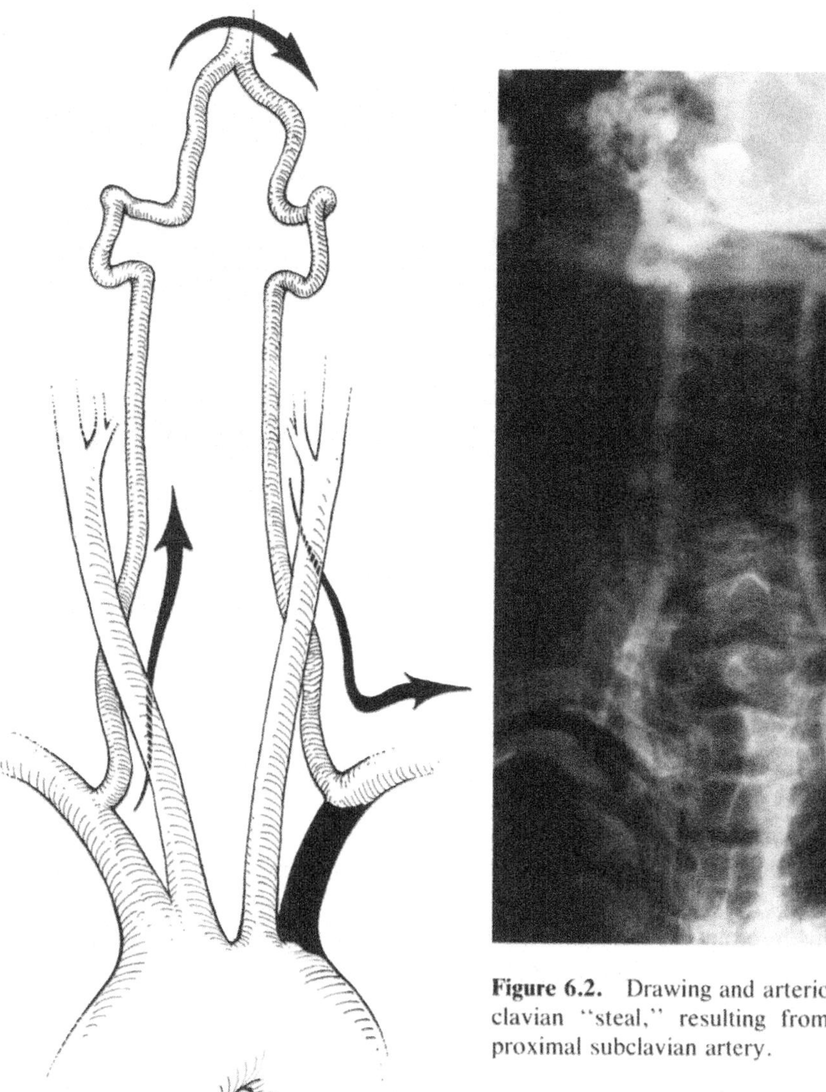

Figure 6.2. Drawing and arteriogram showing subclavian "steal," resulting from occlusion of left proximal subclavian artery.

usually produces symptoms of vertebrobasilar insufficiency. Ischemic manifestations in the arms, such as claudication, rest pain, or gangrene, may develop from occlusive disease of the aortic arch, subclavian artery, or innominate artery. Ophthalmologic symptoms, such as visual field defects, decreased vision, or blindness, may result from retinal arterial emboli or general ischemia.

Of particular importance in the clinical consideration of the anatomic patterns of the disease is the fact that they tend to produce characteristic cerebrovascular manifestations and neurologic disturbances. In a number of patients, however, these symptoms do not always reflect the exact site and extent of disease because of the frequency of multiple arterial involvement and the development of collateral circulation.[6] In some patients, for example, with characteristic ischemic manifestations due to occlusive lesions affecting the internal carotid arteries, arteriography may disclose the responsible, and surgically correctable, lesion to be in the proximal segment of the innominate, common carotid, or vertebral artery. In other patients with characteristic manifesta-

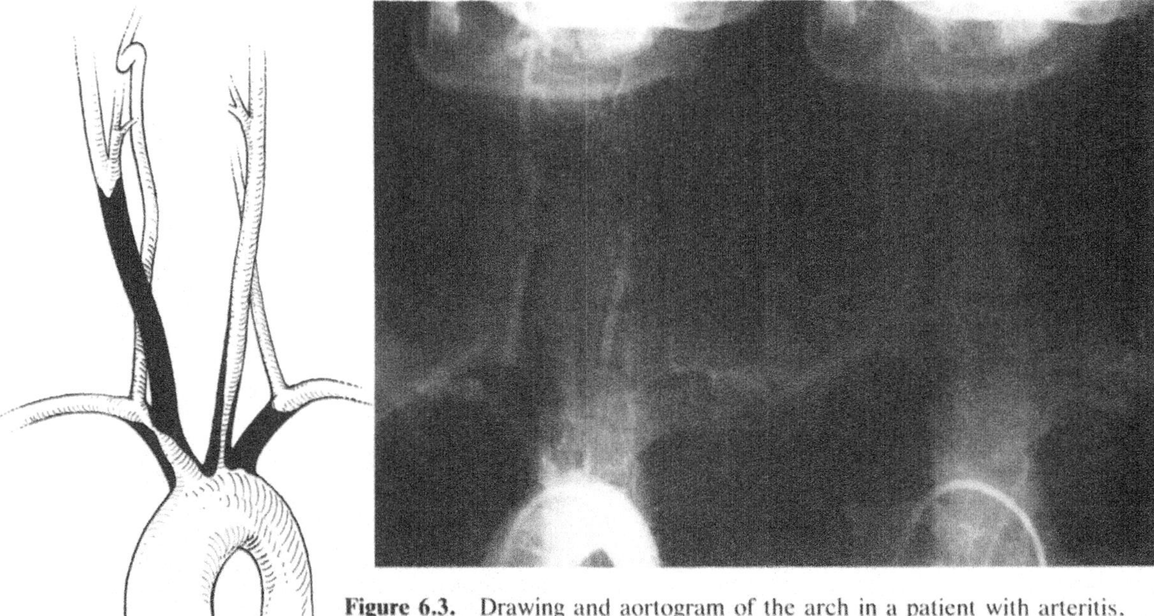

Figure 6.3. Drawing and aortogram of the arch in a patient with arteritis, showing occlusion of origins of brachiocephalic vessels and visualization of the patent distal carotid and subclavian vessels.

tions of vertebrobasilar arterial insufficiency, the responsible, and surgically correctable, lesion may be in the internal carotid or in the proximal segments of the innominate, common carotid, or subclavian artery.

Diagnosis

On physical examination, diminished or absent pulses can be detected in the occluded carotid or subclavian artery. Systolic bruits, which can usually be heard on auscultation over the diseased vessels, diminish or disappear when occlusion is complete or nearly complete. Differential or absent blood pressure in the arms is common.

Results of neurologic examination can be entirely normal in patients who have had transient ischemic attacks that have resolved. On the other hand, a variety of localizing or nonlocalizing neurologic abnormalities may be observed if prolonged, progressive, or permanent neurologic defects have occurred. Serial neurologic examinations are important to establish the evolution of the neurologic disorder.

Funduscopy may disclose emboli in the retinal arteries. Blood pressure differentials or absent pulses in the arms suggest proximal occlusive disease. The blood pressure in the arms and legs should be compared. Distal ischemic changes may occur in the arms. In the presence of the "steal" syndrome, neurologic symptoms may be precipitated by exercise of the limb. Electroencephalography, brain scanning, computerized axial tomography, and roentgenography of the skull are helpful in establishing a baseline for the individual patient with cerebrovascular insufficiency, as well as in screening for nonvascular disorders.

Noninvasive vascular testing is helpful in screening high-risk patients. It is also useful in prearteriographic and preoperative evaluation. Comparison of studies is useful in follow-up. Proximal disease involving the arch vessels is suggested by bruits, diminished or absent pulses, and pressure differentials. The subclavian vessels can be evaluated with Doppler pressures and pulse volume recordings of the arms. The carotid arteries can be examined for flow-reducing lesions with occuloplethysmography, carotid phonoangiography, and Dop-

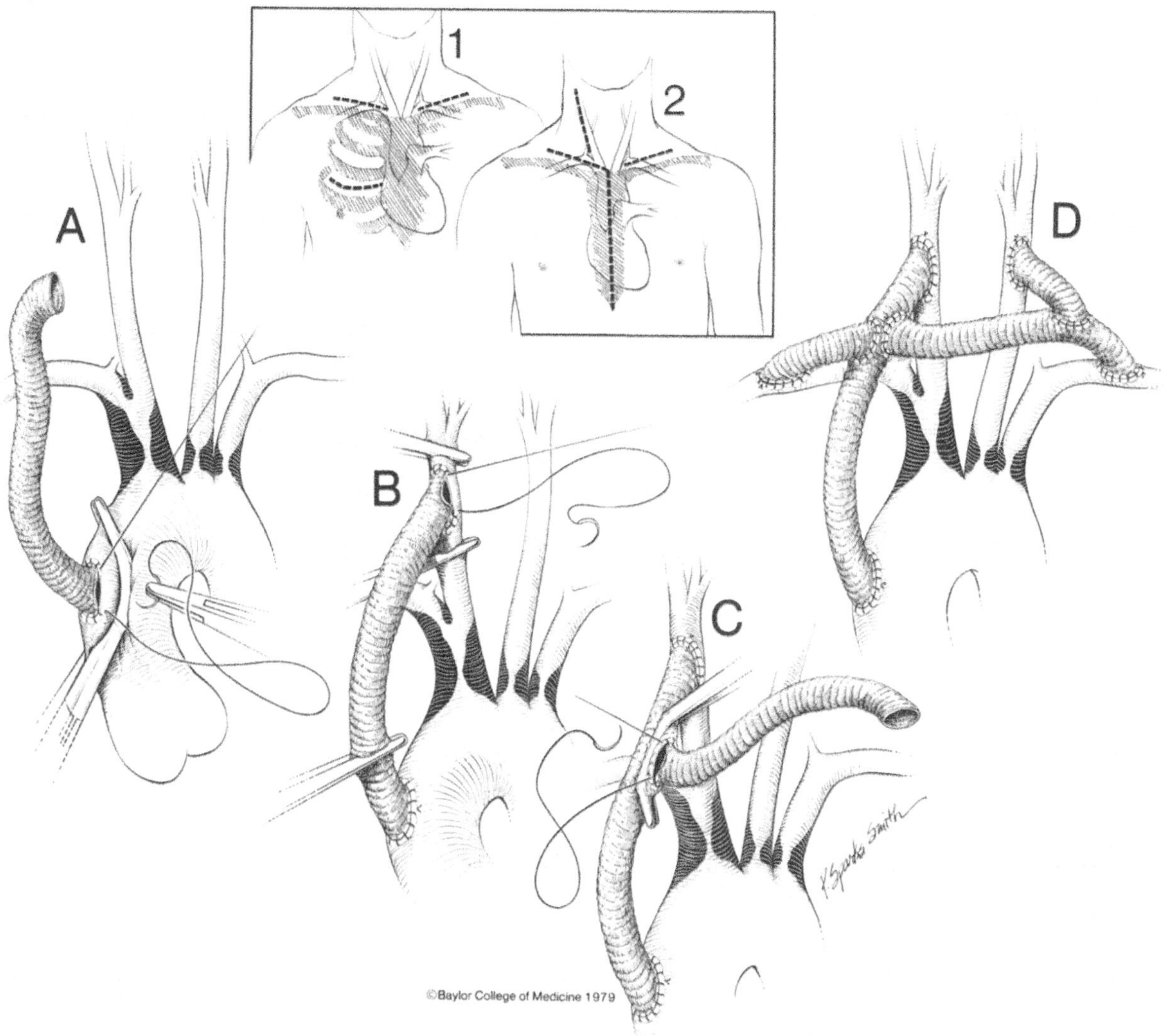

Figure 6.4. Surgical technique for revascularization in patients with occlusive disease of the aortic arch. Exposure is through (1) the right anterior third intercostal space or (2) a median sternotomy. Cervical incisions used with each are shown. Transverse supraclavicular incisions are used to expose proximal carotid and subclavian arteries. Carotid bifurcation is exposed through an incision medial to sternocleidomastoid muscle. **A.** Anastomosis of graft to ascending aorta with use of a partial occluding clamp. **B.** Graft is tunneled to the proximal carotid artery for distal anastomosis and then attached to appropriate carotid or subclavian vessel. It is important to flush the artery and graft before establishing blood flow. **C.** Attachment of side branches to other affected vessels. **D.** Completion of revascularization of all affected vessels.

pler spectral analysis. B-mode scanning will visualize disease in the cervical carotid. The vertebral arteries are not amenable to presently used clinical noninvasive testing. The accuracy and limitations of each of these noninvasive tests must be understood and appropriately considered in their interpretation and application.

Arteriography is the ultimate diagnostic study for localizing the site and determining the extent of the arterial disease. Reconstructive procedures require precise arteriography for proper planning and execution. Properly performed arteriography permits visualization and identification of ulcerative and occlusive disease. The aortic arch can best be studied by

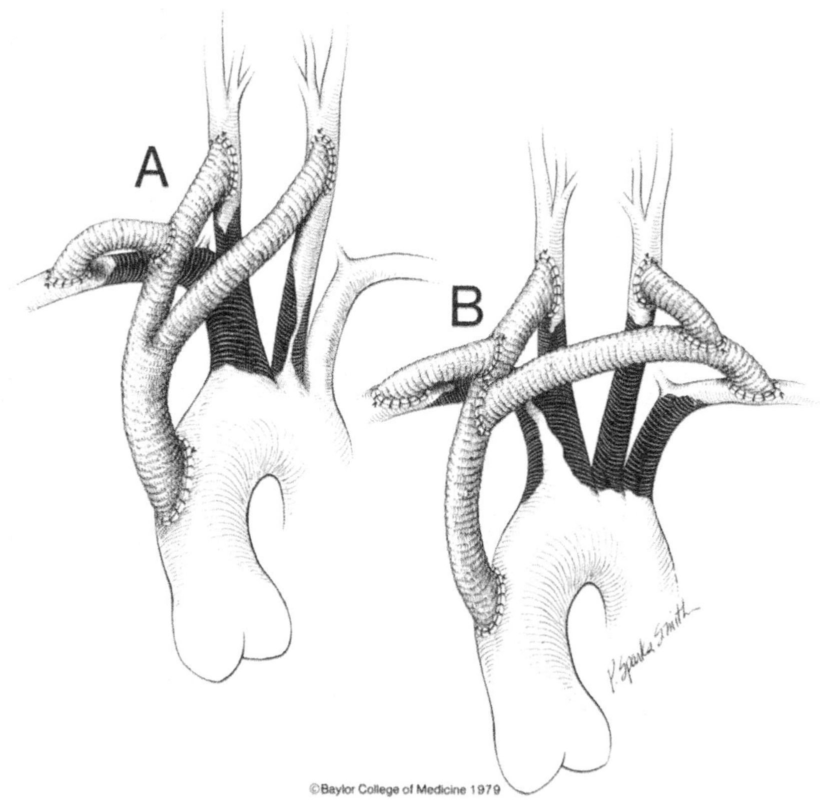

Figure 6.5. Revascularization of aortic arch occlusive disease using **A,** bifurcation graft attached to ascending aorta with additional grafts attached to its limbs to complete revascularization and **B,** tube graft anastomosed to ascending aorta with separate grafts to each of the vessels.

transcutaneous catheter techniques (Fig. 6.1). Flush aortography, selective catheterization, and injection of the vessels can be performed. Serial films permit visualization of the contrast material as it circulates through the vasculature. In this way, collateral filling of occluded vessels and "steals" can be identified (Figs. 6.2, 6.3), and operative procedures can be tailored to the specific needs of the individual. Digital subtraction arteriography is being used more and more for screening and definitive study. The venous injections, which are commonly used, are not as precise as the arterial flush and selective injections.

Surgical Treatment

A variety of surgical procedures is used in the treatment of occlusive disease of the aortic arch and of the innominate, proximal subclavian, carotid, and vertebral arteries.[2-8,9,11-14,23] Bypass is most common for proximal occlusion of these arteries, with the exception of the vertebral artery. During bypass operations, extrathoracic procedures are used, when feasible, to reduce the morbidity and mortality rates. In the presence of occlusion of the carotid bifurcation, carotid endarterectomy can be performed concomitantly and, if necessary, incorporated into the bypass procedure. The vertebral artery is revascularized, with bypass graft to the subclavian artery when proximal subclavian and innominate arterial occlusion are responsible for the diminished blood flow. Localized stenosis of the proximal vertebral artery, however, is treated by dilation or patch-graft angioplasty in selected patients. Dilation is used in only a small percentage of patients. Endarterectomy with or without patch-graft angioplasty of the large proximal vessels is rarely used.

When occlusive disease affects the origin of

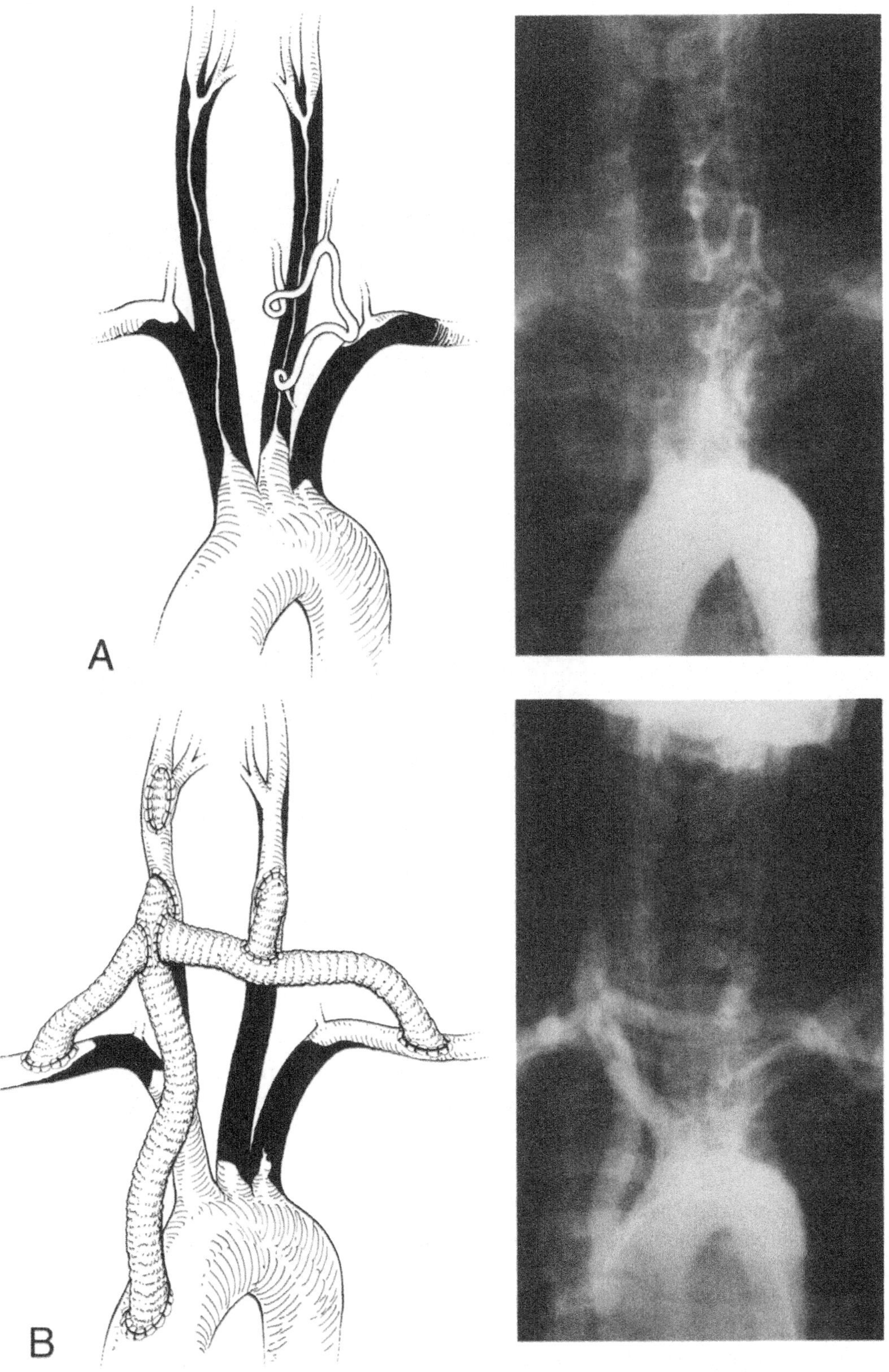

Figure 6.6. Patient with arteritis that produced complete obstruction of proximal brachiocephalic vessels. **A.** Site and extent of lesions. **B.** 12 years after operation, showing operative reconstruction with functioning bypass grafts.

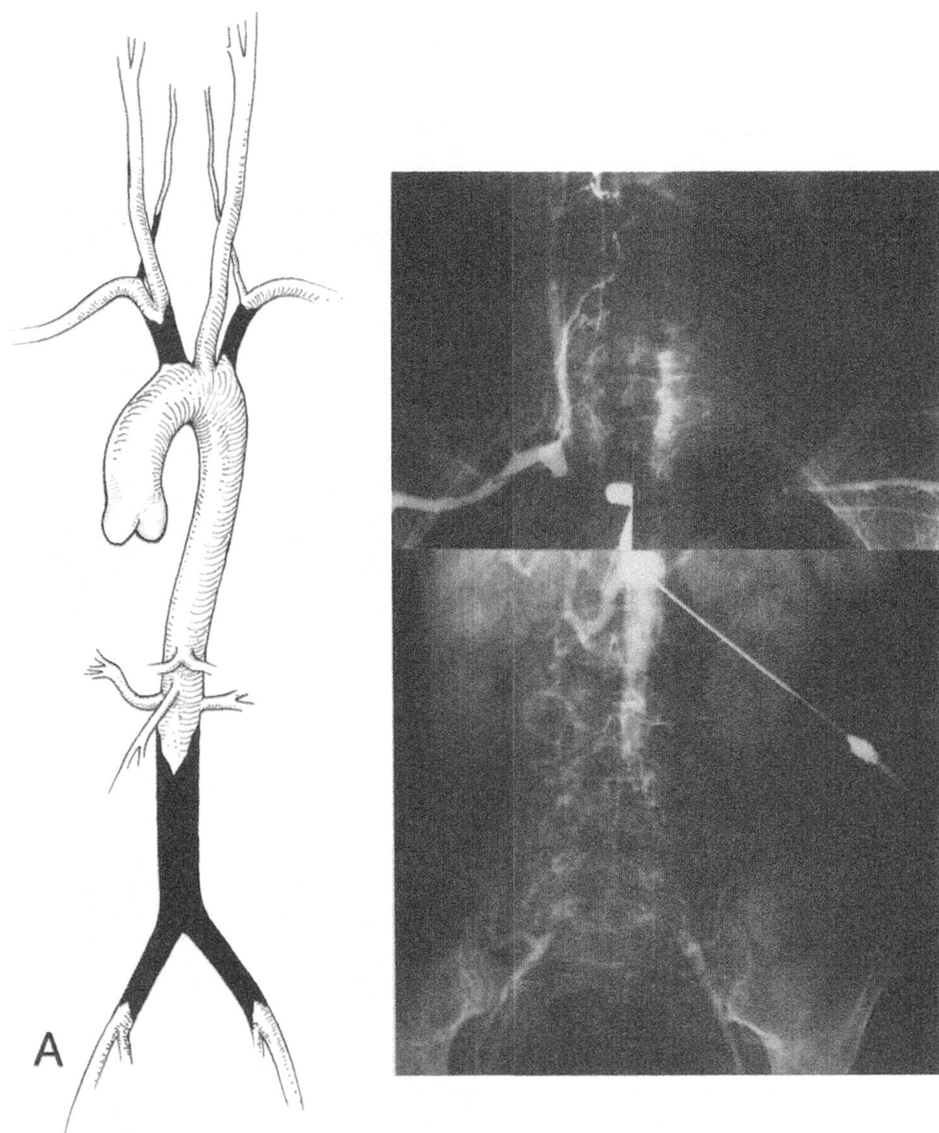

Figure 6.7. Patient with atherosclerotic occlusive disease of aortic arch vessels and distal abdominal aorta. **A.** Site and extent of occlusions. **B.** Operative techniques used in arterial reconstruction and arteriograms showing both bypass grafts functioning 15 years after operation.

all arch vessels, the proximal anastomosis of the bypass graft must be attached to the ascending aorta (Fig. 6.4). An incision is made in the right anterior third intercostal space or through median stenotomy, and the ascending aorta is exposed by incising the pericardium. A partial occluding clamp is applied to the aorta, and a longitudinal arteriotomy is made. An 8-mm to 10-mm DeBakey Dacron® velour tube or a 14-mm to 16-mm bifurcation graft is anastomosed to the ascending aorta with continuous polyester or polypropylene sutures. When completed, the graft and anastomosis are examined for bleeding. When a thoracotomy has been used for the proximal anastomosis, the extrathoracic segments of the carotid and subclavian arteries selected for the distal anastomosis are exposed through transverse cervical and supraclavicular incisions. When a median sternotomy is used, it can be extended to the carotid or subclavian arteries. The common carotid arteries are isolated below the bifurcation unless the disease

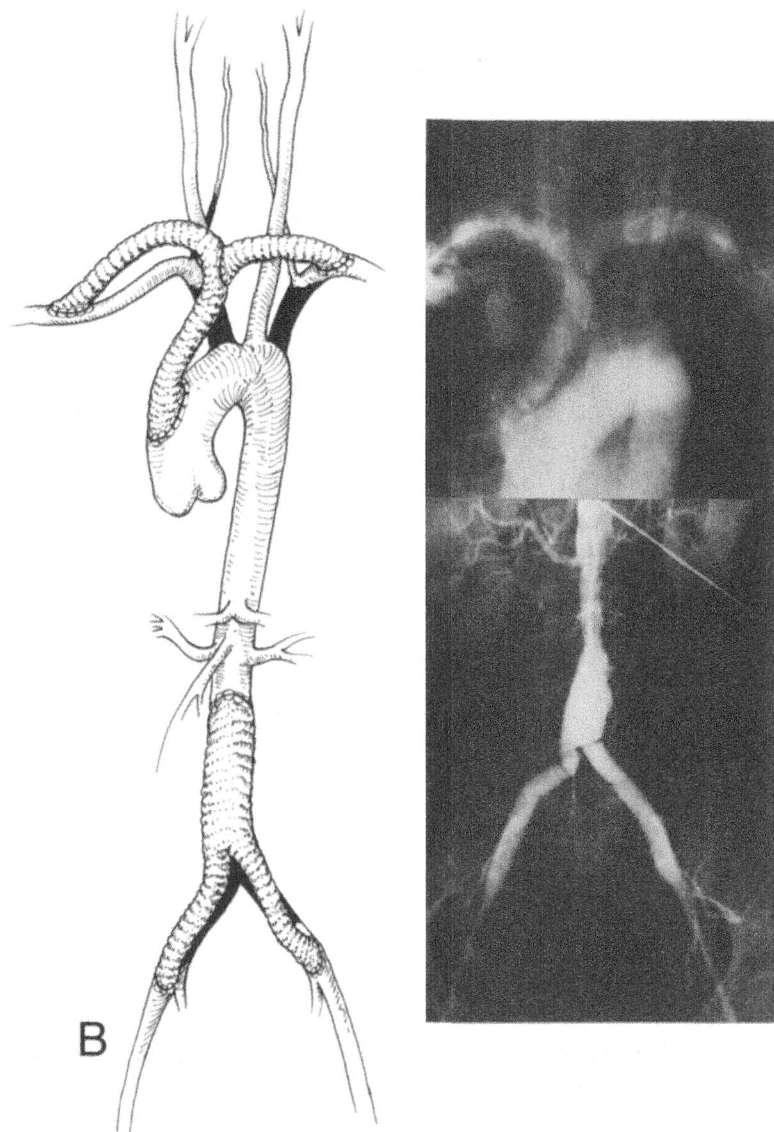

extends to, or involves, the bifurcation. The carotid bifurcation is then exposed through an incision along the medial border of the sternocleidomastoid muscle. The subclavian arteries are best exposed distal to the origin of the vertebral and thyrocervical trunk. The anterior scalene muscle is divided, care being taken to avoid injury to the phrenic nerve along its medial border. Occasionally, the axillary or brachial artery must be isolated for the distal anastomosis. After the extrathoracic vessels have been exposed, the graft is tunneled retrosternally to the appropriate extrathoracic site. When a single-tube graft is anastomosed to the ascending aorta, the right common carotid artery is usually the most accessible vessel for distal anastomosis. The vessel is clamped proximally and distally. A longitudinal arteriotomy is made, and the anastomosis is performed with a continuous suture of polyester or polypropylene. Before completion of the anastomosis, the graft and artery are flushed to remove any clot

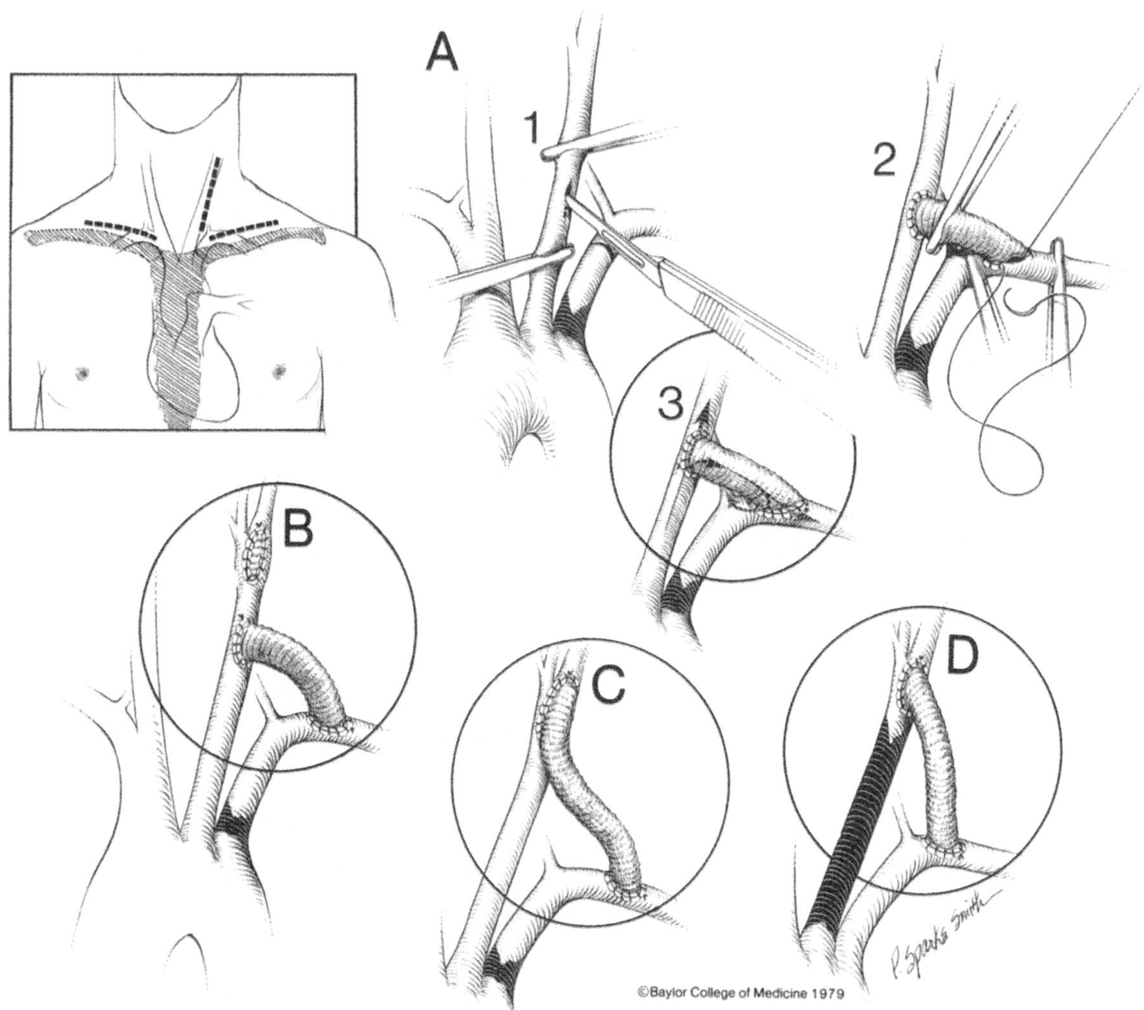

Figure 6.8. Operative techniques for carotid-subclavian and subclavian-carotid bypasses. **A.** Cervical incisions used. A single supraclavicular incision is used for ipsilateral bypass unless it is necessary to expose carotid bifurcation. 1. Anastomosis of the graft to the proximal common carotid artery. 2. After completion of anastomosis, blood flow is reestablished through the carotid, the graft is occluded, and subclavian anastomosis is performed. 3. Completed carotid subclavian bypass. **B.** Technique used for carotid subclavian bypass when there is associated disease of bifurcation using a separated carotid endarterectomy with patch-graft angioplasty. **C.** Carotid subclavian bypass after endarterectomy at carotid bifurcation with proximal anastomosis of graft to opening in carotid artery. **D.** Subclavian carotid bypass.

or debris. Side branches used to bypass the other diseased vessel are then attached to the graft with polyester sutures. The branch grafts are extended to the affected vessels and anastomosed by a technique similar to that described for the carotid artery (Figs. 6.5–6.7).

For isolated carotid or subclavian arterial occlusion, bypass procedures can be performed without use of the ascending aorta. The entire operation is extrathoracic (Fig. 6.8). With subclavian occlusive disease, carotid-to-subclavian, axillary, or brachial artery bypasses are performed. Subclavian-to-carotid artery bypass is used for carotid-artery occlusion. The ipsilateral carotid and subclavian arteries are exposed through a single supraclavicular incision except when the carotid is anastomosed to the carotid bifurcation. Such cases require a second incision along the medial border of the sternocleidomastoid muscle. Dacron® velour tube

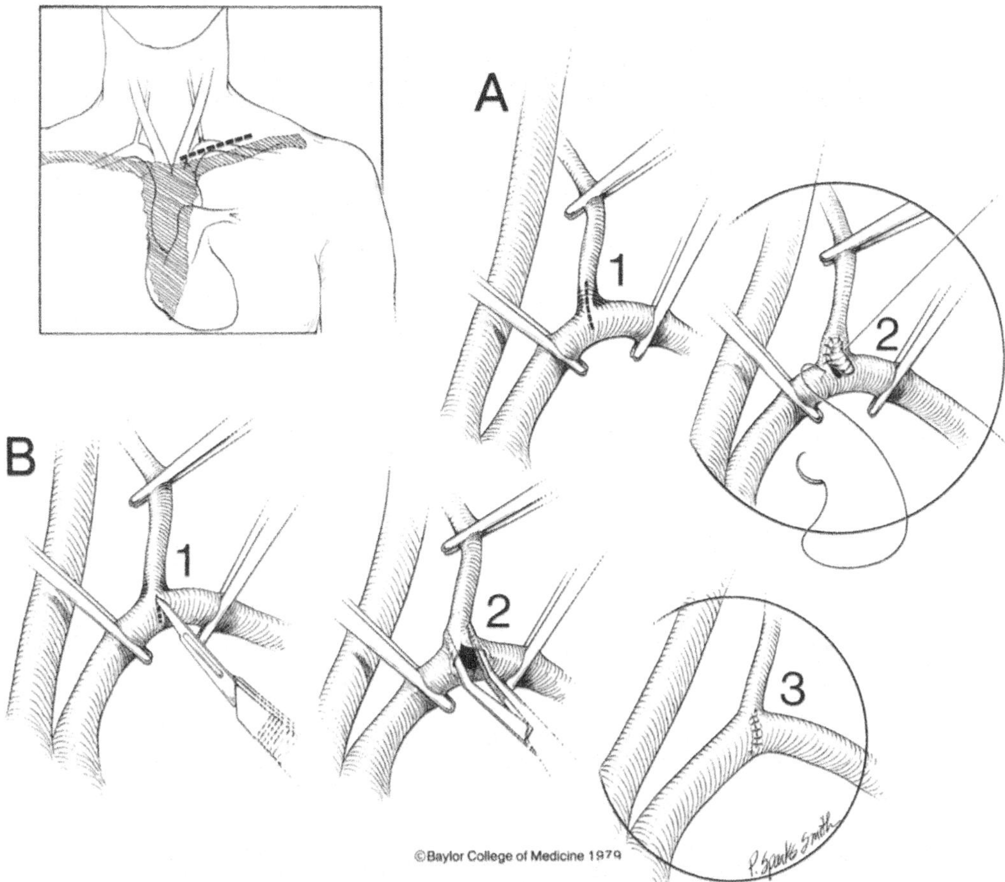

Figure 6.9. Surgical techniques used for reconstruction of vertebral artery. **A.** Incision used for exposure of vertebral and subclavian arteries. 1. Subclavian and vertebral arteries are clamped, and an arteriotomy is extended from subclavian into vertebral artery. 2. Depending on the occlusive lesion, endarterectomy may or may not be performed after which patch-graft angioplasty is performed with Dacron® velour or autogenous saphenous vein. **B.** Dilation technique of vertebral arterial occlusion, which may occasionally be performed. 1. Clamps are applied to vertebral and subclavian arteries, and incision is made in subclavian artery. 2. Blunt-end hemostat is passed through this incision into the vertebral artery and opened to dilate the stenotic lesion. 3. Opening in the subclavian artery is closed with a continuous suture.

grafts, 6 to 8 mm in diameter, are used for the bypass except when the bypass is extended to the axillary or brachial artery. Autogenous saphenous vein is preferred for these distal arteries. Bypasses such as contralateral subclavian-subclavian, subclavian-axillary, or femoral-subclavian are rarely used.

In patients whose neurologic symptoms are considered secondary to stenosis of the proximal vertebral artery, a reconstructive procedure is performed (Fig. 6.9). The vertebral artery is exposed through a transverse supraclavicular incision beginning lateral to the suprasternal notch and extending to the midclavicle. The sternocleidomastoid muscle is partly divided, and the internal jugular vein is retracted medially. Care is taken to avoid injury to the thoracic duct and recurrent laryngeal nerve on the right. The subclavian artery is identified and exposed. The thyrocervical trunk or its branches are divided, if necessary, to facilitate exposure of the origin of the vertebral artery. The vertebral artery is then exposed for several centimeters distal to its origin, and the subclavian and vertebral arteries are clamped. A transverse incision is made in the subclavian

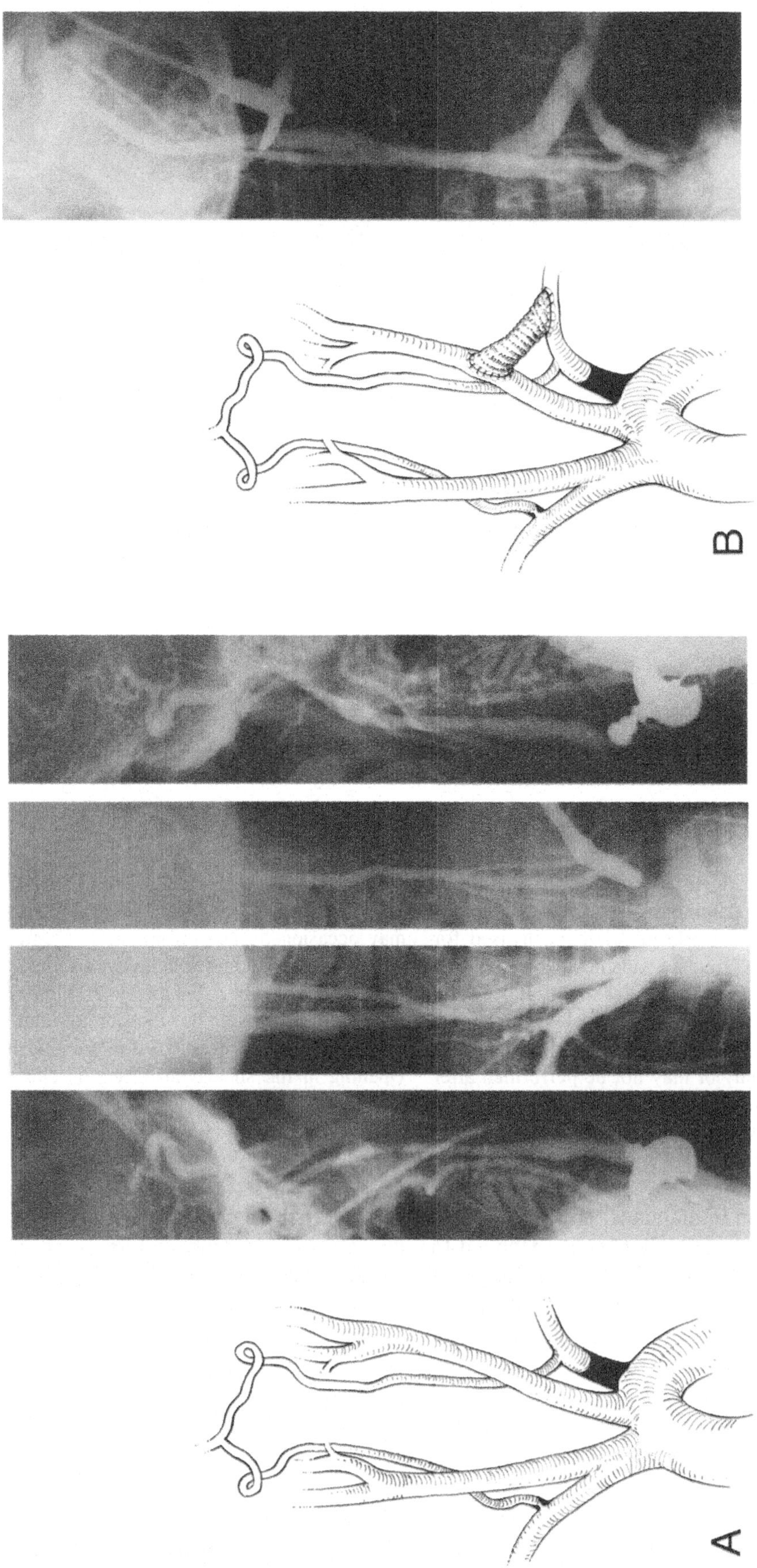

Figure 6.10. Drawing and arteriogram showing **A,** occlusion of left subclavian artery in 58-year-old white man with manifestations of vertebrobasilar insufficiency and weakness of left arm (subclavian "steal" syndrome). **B,** operative reconstruction with carotid subclavian bypass and arteriogram 10 years after operation, showing functioning bypass graft.

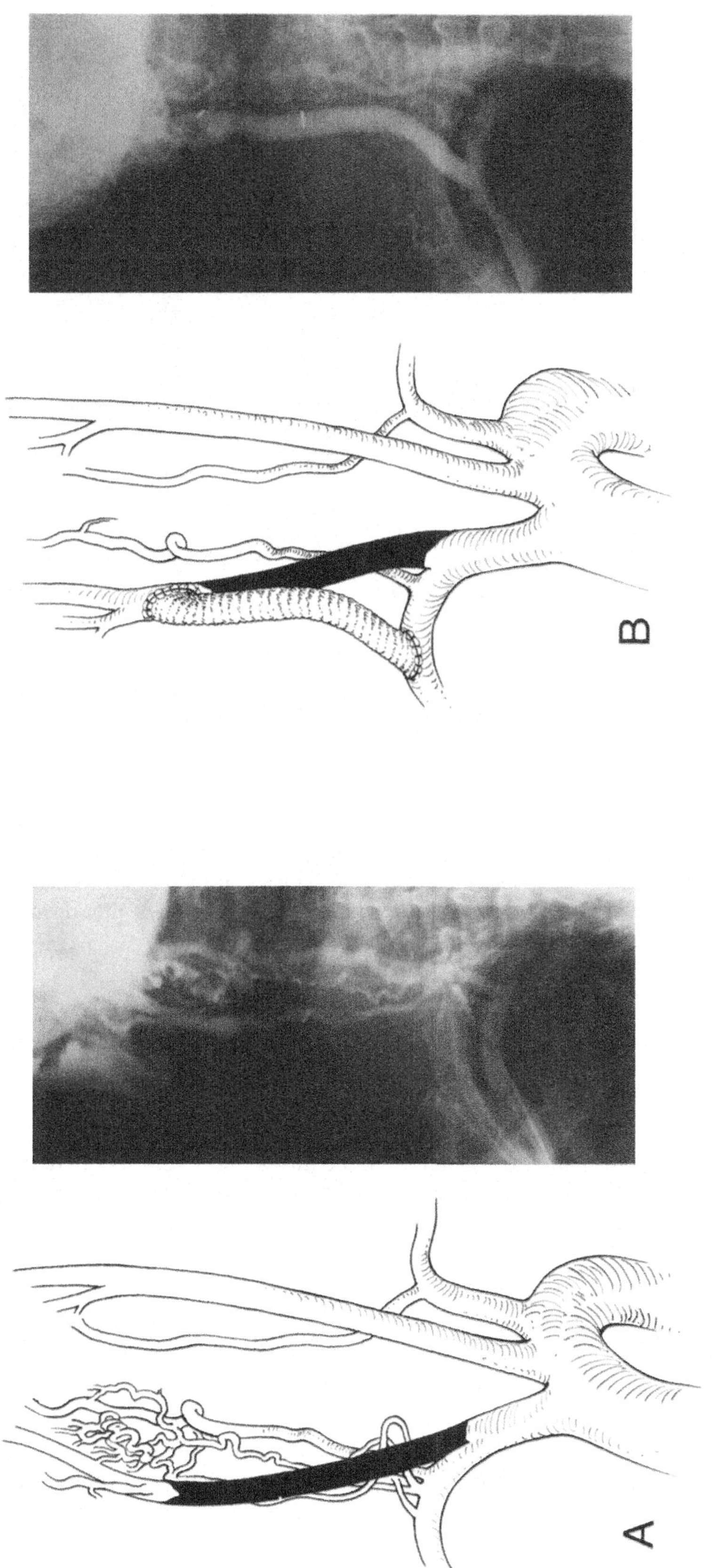

Figure 6.11. Drawing and arteriogram in **A,** 50-year-old man who had several left-sided seizures from occlusion of right common carotid artery; **B,** operative procedure consisting of right subclavian carotid bypass and arteriogram showing functioning bypass graft 12 years after operation.

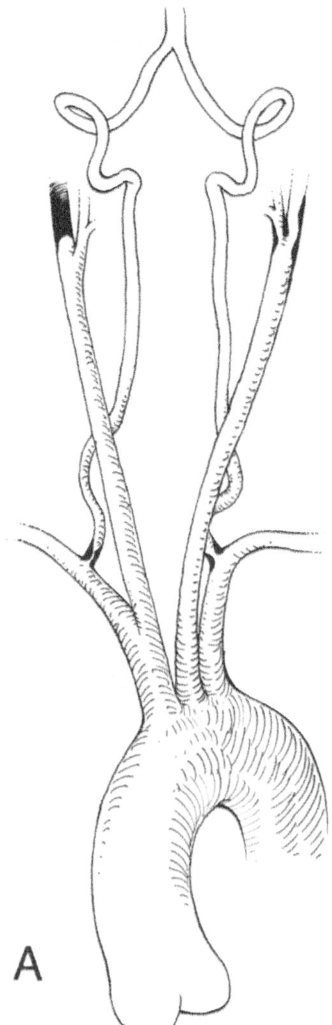

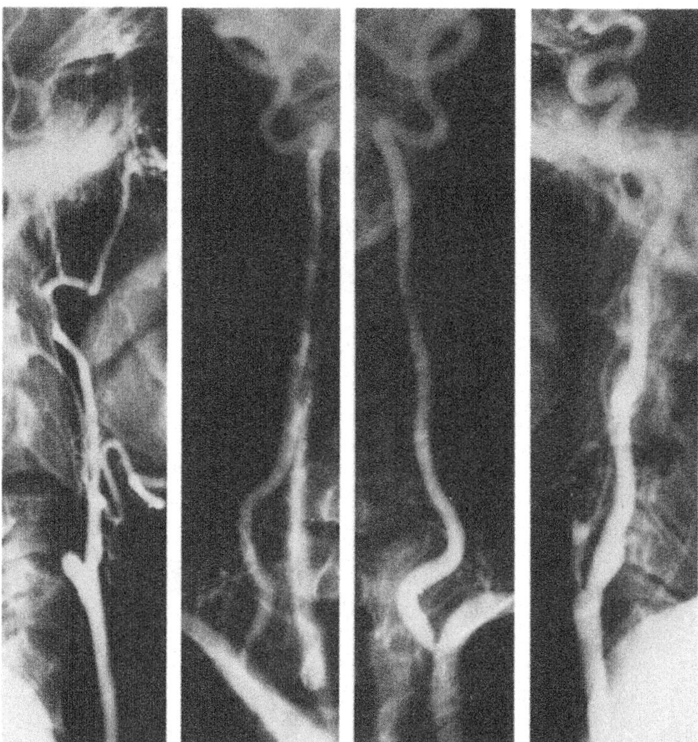

Figure 6.12. Drawing and arteriogram in **A**, patient with occlusive disease of both vertebral arteries and complete occlusion of right internal carotid artery; **B**, method of surgical treatment consisting of endarterectomy with patch-graft angioplasty of both vertebral arteries and arteriogram showing restoration of normal lumen and blood flow through vertebral arteries 15 years after operation. Patient has remained asymptomatic.

artery and carried longitudinally up the vertebral artery beyond the lesion. Patch-graft angioplasty with Dacron® velour or autogenous vein and polypropylene suture is performed.[13] Care is taken to avoid tearing the thin, friable vertebral artery. Endarterectomy is sometimes necessary, but care should be taken in controlling the distal ends of dissection. A rare patient may be treated by dilation of the vertebral artery through an incision made in the subclavian artery but not extended into the vertebral artery (Fig. 6.9). When heparinization is used during the operation, the grafts must be preclotted before the heparin is injected to prevent bleeding through the interstices of the graft.

Patients must be carefully observed during the immediate postoperative period. Since hematomas that develop after operation can produce airway and venous obstruction, hemostasis during operation is important. The patient's head should be elevated at least 30° to facilitate venous return and minimize edema. The arterial blood pressure should be maintained at a normal level; hypotension and hypertension are to be avoided. If there is any sign of cerebral edema or postoperative neurologic deficits, intravenous injection of 6 mg of dexamethasone (Decadron) every six hours, 150 mg of papaverine every six hours, and 100 mg of phenatoin sodium (Dilantin) every eight hours is indicated.

Percutaneous transluminal balloon angioplasty[17] is widely used in the treatment of selected occlusive disease throughout the arterial

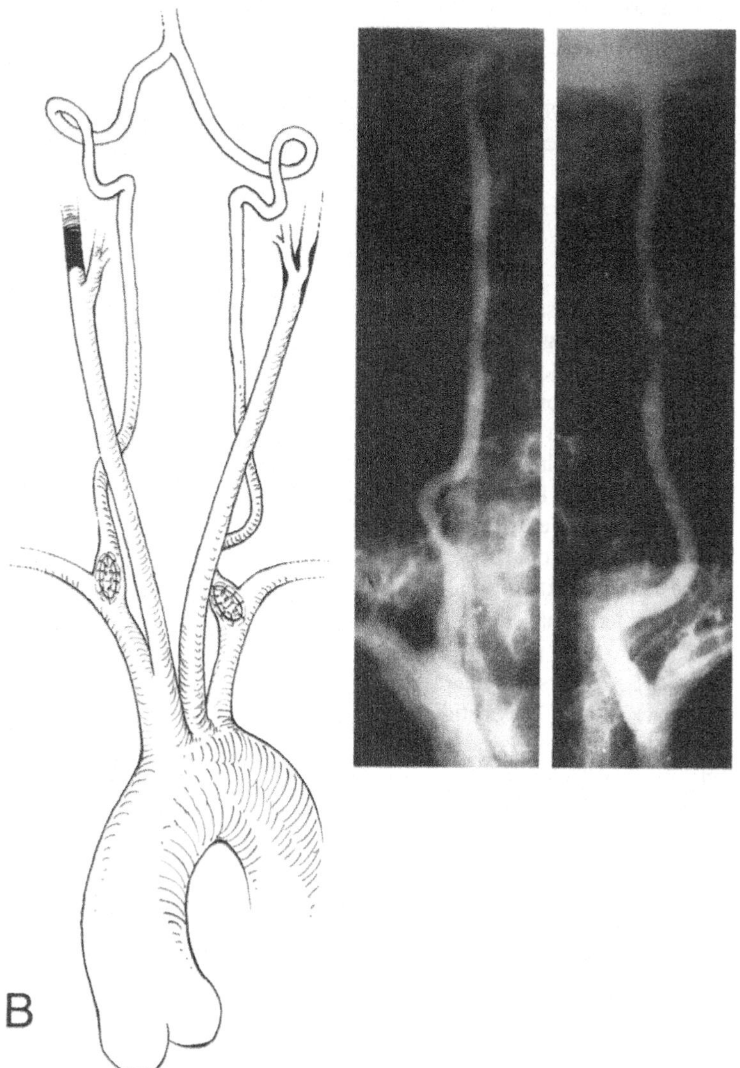

tree. Although this procedure has had limited use in the treatment of diseased innominate, carotid, subclavian, and vertebral vessels, wider application is anticipated.[17,21]

Results

Immediate and long-term results have been gratifying[2,3,7–11] (Figs. 6.6, 6.7, 6.10–6.12). The operative mortality rate is about 3% and is usually caused by associated cardiac or coronary disease rather than neurologic disease. For this reason, proper preoperative studies must be performed to assess cardiac status. Indeed, in recent years patients with associated coronary disease have had careful studies, including angiography, if indicated, and the determination is then made as to whether the aortocoronary bypass operation should be performed first.

Long-term results based on follow-up studies more than ten years after operation have been highly gratifying. More than 90% of patients are asymptomatic or improved, and only 2% are worse. Long-term graft patency is also excellent (Figs. 6.6, 6.7, 6.10–6.12). Occlusion recurs in less than 5% of the patients. Follow-up studies also suggest that surgical treatment prolongs life in these patients. Thus, in patients with no associated cardiovascular disease, the survival rate five years or more after operation is almost equal to that of the normal population.

Since the underlying pathologic lesion in most of these patients is atherosclerosis, proper control of such risk factors as hyperlipidemia, hypertension, and smoking is important. Arteritis may remain stable or may progress. Response to steroid therapy is not predictable, and no specific treatment is available at present.

References

1. Broadbent WH: Absence of pulsation in both radial arteries, the vessels being full of blood. Trans Clin Soc Lond 8:165–168, 1875
2. Crawford ES, DeBakey ME, Morris GC Jr, et al: Surgical treatment of occlusion of the innominate, common carotid, and subclavian arteries: a 10 year experience. Surgery 65:17–31, 1969
3. Crawford ES, DeBakey ME, Weibel J: Surgical treatment of occlusive disease of the vertebral arteries, In Gillespie JA (ed): Extracranial Cerebrovascular Disease and its Management, Chapt 9, Butterworths, London, 1969, pp 145–169
4. Crawford ES, Stowe GL, Powers RW Jr: Occlusion of the innominate, common carotid, and subclavian arteries: long-term results of surgical treatment. Surgery 94:781–791, 1983
5. Davis JB, Grove WJ, Julian OC: Thrombic occlusion of the branches of the aortic arch, Martorell's syndrome: report of a case treated surgically. Ann Surg 144:124–126, 1956
6. DeBakey ME: Concepts underlying surgical treatment of cerebrovascular insufficiency, In Mosberg WH Jr (ed): Clinical Neurosurgery, Vol 10, Williams and Wilkins, Baltimore, 1964, pp 310–340
7. DeBakey ME: Patterns of atherosclerosis and rates of progression, In Paoletti R, Gotto AM Jr (eds): Atherosclerosis Reviews, Vol 3, Raven Press, New York, 1978, pp 1–56
8. DeBakey ME, Crawford ES: Surgical treatment of innominate, common carotid, and subclavian artery occlusions, In Gillespie JA (ed): Extracranial Cerebrovascular Disease and its Management, Chapt 10, Butterworths, London, 1969, pp 170–193
9. DeBakey ME, Crawford ES, Cooley DA, et al: Surgical considerations of occlusive disease of innominate, carotid, subclavian, and vertebral arteries. Ann Surg 149:690–710, 1959
10. DeBakey ME, Crawford ES, Cooley DA, et al: Cerebral arterial insufficiency: one to 11-year results following arterial reconstructive operation. Ann Surg 161:921–945, 1965
11. DeBakey ME, Crawford ES, Fields WS: Surgical treatment of lesions producing arterial insufficiency of the internal carotid, common carotid, vertebral, innominate and subclavian arteries. Ann Intern Med 51:436–448, 1959
12. DeBakey ME, Crawford ES, Morris GC Jr, et al: Arterial reconstructive operations for cerebrovascular insufficiency due to extracranial arterial occlusive disease. J Cardiovasc Surg 3:12–25, 1962
13. DeBakey ME, Crawford ES, Morris GC Jr, et al: Patch graft angioplasty in vascular surgery. J Cardiovasc Surg 3:106–141, 1962
14. DeBakey ME, Morris GC Jr, Jordan GL Jr, et al: Segmental thrombo-obliterative disease of branches of aortic arch: successful surgical treatment. JAMA 166:998–1003, 1958
15. Kalmansohn RB, Kalmansohn RW: Thrombotic obliteration of the branches of the aortic arch. Circulation 15:237–244, 1957
16. Penzoldt F: Ueber Thrombose (autochthone oder embolische) der Carotis. Dtsch Arch Klin Med 28:80–93, 1881
17. Roberts B, Ring EJ: Current status of percutaneous transluminal angioplasty. Surg Clin North Am 62:357–372, 1982
18. Ross RS, McKusick VA: Aortic arch syndromes: diminished or absent pulses in arteries arising from arch of aorta. Arch Intern Med 92:701–740, 1953
19. Savory WS: Case of a young woman in whom the main arteries of both upper extremities and of the left side of the neck were throughout completely obliterated. Trans Med-Chir Soc Lond 39:205–220, 1856
20. Shimizu K, Sano K: Pulseless disease. J Neuropathol Clin Neurol 1:37–47, 1951
21. Sundt TM Jr, Smith HC, Campbell JK, et al: Transluminal angioplasty for basilar artery stenosis. Mayo Clin Proc 55:673–680, 1980
22. Takayasu M: Case of queer changes in central blood vessels of retina. Acta Soc Ophthalmol Jpn 12:554, 1908
23. Wylie EJ, Effeney DJ: Surgery of the aortic arch branches and vertebral arteries. Surg Clin North Am 59:669–680, 1979

7

Subclavian Steal Syndrome

Jim L. Story, Willis E. Brown, Jr., George L. Bohmfalk, and Moustapha Abou-Samra

Introduction

A subclavian steal occurs when blood flows away from the circle of Willis, retrograde down the vertebral artery into the distal subclavian artery. Most cases are due to atherosclerosis, which causes stenosis or occlusion of the subclavian or innominate artery proximal to the origin of the vertebral artery. The subclavian artery distal to the stenosis or occlusion then functions as a sink. Retrograde flow occurs down the left vertebral artery in about 75% of cases.* Other less common causes of this syndrome are trauma and embolization. In a few cases the treatment of a subclavian steal has been followed by the development of a subclavian steal contralaterally.[3,48] Congenital cardiovascular anomalies, or occasionally the surgical procedures used to treat these anomalies, may produce this syndrome.[32,42,50,58] A principal example of this is the Blalock-Taussig procedure (subclavian to pulmonary artery end-to-side anastomosis) for tetralogy of Fallot. The division of the subclavian artery, required in this procedure, may lead to subclavian steal.[25,38]

Historical Review

The first reported case of subclavian steal syndrome and its surgical treatment was that of Mr. William Banks, a patient treated by Dr. Andrew Smyth at the Charity Hospital in New Orleans in 1864.[68] It is of interest that Banks' subclavian steal was iatrogenic. The 32-year-old ship's steward was involved in a collision of ships; he developed a traumatic right subclavian aneurysm after clinging to an anchor with another man, in turn, holding onto him. Smyth employed a variation of Hunterian ligation for treatment of the aneurysm, as recommended by Rogers, a surgeon visiting from New York. He ligated the innominate artery and the common carotid artery in order to "intercept a retrograde current through [the carotid artery], which he supposed had occurred in former cases." Fourteen days later profuse hemorrhage ensued, "causing syncope rapidly." Smyth was struck by the rapid occurrence of syncope during a second bleed weeks later and concluded that the vertebral artery must be carrying blood away from the brain, thereby providing collateral flow to the subclavian artery distal to the aneurysm. This pathway had been described in 1829 by Robert Harrison, in his text *The Surgical Anatomy of the Arteries of the Human Body*.[31] Smyth, therefore, ligated the vertebral artery. Banks survived and worked for 10 years, at which time the aneurysm recurred. Despite ligation of the internal mammary artery and an attempt at packing the sac, he died from postoperative hemorrhage, a result of collateral flow to the aneurysm through the subscapular artery.[72]

*References 19, 22, 29, 32, 37, 38, 56.

Fields,[21] who publicized Smyth's report in 1970, implied that the subclavian steal syndrome would have become generally recognized decades earlier had Smyth's paper been published in a more widely read journal than the first issue of the *New Orleans Medical Record*, in the wake of the War Between the States. However, Contorni[10] later noted that Smyth's "brilliant intuitions" were indeed well disseminated, especially in Europe. Smyth's contributions, nevertheless, were subsequently forgotten as newer surgical techniques for aneurysms were developed near the turn of the century.[10]

In 1960 Contorni first reported, in the Italian literature, angiographic evidence of retrograde flow in the vertebral artery. His patient was neurologically asymptomatic, but had absent left upper extremity pulses.[9] Contrast medium injected into the right subclavian artery passed up the right vertebral and refluxed down the left vertebral into the left subclavian artery. Similar arteriographic findings in four patients, three of whom had symptoms of basilar insufficiency, were presented during the Third Princeton Conference on Cerebral Vascular Disease in January 1961 by Fields[20] and Toole[76]. In a widely recognized article, Reivich et al correlated the reversal of flow in the vertebral artery to cerebral ischemia. This paper appeared in November 1961[61] and included complete descriptions of two patients whose arteriograms had been presented earlier that year by Toole at the Third Princeton Conference. These authors are generally credited as the first to associate reversal of blood flow with brain ischemia. However, at the same Third Princeton Conference, Rob,[62] discussing techniques of surgical therapy for incipient stroke, had clearly recognized that the transient cerebral ischemia in one of his patients was due to right subclavian artery occlusion, which resulted in "blood being withdrawn from the cerebral circulation into the right arm when that limb was exercised." These authors were all apparently unaware of Contorni's publication the previous year and of Smyth's paper published in the previous century. In the editorial accompanying the article by Reivich et al,[61] C.M. Fisher proposed the term "subclavian steal" to describe the syndrome.[24] Shortly thereafter, numerous cases appeared in the literature. Some authors suggested more anatomic terms, such as "brachial-basilar insufficiency syndrome."[56] Contorni recently urged belated recognition of the original contributors by adopting the eponym "Harrison and Smyth's syndrome,"[10] but Fisher's appelation still stands.

Clinical Course and Manifestations

The natural history of subclavian steal syndrome is variable. Although a subclavian steal may be seen by angiography with moderate frequency, it is often asymptomatic.[22,25,38,49,57] When the steal becomes symptomatic, it may be incapacitating. Although most patients complain of neurological symptoms, a small percentage have symptoms of brachial ischemia.[22,23,59] Production of neurological symptoms by exercising the relatively ischemic arm is common in some series and rare in others.[†] The neurological symptoms usually result from brain stem and cerebellar ischemia; however, cerebral symptoms may also occur, even in the absence of carotid artery occlusive disease.[4,5] Completed stroke is uncommon in this syndrome[22]; when stroke does occur, the cerebral hemisphere as well as the brain stem or the cerebellum may be affected.[34,39,44,79] This paradox, i.e., neurological deficit in areas not normally supplied by the vertebral or basilar artery, may result from secondary intracranial steal.[4,77] Finally, there are reports of spontaneous remission of symptoms, and in a case caused by trauma, return of antegrade vertebral artery blood flow was documented angiographically.[44,71,79]

Preoperative Evaluation

Preoperative evaluation of patients suspected of subclavian steal must include appropriate studies to exclude metabolic, cardiovascular, and otologic causes of the symptoms.

Computerized tomography (CT) and radionuclide scanning are important, especially in those patients with cerebral symptoms. When there is clinical and radiographic evidence of infarction, early surgical intervention must be weighed with care because of the possibility of hemorrhage into the infarction.[81]

†References 22, 29, 32, 34, 38, 56, 79.

The cornerstone in the evaluation of patients with subclavian steal is extensive angiography. The aortic arch and subclavian arteries must be seen. Furthermore, not only the origin but the entire course of the carotid and vertebral vascular systems must be visualized in the early, middle, and late angiographic phases.

Highly important in the planning of a surgical procedure for correction of a subclavian steal is a comprehensive understanding of the patient's intracranial and extracranial collateral circulation. This is particularly imperative in procedures that require occlusion of the common carotid artery during an anastomosis. Common carotid artery occlusion does not carry the risks of internal carotid artery occlusion[53,75]; nevertheless, if impaired collateral circulation has been demonstrated, consideration should be given to the use of protective measures such as hypothermia, barbiturates,[35] or temporary shunting.

Surgical Procedures

A variety of operations rapidly evolved as surgeons became aware of the subclavian steal syndrome. We shall review these procedures and discuss vertebral to common carotid artery transposition, a procedure that we have found to be very effective in the management of this syndrome. In the modern era, Rob[62] appears to have been the first to recognize and treat, surgically, a patient with symptomatic subclavian steal. He, like Smyth 100 years before, ligated the vertebral artery. Reivich et al[61] treated one of their patients with subclavian endarterectomy; they did not describe the postoperative results. The subclavian steal of their second patient was not clearly symptomatic. His operation was directed to a carotid occlusion. During 1962 at least four papers appeared and reported experience with the syndrome in 13 patients.[39] Subclavian endarterectomy via sternal splitting was performed with success and failure by Mannick et al,[45] by Simon et al,[66] and by DeBakey's group.[56] The last group introduced extrathoracic reconstruction in the same paper; they reported a supraclavicular subclavian endarterectomy in one patient and a carotid to subclavian artery bypass graft in four others.[56]

Regarding carotid to subclavian artery bypass, it is of interest that Lyons and Galbraith[43] had previously reported the use of subclavian to carotid artery bypass grafts for treatment of common carotid artery occlusion. In subclavian to carotid bypass, blood is shunted directly from the subclavian artery, beyond the occluded common carotid artery, into the internal and external carotid arteries. In contrast, the carotid to subclavian bypass, when used to treat subclavian steal, directs blood away from the common carotid artery into the subclavian artery. Blood flow in the subclavian artery in the latter circumstance is bidirectional, retrograde to the origin of the vertebral artery, and antegrade to an extremity.

Controversy arose, and continues, as to whether or not a carotid to subclavian steal develops after the carotid to subclavian bypass graft procedure. Intraoperative blood pressure and flow measurements in several patients suggested that this steal does not occur,[1,14,18] but in another report a steal was demonstrated.[28] Animal experiments designed to evaluate this point have also produced conflicting results. In one preparation of carotid to subclavian artery bypass, there was no change in proximal or distal common carotid artery blood flow with the upper extremity at rest. When exercise of the extremity was simulated (by creation of a distal subclavian arteriovenous fistula), flow in the common carotid artery proximal to the graft increased, and there was no decrease in flow to the distal carotid artery. The authors concluded that there was no steal from arteries supplying the brain in their experimental model.[41] However, several other animal studies have demonstrated decreases in distal carotid artery flow under similar circumstances,[2,11,30] particularly in the presence of stenosis at the origin of the internal carotid artery.

Although there have been no well-documented reports of symptoms of carotid to subclavian steal in patients, the carotid to subclavian bypass has failed to relieve vertebrobasilar symptoms in some cases.[28] We have seen two cases of such failure. The first was that of a patient whose vertigo recurred following a carotid to subclavian bypass graft. Angiography showed the graft to be patent, but flow was preferential into the arm. There was no longer a steal down the vertebral artery, but the dye column in the vertebral artery was essentially stagnant. The limited antegrade flow on the side of the bypass was coupled with contralateral vertebral artery stenosis at its origin; these factors undoubtedly caused her recurrent symptoms. The second of our patients, who was previously treated by carotid subclavian bypass, developed recurrent symptoms caused by progressive stenosis of the subclavian artery distal to the origin of the vertebral artery and proximal to the subclavian graft site. Additionally, stenosis of the contralateral vertebral artery origin had progressed, further aggravating the brain stem ischemia. Thus, regarding the brain, the hemodynamic effect of the carotid to subclavian bypass was—in these two cases, at least—hardly better than vertebral artery ligation. This problem, i.e., the failure of a carotid to subclavian bypass to restore adequate vertebral flow, has also been demonstrated in animal preparations in which retrograde flow in the vertebral artery has been induced by subclavian artery ligation. In several such animals the retrograde flow was only diminished or arrested, never reversed, upon opening a carotid to subclavian bypass graft.[2,30] The appropriate criterion for success in this and other indirect bypass procedures is, therefore, not merely equalization of brachial blood pressures, but restoration of antegrade flow in the vertebral artery. Although carotid to subclavian bypass graft currently appears to be the most frequently used method for treating subclavian steal syndrome, these instances of failure to normalize vertebral perfusion indicate the need for more effective extrathoracic techniques that are equally safe.

Variations on the carotid to subclavian artery bypass procedure have been reported. A more lateral graft placement (anastomosis of the graft to the axillary artery rather than the subclavian artery) is thought by some to be technically easier and equally effective with regard to hemodynamics.[65] Direct common carotid to vertebral artery side-to-side anastomosis is a variant of carotid to subclavian artery bypass that requires only one anastomosis. This procedure was facilitated by an elongated, tortuous vertebral artery in the one case reported.[67] The simplicity of a single anastomosis lead Edwards and Wright[17] to favor direct side-to-side or end-to-side subclavian to carotid artery anastomosis. Mehigan et al[51] also recommended subclavian to common carotid artery transposition and stressed the additional advantage of concomitant eversion endarterectomy of the subclavian artery and vertebral artery origin. The dissection required, however, is deep and potentially hazardous. Excision of the medial third of the clavicle, which may produce disabling symptoms,[22] is occasionally required for exposure in this procedure.[17,64]

The subclavian to subclavian artery bypass was introduced in 1968 to avoid manipulation of the carotid artery.[23] Experimental studies in dogs indicate that this procedure, like carotid to subclavian artery bypass, is usually effective in restoring antegrade flow in the vertebral artery.[26] Criticisms of this procedure include the possibility of injury to the thoracic duct, to the phrenic nerve, and to the recurrent laryngeal nerve. Some critics believe that the dissection is technically difficult.[36,47] Others object to the subcutaneous location of the graft.[33]

Axillo-axillary bypass has been promoted as having the same benefits as subclavian to subclavian bypass and as being easier to perform.[13,36,47] Additionally, the procedure can be done under local anesthesia, as can some of the other operations, and two operating teams can complete the procedure in less than one hour.[70] There have been isolated reports of graft occlusion, both spontaneous and as a result of compression of the graft.[60,70] Problems with injury to the surrounding brachial plexus have also been reported.[40,70] Herring[33] raised the interesting consideration that inasmuch as 10% of patients with subclavian steal develop coronary artery occlusion during an extended follow-up,[22] the presternal graft might interfere with the approach for a coronary bypass operation. Nonetheless, axillo-axillary bypass has a good clinical record.[40] It is supported by data demonstrating restoration of antegrade blood flow in the vertebral artery and has a mortality approaching zero.[54]

The vertebrobasilar symptoms of subclavian steal have been relieved by treatment of coincidental carotid artery stenosis.[22,55,64,67,80] Carotid endarterectomy presumably increases the intracranial collateral flow to the posterior circulation. Najafi et al,[55] however, reported several patients treated with carotid endarterectomy alone whose vertebrobasilar insufficiency symptoms persisted. A second operation directed to the subclavian steal was required. His group therefore began performing, in selected patients with ipsilateral disease, concomitant carotid endarterectomy and carotid to subclavian artery bypass grafts. Their results were satisfactory.[55]

The operation of least magnitude for symptomatic subclavian steal is vertebral artery ligation. Rob did this and described its success in his early report, as mentioned previously. Despite this success, in 1964 Rob[63] recommended using this "inferior" procedure only "exceptionally in poor risk patients." We have found 20 instances of vertebral artery ligation for symptomatic subclavian steal in the literature. Useful clinical information is available from ten.[4,5] Neurological symptoms were relieved or improved in ten instances. None of the described patients suffered neurological deficit as a result of the ligation. Although radial pulses disappeared in two cases after the ligation, and in one case the arm briefly appeared threatened, these signs universally cleared, and the patients regained good use of their extremities.[6,69]

Although vertebral artery ligation can relieve the symptoms of subclavian steal, there are at least three advantages of bypass procedures that restore antegrade flow in the vertebral artery. First, flow to the brain is increased. Second, the potential ischemic consequences of progressive occlusive disease in the contralateral vertebral artery may be avoided. Third, it is not uncommon for collateral channels to the subclavian artery to develop between the distal vertebral artery and branches of the thyrocervical trunk. After vertebral artery ligation, these channels remain open and continue to supply collateral flow to the upper extremity. This persistent collateral flow, however, is compensated by those bypass operations that restore adequate antegrade flow in the vertebral artery or reduce the demand for collateral flow.

Although most of the available procedures thus far described have a good record, they vary in complexity, in technical difficulty, and in the amount of antegrade blood flow restored in the vertebral artery.[4,5] Therefore, we looked for a procedure that is conceptually simple, that can be performed on very ill patients, and that provides high-volume antegrade flow in the vertebral artery. Vertebral to carotid transposition appears to fulfill these objectives.[4,5]

The historical groundwork that led to the use of vertebral to carotid artery transposition for the treatment of the neurological symptoms of subclavian steal was laid in several papers.

In 1966 Clark and Perry[8] reported success in one case of subclavian steal syndrome managed by anastomosis of the external carotid artery to the distal vertebral artery. The patient was asymptomatic following surgery, and there was no reduction of blood pressure in the involved arm. Their procedure required an extensive dissection to remove the vertebral artery from the upper cervical transverse processes. In 1977 Corkill et al[12] reported external carotid to vertebral artery anastomoses in two patients with vertebrobasilar insufficiency due to vertebral artery stenosis. In their cases the external carotid was attached end-to-side to the vertebral artery between a pair of transverse processes.

A more proximal carotid system to vertebral artery anastomosis was first reported by Galbraith and McDowell in 1969.[27] They treated a patient with vertebrobasilar insufficiency due to vertebral origin stenosis by end-to-side proximal vertebral artery to common carotid artery transposition. Wylie and Ehrenfeld[80] reported a patient with stenosis of one vertebral artery origin and occlusion of the contralateral vertebral artery. They also transposed the proximal vertebral artery, just above the stenosis, to the common carotid artery. This procedure relieved the patient's symptoms. (Recently, Edwards et al[15,16] successfully treated symptomatic vertebral artery stenosis with this transposition. We also have found this to be a useful procedure for dealing with vertebrobasilar insufficiency due to proximal vertebral artery stenosis.)

Stimulated by these reports, and reassured by the literature that transposition of the vertebral artery would not jeopardize the upper extremity, we undertook a series of vertebral to carotid transpositions in patients with neurological symptoms of subclavian steal.[4,5] The results have been gratifying, and vertebral to carotid transposition has become our preferred method in treating these patients.

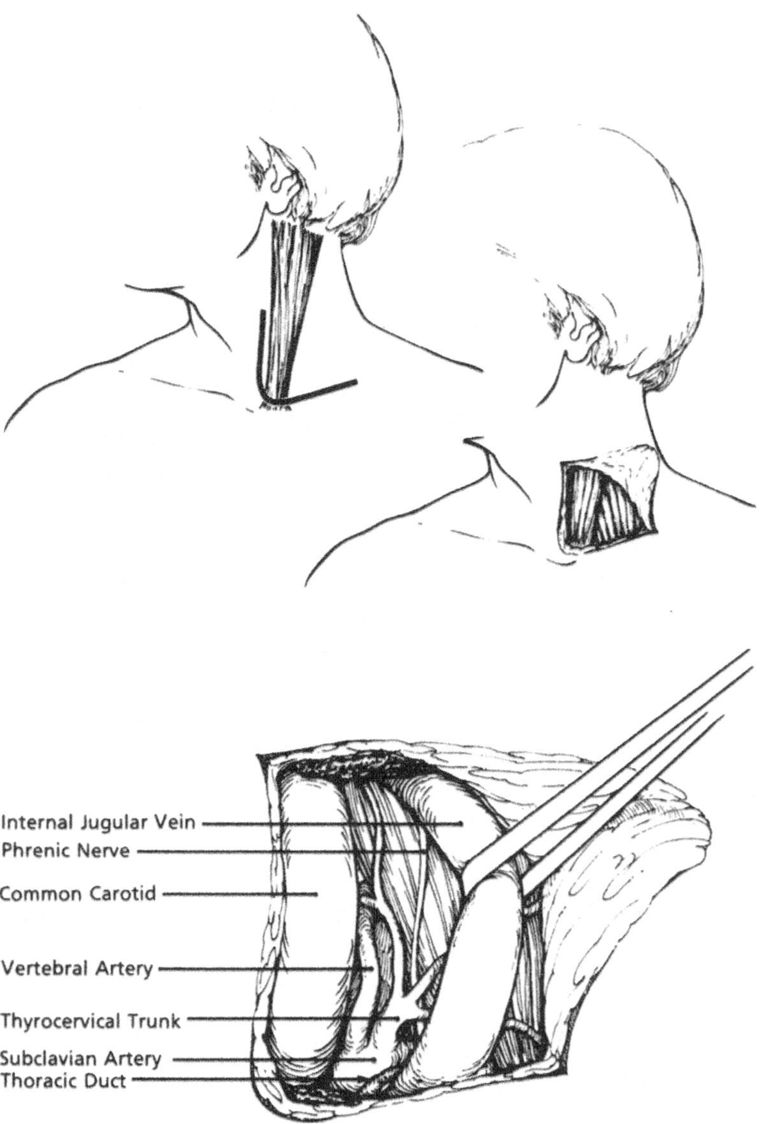

Figure 7.1. Vertebral to carotid transposition: the incision and skin flap.

Figure 7.2. Vertebral to carotid transposition. The dissection exposes the common carotid artery and the origin of the vertebral artery.

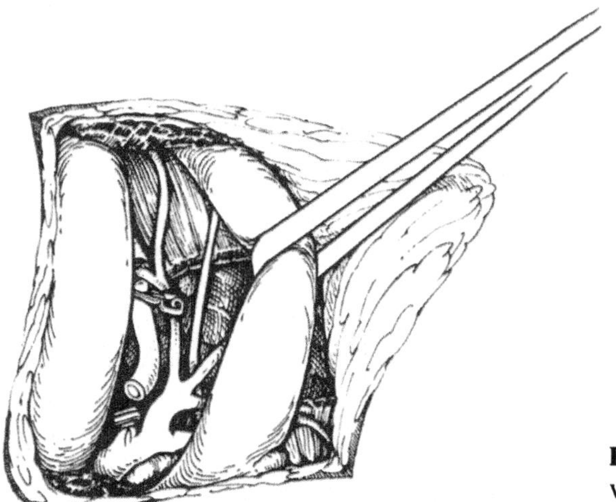

Figure 7.3. Vertebral to carotid transposition. The vertebral artery is divided as proximally as possible to provide maximum length for transposition.

Surgical Procedure for Vertebral to Common Carotid Artery Transposition

The technical aspects of proximal vertebral to common carotid artery transposition are relatively strightforward. General endotracheal anesthesia is employed. Maintenance of a normal or slightly elevated mean systemic arterial blood pressure to ensure effective cerebral blood flow is imperative.[80] Further, the PaO_2 should be maintained higher than 100 torr, and the $PaCO_2$ should be maintained at a normal level.

The skin and subcutaneous incisions are made along the medial margin of the sternocleidomastoid toward the suprasternal notch and then carried laterally about 2 cm above and parallel to the clavicle. The skin flap is then undermined and reflected (Fig. 7.1). The clavicular head of the sternocleidomastoid and the anterior scalene muscle are divided to expose the subclavian, the vertebral, and common carotid arteries. On the left side the thoracic duct may be encountered medially; either it should be protected or, if entered, it should be ligated (Fig. 7.2). After dissection of the vertebral artery, 3,500 units of heparin are given intravenously, a temporary clip is placed high on the vertebral artery, and the artery is doubly clipped just above its origin. When applying the proximal clips, care must be taken to prevent a vascular tear that might extend into the subclavian artery. The vessel is then divided as proximally as is convenient (Fig. 7.3). The common carotid artery is then briefly occluded, its wall is incised, and an eliptical arteriotomy is created with a 4- to 5-mm aortic punch. A partially occluding vascular clamp is applied to the common carotid artery to allow carotid flow to continue during the anastomosis. The end-to-side anastomosis is performed with a continuous 7-0 suture under the operating microscope or magnifying loops (Fig. 7.4 and 7.5).

Occasionally the length of the vertebral artery may be insufficient for a direct transposition to the carotid artery. A saphenous vein graft may be sutured end-to-end to the vertebral artery and end-to-side of the common carotid artery to provide additional length. In one of our patients we utilized a short segment of a 3- to 4-mm internal diameter expanded polytetrafluoroethylene (PTFE) (Gore-tex, W.L. Gore and Associates, Flagstaff, Arizona) as an interposition tube graft (Fig. 7.6).[7,46,52,73,74,82] Although the results with expanded PTFE as a small vascular conduit are encouraging, a greater experience and longer follow-up for patency is necessary before these grafts can be recommended for use in preference to autogenous vein grafts.

Carotid endarterectomy, when performed at the same operation, usually follows the vertebral to common carotid artery anastomosis for two reasons: this sequence permits the restored antegrade flow in the vertebral artery to contribute to, and not steal from, the cerebral circulation during the endarterectomy; it prevents an opportunity for thrombus formation at the fresh endarterectomy site if internal carotid blood flow is reduced during partial occlusion of the proximal common carotid artery.

Intraoperative blood flow measurement is useful although not required. It permits determination of the direction and rate of flow in the vertebral artery before and after procedures performed to correct a symptomatic subclavian steal. The technique is of additional value in monitoring blood flow in the distal common or internal carotid artery during procedures that may require prolonged complete or partial occlusion of the common carotid artery. We have used such flow data to evaluate the effectiveness of various operative procedures and have found that antegrade flow following vertebral to carotid transposition in two patients exceeded that reported after other procedures for correction of subclavian steal.[5]

Illustrative Cases

We shall summarize four case histories to emphasize the clinical manifestations of the syndrome as well as the following points:

1. Symptomatic carotid artery disease and symptomatic subclavian steal may occur simultaneously and require combined vertebral to carotid transposition and carotid endarterectomy (Case 2).
2. Cerebral symptoms in the absence of carotid system disease can be caused by an intracranial steal from the anterior circulation (Case 3).
3. Vertebral to carotid artery transposition can

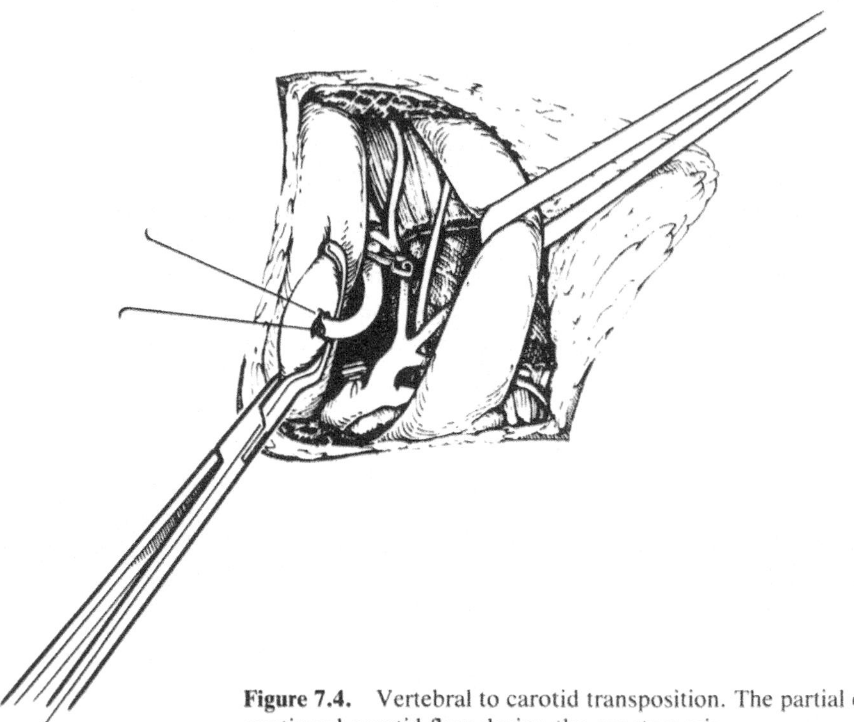

Figure 7.4. Vertebral to carotid transposition. The partial occlusion clamp permits continued carotid flow during the anastomosis.

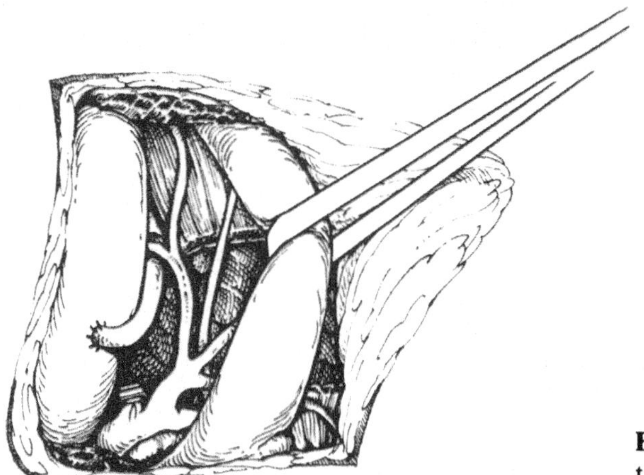

Figure 7.5. Vertebral to carotid transposition. The completed anastomosis permits return of antegrade flow in the vertebral artery.

relieve persistent or recurrent neurological symptoms when bypass procedures, such as the popular carotid to subclavian bypass, have failed (Case 4).

Case 1

A 57-year-old, right-handed high-school maintenance foreman experienced progressively severe episodes of vertigo and disequilibrium for two years. These episodes prevented him from working. He could not relate the episodes to arm exercise, but he noted that they frequently followed arising from a squatting position.

Examination. Both radial pulses were diminished, but they were easily felt, and there was no pulse delay. His brachial blood pressures

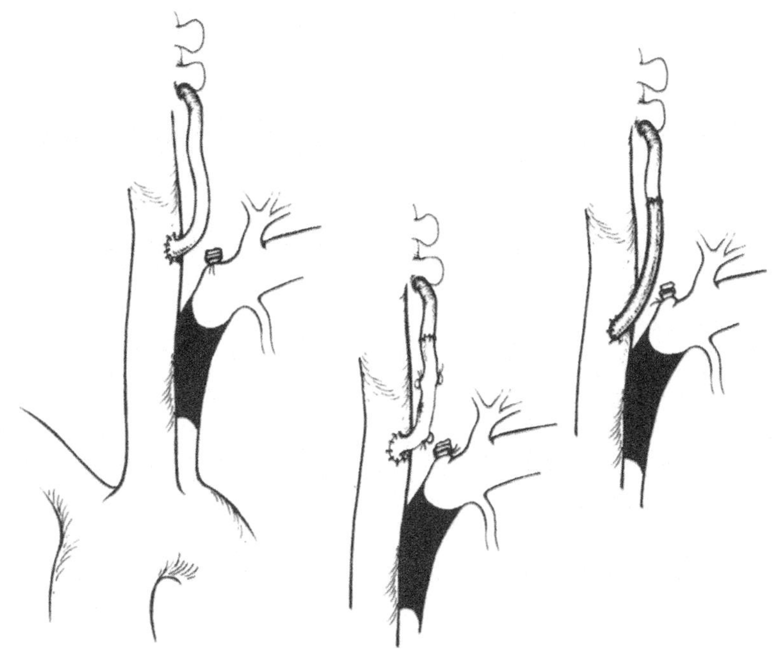

Figure 7.6. Vertebral to carotid transposition. In most cases direct transposition is possible (*left*). When extra length is needed, a saphenous vein graft may be interposed (*middle*) or, on occasion, a PTFE tube graft may be utilized (*right, see text*).

were 74/40 bilaterally. At the level of the thigh, blood pressures were 150/90 bilaterally. There were soft bilateral carotid bruits. Arm exercise did not precipitate symptoms. His general and neurological examinations were otherwise unremarkable.

Angiograms of the aortic arch demonstrated complete occlusion of the proximal left subclavian artery (Fig. 7.7) with rapid appearance of contrast medium flowing retrograde down the left vertebral artery to the subclavian artery (Fig. 7.8). Numerous collateral channels to the left subclavian artery were demonstrated. Among these were left external carotid to thyrocervical trunk anastomoses and distal vertebral to thyrocervical trunk anastomoses. (Fig. 7.8). A right retrograde brachial angiogram confirmed the rapid left subclavian steal and a proximal subclavian stenosis on the right side. The intracranial circulation was unremarkable.

Operation and Postoperative Course. The proximal left vertebral artery was transposed to the left common carotid artery. The patient has experienced no neurological symptoms in three years since the operation, even with manuevers that readily produced symptoms preoperatively. Blood pressure in the left arm was unchanged by the procedure, and the left radial pulse remains readily palpable. The patient has returned fulltime to his previous job. An angiogram three years postoperatively demonstrated prompt antegrade filling of the left vertebral artery from the common carotid artery (Fig. 7.9). The left subclavian artery received collateral flow from the distal vertebral through the thyrocervical trunk (Fig. 7.9). However, the chief collateral flow to the subclavian artery was derived from the external carotid system, which had extensive anastomoses with the thyrocervical trunk (Fig. 7.10). Abundant filling of the basilar artery circulation was seen. There was a stenosis in the right subclavian artery, and a moderate contralateral steal was demonstrated down the right vertebral artery (Fig. 7.10).

Case 2

This 64-year-old, right-handed woman experienced vertigo, staggering, and multiple falls for five months. During one of these episodes, she fractured her wrist. She had no symptoms of brachial ischemia, and she could not relate her spells to arm exercise.

Examination. Blood pressure in her upper extremities was 200/100 on the right and 150/90 on the left. She had soft left carotid and supraclavicular bruits. The remainder of her general and

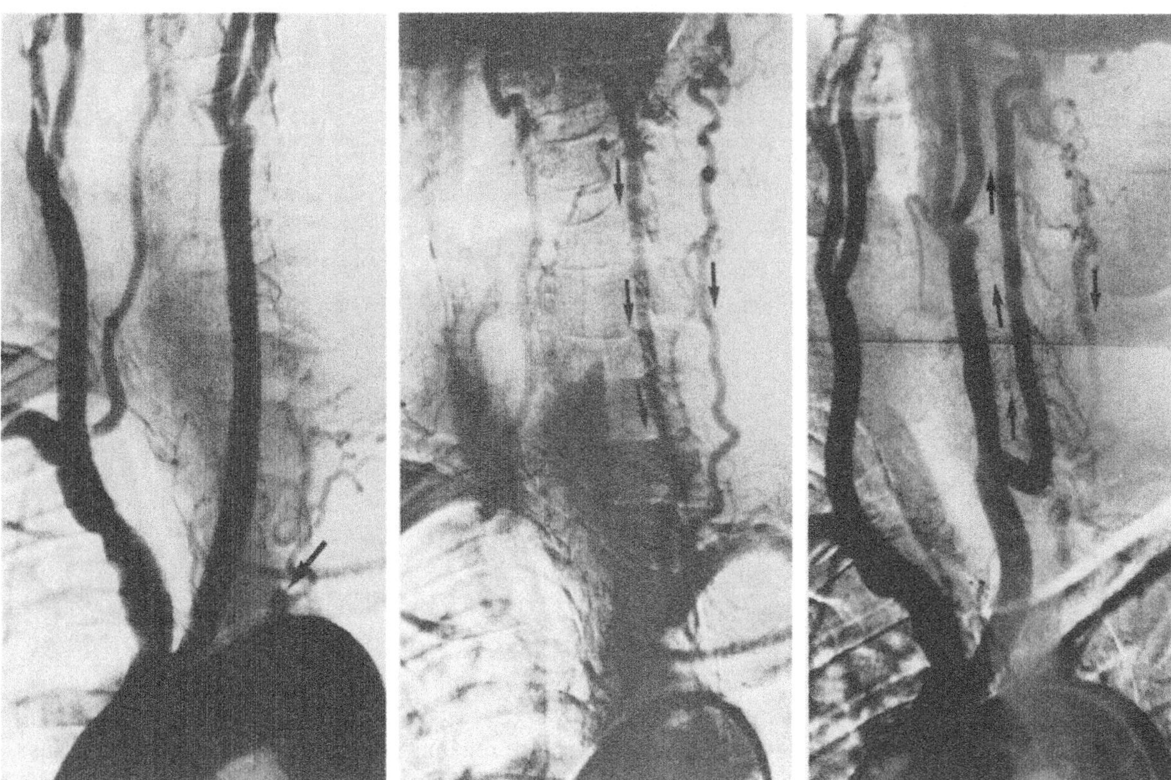

Fig. 7.7 Fig. 7.8 Fig. 7.9

Figure 7.7. Case 1. Preoperative angiogram of the aortic arch demonstrating occlusion of the proximal subclavian artery on the left and nonfilling of the left vertebral artery.

Figure 7.8. Case 1. A film later in the angiographic sequence showing retrograde flow in the left vertebral artery (*triple arrow*) and filling of the left subclavian artery from the vertebral artery and from external carotid and vertebral artery collaterals to the thyrocervical trunk (*single arrow*).

Figure 7.9. Case 1. Postoperative angiogram of the aortic arch three years following a left vertebral to common carotid artery transposition. The *arrows* denote antegrade flow through the left vertebral artery and retrograde flow down the thyrocervical trunk.

neurological examinations was normal. Arm exercise did not produce neurological symptoms.

Transfemoral aortic arch and selective cerebral angiograms demonstrated significant stenosis at the origin of the left subclavian artery and revealed minimal proximal left internal carotid artery stenosis (Fig. 7.11). There was generalized intracranial vascular disease. Following right vertebral injection, there was retrograde flow in the left vertebral artery (Figs. 7.12A,B). Surgical correction was recommended, but the patient minimized her symptoms and refused the operation.

Eight months later she returned. Her symptoms had intensified, they recurred daily, and she was unable to do her housework. She also experienced occasional paresthesias in the right extremities. Her blood pressures were unchanged from before. There was a pulse delay at the left wrist. The left carotid bruit was definitely louder and higher in pitch than earlier. She had no neurological deficits. A second angiogram showed marked progression of the stenosis in both left internal and external carotid arteries (Fig. 7.13). The left subclavian artery was more stenotic. The left vertebral to left subclavian steal was unchanged.

Operation and Postoperative Course. Because the patient had symptoms of both vertebrobasilar and left carotid artery insufficiency, the proximal left vertebral artery was trans-

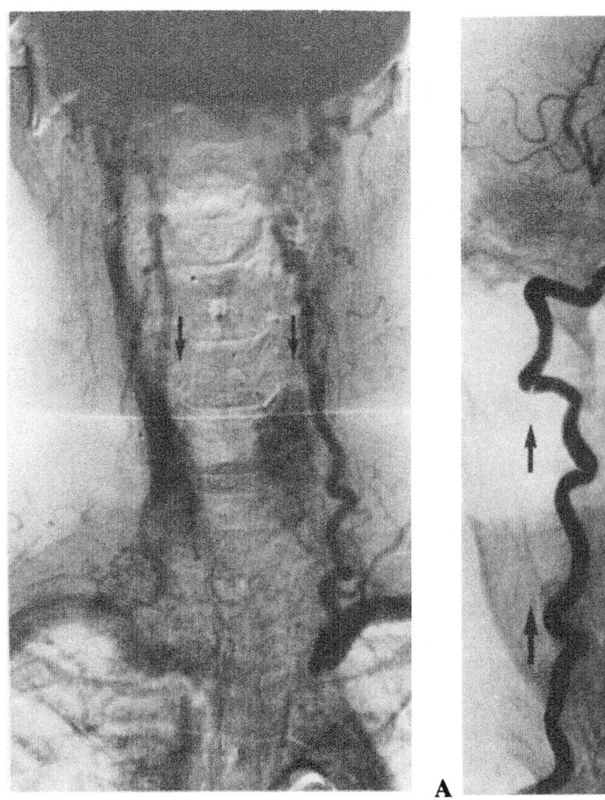

Fig. 7.10

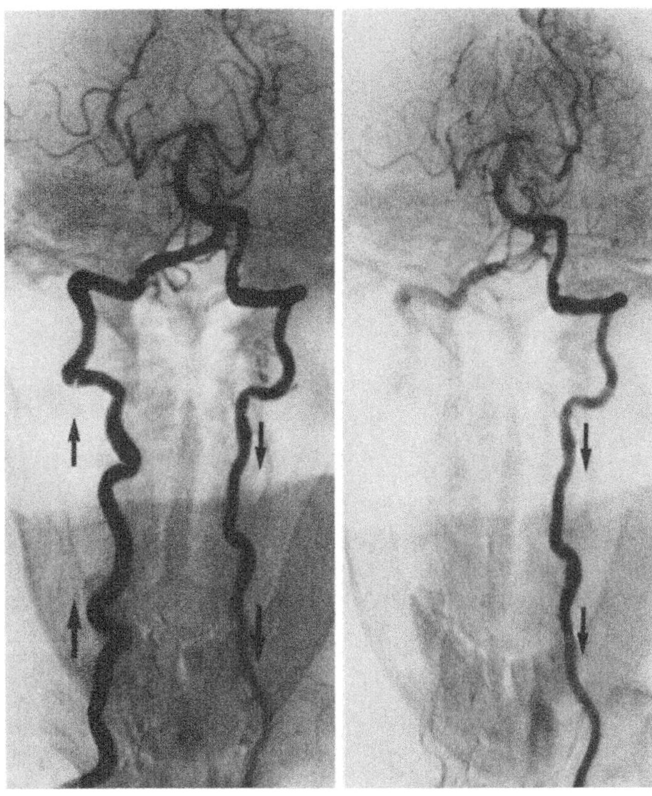

Fig. 7.12

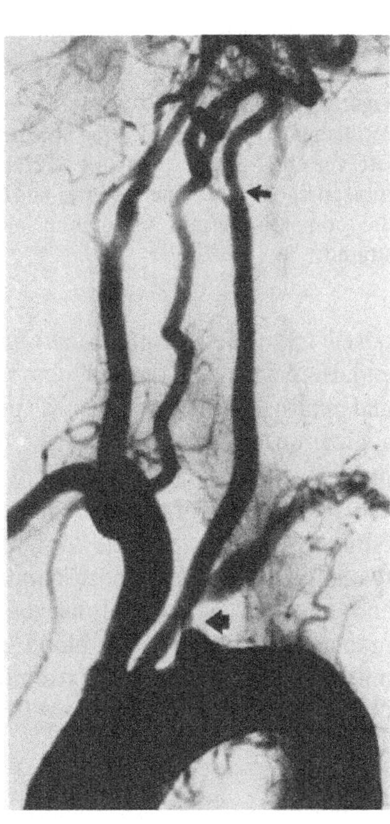

Fig. 7.11

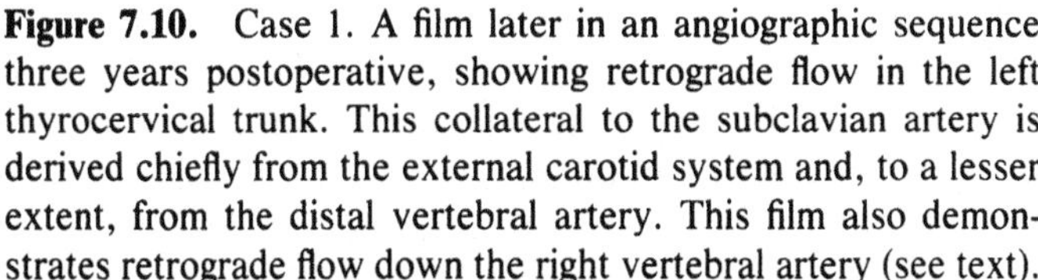

Figure 7.10. Case 1. A film later in an angiographic sequence three years postoperative, showing retrograde flow in the left thyrocervical trunk. This collateral to the subclavian artery is derived chiefly from the external carotid system and, to a lesser extent, from the distal vertebral artery. This film also demonstrates retrograde flow down the right vertebral artery (see text).

Figure 7.11. Case 2. Preoperative aortic arch angiogram demonstrating significant proximal stenosis of the left subclavian artery and a minimally stenotic origin of the left internal carotid artery.

Figure 7.12. Case 2. Preoperative angiogram with selective right vertebral injection demonstrating early (**A**) and persistent retrograde flow in the left vertebral artery (**B**).

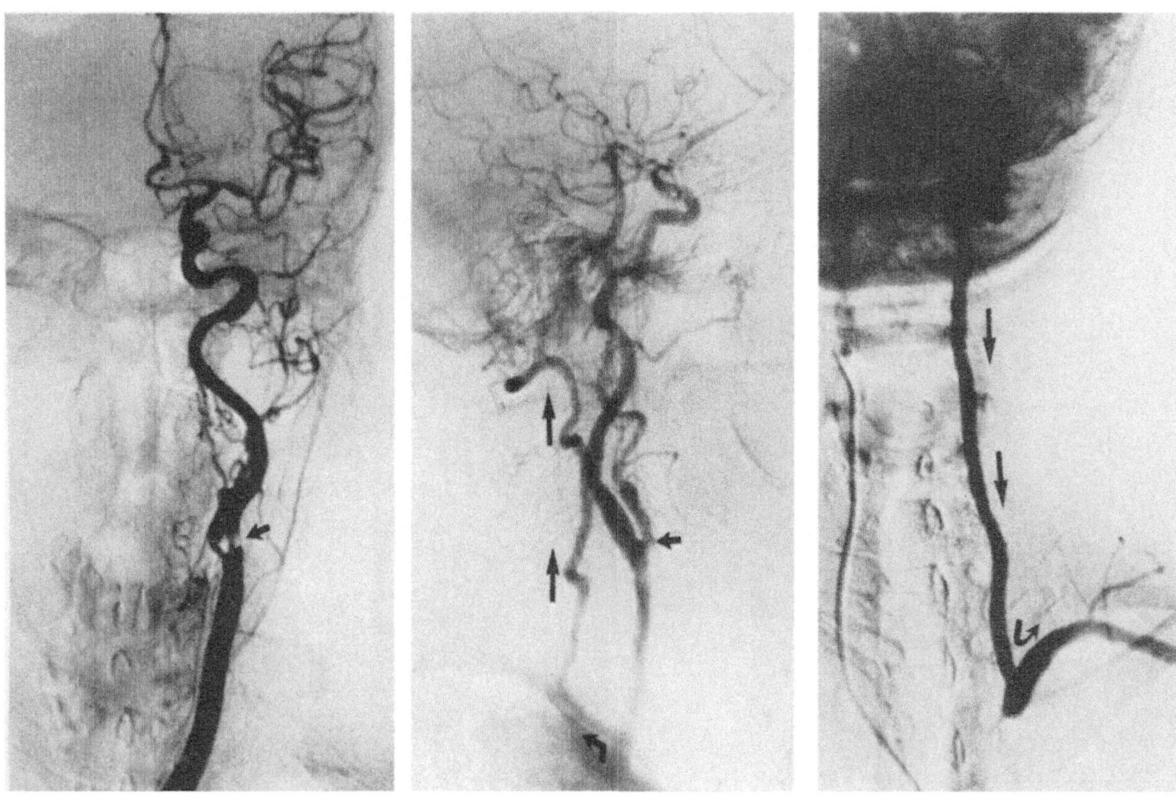

Fig. 7.13 Fig. 7.14 Fig. 7.15

Figure 7.13. Case 2. Left common carotid angiogram demonstrating a high-grade internal carotid artery stenosis that was not present eight months earlier (compare Fig. 7.11).

Figure 7.14. Case 2. Postoperative left common carotid angiogram demonstrating antegrade flow in the left vertebral artery following vertebral to carotid transposition. The result of the endarterectomy of the common carotid bifurcation also is demonstrated.

Figure 7.15. Case 3. Preoperative right vertebral angiogram demonstrating left subclavian artery steal: the retrograde flow in the left vertebral artery fills the subclavian artery.

posed to the left common carotid artery, and endarterectomy of the left common, internal, and external carotid arteries was performed. An angiogram before discharge demonstrated prompt antegrade flow in the left vertebral artery and patency of the entire left carotid distribution (Fig. 7.14). She has done well during the two and one-half years postoperative follow-up and has had no central nervous system or brachial symptoms. The blood pressure and pulse in the left upper extremity were unchanged by the procedure.

Case 3

This 48-year-old, right-handed woman was aware of asymmetric brachial blood pressures for at least 10 years; her pulse and blood pressures were difficult to obtain on the left. She complained of frequent episodes of vertigo, often accompanied by dysarthria and numbness in the hands and in the perioral region. Six months before admission she experienced a frightening episode described as "other worldliness." The episode lasted 24 hours and was associated with vertigo, dysarthria, and lightheadedness. Diplopia persisted for another 24 hours. Her admission to the hospital was prompted by a sudden left upper extremity paresis, followed within minutes by complete left hemiparesis. She had no symptoms of brachial ischemia, and she could not relate her spells to arm exercise.

Examination. The brachial blood pressures were 130/80 on the right and 90/50 on the left. Comparison of radial pulses revealed a definite delay on the left. No arterial bruits were heard. The patient was irritable and lethargic. She had a left central facial paresis. Visual fields were full to confrontation. She retained only antigravity power in the left upper extremity. The left lower extremity was mildly paretic. Sensory perception was impaired to all modalities on the left side. Manipulation of her left arm by passive exercise and by compression with a blood pressure cuff to levels above systolic pressure neither aggravated nor alleviated her findings.

Transfemoral arch and selective cerebral angiograms revealed proximal occlusion of the left subclavian artery and no other occlusive or ulcerated lesions. Injection of her right vertebral artery demonstrated that contrast medium promptly refluxed down the left vertebral artery into the left subclavian artery (Fig. 7.15). The right vertebral artery injection briefly and incompletely filled the superior cerebellar arteries, but the posterior cerebral arteries did not fill (Figs. 7.16A,B). On common carotid artery injection, the right posterior cerebral artery filled persistently from the right internal carotid artery. An early draining vein emerged from the upper region of the right frontoparietal area in the midst of a faint vascular blush and suggested luxury perfusion in this area (Fig. 7.17). No occluded vessel was seen on the right; the carotid system was entirely normal. The left common carotid artery injection showed prompt, persistent, bilateral filling of the posterior cerebral and superior cerebellar arteries via the left posterior communicating artery (Figs. 7.18A,B). The left vertebral artery and cervical muscular branches were faintly opacified, in a retrograde manner, by collateral flow from the left external carotid artery. CT scans without and with contrast enhancement on the second and seventh hospital days did not demonstrate cerebral infarction.

The cause of the patient's acute left hemiparesis was not entirely clear. Her past history indicated chronic vertebrobasilar insufficiency. However, angiographic findings indicated that an intracranial steal had also developed from the internal carotid to the vertebrobasilar distribution in response to the vertebral to subclavian artery steal. Two points of angiographic evidence supported this concept of anterior to posterior circulation intracranial steal: first, the prompt and persistent bilateral filling of the posterior cerebral and superior cerebellar arteries from the internal carotid arteries; and second, nonfilling of the posterior cerebral vessels and the distal basilar artery by the vertebral arteries. The expression of this intracranial steal by way of right hemispheral symptoms and signs may be related to the fact that both anterior cerebral arteries filled from the right internal carotid artery. These flow patterns—i.e., dependence of both anterior cerebral circulations on the right internal carotid artery and dependence of the posterior cerebral and superior cerebellar arteries on the anterior circulation—placed abnormal demands on the right internal carotid artery circulation. As a result of this intracranial steal, the watershed area of perfusion between the right anterior and middle cerebral arteries may have become underperfused and subsequently ischemic. This explanation is supported by the location of the early draining vein and vascular blush in the watershed area, the absence of a visible occluded vessel on the angiogram, and the absence of a cause for emboli from the proximal carotid arteries or from the heart.

Operation and Postoperative Course. The patient's left hemiparesis improved steadily. However, by the second week she still had only fair finger movement. On the 12th hospital day the proximal left vertebral artery was transposed to the left common carotid artery. Two years postoperatively, the left brachial blood pressure is 90/60, and the left radial pulse is unchanged. There have been no new neurological symptoms and neurological function has improved and stabilized. The patient has useful function in the left hand and minimal paresis in the left lower extremity.

Case 4

A 50-year-old, right-handed man developed transient symptoms of vertebrobasilar insufficiency at age 42. The symptoms were described as severe dizzy spells, a feeling of impending syncope, and a feeling of extreme weakness in the lower extremities. At age 44, at another hospital, angiographic examination revealed proximal stenosis of the left subclavian artery and a left vertebral to left subclavian artery steal. Ul-

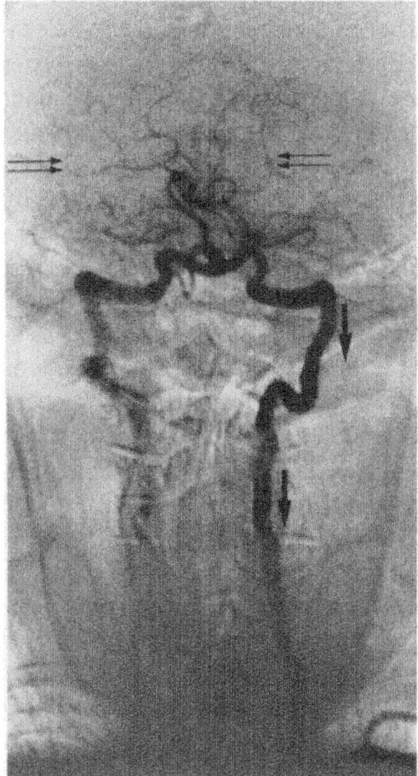

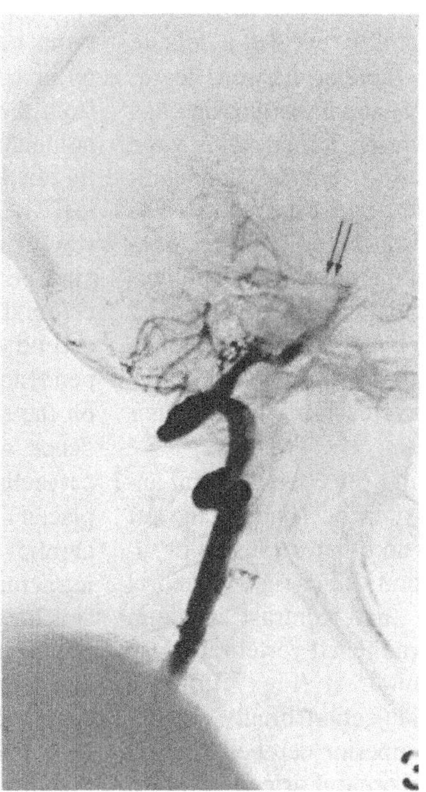

Figure 7.16. Case 3. Preoperative right vertebral angiogram demonstrating that the left subclavian steal precludes filling of the posterior cerebral arteries and permits only transient partial filling of the superior cerebellar arteries (*double arrows*).

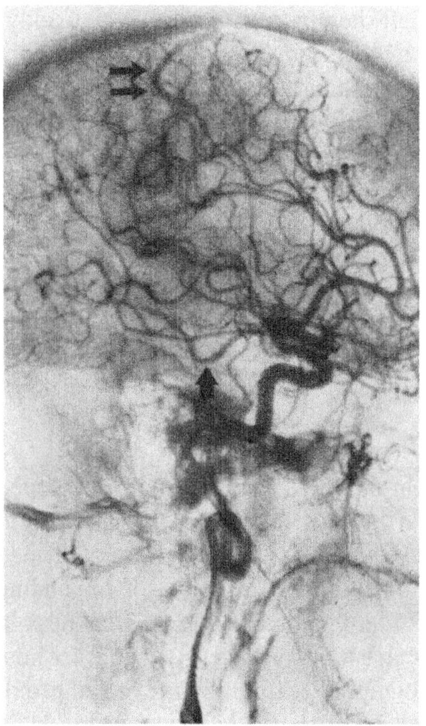

Figure 7.17. Case 3. Postoperative right common carotid angiogram demonstrating filling of the right posterior cerebral artery by way of the right posterior communicating artery (*single arrow*) and an early draining vein in the right frontoparietal area suggesting luxury perfusion (*double arrow*).

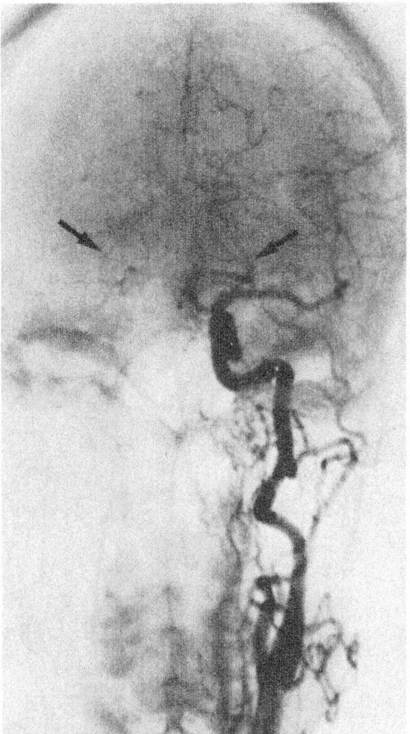
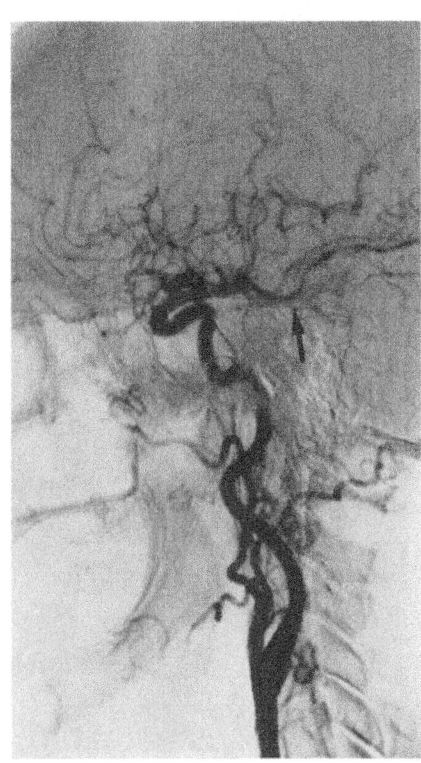

Figure 7.18. Case 3. Preoperative left common carotid artery angiogram demonstrating filling of the posterior cerebral arteries and the superior cerebellar arteries. Although the basilar artery was patent, the subclavian steal—by reversing flow in the distal basilar artery—caused prompt and persistent filling of the posterior cerebral and superior cerebellar arteries from the anterior circulation.

cerated plaques at the bifurcation of the common carotid artery were seen bilaterally. An endarterectomy of the right common and right internal carotid artery was performed. At another operation a left common and left internal carotid endarterectomy was combined with common carotid to subclavian artery bypass, utilizing a Dacron graft (E.I. du Pont de Nemours & Company, Wilmington, Delaware). The patient awoke from the second procedure with a right hemiparesis without aphasia. He recovered over a period of seven months.

Thereafter, he was well, and he experienced only an occasional dizzy spell. At age 47, however, he experienced a severe episode of vertigo and fell. Repeat angiography was said to show occlusion of the origin of the subclavian artery. There was no description, however, of the intracranial vertebrobasilar circulation.

At age 50 the patient came to our attention and was suffering from progressive and more frequent episodes of dizziness and feelings of impending syncope. These symptoms became incapacitating and they occurred as often as twice daily. He also described a transient episode of right facial paresthesias and two transient episodes of right hemiparesis and aphasia.

Examination. Despite all of his antecedent problems, the patient appeared to be in good general condition. His blood pressure was 190/110 in both upper extremities. Bilateral carotid and left subclavian artery bruits were present. The Dacron bypass graft was pulsatile. The neurological examination was essentially normal.

Angiographic examination revealed normal cervical carotid arteries. The posterior cerebral and superior cerebellar arteries and the distal basilar artery filled persistently from either carotid artery injection. Aortic arch injection revealed stenosis of the right vertebral artery at its origin and opacification of the right posterior inferior cerebellar artery and of both anterior

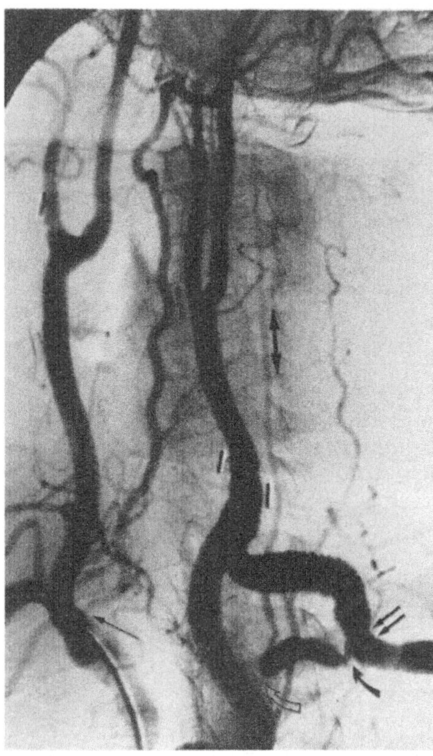

Figure 7.19. Case 4. Preoperative arch angiogram demonstrating stenosis of the right vertebral artery origin (*thin arrow*), occlusion of the proximal left subclavian artery (*open curved arrow*), marked stenosis of the subclavian artery (*closed curved arrow*) proximal to the distal anastomosis of the carotid subclavian bypass graft (*double solid arrow*), and faint filling of the left vertebral artery (*double-headed arrow*). Note that the left vertebral artery arises from a segment of the subclavian artery that is essentially isolated from the circulation. Additional films from this angiographic series confirmed that the dye column in the left vertebral artery never extended intracranially.

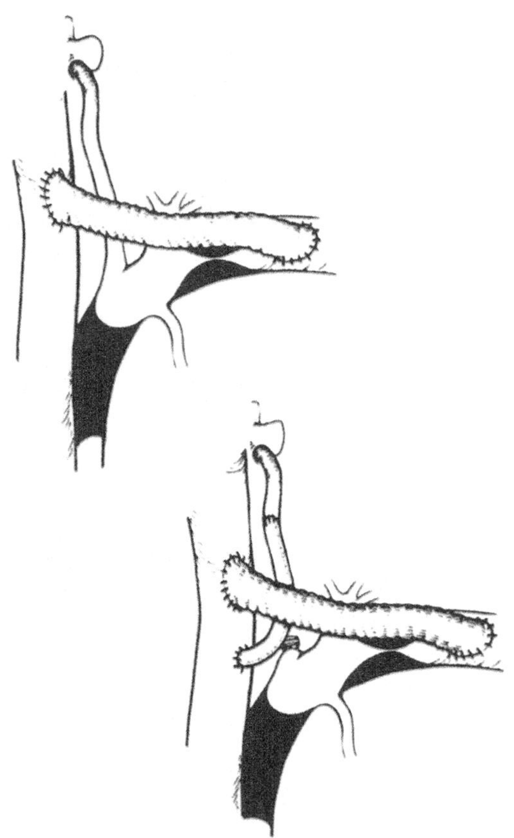

Figure 7.20. Case 4. *Left:* Progressive subclavian stenosis between the vertebral artery origin and the carotid to subclavian graft precluded adequate flow to the left vertebral artery. *Right:* Transposition of the left vertebral artery to the carotid artery restored flow in the vertebral artery. An interposition graft facilitated the procedure.

inferior cerebellar arteries. Occlusion of the mid portion of the basilar artery was demonstrated and explained the filling of the distal basilar artery and its branches from the anterior circulation. There was slight reflux of dye into the distal left vertebral artery. A left retrograde brachial artery injection demonstrated excellent opacification of the carotid subclavian bypass and the extracranial and intracranial carotid circulation. The proximal subclavian artery was, indeed, occluded, and the subclavian artery distal to the origin of the vertebral artery and proximal to the Dacron graft site was markedly stenotic. There was minimal antegrade flow in the vertebral artery, and this flow never reached the intracranial circulation (Fig. 7.19).

It was concluded that occlusion of the mid portion of the basilar artery had probably occurred at the time of the drop attack three years earlier. The recurrent symptoms of basivertebral insufficiency were felt to be caused by decreased blood flow in both vertebral arteries. This diminished flow was due to progressive vertebral origin stenosis on the right and to a shortcoming of the carotid subclavian bypass: A marked stenosis of the subclavian artery had developed between the origin of the left vertebral artery and the subclavian artery graft (Fig.

7.20). The left vertebral artery, the thyrocervical trunk, and the internal mammary artery were derived from a virtually isolated segment of subclavian artery.

Operation and Postoperative Course. A left vertebral to common carotid artery bypass was performed. A 3 mm internal diameter interposition PTFE tube graft 3 cm in length was sutured end-to-end to the vertebral artery and end-to-side of the common carotid artery. The graft facilitated the transposition by providing added length to the vertebral artery (Fig. 7.20).

At the time of this writing the patient has been followed for four months postoperatively and has experienced only one transient episode of dizziness and another episode of paresthesias in the right hand. Left reflux brachial angiography, six weeks postoperative, revealed excellent opacification of the carotid system and the transposed vertebral artery (Fig. 7.21). There was intracranial filling of the basilar artery to the point of previous occlusion and opacification of the posterior and anterior inferior cerebellar arteries (Fig. 7.22).

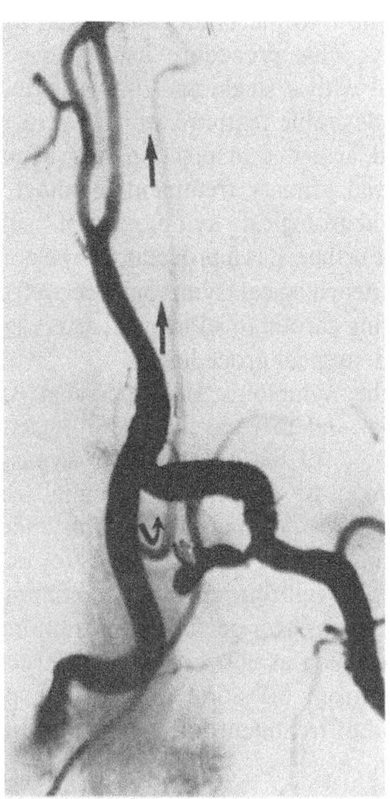

Figure 7.21. Case 4. Postoperative left retrograde brachial angiogram demonstrating transposition of the left vertebral artery to the left common carotid artery. The flow in the left vertebral artery now extends intracranially.

Comment on Vertebral to Carotid Artery Transposition

Immediately after the vertebral to carotid transposition, brachial blood pressures in all of our patients were unchanged from preoperative levels. None of the patients has any symptoms of brachial ischemia, even with exercises designed to increase blood flow to the upper extremity.[5,78] The incapacitating intermittent neurological symptoms in all patients have ceased.

An interposition vascular graft may occasionally be required in vertebral to carotid artery transposition. Saphenous vein may be effectively used for this purpose. We have used a short segment of expanded PTFE tube graft 3 to 4 mm in diameter.[7,46,52,73,74,82] As pointed out earlier, a greater experience with synthetic materials is necessary before they can be recommended in preference to autogenous vein grafts.

Vertebral to common carotid artery transposition is a relatively simple procedure. It is safe and does not require prolonged common carotid artery occlusion. It is a procedure that emphasizes restoration of high-volume antegrade

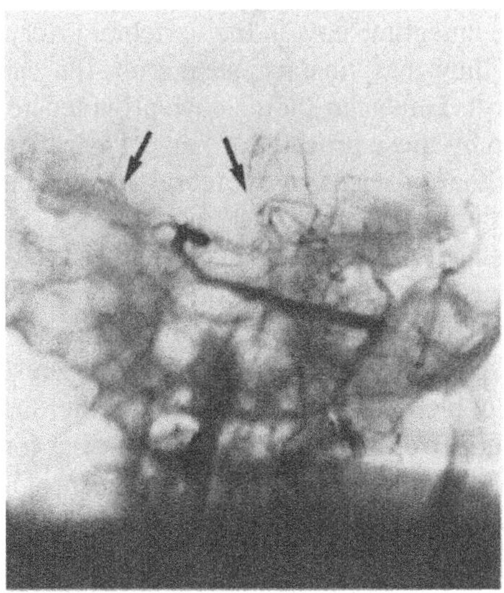

Figure 7.22. Case 4. Postoperative left retrograde brachial angiogram with carotid compression demonstrating opacification of the posterior and anterior inferior cerebellar arteries by way of the transposed left vertebral artery.

blood flow to the brain rather than to the extremity. This procedure usually can be performed with a single anastomosis. Because of these desirable features, vertebral to common carotid artery transposition has become our preferred primary treatment for most patients with neurological symptoms of subclavian steal. Further, it is a procedure to be considered when neurological symptoms persist or recur following carotid to subclavian artery bypass or related surgical procedures.

If the symptoms of subclavian steal are brachial and there are no neurological symptoms, one of the extrathoracic bypass procedures may be selected as an initial treatment. Under rare and unusual circumstances, e.g., when innominate artery stenosis (or occlusion) is coupled with proximal left common carotid artery stenosis (or occlusion), intrathoracic procedures such as subclavian endarterectomy or bypass from the aorta may be the preferred method of treatment for subclavian steal.

Conclusion

Symptomatic subclavian steal syndrome may be treated successfully by a number of procedures. The literature suggests that the commonly used carotid to subclavian artery bypass and other related extrathoracic procedures are generally safe and effective. There is evidence, however, that these bypasses may fail to restore antegrade flow in the vertebral artery and that they may, in fact, steal from the carotid artery. Thus, the blood flow provided to the brain by these procedures may be hardly more than that provided by vertebral artery ligation. Further, vertebrobasilar insufficiency symptoms have been noted to continue or recur following such bypass procedures.

Vertebral artery to common carotid artery transposition, a procedure emphasizing restoration of blood flow to the the brain rather than to the upper exremity, may be preferable for the management of most patients with neurological symptoms of subclavian steal syndrome.

References

1. Barner HB, Kaiser GC, Willman VL: Hemodynamic of carotid-subclavian bypass. Arch Surg 103:248–251, 1971
2. Barner HB, Rittenhouse EA, Willman VL: Carotid-subclavian bypass for "subclavian steal syndrome." The concept of secondary relative carotid stenosis. J Thorac Cardiovasc Surg 55:773–782, 1968
3. Berger RL, Sidd JJ, Ramaswamy K: Retrograde vertebral-artery flow produced by correction of subclavian steal syndrome. N Engl J Med 277:64–69, 1967
4. Bohmfalk GL, Story JL, Brown WE Jr, Marlin AE: Subclavian steal syndrome. Part 1: Proximal vertebral to common carotid artery transposition in three patients, and historical review. J Neurosurg 51:628-640, 1979
5. Bohmfalk GL, Story JL, Brown WE Jr, Marlin AE: Subclavian steal syndrome. Part 2: Intraoperative vertebral artery blood flow measurement. J Neurosurg 51:641-643, 1979
6. Cameron DJ, Wright IS: Subclavian steal syndrome with olfactory hallucinations. Ann Intern Med 61:128–133, 1964
7. Campbell CD, Brooks DH, Siewers RD, Peel RL, Bahnson HT: Extra-anatomic bypass with expanded polytetrafluoroethylene. Surgery 148: 1–6, 1979
8. Clark K, Perry MO: Carotid vertebral anastomosis: an alternate technic for repair of the subclavian steal syndrome. Ann Surg 163:414–416, 1966
9. Contorni L: (The vertebro-vertebral collateral circulation in obliteration of the subclavian artery at its origin.) Minerva Chir 15:268–271, 1960 (Italian)
10. Contorni L: The true story of the "subclavian steal syndrome" or "Harrison and Symth's syndrome." J Cardiovasc Surg 14:408–417, 1973
11. Cook CH, Stemmer EA, Connolly JE: Effect of peripheral resistance on carotid blood flow after carotid-subclavian bypass. Arch Surg 105:9–13, 1972
12. Corkill G, French BN, Michas C, Cobb CA III, Mims TJ: External carotid-vertebral artery anastomosis for vertebrobasilar insufficiency. Surg Neurol 7:109–115, 1977
13. Dardik H, Dardik I: Axillo-axillary bypass with cephalic vein for correction of subclavian steal syndrome. Surgery 76:413–418, 1974
14. DeBakey ME, Crawford ES, Cooley DA, Morris GC Jr, Garrett HE, Fields WS: Cerebral arterial insufficiency: one to 11-year results following arterial reconstructive operation. Ann Surg 161:921–945, 1965
15. Edwards WH, Mulherin JL Jr: The surgical approach to significant stenosis of vertebral and subclavian arteries. Surgery 87:20, 1980
16. Edwards WH, Mulherin JL Jr: The surgical man-

agement of proximal subclavian-vertebral artery stenosis. Contemp. Surg 17:11–19, 1980
17. Edwards WH, Wright RS: Surgical therapy in subclavian occlusive disease. Am J Surg 123:689–693, 1972
18. Ehrenfeld WK, Harris JD, Wylie EJ: Vascular "steal" phenomenon: an experimental study. Am J Surg 116:192–197, 1968
19. Ewing DD, Campbell DW, Kartchner MM, Lovett VF: Subclavian steal syndrome. Vasc Surg 5:137–141, 1971
20. Fields WS: Discusion in Baker HL Jr: Arteriography: technique and complications, In Siekert RG, Whisnant JP (eds.): Cerebral Vascular Diseases, Third Princeton Conference. Grune and Stratton, New York, 1961, pp 26–39
21. Fields WS: Reflections on "the subclavian steal." Stroke 1:320–324, 1970
22. Fields WS, Lemak NA: Joint study of extracranial arterial occlusion. VII. Subclavian steal: a review of 168 cases. JAMA 222:1139–1143, 1972
23. Finkenstein NM, Byer A, Rush BF Jr: Subclavian-subclavian bypass for the subclavian steal syndrome. Surgery 71:142–145, 1972
24. Fisher CM: A new vascular syndrome: "the subclavian steal." N Engl J Med 265:912–913, 1961 (Editorial)
25. Folger GM Jr, Shah KD: Subclavian steal in patients with Blalock-Taussig anastomosis. Circulation 31:241–248, 1965
26. Forestner JE, Ghosh SK, Bergan JJ, Conn J Jr: Subclavian-subclavian bypass for correction of the subclavian steal syndrome. Surgery 71:136–141, 1972
27. Galbraith JG, McDowell HA Jr: Stroke and occlusive cerebrovascular disease. Review and surgical results in 265 cases. J Med Assoc. State Ala 38:1107–1111, 1969
28. Golding AL, Cannon JA: Application of electromagnetic blood flowmeter during arterial reconstruction. Results in conjunction with Papavarine in 47 cases. Ann Surg 164:662–677, 1966
29. Hafner CD: Subclavian steal syndrome. A 12-year experience. Arch Surg 111:1974–1980, 1976
30. Harper JA, Golding AL, Mazzei EA, Cannon JA: An experimental hemodynamic study of the subclavian steal syndrome. Surg Gynecol Obstet 124:1212–1218, 1967
31. Harrison R: The Surgical Anatomy of the Arteries of the Human Body. Hodges and Smith, Dublin, 1829
32. Herring M: The subclavian steal syndrome: a report of 14 cases. J Indiana State Med Assoc 67:641–646, 1974
33. Herring M: The subclavian steal syndrome. A review. Am Surg 43:220–228, 1977
34. Heyman A, Young WG Jr, Dillon M, Goree JA, Klein LJ, Tindall G: Cerebral ischemia. Caused by occlusive lesions of the subclavian or innominate arteries. Arch Neurol 10:581–589, 1964
35. Hoff JT, Smith AL, Hankinson AL, Nielsen SL: Barbiturate protection from cerebral infarction in primates. Stroke 6:28–33, 1975
36. Jacobson JH II, Mozersky DJ, Mitty HA, Brothers MJ: Axillary-axillary bypass for the "subclavian steal" syndrome. Arch Surg 106:24–27, 1973
37. Julian OC, Javid H: Surgical management of cerebral arterial insufficiency. Curr Probl Surg (March) 1–42, 1971
38. Killen DA, Foster JH, Gobbel WG Jr, Scott HW Jr: The subclavian steal syndrome: clinical experiences. Am Surg 33:128–138, 1967
39. Killen DA, Foster JH, Gobbel WG Jr, Stephenson SE Jr, Collins HA, Billings FT, Scott HW Jr: The subclavian steal syndrome. J Thorac Cardiovasc Surg 51:539–560, 1966
40. Lamis PA, Stanton PE Jr, Hyland L: The axillo-axillary bypass graft. Further experience. Arch Surg 111:1353–1356, 1976
41. Lord RSA, Ehrenfeld WK: Carotid-subclavian bypass: a hemodynamic study. Surgery 66:521–526, 1969
42. Love JW: Varieties of congenital subclavian steal with and without the syndrome. J Cardiovasc Surg 9:358–364, 1968
43. Lyons C, Galbraith G: Surgical treatment of atherosclerotic occlusion of the internal carotid artery. Ann Surg 146:487–498, 1957
44. Mandelbaum I, Nahrwold DL, Dzenitis AJ: Spontaneous resolution of traumatic subclavian steal syndrome. Ann Surg 164:314–317, 1967
45. Mannick JA, Suter CG, Hume DM: The "subclavian steal" syndrome: a further documentation. JAMA 182:254–258, 1962
46. Matsumoto H, Hasegawa T, Fuse K, Hamamoto J, Saigusa M: A new vascular prosthesis for a small caliber artery. Surgery 74:519–523, 1973
47. Maxwell TM, Pollak E, Alexander JL, Mandall AK: Axillary-axillary by-pass graft: an alternative technique for repair of the subclavian steal syndrome. Vasc Surg 9:58–62, 1975
48. McDowell HA Jr: Surgical correction of vertebral steal followed by contralateral retrograde vertebral flow. Ann Surg 168:154–156, 1968
49. McLaughlin JS, Linberg E, Attar S, Wolfel D, Cowley RA: Cerebral vascular insufficiency. Syndromes of reversed blood flow in vessels supplying the brain. Am Surg 33:317–324, 1967
50. McMullan MH, Hardy JD: Lesions of the subclavian artery: survey of 31 cases with emphasis on steal syndrome. Ann Surg 178:80–86, 1973

51. Mehigan JT, Buch WS, Pipkin RD, Fogarty TJ: Subclavian-carotid transposition for the subclavian steal syndrome. Am J Surg 136:15–20, 1978
52. Molina JE, Carr M, Harnoz MD: Coronary bypass with gore-tex graft. J Thorac Cardiovasc Surg 75:769–771, 1978
53. Mount LA: Results of treatment of intracranial aneurysms using the selverstone clamp. J Neurosurg 16:611–618, 1959
54. Mozersky DJ, Sumner DS, Barnes RW, Callaway GP, Strandness DE Jr: The hemodynamics of the axillary-axillary bypass. Surg Gynecol Obstet 135:925–929, 1972
55. Najafi H, Dye WS, Javid H, Hunter JA, Ostermiller WE, Julian OC: A one-stage surgical correction. Arch Surg 99:289–292, 1969
56. North RR, Fields WS, DeBakey ME, Crawford ES: Brachial-basilar insufficiency syndrome. Neurology 12:810–820, 1962
57. Piccone VA Jr, Karvounis P, Leveen HH: The subclavian steal syndrome. Angiology 21:240–259, 1970
58. Pifarre R, Rouse RG: Congenital subclavian steal syndrome: anatomy, physiology, pathology and surgical correction. Chest 66:299–302, 1974
59. Ponsdomenech ER, Lepere RH, Heaney JP: Proximal subclavian artery occlusion and the steal syndrome. Ann Thorac Surg 4:551–558, 1967
60. Poulos E, Dammert W, Chandler ER, Lindsey TM: Experience with subclavian steal syndrome. Tex Med 71:74–79, 1975
61. Reivich M, Holling HE, Roberts B, Toole JF: Reversal of blood flow through the vertebral artery and its effect on cerebral circulation. N Engl J Med 265:878–885, 1961
62. Rob C: Technique of surgical therapy. In Siekert RG, Whisnant JP (eds.): Cerebral Vascular Diseases, Third Princeton Conference. Grune and Stratton, New York, 1961, pp 110–112
63. Rob C: Subclavian occlusive disease and reversal of the flow in the ipsilateral vertebral artery: treatment, in Siekert RG, Whisnant JP (eds.): Cerebral Vascular Diseases, Fourth Princeton Conference. Grune and Stratton, New York, 1965, pp 122–124
64. Rutledge RH, Freese JW: Subclavian steal syndrome: diagnosis and treatment. Tex Med 63:56–63, 1967
65. Shumacker HB Jr: Carotid axillary bypass grafts for occlusion of the proximal portion of the subclavian artery. Surg Gynecol Obstet 136:447–448, 1973
66. Simon M, Rabinov K, Horenstein S: Proximal subclavian artery occlusion and reversed vertebral blood flow to the arm. Clin Radiol 13:201–206, 1962
67. Smith JW: Management of the "subclavian steal" syndrome in the poor-risk patient. Nebr Med J 52:361–366, 1967
68. Smyth AW: Successful operation in a case of subclavian aneurism. New Orleans Med Rec 1:4–7, 1866
69. Smyth AW: A case of successful ligature of the innominate artery. New Orleans J Med 22:464–469, 1869
70. Snider RL, Porter JM, Eidemiller LR: Axillary-axillary artery bypass for the correction of subclavian artery occlusive disease. Ann Surg 180:888–891, 1974
71. Snyder EN Jr: Discussion in Lee RH, Kieraldo JH, Jamplis ER: Surgical treatment of the subclavian steal syndrome. Am J Surg 114:308–313, 1967
72. Souchon E: Reminiscences of Dr. Andrew W. Smyth of subclavian aneurism fame. New Orleans Med Surg J 73:352–358, 1920
73. Story JL, Brown WE Jr, Eidelberg E, Arom KV, Stewart JR: Cerebral revascularization: proximal external carotid to distal middle cerebral artery bypass with a synthetic tube graft. Neurosurgery 3:61–65, 1978
74. Story JL, Brown WE Jr, Eidelberg E, Arom KV, Stewart JR, Smith BD: Cerebral revascularization: cervical carotid artery-intracranial arterial long graft bypass. In Marguth F, Brock M, Kazner E, Klinger M, Schmiedek P (eds.): Advances in Neurosurgery, Volume 7, Neurovascular Surgery—Specialized Neurosurgical Techniques. Springer-Verlag, Berlin, Heidelberg, New York, 1979, pp 15–23
75. Tindall TG, Odom GL, Dillon ML, Cupp HB Jr, Mahaley JS Jr, Greenfield JC Jr: Direction of blood flow in the internal and external carotid arteries following occlusion of the ipsilateral common carotid artery. J Neurosurg 20:985–994, 1963
76. Toole JF: Discussion in Baker HL Jr: Arteriography: technique and complications. In Siekert RG, Whisnant JP (eds.): Cerebral Vascular Diseases, Third Princeton Conference. Grune and Stratton, 1961, pp 26–39
77. Toole JF, McGraw CP: The steal syndromes. Annu Rev Med 26:321–329, 1975
78. Toole JF, Tulloch EF: Bilateral simultaneous sphygmomanometry: a new diagnostic test for subclavian steal syndrome. Circulation 33:952–957, 1966
79. Wheeler HB: Surgical treatment of subclavian-artery occlusions. N Engl J Med 276:711–717, 1967

80. Wylie EJ, Ehrenfeld WK: Extracranial Occlusive Cerebrovascular Disease: Diagnosis and Treatment, WB Saunders, 1970, Philadelphia, London, Toronto, 231 pp
81. Wylie EJ, Hein MF, Adams JE: Intracranial hemorrhage following surgical revascularization for treatment of acute strokes. J Neurosurg 21:212–215, 1964
82. Yokoyama T, Gharavi MA, Lee Y, Edmiston WA, Kay JH: Aorta-coronary artery revascularization with an expanded polytetrafluoroethylene vascular graft. A preliminary report. J Thorac Cardiovasc Surg 74:552–555, 1978

8

Extracranial-Intracranial Bypass Surgery

Jack M. Fein

Introduction

Surgical treatment of cerebrovascular occlusive disease was initially confined to reconstructive procedures on the extracranial carotid and vertebral arteries. Extracranial-intracranial bypass (EC-IC) procedures have now been developed to manage selected patients with intracranial vascular occlusive lesions.

Approximately 20% of patients with symptoms of cerebrovascular insufficiency have occlusive lesions of the intracranial carotid or middle cerebral arteries.[61] Earlier attempts at direct repair of these lesions were not very fruitful. In 1955 Welch[88] described two patients in whom intracranial surgical procedures were performed to remove emboli. The first patient was operated on 28 days following the onset of symptoms; an obstruction of the posterior temporal branch of the middle cerebral artery was removed. However, postoperative angiography disclosed that there was no significant filling of that branch. The second patient had an occlusion beyond the intracranial bifurcation of the internal carotid artery and was operated on acutely. However, the patient remained hemiplegic, and angiography demonstrated recurrent occlusion. Scheibert[80] described five patients in whom attempts were made to open an occluded middle cerebral artery. In only one of these five cases was patency reestablished. Piazza and Geist[67] described a patient with a shotgun pellet that had embolized to the middle cerebral artery. This patient was operated on by Meletti in Bologna, who was able to milk the pellet down to the internal carotid artery and ligate the artery distal to this point. Cross flow from the opposite carotid circulation supplied the symptomatic side. Other reports[13,23,54,58,81] appeared. Zlotnick[95] removed a thrombus of the middle cerebral artery by way of one of its side branches, which was subsequently clipped. In this manner patency of the parent artery was maintained. These procedures utilized conventional neurosurgical techniques to open intracranial arteries that were less than 2 mm in diameter. Furthermore, prolonged retraction of acutely swollen brain was sometimes required to expose the major arteries at the base. Such procedures were considered impractical approaches to the problem of intracranial occlusive lesions.

Denny-Brown[17] and others[47] underscored the importance of the collateral circulation in determining the neurologic consequences of occlusive arterial lesions. In this context it is not the size or the site of an arterial occlusive lesion that predetermines the resulting neurologic deficit. The ability to recruit collateral sources of blood flow is an important factor in outcome. Several investigators then attempted to revascularize the cerebral hemispheres by augmenting the collateral circulation rather than by reconstructing the occluded artery. In 1942 Henschen[42] attempted to increase the collateral circulation over the cerebral hemisphere in a patient with progressive neurologic deficit due to bilateral internal carotid artery occlusions. He transplanted a temporalis muscle pedicle to the surface of the brain and described clinical improvement in the patient thereafter. Unfortunately, postoperative angiography was not performed so that it is unclear if this reported improvement was related to an increase in the transcortical collateral circulation. Pool[68] in 1951 described a shunt, consisting of a plastic tube, between the superficial temporal artery and the distal portion of the left anterior cerebral artery after trapping a calloso-marginal artery aneurysm. However, this appeared to be a temporizing measure and postoperative angiography performed 10 days later showed that the shunt was occluded. Woringer and Kunlin[90] in 1963 described an operation for bypass of an internal carotid artery occlusion in which a saphenous vein graft was interposed between the common carotid artery and the intracranial portion of the internal carotid artery. Postoperative angiography was not performed and the results are unclear.

A practical means for reconstructing the collateral circulation awaited the development of microvascular surgical techniques. Jacobson[48] demonstrated that arteriotomy and anastomosis of 1-mm arteries were possible using microsurgical techniques for incision and manipulation of the vessels. During the period between 1960 and 1967 adaptations were also made in microsurgical instruments, sutures, and the operating microscope for use in microvascular neurosurgery.[91] Donaghy developed the microsurgical laboratory to foster the skills required for microvascular surgery.[19–21] Arteriotomy repair as well as end-to-end and end-to-side anastomoses was performed in arteries 1 to 2 mm in diameter with patency rates of more than 90%. Donaghy[19] and Yasargil[91] together developed the procedure of superficial temporal artery to middle cerebral artery (STA-MCA) anastomosis and operated on the first two patients simultaneously in Burlington, Vermont, and Zurich, Switzerland, on June 7, 1967. These procedures stimulated widespread interest in the management of patients with intracranial occlusive lesions. This review describes cerebral hemodynamic factors pertinent to EC-IC bypass, a consensus regarding patient selection, as well as the author's technique and experience.

Hemodynamic Basis for Bypass Surgery

The mechanism by which vascular occlusive lesions produce ischemic symptoms is not well understood. However, hemodynamic insufficiency and thromboembolism to the distal arterial circulation are the most likely factors responsible. Occasionally viscosity changes in blood may play a role. To assess the role of hypoperfusion in patients with intracranial occlusive lesions, cortical artery pressures were measured during bypass in 115 patients.[26,27] The relative pressure drop between systemic blood pressure and pressure in 1.0 to 1.5-mm cortical arteries in patients with aneurysms who are otherwise free of cerebrovascular disease is 12 ± 3.2%. Cortical artery pressure was reduced in patients with intracranial arterial lesions compared with patients free of cerebrovascular disease. The lowest cortical artery pressures were found in patients who had the most extensive number of occlusive lesions. Patients with middle cerebral artery occlusive lesions had lower mean cortical artery pressures than those with internal carotid artery lesions and those with multiple lesions had lower mean cortical artery pressure than those with single lesions. Selective pressures were measured from the proximal and distal limbs of the cortical artery. The failure of the collateral circulation was indicated by the low ratio of distal to proximal cortical artery pressures. Hypoperfusion may therefore be an important mechanism for the production of symptoms and may be responsive to augmentation of blood flow. However, volume flow in the superficial temporal artery (24–74 mL/min) is significantly less than that in the middle cerebral artery (120–170 mL/min), and this has caused concern regarding the ability of an STA-MCA bypass to augment flow significantly. However, regional cerebral blood flow studies indicate that neurophysiologic dysfunction does not occur until regioinal cerebral blood flow (CBF) is decreased to levels of 18 to 22 mL/min. It may be necessary, therefore, only to keep regional blood flow values above this threshold to provide clinically effective augmentation of flow by bypass surgery.

There is substantial evidence that hemodynamic insufficiency may be influenced by bypass procedures.[5,30,37,38,41] In experimental animals with middle cerebral artery occlusion, an increase in regional CBF of 20% to 35% was seen after EC-IC bypass.[28] This was confirmed in a later study by Hitchon et al.[43] Gratzl et al[37] studied a group of patients with transient ischemic attacks (TIAs) with preoperative and postoperative measurement of CBF. In patients with relative focal ischemia, bypass resulted in significant improvement in postoperative CBF. Heilbrun et al[41] performed CBF studies in 16 patients after bypass. They found a global reduction in all patients with no significant difference between patients with TIA and minor strokes and those with completed strokes. They concluded that hypoperfusion rather than embolism was the more important mechanism for symptoms in this group. In another study[56] the greatest increase in postoperative blood flow values (of up to 30%) were found in patients with the lowest preoperative flow values. Meyer et al[64] studied 33 patients who were treated with bypass and 13 patients who were suitable for bypass but were treated medically. Both the xenon 133 inhalation and stable xenon computed tomography (CT) methods were used. In all groups gray matter blood flow values were reduced in both ischemic and opposite hemispheres, with the former also showing impaired vasomotor reactivity to 5% CO_2 or 100% O_2 inhalation. After surgery mean hemispheric gray matter blood flow values increased by 12.8% on the bypassed side and by 10.5% on the contralateral side. Maximal increases were seen ipsilateral frontal regions of 24.2% at three months after bypass. Medically treated cases did not show similar increases. These results are in agreement with the results reported by Halsey et al[38] of +10.5% on the operated side and +8% on the nonoperated side and +13% on the bypassed side reported by Hungerbuhler et al.[46] These results are similar to those found by others.[1,2]

Significant correction of intracerebral and interhemispheric steal after bypass was found in three studies. Fein et al[24] demonstrated reversal of an intracerebral steal by cineangiography. Laurent[56] studied 27 patients preoperatively and within eight weeks postoperatively. STA-MCA anastomosis resulted in reversal of an apparent "intracerebral steal" and increased contralateral hemispheric flow by 23% while increasing flow ipsilaterally by 24%. These interhemispheric shifts are, of course, dependent on a competent circle of Willis.

Preoperative Evaluation

A detailed history of the onset, time course, and resolution of each ischemic attack is obtained. Since regional cerebral dysfunction may be secondary to proximal extracranial or more distal intracranial lesions, there are no specific complaints that help identify patients suitable for bypass. A thorough neurologic examination is carried out. If intellectual function is affected, detailed psychometric studies should be carried out.[89] Deficits found on motor examination are detailed for comparison during postoperative follow-up. Neurovascular examination will elicit evidence of pulse asymmetry, bruits, or thrills in the carotid and scalp arteries. Retinal artery pressures are measured bilaterally.[53] General physical examination and review of systems will reveal evidence of cardiac, general circulatory, or respiratory problems. Coronary insufficiency, hypertension, and a history of smoking are common findings in patients with cerebrovascular insufficiency. Cardiac evaluations should include an ECG examination and 24-hour study with a Holter monitor to rule out significant arrhythmias. Hematologic abnormalities and coagulopathies should be sought with a blood count, platelet studies, prothrombin time, lipid and lipoprotein determinations.

Several noninvasive studies are useful for evaluating patients with cerebral ischemia. These include CT scan, CBF studies, and digital subtraction angiography. CT scan is useful to determine the extent of cerebral infarction and the presence of areas of brain edema. If infarction is extensive, the value of any surgical procedure is questionable. If cerebral edema is present, it is best to delay surgery until this resolves. Noninvasive regional CBF studies using the inhalation of ^{133}Xe can identify asymmetric hemisphere perfusion, areas of relative focal ischemia, and evidence of loss of autoregulation. It should be recognized however, that regional CBF rates may be normal between TIAs.

Digital subtraction angiography (DSA) is one of the more effective screening tests in patients with cerebrovascular disease. Stenosis or occlusion of the cervical carotid arteries as well as occlusive lesions of the largest intracranial arteries may be visualized. Once a significant lesion is found on the DSA study, an arterial angiogram should be performed prior to surgery to visualize details of the intracranial circulation that are not resolved adequately by DSA.

Nuclear magnetic resonance study is rapidly becoming a clinically useful imaging technique. In acute cerebral infarction, changes may be seen within several hours, whereas such evidence may not be seen on CT scan for 24–48 hours.

Arterial angiography is carried out by transfemoral selective catheterization to assess the presence of specific lesions of the internal carotid and middle cerebral arteries. If symptoms are clearly hemispheric in nature, selective injection of both carotid arteries and one vertebral artery is performed. High-quality serial studies are often necessary to visualize the contribution of ophthalmic collaterals to the carotid siphon are and the contribution of leptomeningeal collaterals to the middle cerebral areas.[61] A lateral view will visualize the carotid siphon area, and transorbital or base views will visualize the horizontal portion of the middle cerebral artery.

Clinical Indications for Bypass Surgery

The natural history and prognosis of patients with cerebrovascular insufficiency is variable and depends on the initial clinical syndrome and specific arterial lesion. Recognizing these limitations, tentative clinical and angiographic criteria were developed to select patients at risk, for bypass surgery.[92–94] Candidates for surgery[65] include patients who have experienced either recurrent TIAs, reversible ischemic neurologic deficits (RIND), progressive strokes despite medical therapy, or nondebilitating completed stroke.

After TIA in the anterior circulation the risk of a new completed stroke within four years of the first event varies from 32% to 43%.[22,39,47] The majority of patients who have undergone bypass have had TIAs. In most of the reported series the authors noted a dramatic reduction or abolition of TIAs in the postoperative period. In the larger reported series with follow-up periods of one to nine years, transient ischemic episodes were abolished after surgery in 85% to 95% of patients, and 5% to 8% experienced reduction in the frequency of their TIAs.[69,72,73,85]

In patients who have suffered a mild nondebilitating stroke, the risk of a second stroke may be as high as 67% within two years.[47] In five reported series[21,72,77,78,85] the incidence of subsequent stroke after bypass was only 1.7%. On the other hand, the treatment of patients with severe and extensive stroke in an effort to improve neurologic function has generally been unrewarding. Isolated cases of improved neurologic function after long-standing deficits have appeared.[49,75] Several authors have described test situations designed to predict which patients will improve after bypass. Holbach et al[44] suggested use of hyperbaric oxygenation to determine if clinical improvement is associated with increased tissue nutrition in such patients. Although the use of such screening examinations may theoretically identify patients with completed stroke who are suitable candidates for revascularization, data to date are unconvincing, and bypass is not recommended in this setting.

It has been suggested that revascularization during the course of a progressing stroke or within 8 to 10 hours of onset of an acute stroke may favorably influence the outcome. This presupposes that part of the neurologic deficit associated with cerebral infarction is related to a zone of ischemic but viable neural tissue. Augmentation of blood flow to these areas may improve the function of these so-called "idling neurons." Several surgical series suggest that the recovery rate may be enhanced by this intervention.[18,76] The efficacy of flow augmentation under these circumstances is unknown, however, and the risk of converting an ischemic infarction to a hemorrhagic infarction is significant. Management of such patients should be based primarily on providing optimal cerebral hemodynamics and arterial blood gas concentrations. Cerebral edema is treated with steroids and if this is severe and progressive, intracranial pressure monitoring in conjunction with intravenous mannitol is used.

Arterial Lesions

Angiography will demonstrate the presence of arterial occlusive lesions that are not amenable to direct repair in 20% to 30% of patients with cerebrovascular insufficiency. In the Joint Study of Extracranial Arterial Occlusions 4,748 patients were studied.[40] Internal carotid artery occlusion (extracranial plus intracranial) accounted for 52.5% of the angiographic lesion, intracranial internal carotid artery (IICA) stenosis accounted for 13.3% of the lesions and middle cerebral artery (MCA) stenosis or occlusions for 11.9%.

In a postmortem series by Fisher[33] 67% of patients with internal carotid artery occlusion were symptomatic. The future risk of stroke in patients with internal carotid artery occlusion, however, varies in different series.[36,35,39] McDowell, et al[63] found that 8% of 38 patients with internal carotid occlusion had a new stroke within two years of diagnosis. Dyken[23] found that 7% of 143 patients with carotid artery occlusion had a second stroke within 16.5 months. In the Joint Study of Extracranial Arterial Occlusion[31] 10% of 359 patients with unilateral carotid artery occlusion had an ipsilateral stroke within 44 months of diagnosis.

Internal carotid artery occlusion is usually inoperable by carotid endarterectomy. Occasionally, however, collateral circulation through the ophthalmic artery or through tympanic and cavernous branches shows reflux of contrast down to the petrous portion.[15] In five such cases in the author's series, back flow was reestablished by carotid endarterectomy. Two of these patients, however, developed recurrent thrombosis by the third postoperative day. The majority of patients with internal carotid occlusion have some degree of collateral circulation to the ipsilateral hemisphere from the contralateral side across the anterior circle of Willis or from the posterior circulation through the posterior communicating artery. Visualization of these collaterals after the occlusion has progressed to completion, however, does not facilitate predictions of future risk, since these collateral channels were inadequate to prevent the primary ischemic event. In the presence of collateral flow via the external carotid, internal maxillary, and ophthalmic arteries, embolization from the proximal stump of the internal carotid artery may be responsible for ischemic symptoms.[7] Our current state of knowledge suggests that patients who have recurrent ischemic episodes related to internal carotid occlusion should undergo EC-IC bypass, unless ophthalmic collateral channels are prominent.

The distal portion of the internal carotid artery may be involved by severe atherosclerotic narrowing. Occasionally the distal extracranial artery may be involved, but more commonly the intracranial internal carotid artery may be stenotic. Long-term prognosis for patients with intracranial internal carotid stenosis is worse than for patients with internal carotid occlusion. In a series from the Cleveland Clinic[62] 18 patients (27.3%) experienced further ischemic events; 8 (12.1%) had isolated TIA, and 10 (15.2%) had a stroke during an average follow-up of 3.9 years. The patients with tandem lesions of the extracranial internal carotid artery had an even greater risk of stroke than those with isolated intracranial internal carotid stenosis. The risk of future stroke in patients older than 35 years was 13 times that expected for a normal population. In another review of 58 patients followed by 2.5 years, the prognosis was even worse.[16] Most of these patients were treated with antiplatelet aggregating agents or anticoagulants. Only 33% of the patients were alive and free of subsequent cerebrovascular events at the end of the follow-up period; 43% suffered cerebrovascular events; 29% suffered a stroke of which 65% were appropriate to the involved artery. The asymptomatic patients had as poor a prognosis as the symptomatic ones, and the degree of stenosis did not appear to affect the prognosis.

Patients with segmental stenosis of the distal cervical portions of the internal carotid artery may be suitable candidates for bypass. The exposure for carotid endarterectomy is usually inadequate for stenotic lesions located more than 2 cm distal to the carotid bifurcation. Low flow rates associated with any high-grade stenosis may produce a "slim" sign in the proximal internal carotid artery because of pooling of slowly flowing contrast in the supine position.

This must be differentiated from longitudinal narrowing of the arterial walls seen with inflammatory processes or with a traumatic or spontaneous dissection. Similarly low flow rates and a miniscule column of contrast distal to a high-grade stenosis at the origin of the internal carotid artery may give the appearance of a complete occlusion. The "pseudo-occlusion" should be suspected when a tapered narrowing of contrast is seen and can be better visualized with a larger dose of contrast coupled with a more rapid frame sequence. Endarterectomy rather than bypass should be offered such patients. Tandem lesions of the origin and distal segments of the extracranial internal carotid artery occurred in 8% of the patients in our series. Under such circumstances, poor back flow is seen during carotid endarterectomy and may lead to postoperative thrombosis at the arteriotomy site. The distal lesion is usually most critical and such patients should be selected for bypass. If symptoms recur and proximal plaque shows ulcerative changes, an endarterectomy may be subsequently performed.

Stenosis or occlusion of the middle cerebral artery occurs in 7% of patients with cerebrovascular insufficiency in North America, but is more frequent in Japan. In a postmortem study Fisher[32] found that 86% of patients with middle cerebral occlusion were symptomatic from the occlusion. Lesions of the middle cerebral artery from its origin to the major branch points in the sylvian fissure, which are hemodynamically significant, are suitable for bypass.

Patients with bilateral internal carotid occlusion or a combination of occlusion and contralateral stenosis may have severe postural symptoms. Patients with internal carotid occlusion ipsilateral to the symptoms and contralateral internal carotid stenosis may benefit from bypass, particularly if cross flow is poor. In Moya Moya disease, progressive occlusion of cerebral arteries evokes an exuberant proliferation of small intradural collateral channels at the base of the brain.[8,50] Persistent ischemic events may be eliminated by the additional collaterals provided by a bypass.

Other Indications

In addition to atherosclerotic lesions, bypass may be utilized in certain cases where ligation of the internal carotid or middle cerebral artery is planned. Large unclippable internal carotid aneurysms may be treated more effectively by internal carotid ligation than by common carotid ligation.[10] The risks of delayed hemispheric stroke attendant upon internal carotid ligation may be reduced by simultaneous EC-IC bypass.[25,45,74] Bypass has been employed in relatively few patients with basal tumors. The risks of trapping or ligation of the internal carotid or middle cerebral artery during these resections may be reduced by increasing collateral blood flow. Its use in other situations has been advocated but is unproven.[14,34]

Contraindications

Bypass surgery is primarily a prophylactic procedure and is not appropriate for patients with extensive infarction. Patients with other life-limiting diseases are generally unsuitable candidates. Conditions that increase the perioperative risk such as severe coronary ischemia, acute or chronic pulmonary disease, or other advanced diseases are all relative contraindications to surgery.[11] Prophylactic therapy for a future stroke should not be offered to a patient who is threatened by another more pressing disorder. Occlusive lesions caused by cardiac emboli and hemodynamic failure related to cardiac arrhythmias require attention to the sources of the disorder.

Most of the patients selected for bypass are evaluated by a cardiologist to assess the role of these cardiac factors in the cerebral syndrome as well as to assess the risks of surgery. In our series 35% of the patients had essential hypertension preoperatively. Decisions should be made regarding the selection of antihypertensive medication which may be required intraoperatively or postoperatively. Ten percent of the author's patients had a history of previous myocardial infarction and 15% have had cardiac arrhythmias.

Timing of Bypass Surgery

Bypass procedures should be carried out after acute ischemic changes have subsided, but before the development of cerebral infarction.

There may be no deficit after a TIA but the CT scan in some patients may show evidence of a small cerebral infarction in clinically silent areas of the brain. Under such circumstances it is worthwhile waiting several weeks before proceeding with revascularization.

In patients with frequently recurring ischemic attacks or progressive stroke despite heparin therapy, bypass surgery may be necessary despite the risks of producing a hemorrhagic infarction. After an acute but nondebilitating stroke, plans for prophylactic bypass surgery should be delayed three to six weeks, depending on the severity and extent of the cerebral infarction.

Sequence of Procedures

A significant number of patients have multiple lesions that may require separate procedures. The most common combination of lesions is an internal carotid occlusion and a contralateral internal carotid stenosis. In the Joint Stroke Study 55% of patients with this combination of lesions had symptoms referable to the occluded side, 10% had lesions referable to the stenotic side, and 16% had bilateral symptoms.[31] In the author's series, 70 patients had this combination of lesions. Bypass had the advantage of producing increased flow without the risks of temporary clamping of the major blood supply to the cerebral hemisphere. Bypass preceded endarterectomy in 30 patients; whereas endarterectomy was first performed in 20 patients. Only four of the 30 patients with a previous bypass had significant EEG slowing over the occluded hemisphere and required an intraoperative shunt, whereas all 20 patients who underwent endarterectomy primarily had such changes and required shunts. Ten of the latter patients had a bypass performed. After a mean follow-up of three years, there was one minor ischemic event in the ipsilateral hemisphere in the patients who had both precedures. Three of 10 patients with endarterectomy alone had transient ischemic events referable to the occluded side, and one of these three also had a completed stroke.

In a number of patients with lesions suitable for bypass there is also disease of the external carotid artery. Where this is felt to be significant, bypass is preceded by external carotid endarterectomy. In patients with bilateral intracranial lesions and bilateral symptoms, bypass should first be performed on the dominant hemisphere. In patients with symptomatic ischemic lesions and asymptomatic aneurysms, we have treated the ischemic lesion first and then clipped the aneurysm either at the same time or at a separate procedure.

Technique of EC-IC Bypass

Different bypass procedures are possible in the anterior circulation and depend on the choice of extracranial and intracranial arteries.[86] The most commonly performed procedure is a bypass between the superficial temporal artery and a cortical branch of the middle cerebral artery.

Anesthetic Technique

After induction with sodium thiopental and endotracheal intubation, an arterial catheter is placed percutaneously in the radial artery to monitor the blood gas concentration as well as the blood pressure. Arterial PCO_2 is kept between 34 and 40 mm Hg. Arterial PO_2 is kept between 120 and 150 mm Hg, and a high normal blood pressure is maintained throughout the procedure. A Foley catheter is placed simultaneously and the head is shaved. The patient is placed in the three-quarter supine position with the head turned contralaterally into the full lateral position (Fig. 8.1). Severe rotation of the cervical spine should be avoided. This is particularly important in patients with severe osteoarthritis or contralateral carotid or vertebral atherosclerosis. Such patients are placed in the full lateral decubitus position. The head is then fixed in the pinion headholder.

Surgical Technique (STA-MCA Bypass)

Magnification and illumination are provided with the Zeiss OPMI 6 microscope fitted with 12.5× eyepieces, the inclined binocular tube, and the 200-mm objective. A Hitachi television camera and a 35-mm Cannon high-lens reflex camera are mounted on the Designs for Vision Optical switch. A binocular observer tube is used by the first assistant.

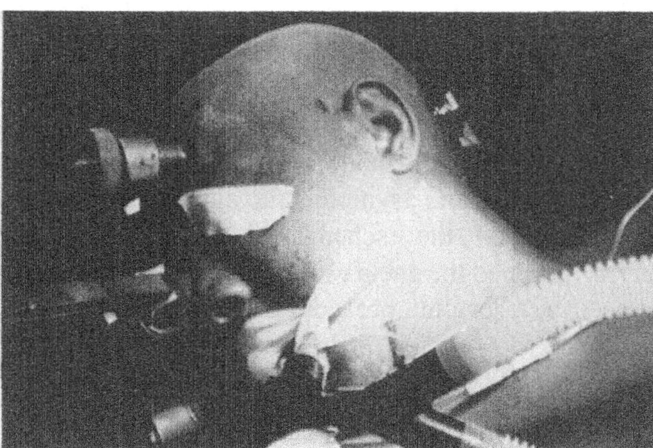

Figure 8.1. Patient is positioned in the three-quarter supine position with a support under the ipsilateral shoulder. Head is placed in full lateral position and fixed in pinion headholder.

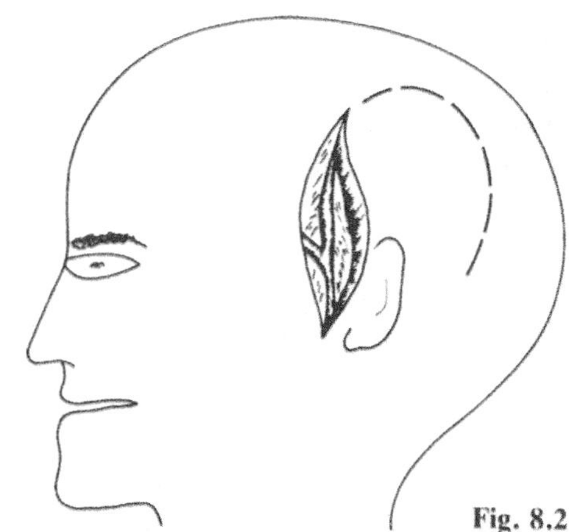

Figure 8.2. Exposure of the STA anterior to the ear. A supra-auricular flap is then turned for the craniotomy.

The superficial temporal artery (STA) divides into a frontal and parietal branch approximately 1 cm anterior and superior to the external auditory meatus. The position of the scalp artery is localized anterior to the tragus by palpation or with a Doppler stethoscope if necessary. With the microscope in position over the temporal region, an incision is made with a #15 scalpel blade directly over the proximal portion of the scalp artery (Fig. 8.2). The skin edges are retracted with Adson forceps to minimize bleeding. Subcutaneous bleeding vessels are individually coagulated with an angled bipolar microcautery forceps. Skin edge bleeding, however, should be controlled by retraction of the edges with forceps and dural hooks. The scalp artery is exposed on its superficial aspect, but left undisturbed in its fascial bed (Fig. 8.3). The dissection continues in the plane between the adventitia and the overlying subcutaneous fascia. Although the frontal branch is usually larger than the parietal branch, it is not dissected if it provides collateral channels to the orbit. The appropriate branch is exposed progressively by sharp dissection of the skin and the fascia overlying the artery for 5 to 6 cm. This length is necessary, bearing in mind the new course of the vessel through the cranial layers and across the subdural space. Incisions are then made through the galea on either side of the artery and down to the temporalis fascia. This provides a cuff of fascia on three sides of the scalp artery. The distal 1 cm of the scalp artery is then prepared and cleaned of its surrounding fascia and fat by a sharp dissection technique.

The skin incision is then extended posteriorly approximately 3 cm above the ear. Scalp flaps are raised and held apart by dural hooks. A stellate incision is made in the muscle using the electrocautery. Muscle flaps are then elevated by subperiosteal dissection, but the muscle fascia should be preserved for later closure. A craniectomy 4 cm in diameter is made in the posterior temporal region using the craniotome (Fig. 8.4). Unless the dura is tightly adherent to the inner table, the edges are lined with strips of Gelfoam, and 4-0 neurolon tenting sutures are placed along the bone edge. The dura is then opened in stellate fashion, and the dural edges are thoroughly coagulated and held back with sutures. The subarachnoid space may bulge against the craniotomy edges, in which case the arachnoid is opened sharply to release cerebrospinal fluid. This is sufficient to relax the brain.

The angular artery is usually the largest cortical branch of the middle cerebral artery, with a mean diameter of 1.2 mm. The posterior temporal artery and the posterior parietal branches are also usually larger than 1.0 mm. When an appropriate recipient artery is selected, the investing arachnoid directly over the artery is elevated with Dumont forceps and cut sharply with a curved microscissor under 16× magnification (Fig. 8.5). Traction on the periarterial chordae, which suspend the arteries in the sub-

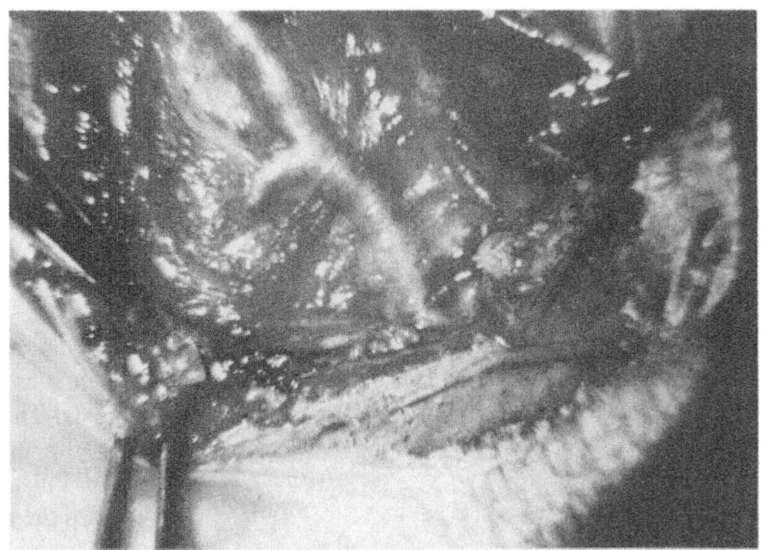

Figure 8.3. Microscope is used at 6× to allow sharp dissection along the course of the parietal branch of the STA.

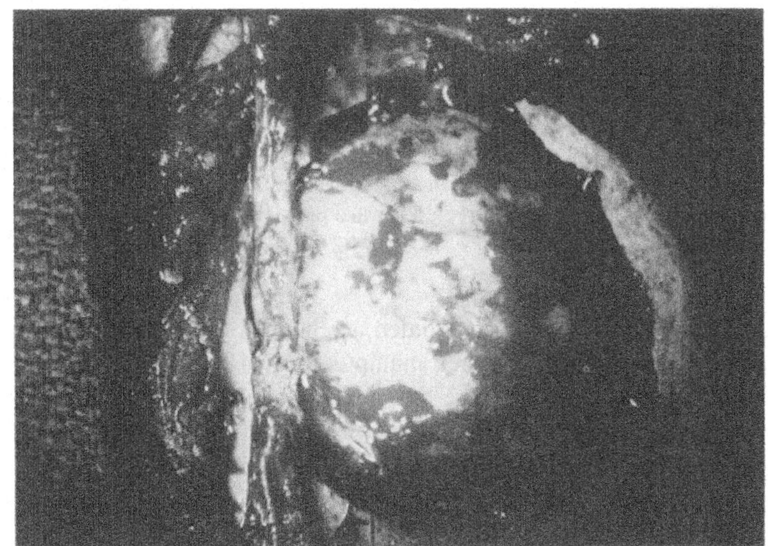

Figure 8.4. Intraoperative photograph demonstrates the vascular pedicle graft containing the STA and its surrounding fascia. Muscle flaps have been raised, and the craniotome is used to remove a circular bone flap in the supra-articular region.

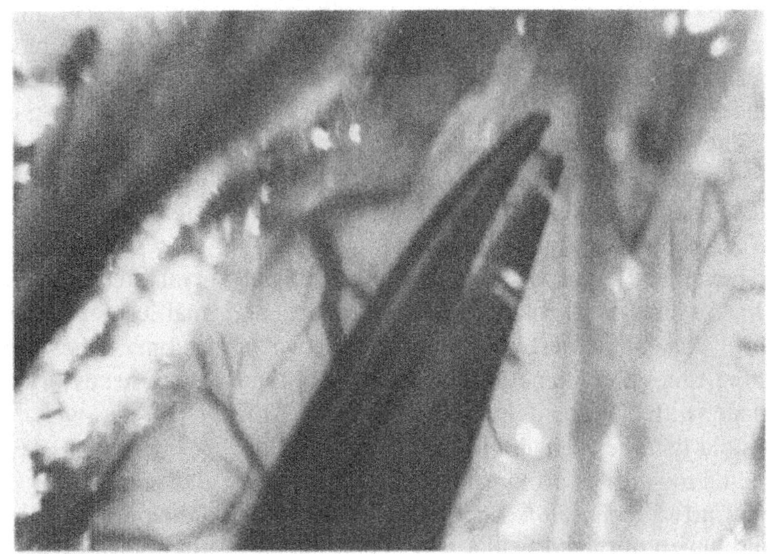

Figure 8.5. After opening the dura, a suitable cortical recipient artery is chosen. The arachnoid over the artery is sharply incised with a curved microscissor for approximately 1 cm.

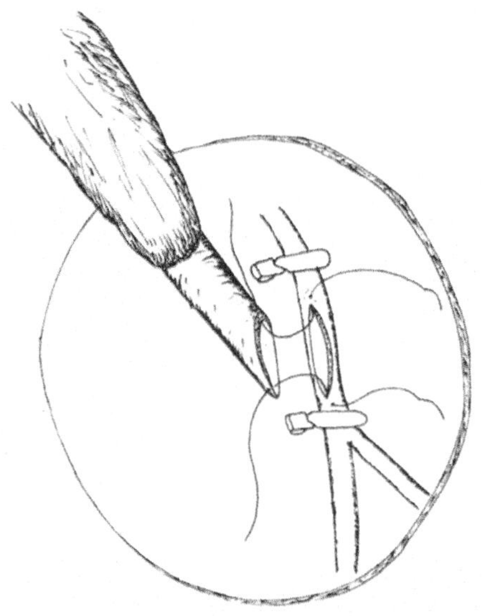

Figure 8.6. Intraoperative sketch demonstrates the bevel placed on the end of the STA. The artery is transposed intracranially and then aligned so that the leading edge of the bevel is directed toward proximal side of cortical arteriotomy.

arachnoid space, should be avoided, as this will produce vasospasm. Further manipulation of the artery may then be more difficult. If vasospasm occurs, a few drops of papavarine solution may be applied to the vessel. The cortical artery is mobilized from the cortical surface by coagulating and cutting two to three penetrating branches. This should provide a 1.5-cm length of the cortical artery for bypass. After the cortical artery is mobilized, a small rubber dam is cut and placed under the artery to protect the underlying cortex.

The proximal portion of the STA is temporarily occluded with a long Biemer clip, and the distal portion is permanently occluded with a Weck clip. The distal STA is then transected on a bevel and transposed intracranially. Small Biemer clips are then applied to the cortical artery. An eliptical arteriotomy incision two to three times the diameter of the artery is then made with a curved microscissor. The STA should then be aligned with its leading edge directed toward the proximal segment of the cortical artery (Fig. 8.6). The lumen of the STA and lumen of the cortical artery should be perfectly opposed. The lumen of the STA can be enlarged by a simple extension of the incision along the shorter wall if necessary (fish-mouth opening). Separate tacking sutures (10-0 ethilon) are then placed 180° apart and used as a continuous suture on either side of the anastomosis (Figs. 8.7, 8.8). Each suture is tied to itself and remains independent of the other suture (Fig. 8.9). This partially continuous suture allows delayed expansion of the graft. After completing the anastomosis, the distal cortical clip is opened first to allow back bleeding at the anastomosis. The proximal cortical clip and finally the clip on the STA are then removed (Fig. 8.10). Pulsations should progress from the STA toward the proximal portion of the cortical artery. There may be some persistent ooze from the fascia of the STA and these points are identified with gentle irrigation and controlled with microbipolar cautery. Absolute hemostasis is required before closure. The dura is left open and a disk of Gelfoam is placed over the craniectomy defect. The temporalis muscle is partially closed so that the artery is not kinked. The galea is usually deficient where the STA was dissected, and special care is needed to close this layer with inverted Vicryl suture. The skin edges are then gently opposed with nylon suture.

Rheomacrodex (low molecular weight dextran) is infused intravenously at a rate of 50 cc/h beginning about two hours after surgery. This is maintained for the first 24 hours postoperatively and is followed by aspirin 5 g twice daily.[9,82,87] The patient is observed in the intensive care unit to be certain that the blood pressure, pulse, and arterial blood gases are monitored frequently. Liberal fluid replacement at approximately 100 cc/h is employed; after 24 hours the patient is gradually elevated, and he may sit out of bed with continuous blood pressure monitoring. Scalp sutures are removed seven days after surgery. Patency of the bypass can often be evaluated by palpating the pulse from the proximal segment of the STA to the edge of the craniectomy. The Doppler stethoscope is also used when necessary to assess patency.

Alternative Bypass Grafts

Other arteries or graft materials have been used for bypass when the caliber of the STA was inadequate. The occipital branch of the external carotid artery was used by Spetzler.[83] The middle meningeal arteries have been used by Nishi-

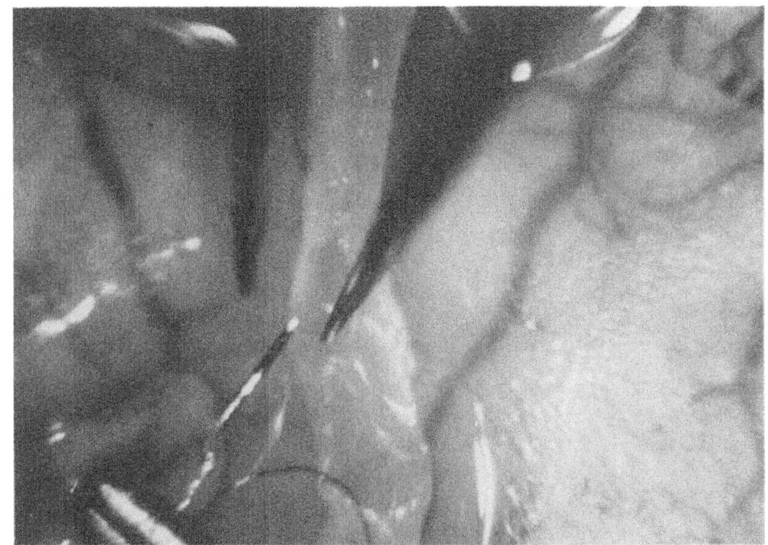

Figure 8.7. Intraoperative photography demonstrating the first suture. This was passed from the outer wall to the inner wall of the cortical artery and then from the inner wall to the outer wall of the STA.

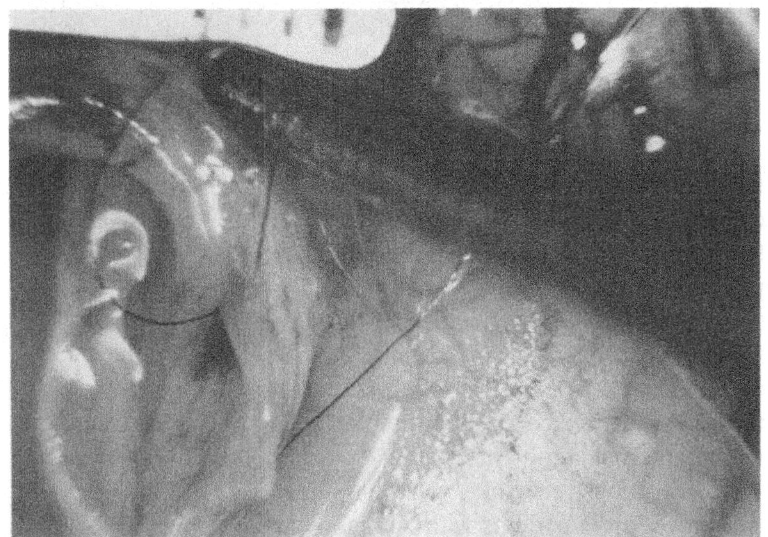

Figure 8.8. The second stay suture has been passed from the cortical artery to the STA. Lumen of the STA was slightly enlarged by a fish-mouth opening, which allows for better alignment.

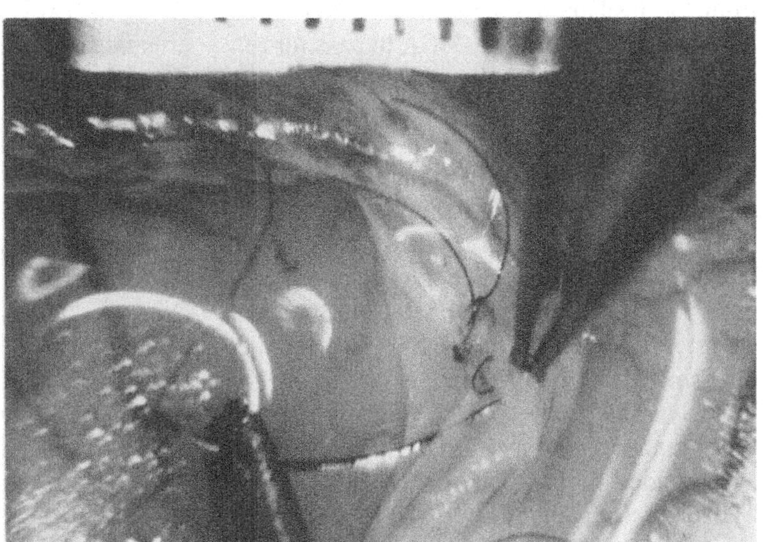

Figure 8.9. Each stay suture is then used in a continuous suture technique on each side of the anastomosis.

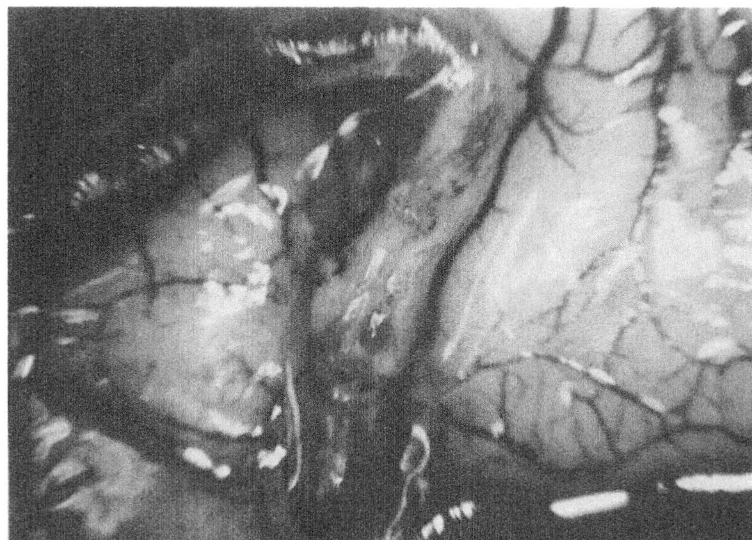

Figure 8.10. After completion of anastomosis, the STA overlies the cortical artery, temporary clips have been removed, and hemostasis has been obtained.

kawa[66] for bypass in a patient with Moya Moya disease. Lougheed et al[60] described the use of a free vein graft harvested from the leg and interposed between the common carotid and intracranial carotid artery in a patient with recurrent symptoms secondary to a right internal carotid occlusion. Attempts in two other patients were unsuccessful because of atheroma in the intracranial internal carotid artery.

Interposition free grafts were employed by Ausman et al[3] in patients with common carotid artery occlusion. A long vein graft was placed from the ipsilateral subclavian to external carotid followed by an STA-MCA bypass for retinal ischemia. Radial artery grafts were used between the external carotid artery and middle cerebral branches by a number of surgeons but have been complicated by intimal hyperplasia. We have utilized long saphenous vein grafts to the cortical artery in five patients with inadequate STAs. A short saphenous vein graft was used between the proximal STA and the cortical artery in patients with an STA that ramified into small branches that were inadequate for use. Synthetic materials have been used by other authors. Story et al[84] described the use of expended polytetrafluoroethylene (Gortex). The long-term patency rates using these materials are not as good as with the STA. All free grafts require both proximal and distal anastomosis and are devoid of an intrinsic blood supply. In addition, vein grafts tend to react to arterial blood pressure surges with intimal hyperplasia.

Results of Bypass Surgery

The technical results of bypass have been evaluated by percutaneous palpation and auscultation of the scalp artery as it enters the craniectomy defect. A Doppler stethescope is placed over the defect, and the underlying bruit is heard. If compression of the scalp artery anterior to the ear eliminates the bruit, then the flow originates from the STA. The only runoff of the STA distal to its entry into the craniectomy is through the anastomosis, and it is presumed that the bypass is patent.

Postoperative angiography has been described by Latchaw et al[55] and others.[50,78] Within several weeks of surgery there is a significant enlargement of the STA. The degree of filling of the cortical arteries may be related to the transcranial pressure gradient between the extracranial and intracranial arteries.[26] The clinical results of surgery are most often described in terms of the rate of stroke postoperatively. These results are often compared with the stroke rate in an untreated group of patients. Most reports describe the results within a group of patients characterized by their clinical syndrome rather than by their vascular lesion.

Samson et al[77–79] found that in patients with completed stroke who subsequently develop TIA in the territory of an occluded carotid artery bypass is associated with a lower incidence (7%) of subsequent stroke compared with the rate expected (40%) from previously published studies.

A cooperative randomized study to compare the frequency of future ischemic events in patients treated with aspirin and in those treated with aspirin and bypass is in progress. The aim of the study is to see if there is a 50% reduction in the frequency of stroke. It is unlikely that this degree of risk reduction can be found in a heterogeneous population of patients with a variable intrinsic risk for stroke. It is unclear whether statistically significant trends can be expected in smaller subgroups of patients that might benefit from bypass.

Clinical Results

One hundred eighty one procedures were performed in 170 patients. These were 121 males and 49 females. The average age of the patients was 56 years and ranged between 24 years and 78 years of age. Most patients who had multiple ischemic episodes had stereotyped events; however, many had a variety of syndromes. The patients are described in Table 8.1 according to the most severe clinical syndrome experienced preoperatively and according to their angiographic lesions.

Internal carotid occlusion was the most common lesion. This was followed by middle cerebral stenosis. Multiple lesions occurred in 76 patients and included cases with bilateral lesions as well as patients with tandem ipsilateral lesions. Multiple procedures were performed in 42 patients. The most common combination of multiple lesions was internal carotid occlusion and contralateral internal carotid stenosis. This occurred in 49 patients. In 31 patients symptoms were referable to the occluded side only or to both sides. All 31 patients were treated with ED-IC bypass followed by a contralateral carotid microendarterectomy in 28.

The major goal of bypass surgery is to reduce the risk of recurrent ischemic events and in particular the risk of completed stroke in patients at risk. The postoperative frequency of all ischemic vascular events was 1.4% per year, and the frequency of completed stroke was .82% per year.

Postoperative Angiography

There are various techniques for measuring the quality and degree of cerebral perfusion achieved through the bypass graft. However, none is as informative as selective angiography.

Angiography provides detailed visualization of the bypass and its relative contribution to cerebral perfusion. In 52 patients postoperative angiography was performed between one week and four years after surgery. The patency rate in this group was 95%. The diameter of the STA increased in time. In the initial study there was an increase of at least 25% in the diameter of the STA in 40% of patients.

Digital Angiography

Digital subtraction angiography (DSA) is a noninvasive method for assessing patency. Oblique views may demonstrate the bypass. Details of intracranial filling patterns are not as good, however, as with conventional arterial angiography. In 87 cases in which postoperative DSA studies were performed, 82 showed a definitely patent bypass. Three studies were equivocal and two suggested an occluded graft. Arterial angiography disclosed that all of the three equivocal cases were actually patent.

Complications

EC-IC bypass is a low-risk procedure in properly selected patients. Surgical mortality rates have varied from 0% to 7.7%.* Ischemic complications are more frequent in patients operated on for stroke in evolution. The only stroke-related death in our series occurred in a 38-year-old woman with bilateral carotid occlusive disease who had surgery during a stroke in evolution. She developed a hemorrhagic infarction 24 hours after surgery and rapidly deteriorated thereafter. The other surgical mortality

*References 4, 12, 29, 34, 52, 55, 57, 59, 69, 70, 72.

was the result of an acute myocardial infarction in a 72-year-old patient occurring 25 days postoperatively. In the author's series the mortality rate was 0.71%.

Ischemic complications during surgery or immediately thereafter are unusual.[51,71] None of the patients in our series have had an intraoperative stroke. The frequency of local complication was 7%. Scalp necrosis developed at the junction of the T-shaped incision in 14 patients. This most often involved the skin and healed with no specific treatment. Surgical revision consisting of debridement and reapproximation of the edges was required in two patients. Since the muscle and dural closure is incomplete, a superficial infection may rapidly communicate with subdural or intracerebral compartments through the open dura. Subgaleal and subdural empyema was seen in two patients. Both patients developed fever and focal seizures. Both required reoperation, irrigation, and debridement followed by a single layer closure of the scalp flap. There were no long-term sequelae in these patients. Cellulitis of the skin overlying the bypass occurred in one patient and responded to intravenous penicillin and chloramphenicol. There were no lasting effects from this. Since tight dural closure cannot be achieved, a very meticulous and complete closure of the galea is employed in anticipation of a CSF leak.

The rate of cardiac and systemic complications was low. Four patients developed new cardiac arrhythmias and two had recurrence of perioperative arrhythmias that were successfully treated. One patient had a myocardial infarction two weeks postoperatively with no sequelae. Three patients developed transient pneumonia, and 11% had transient urinary tract infections.

Future Prospects

The feasibility of using other techniques for bypass are under study. Interposition vein grafts have the advantage of a greater flow capacity, but are technically more difficult to use and have a lower long-term patency rate. The limitation on their function is usually related to the small size of the distal anastomosis, which can only be partially overcome by the onlay graft techniques described above. Anastomosis to one of the main divisions of the middle cerebral artery through the sylvian fissure may be more successful. Preoperative and postoperative evaluations of these patients may be more fruitful with the development of tomographic techniques for studying CBF.

References

1. Ausman JI, Lee MC, Geiger JD, Klassen AC, Chou SN: Clinical results of middle cerebral artery anastomosis in ischemic stroke patients. In Internal Carotid Artery Distribution. AANS Ann Mtg, New Orleans, La, 1978
2. Ausman JI, Lindsay W, Ramsey RC, Chou SN: Ipsilateral subclavian to external carotid and STA-MCA bypass for retinal ischemia. Surg Neurol 9:508, 1978
3. Austin G, LaManna J, Jobsis F: Measurement of Oxidative Metabolism During Microanastomosis for Cerebral Ischemia. Section of Neurological Surg. and Dept. of Physiology & Pharmacology, Loma Linda Univ. School of Med. and Duke Univ. Univ. of California Press, San Diego, Ca. 1977
4. Austin G, Luffin D, Haywood W: Cerebral blood flow in patients undergoing microanastomosis for modification or prevention of stroke. Ann Clin Lab Sci 5:229–235, 1975
5. Austin GM, Zimmerman D: Prediction of relative flow deficit and EC-IC effectiveness by computer model of circle of Willis: J CBF Metab 1:497–498, 1981
6. Barker WF, Gurdjian ES: Intra- and Extracranial Procedures for Cerebral Ischemia, Amer. Coll of Surg, 61st Ann Clinical Congress, San Francisco, Oct. 13–17, 1975
7. Barnett HJM, Peerless SJ, Kaufman JCE: The "stump" of the internal carotid artery—a source of further cerebral embolic ischemia. Stroke 9:448–456, 1978
8. Boone SC, Sampson DS: Observations on Moyamoya Disease: A case treated with superficial temporal middle cerebral artery anastomosis. Surg Neurol 9:189–193, 1978
9. Bousser MG, Eschwege E, Hagvenau M, Lefauconnier JM, Thibult N, Touboul D, Touboul PJ: "AICLA" controlled trial of aspirin and Depyramidole in the secondary prevention of atherothrombotic cerebral ischemia. Stroke 14:5–14, 1983
10. Bushe KA, Bockhorn J: Extracranial-intracranial arterial bypass for giant aneurysms. Acta Neurochirurgica, 54:107–115, 1980

11. Cassidy JE: Management of risk factors and other disease in candidates for microneurosurgical anastomosis in cerebral ischemia. In Fein JM, Reichman OH (eds.): Microvascular Anastomoses for Cerebral Ischemia. Springer-Verlag, New York, 1978
12. Chater N, Popp J: Microsurgical vascular bypass for occlusive cerebrovascular disease. Review of 100 cases. Surg Neurol 6:115–118, 1976
13. Chou SN: Embolectomy of middle cerebral artery; report of a case. J Neurosurg 20:161–163, 1963
14. Cobb CA, Keller T: Microsurgical vascular anastomosis for traumatic middle cerebral artery occlusion. J Trauma 16:738–741, 1978
15. Countee RW, Vijayanathan T: Reconstitution of "totally" occluded internal carotid arteries. J Neurosurg 50:747–757, 1979
16. Craig DR, Meguro K, Watridge C, Robertson JT, Barnett HJ, Fox AJ: Intracranial internal carotid artery stenosis. Stroke 13:825–828, 1983
17. Denny-Brown D: Recurrent cerebrovascular episodes. Arch Neurol 2:194–210, 1960
18. Diaz FG, Ausman JI, de los Reyes RA, Dujovny M: Successful application of acute cerebral revascularization to stroke in evolution. Presented at American Heart Assoc., 55th Scientific Session, Oct. 1982
19. Donaghy RMP: Patch and bypass in microangional surgery. In Donaghy RMP, Yasargil MG (eds.): Microvascular Surgery. Thieme Verlag, Stuttgart, 1967, pp 75–86
20. Donaghy RMP: Surgery of Cerebrovascular Disease. Ann AANS Meeting, San Francisco, CA, 1976
21. Donaghy RMP, Yasargil G: Microangional Surgery and Its Techniques. Progress in Brain Research. W Luyendijk (ed.). Elsevier Publishing Co, pp 263–264
22. Driesen W: Erfolgreiche Naht der linken A. cerebri media nach Verletzung bei Tumorresektion. Acta Neurochir (Wein), 10:462–465, 1962
23. Dyken ML, Klatte E, Kolar OJ, et al: Complete occlusion of common or internal carotid arteries: Clinical significance. Arch Neurol 30:343–346, 1974
24. Fein JM: Reversal of intracerebral nutrient steal phenomenon after extracranial-intracranial (EC-IC) bypass graft. Neurosurgery 2:158, 1978
25. Fein JM, Flamm E: Planned revascularization prior to proximal ligation for traumatic aneurysm. Neurosurgery 5:254–258, 1979
26. Fein JM, Lipow KI: Cortical artery pressure measurements in cerebrovascular occlusive disease. Neurosurgery (Submitted for publication)
27. Fein JM, Lipow KI, Marmarou A: Cortical artery pressure measurements in normotensive and hypertensive aneurysm patients. J Neurosurgery 59:51–56, 1983
28. Fein J, Molinari G: Experimental augmentation of regional cerebral blood flow by microvascular anastomosis. J Neurosurgery 35:128–140, 1971
29. Fein JM, Reichman OH: Microvascular Anastomosis for Cerebral Ischemia. Springer-Verlag, New York, 1979
30. Fein JM, Veith F: Relationship of internal carotid artery stump pressure to ipsilateral and contralateral superficial temporal artery-middle cerebral artery bypass graft function. Neurosurgery 3:231, 1978
31. Field WS, Lemak NA: Joint study of extracranial arterial occlusion. X. Internal carotid artery occlusion. JAMA 235:2734–2738, 1976
32. Fisher CM: The natural history of middle cerebral artery stem occlusion. In Austin G (ed.): Microneurosurgical Anastomoses for Cerebral Ischemia. Charles C Thomas Publisher, Springfield, Ill, 1974.
33. Fisher M: Occlusion of the internal carotid artery. Arch Neurol Psychiatry 65:346–377, 1951
34. Fox J: Part I: Personnel, equipment, extracranial-intracranial anastomosis. Neurosurgery 2: 287–304, 1978
35. Furlan AJ, Whisnant JP: Long prognosis following carotid artery occlusion. Neurology 30: 986, 1980
36. Furlan AJ, Whisnant JP, Baker HL Jr: Long term prognosis after carotid artery occlusion. Neurology 30:986–988, 1980
37. Gratzl O, Schmiedek P, Spetzler R, Steinhoff H, Marguth F: Clinical experience with extra-intracranial arterial anastomosis in 65 cases. J Neurosurg 44:313–324, 1976
38. Halsey JH Jr, Morowetz RB, Baluenstein U: The hemodynamic effect of STA-MCA bypass. Stroke 13:163–166, 1982
39. Hardy WG, Lindner DW, Thomas LM, Gudjian ES: Anticipated clinical course in carotid artery occlusion. Arch Neurol 6:138–150, 1962
40. Hass WK, Fields WS, North RR, et al: Joint study of extracranial arterial occlusion II. Arteriography techniques, sites and complications. JAMA 203:159–166, 1968
41. Heilbrun MP, Reichman OH, Anderson RE, Roberts TS: Regional cerebral blood flow studies following superficial temporal-middle cerebral artery anastomosis. J Neurosurg 43:706–716, 1975
42. Henschen C: Operative revasklarisation des zirkulatorisch geschadigten Gehirns durch Autlage gestielter Muskellappen (Encephalo-Myo Synangiose). Langenbecks Arch Klin Chir 264:392–401, 1950
43. Hitchon PW, Kassel NF, Gross CE, Adams HP, Hill TR: Influences of superficial temporal artery

to middle cerebral artery bypass on cerebral blood flow in dogs with middle cerebral artery occlusion. Stroke 12:224–228, 1981

44. Holbach KH, Wassmann H, Hoheluchter KL, Jain KK: Differentation between reversible and irreversible post-stroke changes in brain tissue: Its relevance for cerebrovascular surgery. Surg Neurol 7:325–331, 1977
45. Hopkins LN, Grand W: Extracranial-intracranial arterial bypass in the treatment of aneurysms of the carotid and middle cerebral arteries. Neurosurgery 5, 1: I:21–31, 1979
46. Hungerbuhler JP, Younkin D, Reivich M, Obrist WD, O'Connor M, Goldberg H, Gordon J, Gur R, Hurtig H, Amarneck W: The effect of STA-MCA anastomosis on rCBF, neurologic and neuropsychologic function in patients with completed strokes. In Meyer JS, Lechner H, Reivich LM, Ott EO, Aranibar A (eds.): Cerebral Vascular Disease 3. Excerpta Medica, Amsterdam, 1981, pp 73–75
47. Hutchinson EC, Acheson EJ: Strokes; natural history, pathology and surgical treatment. B Saunders Co, London, 1975
48. Jacobson JH, Wallman LJ, Schumacher GA, Flanagan M, Suarez FL, Donaghy RMP: Microsurgery as an aid to middle cerebral artery endarterectomy. J Neurosurg 19:108–115, 1962
49. Jacques S, Garner JT: Reversal of Aphasia with superficial temporal artery to middle cerebral artery anastomosis. Surg Neurol 5:143–145, 1976
50. Karasawa J, Kikuchi H, Furuse S, Kawamura J, Sakaki T: Treatment of Moyamoya disease with STA-MCA anastomosis. J Neurosurg 49:679–688, 1978
51. Khodadad G: Transient postoperative occlusion of the superficial temporal-middle cerebral artery branch anastomosis: Spasm, swelling or thrombosis. Surg Neurol 3:341–345, 1975
52. Kikuchi H, Karasawa J: Clinical experiences with STA cortical MCA anastomosis in 46 cases. In Fein JM, Reocj am OH (eds.): Microvascular Anastomosis for Cerebral Ischemia. Springer-Verlag, New York, 1979
53. Kobayashi S, Hollenhorst RW, Sundt TM Jr: Retinal arterial pressure before and after surgery for carotid artery stenosis. Stroke 2:569–575, 1971
54. Konavalov AN, Serbienko FA: A case of succesful removal of a middle cerebral artery thrombosis developed after occlusion with balloons of different vessels of the arteriovenous aneurysm. Vop Neirokhir, 4:29–34, 1973 (Rus)
55. Latchaw RE, Ausman JI, Lee M: Superficial temporal-middle cerebral artery bypass. J Neurosurg 51:455–465, 1979
56. Laurent JP, Lawner PM, O'Connor M: Reversal of intracerebral steal by STA-MCA anastomosis. J Neurosurg 57:629–632, 1982
57. Lazar ML, Clark K: Microsurgical cerebral revascularization: Concepts and practice. Surg Neurol 1:355–359, 1973
58. Lecuire J, Lapras C, Dechaume J, et al: L'embolectomie arterielle intra-cranienne: donnees experimentales et cliniques. Lon Chir 69:3–8, 1973
59. Lee MC, Ausman JI, Geiger JD, Latchaw RE, Klassen AC, Chou SN, Resch JA: Superficial temporal to middle cerebral artery anastomosis. Arch Neurol 36:1–4, 1979
60. Lougheed WM, Marshall BM, Hunter M, Michel ER, Sandwith-Smyth H: Common carotid to intracranial carotid bypass venous graft. J Neurosurg 34:114–118. 1971
61. Marshall J: Angiography in the investigation of ischemic episodes in the territory of the internal carotid artery. Lancet 1:719–721, 1971
62. Marzewski DJ, Furlan AJ, St. Louis P, Little J, Modic MT, Williams G: Intracranial internal carotid artery stenosis: Long term prognosis. Stroke 13:821–824, 1982
63. McDowell FH, Potes J, Groch S: The natural history of internal carotid and vertebral-basilar artery occlusion. Neurology 11:153–157, 1961
64. Meyer JS, Nakajima S, Okabe T, Amano T, Centeno R, Lee YY, Levine J, Levinthal R, Rose J: Redistribution of cerebral blood flow following STA-MCA bypass in patients with hemispheric ischemia. Stroke 13, 774–784, 1982
65. Millikan C: Treatment of occlusive cerebrovascular disease in cerebrovascular survery report. Joint Council subcommittee on cerebrovascular research. National Institute of Neurological and communicative disorders and stroke. Jan. 1980, pp 244–289
66. Nishikawa M, Hashi K, Shiguma M: Middle meningeal middle cerebral artery anastomosis for cerebral ischemia. Surg Neurol 12:205–207, 1979
67. Piazza G, Geist G: Occlusion of middle cerebral artery by foreign body embolus. Report of a case. J Neurosurg 17:172–176, 1960
68. Pool JL: Aneurysms and arteriovenous anomalies of the brain. Hoeber NYC 1964
69. Reichman OH: Extracranial-intracranial arterial anastomosis. In Whisnant JP, Sandkok BA (eds.): Cerebral Vascular Diseases: Ninth Conference. Grune and Stratton, New York, 1975 pp 175–185
70. Reichman OH: Comments on cerebral revascularization. Presented at Cerebrovascular Symposium, July 7, 1976. Kanton Hospital, Zurich, Switzerland
71. Reichman OH: Complications of cerebral revascularization. Clin Neurosurg 23:318–335, 1976
72. Reichman OH: Neurosurgical microsurgical

anastomosis for cerebral ischemia: Five year's experience. In Scheinberg P (ed.): Cerebrovascular Diseases. Raven Press, New York, 1976, pp 311–330

73. Reichman OH, Davis DO, Roberts TS, Satovick RM: Collateral circulation to the middle cerebral territory by surgical anastomosis. Annual AANS Meeting, 1971
74. Robertson JH, Robertson JT: The relationship between suture number and quality of anastomoses in microvascular procedures. Surg Neurol 10:241–246, 1978
75. Roski RA, Spetzler RF, Nulsen FE: Late ischemic complications of carotid ligation in the treatment of intracranial aneurysm. Presented AANS Annual Meeting, New York, April 1980
76. Roski RA, Spetzler RF, Owen M, Chandar K, Sholl JG, Nulsen FE: Reversal of seven-year-old visual field defect with extracranial-intracranial arterial anastomosis. Surg Neurol 10:267–268, 1978
77. Samson DS, Boone S: Extracranial-intracranial (EC-IC) arterial bypass: past performance and current concepts. Neurosurgery 3:79–86, 1978
78. Samson DS, Hodosh RM, Clark WK: Microsurgical treatment of transient cerebral ischemia. Preliminary results in 50 cases. JAMA 241, 4:376–378, 1979
79. Samson DS, Watts D, Clark K: Cerebral revascularization for transient ischemic attacks. Neurology 27:767–771, 1977
80. Scheibert CD: Middle cerebral artery surgery for obstructive lesions. Presented 27th Ann. Meeting of the Harvey Cushing Society, New Orleans, May 1959
81. Shillito J: Intracranial arteriotomy in three children and three adults. In Donaghy RMP, Yasargil MG (eds.): Microvascular Surgery. Georg Thieme Verlag, Stuttgart, 1967, pp 138–142
82. Sorensen PS, Pedersen H, Marquardsen J, Petersson H, Helteberg A, Simonsen N, Munch O, Andersen LA: Acetylsalicylic acid in the prevention of stroke in patients with reversible central ischemic attacks. A Danish Cooperative study. Stroke 14:15–21, 1983
83. Spetzler R, Chater N: Occipital artery-middle cerebral artery anastomosis for cerebral artery occlusive disease. Surg Neurol 2:235–238, 1974
84. Story JL, Brown WE Jr, Eidelberg E, Arom KV, Stewart JR: Cerebral revascularization: Proximal external carotid to distal middle cerebral artery bypass with a synthetic tube graft. Neurosurgery 3:61–65, 1978
85. Sundt TM Jr, Siekert RG, Piepgras DG, Sharbrough TW, Houser OW: Bypass surgery for vascular disease of the carotid system. Mayo Clin Proc 51:677–692, 1976
86. Tew JM: Reconstructive intracranial vascular surgery for prevention of stroke. Clin Neurosurg 22:264–280, 1975
87. The Canadian Cooperative Study Group. A randomized trial of aspirin and sulfinpyrazone in threatened stroke. N Engl J Med 299:53–59, 1978
88. Welch K: Excision of occlusive lesions of the middle cerebral artery. J Neurosurg 13:73–80, 1956
89. Wolff HG: Concluding summary. In Millikan CH, Siekert RG, Whisnant JP (eds.): Cerebral Vascular Disease. Third Conference. Grune & Stratton, New York, 1961, pp 240–242
90. Woringer E, Kunlin J; Anastomose entre la carotide preimitive et la carotide intra-cranienne ou la sylvienne par greffon selon la technique de la suture suspendue. Neuro-Chirurgie Paris 9, 2:181–188, 1963
91. Yasargil MG: Suturing Techniques in Microsurgery Applied to Neurosurgery. Georg Thomas Verlag, Academic Press, New York, 1969
92. Yasargil MG, Krayenbuhl HA, Jacobson JH: Microneurosurgical arterial reconstruction. Surgery 67:221–233, 1970
93. Yasargil MG, Yonehawa Y: Results of microsurgical extra-intracranial arterial bypass in the treatment of cerebral ischemia. Neurosurgery 1:22–24, 1977
94. Yonehawa Y, Yasargil MG: Extra-intracranial arterial anastomosis. Clinical and technical aspects, results. In Krayenbuhl H (ed.): Advances and Technical Standards in Neurosurgery. Vol 3, Springer-Verlag, Wien, 1976, pp 47–78
95. Zlotnick EI: Thrombectomy of the middle cerebral artery. Case report. J Neurosurg 42:723–725, 1975

9

Intracranial Bypass Grafts for Vertebrobasilar Ischemia

Thoralf M. Sundt, Jr., and David G. Piepgras

Introduction

Ischemic symptomatology in the posterior circulation is very frequently related to vascular disease in the penetrating vessels with the production of lacunar infarcts. However, there does remain a large number of patients with symptomatology related to large-vessel occlusive disease in the posterior circulation. Very commonly this symptomatology is on the basis of hemodynamic changes from high-grade stenotic lesions rather than from emboli. We will consider in this chapter the surgical approach to large-vessel occlusive disease in the posterior circulation. It should be emphasized that these are major procedures and should not be undertaken unless it is clear that the patient's symptomatology is progressing on conservative management.

The operating microscope has revolutionized some surgical specialities of which neurosurgery is one. Use of this instrument helped to improve dramatically the results of surgery for intracranial aneurysms and arteriovenous malformations. Then, following demonstration of the feasibility of extracranial to intracranial bypass procedures by Yasargil,[39,40] an entirely new form of management evolved for patients with ischemic cerebral vascular disease.[24–26,27] The application of bypass procedures to occlusive disease in the posterior circulation was a natural extension of this major achievement.[3,20,21,36] To understand the role of operative procedures, it is necessary to correlate the pathophysiology of ischemic stroke syndromes with the normal physiology of cerebral circulation. Thereafter we will review some typical cases, describe the operative technique, and consider the surgical indications, results, and complications of the procedures.

Anatomic Considerations and Cerebral Blood Flow

The cerebral circulation can be divided into a conducting system and a penetrating system.[34] The conducting vessels are the carotid, middle cerebral, anterior cerebral, vertebral, basilar, and posterior cerebral arteries in addition to their major (named) and minor (unnamed) branches on the surface of the brain. These branches form a vast network of interconnecting and anastomosing vessels on the surface of the brain. The conducting vessels may be regarded as nonresistance-type vessels because there is only a 10% drop in perfusion pressure from the aorta to major branches of the middle cerebral artery and a similar gradient from these large branches to the level of the penetrating arterioles. The latter enter the brain parenchyma at right angles to the surface vessels from which they are derived. The system of conducting vessels serves as a pressure head or pressure equalization reservoir to furnish an adequate perfusion pressure to the penetrating or nutrient arterioles wherein primary autoregulation probably resides. The conducting vessels, the recipients of emboli and the sites of primary atherosclerosis, form a low-resistance bed that is ideal for bypass surgery. The penetrating vessels, when involved with arteriolar sclerosis, cause lacunar infarcts.[11,14]

The rate of normal blood flow to the brain is about 50 to 55 mL/100 g/min.[19] However, the brain can accommodate a substantial reduction in flow and still function.[32] Laboratory and clinical studies indicate that the minimal amount of blood flow required to sustain normal electrical activity in the brain approximates 15 mL/100 g/min.* This type of activity cannot be equated with normal function, but extensive studies during carotid endarterectomy[33] have proved that this degree of marginal flow is entirely reversible. Reductions of flow below this critical level are associated with physiologic paralysis and if prolonged, cerebral infarction. Ischemic tolerance of neural tissue depends both on the duration and the severity of ischemia, but the elegant studies of Branston and co-workers have demonstrated that flows of 5 mL/100 g/min are associated with electrolyte shifts and cellular membrane changes that are probably not reversible.[5] Fortunately, many patients with ischemic symptomatology have marginal flows that, although inadequate to sustain physiologic function, are nevertheless adequate to prevent anatomic infarction.

Patterns of Large-Vessel Occlusive Disease

Fisher and his colleagues reported that in contrast to the carotid arteries where symptomatic occlusions are often extracranial, in the vertebral arteries symptomatic occlusions are intracranial.[12,15,16] This observation, later confirmed by other workers,[9] is of considerable importance because the commonest site for stenosis or occlusion of the vertebral artery is at its origin from the subclavian artery.[27] However, stenotic lesions at this location are usually protected by a collateral system of vessels arising from deep muscular branches of the thyrocervical and costocervical arteries so that cerebral infarction from this source is uncommon. Atherosclerotic plaques are diffusely distributed throughout the vertebral arteries, but ulceration of these plaques is not common.[9] Again, this is in contrast to the carotid system where plaques are often near the bifurcation of the common carotid artery, and ulceration with secondary embolization is common.

Emboli (from the heart or common carotid artery bifurcation) are thought to be the chief cause of occlusion of the major branches of the internal carotid artery intracranially.[22] This does not seem to be the case in the vertebrobasilar systems where Castaigne and associates[9] found thrombosis on a preexisting stenosis to be the cause of 90% of basilar artery occlusions and 70% of the intracranial vertebral artery occlusions. (The correlation of infarction with basilar artery occlusion was 100% and with vertebral artery occlusion 50%.) These workers thought that occlusion on a preexisting stenosis was uncommon in the extracranial vertebral artery but common in the intracranial portion of that vessel. In that study occlusions of the posterior cerebral artery were thought to be embolic in origin in 94% of their cases; this finding indicated that these vessels, the terminal branches of the basilar artery, were the likeliest recipients of emboli and in this respect were similar to the major branches of the internal carotid artery.

Although the cause of infarction in the carotid and vertebrobasilar systems can be evaluated pathologically, the cause of transient ischemic attacks (TIA) are more difficult to assess. Various causes are proposed, two are most often considered; namely, emboli from ulcerated plaques of large vessels to more distal arteries and hemodynamic changes distal to the site of stenosis or occlusion of an artery. Hemodynamic changes may result either from variations in systemic perfusion pressure or from failure of collateral flow. The former seems to

* References 1, 2, 4, 10, 17, 18, 28, 29, 33, 38.

occur more often in the carotid circulation, the latter (in the author's judgment) in the vertebrobasilar circulation.

Ischemic Syndromes

Correlation of clinical symptoms, angiogram, and cerebral blood flow studies indicate that flows between 20 and 30 mL/100 g/min are borderline.[18] Patients with flow rates this low are often neurologically unstable and particularly vulnerable to the effects of emboli. Development of infarction is related to both degree and duration of ischemia. It occurs within minutes in areas of zero flow but may take hours in regions of marginal flow.[29] Blood flows in zones of incomplete focal ischemia is nonhomogeneous, with areas of reactive hyperemia and zones of decreased perfusion often being adjacent to infarcted tissue.[29,38]

A transient focal neurologic deficit due to ischemia less than 24 hours in duration represents a TIA.[13] In the vertebrobasilar system, TIAs are less stereotyped than those in the carotid system.[8,36] Vertigo is a common component of TIA in the vertebrobasilar system; however, vertigo alone is most commonly a manifestation a labyrinthine disorder and, therefore, unless associated with some other manifestation of brainstem ischemia, should not be regarded as a TIA.[23] A transient hemiparesis, hemisensory deficit, or homonymous hemianopsia can arise from ischemia in either the anterior or the posterior circulatory systems. However, they usually represent a carotid TIA unless symptoms occur on alternating sides in different episodes or there is a history of cranial nerve dysfunction or contralateral sensory dysfunction. The occurrence of alternating sides with ischemic events or a transient quadriparesis is most commonly of brainstem origin.

Dysarthria and dysphagia, which are symptoms of bulbar ischemia, may be seen in patients with pseudobulbar palsy from supratentorial lesions, but they are most commonly brainstem in origin. Transient impairment of function of the extraocular muscles may be of definite localizing value, but if diplopia is due to a TIA, it will usually be associated with other symptoms. Ataxia of gait or of the extremities is also of localizing value but must be distinguished from a transient paresis. This is often most difficult to determine on the basis of history alone. Nausea, vomiting, and vertigo may occur with brainstem TIA, but this combination is not useful for distinguishing brainstem from labyrinthine dysfunction.

A reversible ischemic neurologic deficit (RIND) persists longer than 24 hours but nevertheless is fully reversible. In the past it was considered a small infarction, but in the light of laboratory studies it is probable that this is a prolonged ischemic event with a physiologic paralysis that has not progressed to anatomic infarction.

A progressing stroke is a stepwise or gradually progressing neurologic deficit evolving during hours or a few days.[36] The dysfunction begins as a relatively minor deficit that culminates in a major deficit in the absence of treatment. Progressing strokes involving the vertebrobasilar system are often severe and may cause pronounced incapacity leading to death.

Primary orthostatic cerebral ischemia describes a generalized, nonfocal, cerebral ischemia related to erect posture in a patient with multiple occlusions of major extracranial vessels.[34,36] We had described this in an earlier report, but credit for the initial analysis of this syndrome goes to Caplan and Sergay.[6,7] Postural light-headedness or syncope, dimming or blurring of vision, ataxia, and altered mentation or memory are prominent symptoms.

Syncope alone is most commonly related to systemic orthostatic hypotension. However, patients with major extracranial vessel occlusions often have syncope associated with upright position without a drop in the peripheral blood pressure. Perhaps this syndrome can arise from localized ischemia in the brainstem, but, in general, syncope appears to represent a generalized or nonfocal form of cerebral ischemia.

Ischemic pain related to vertebrobasilar occlusive disease is most often referred to the occipital area. Obviously, headaches alone are more commonly due to causes unrelated to ischemia so that one must be careful and cautious in attributing this relatively common complaint to the relatively rare syndrome of vertebrobasilar occlusive disease.[36] The mechanism of this complaint with ischemia in the posterior circulation remains obscure.

Selected Cases

Occipital Artery Pedicle to Posterior Inferior Cerebellar Artery Bypass Procedure

Case 1

A 55-year-old retired farmer came to the Mayo Clinic in February 1976 with complaints of "dizziness and roaring in his ears" of 14 months' duration. In January 1975 he had begun to experience intermittent vertigo associated with blurred vision and a sensation that he was losing consciousness. These episodes occurred daily and were usually associated with exercise or standing up from a sitting position. In April 1975 more severe vertigo developed together with the sensation of a "pounding" in his head. Symptoms progressed to the point where the patient was forced to retire from active employment. Anticoagulants and aspirin were unsuccessful in relieving the patient's symptomatology. Angiograms performed at the local hospital demonstrated symmetrically placed, high-grade stenotic lesions of both vertebral arteries just proximal to the origin of the posterior inferior cerebellar arteries.

At the time of medical and neurologic examination at the Mayo Clinic, loud systolic bruits were heard on auscultation over the mastoid processes bilaterally. Peripheral blood pressures were 136/82 mm Hg; there was no orthostatic decrease. The results of the remainder of the examination were normal.

A relatively large occipital artery originating from the vertebral artery at the level of C-1 rather than the external carotid artery was anastomosed to the left posterior inferior cerebellar artery in April 1976. The patient had an uncomplicated recovery. The pounding sensation ceased, and the bruits were no longer heard on auscultation. Postoperative angiography of the patient before dismissal demonstrated good patency of the graft.

Repeat angiography in September 1976 showed further enlargement of the bypass graft (Fig. 9.1). The vertebral artery stenotic lesions had progressed to total occlusion, and the entire posterior circulation filled through the bypass graft. The patient had returned to normal activities and was essentially asymptomatic.

Case 2

A 47-year-old steelworker from Gary, Indiana, came to the Mayo Clinic in November 1976. He had been in excellent health before 1974, after which time he began to experience intermittent episodes of vertigo, diplopia, diaphoresis, nausea, and vomiting. These were always related to assuming an upright posture. On several occasions he had lost consciousness and had been taken to a local hospital and treated for a "heart attack." On two occasions the patient had experienced numbness in the right side of the face during an attack. In February 1976 he had been hospitalized for severe headache of a nonspecific nature, bifrontal in location. The episodes increased in frequency and were not improved by anticoagulant therapy. At the time he came to the Mayo Clinic, the headaches were occurring on an average of one to two times per week. Between the attacks the patient was asymptomatic except for a subjective sensation of disequilibrium and recent impairment of memory, which were prominent symptoms according to his wife.

Neurologic examination revealed left internuclear ophthalmoplegia. Retinal artery pressures while sitting were 102/50 mm Hg. Blood pressure was 114/98 mm Hg sitting, and no orthostatic decrease was noted.

Angiography demonstrated diffuse stenosis and narrowing of both vertebral arteries, suggestive of fibromuscular disease, from the region of the foramen magnum to an area near their junction to form the basilar artery. A rudimentary left posterior inferior cerebellar artery originated proximal to the beaded segment. A dominant right posterior inferior cerebellar artery originated distal to the beaded segment of the right vertebral artery.

Anastomosis of the right occipital artery to the right posterior inferior cerebellar artery was accomplished in November 1976. Postoperative angiography showed pronounced enlargement of the occipital branch of the right external carotid artery with filling of the vertebral-basilar system through the bypass graft (Fig. 9.2). There was still some retrograde filling of the distal portion of the basilar artery through the

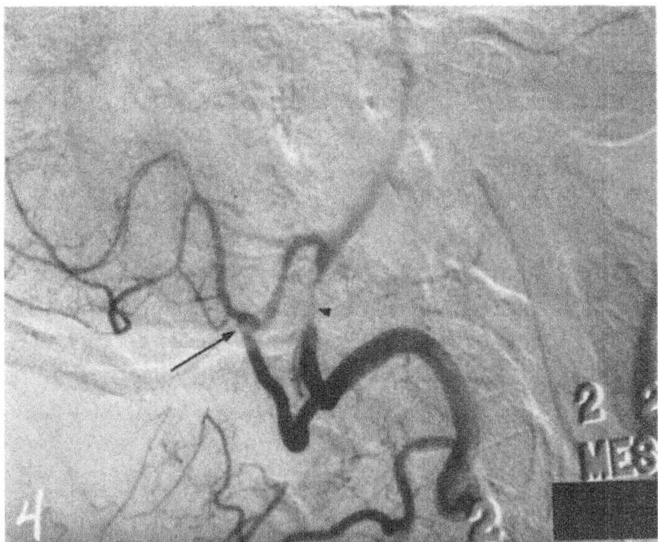

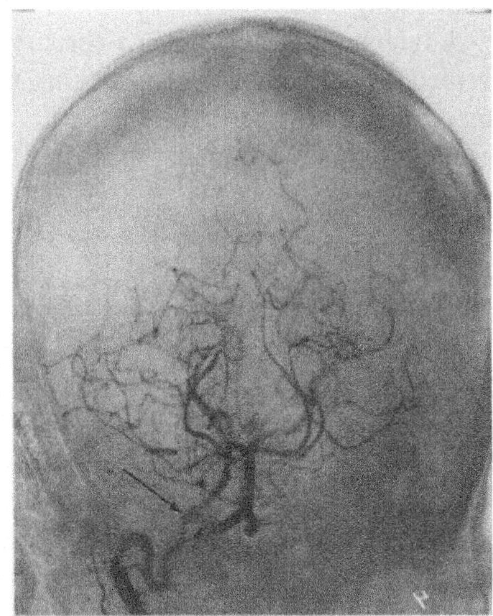

Figure 9.1. Postoperative angiogram six months after bypass graft in patient (case 1; see text). Further enlargement of bypass graft and occlusion of vertebral artery at site of previous stenosis are seen. *Arrow* points to area of anastomosis between occipital artery and posterior inferior cerebellar artery (PICA); *arrowheads* point to proximal and distal segments of PICA. Entire vertebrobasilar system, together with distal segment of opposite vertebral artery (distal to site of opposite vertebral artery stenosis), fills from bypass graft.

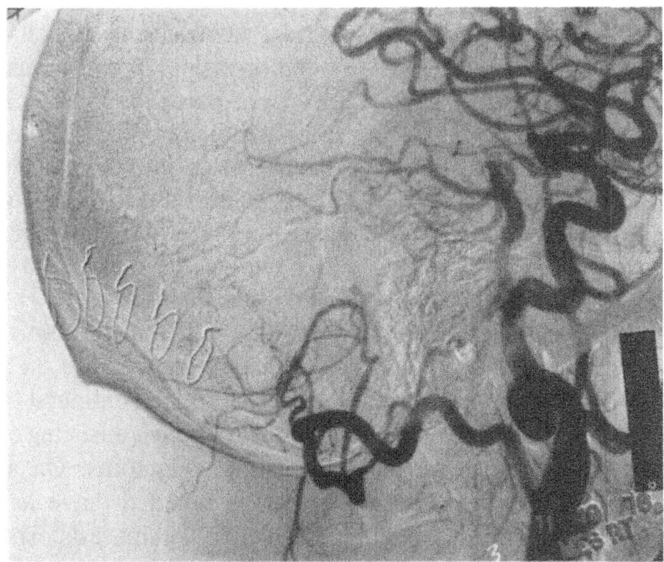

Fig. 9.2

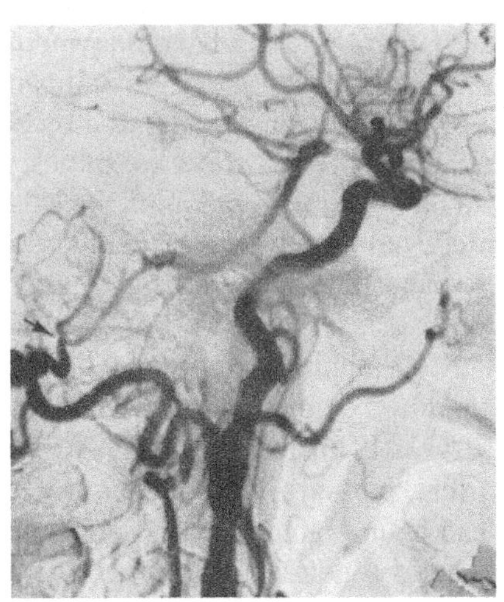

Fig. 9.3

Figure 9.2. Postoperative angiography in Case 2 shows proximal filling of the vertebral basilar system through bypass graft. Distal basilar artery still receives its primary perfusion via retrograde flow through the posterior communicating artery.

Figure 9.3. Postoperative angiography in Case 3, two weeks following placement of the occipital to posterior inferior cerebellar artery bypass pedicle reveals that the primary flow into the posterior circulation is derived through the arterial pedicle.

carotid system via an enlarged posterior communicating artery.

A telephone follow-up in February 1977 revealed that the patient was seeking reemployment. He was having no more "blackout spells"; impaired memory persisted. He considered himself normal.

Case 3

A 55-year-old carpenter was first seen at the Mayo Clinic on January 20, 1976, with signs and symptoms of brainstem ischemia. The patient had had occasional "blackout spells" in 1973 and 1974. Five weeks before admission the patient had experienced blurring vision and complained of dizziness when looking upward with neck extension. Four weeks before admission the patient had had progressive problems with visual focus. He was lethargic during the Christmas holidays but returned to work after the holidays.

Two weeks before admission the patient had an episode of severe dizziness at work and difficulty with balance; he required assistance in walking. This episode was associated with nausea and vomiting. By January 7, 1976, the patient was unable to feed himself and he was admitted to the local hospital. Slurring of speech developed shortly thereafter, and these symptoms became worse.

When he was first seen at the Mayo Clinic, the patient had a left homonymous hemianopsia, skew deviation of eyes and paralysis of upward gaze, nystagmus in all directions of gaze, severe ataxia of the extremities, and severe ataxia of gait with falling to the left. The patient preferred to sleep but he could be aroused with verbal stimuli. Blood pressure was 140/80 mm Hg.

After admission to the hospital, the patient's condition continued to deteriorate and by January 22, 1976, he was unable to speak. Retinal artery pressure was 90/54 mm Hg bilaterally. The main features at this point included headache, dysmetria, dysarthria, ataxia of gait and extremities, skew deviation, nystagmus, paralysis of upward gaze, mild left facial weakness, decreased alertness, and mild confusion. The neurologic diagnosis was progressing ischemic stroke in the vertebral-basilar system.

Angiograms demonstrated a small left vertebral artery that terminated in a posterior inferior cerebellar artery. The right vertebral artery was prominent and was 99% stenosed just proximal to the origin of the right posterior inferior cerebellar artery.

The right occipital artery was anastomosed to the right posterior inferior cerebellar artery on January 28, 1976. Postoperatively, the patient's recovery was slow, but progressive improvement was noted. Angiograms performed on February 10, 1976, demonstrated filling of the entire posterior circulation through the bypass graft (Fig. 9.3).

The patient's speech was slow but clear at the time of postoperative follow-up, by telephone, in February 1977. He reported that he was walking without a cane and that most activities of daily living were normal. He has been unable to return to work as a carpenter because he does not have adequate coordination in his hands. He does not drive his car.

Interposition Saphenous Vein Graft

Case 1

A 69-year-old retired salesman was admitted to the local hospital on August 7, 1980, with a one-week history of intermittent attacks of vertigo, light-headedness, diaphoresis, dysarthria, right hemiparesis, right hemisensory deficits, and occasional diminution or loss of consciousness. These attacks were particularly associated with sitting up or standing up from the supine position and lasted 30 to 45 minutes. He had no previous history of cerebral vascular insufficiency. He was not a diabetic. He had undergone a successful two-vessel coronary bypass procedure seven years previously.

A computed tomography (CT) scan on admission was normal. The patient was placed on a course of heparin and bedrest. He continued to have two to three episodes per day consisting of several or all of the above symptoms. On at least one occasion he was noted to have left hemiparesis rather than right hemiparesis. The extreme orthostatic nature of his problem was noted on at least two occasions when he sat up for one reason or another in bed and promptly had an ischemic attack. Angiograms on August 18, 1980, identified total occlusion of the left vertebral artery up to the level of a small posterior inferior cerebellar artery. The right vertebral artery was small and ended in a large posterior inferior cerebellar artery. The carotid systems were essentially normal.

On August 19 the patient was transfered by air ambulance to St. Mary's Hospital, a distance of some 300 miles, without incident. However, it was necessary to keep him in the supine position on arrival, because his attempts to sit on the edge of the bed or assume the upright position resulted in ischemic events. The neurologic examination revealed no major fixed deficit.

On August 22 surgery was performed under general anesthesia through a modified pterional approach. The right saphenous vein, which had been harvested between the groin and the knee, was anastomosed end-to-end between the resected stump of the right external carotid artery and the proximal posterior cerebral artery just distal to the third nerve. This graft was brought through a tunnel in the neck and ran from the carotid bifurcation in the subcutaneous tissue anterior to the ear and then through the lower margin of the craniotomy in the inferior aspect of the temporal fossa just superior to the zygoma. The intracranial anastomosis was completed using a running 7-0 prolene suture, and the proximal anastomosis was constructed using interrupted 5-0 prolene sutures. Blood flow through the graft was recorded at 140 mL/min.

The patient awoke from the operative procedure with no neurologic deficit and had an uncomplicated postoperative recovery. He was discharged from the hospital on September 3, 1980. Postoperative angiograms (Fig. 9.4) demonstrated excellent flow through the bypass graft. He has remained well since discharge and is taking aspirin and dipyridamole.

Surgical Technique

Occipital Artery Pedicle-Posterior Inferior Cerebellar Artery Bypass Procedure

The operative technique is illustrated in Fig. 9.5. The patient is placed in the sitting position with the head flexed anteriorly and secured in a pinion headholder.[30] A hockey-stick incision is preferred with the longitudinal component of the incision positioned over the midline avascular plane. The musculature is swept unilaterally from the arch of C-1 in the occiput. The cutting current is not used for the scalp incision but is useful to reflect the deep neck muscles from the occiput as far laterally as the mastoid process. The occipital artery is identified in its fascial plane and is thus located by palpation in the mastoid groove just posterior and medial to the mastoid process. This vessel is then dissected free from the surrounding tissue using small blunt scissors. Small branching vessels are coagulated with the bipolar coagulator before division. This is perhaps the most difficult part of the operation as the vessel is intimately adherent to the surrounding tissue and is much more difficult to isolate than is the superficial temporal artery for anterior circulation bypass procedures. It is surrounded by a venous plexus and distally joins a fascial sheath shared by the occipital nerve. The vessel is followed to its point of entrance into the muscular bed at the mastoid groove. In its transplanted course it lies at the base of the occipital and follows a straight path from the mastoid groove to the point of anastomosis. It is important to mobilize this vessel as far proximally as possible to obtain adequate length for the graft. Proximal dissection often permits the resection of the distal 1 to 2 cm of the graft, allowing one to use a larger component of the graft for the anastomosis.

A small unilateral suboccipital craniectomy is effected with a unilateral resection of the arch of C-1. The dura is then opened in a linear fashion and the margins sutured to adjacent tissue. The medullary loop with the posterior inferior cerebellar artery is identified as this vessel passes around the brainstem on its way to the vermis. A small rubber dam is then temporarily placed into this artery and the vessel elevated by suturing the superior end of the rubber dam to the margin of the bone and the inferior end of the dam to muscle or reflected dura. Miniature Mayfield clips or temporary Sugita clips are placed on either side of the area selected for arteriotomy. A small linear incision is made in the posterior inferior cerebellar artery with a broken razor blade on an appropriate holder. The arteriotomy is extended in both directions with small microscissors. The donor vessel (previously prepared for the anastomosis by resection of excess length, removing excessive soft tissue, and spatulating the end) is sewn to the apex of the arteriotomy with a double armed

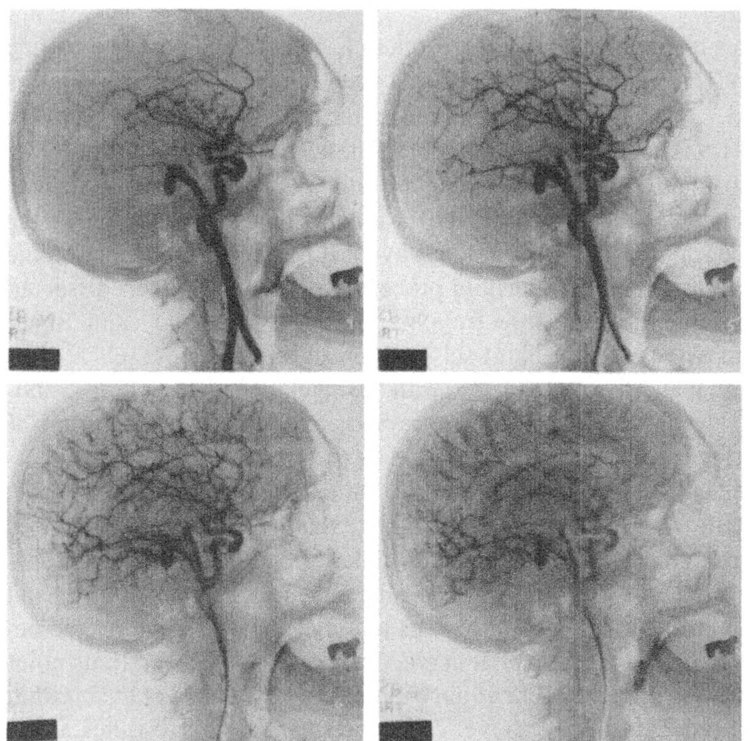

A

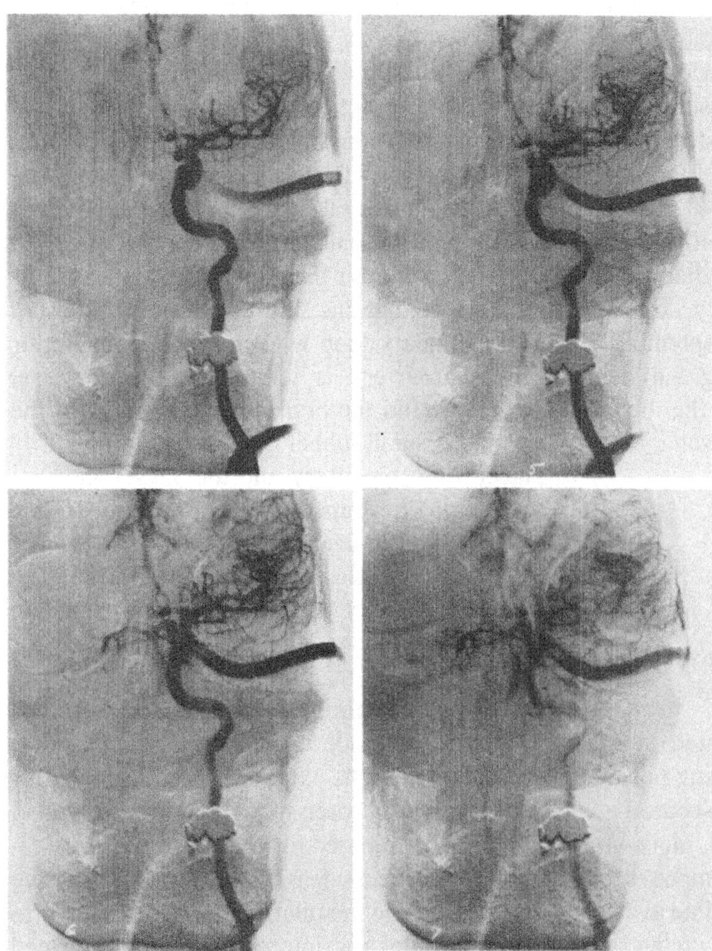

B

Figure 9.4. Postoperative series of angiograms, subtraction technique. **A.** Lateral view revealing good flow through the bypass graft, with retrograde filling of basilar artery to the point of its origin from junction of vertebral arteries. **B.** Anteroposterior projection indicating contour and shape of saphenous vein bypass graft. There is filling of the opposite posterior cerebral artery.

9-0 monofilament nylon suture. This initial suture is an important one and is placed in both vessels from the inside to the outside. The remaining portion of the vessel is then anastomosed in a routine fashion by techniques previously described. Interrupted sutures are used in most cases, but on occasion we have used a running suture. The 9-0 monofilament nylon suture is preferred to the 10-0 monofilament nylon suture because the wall of the occipital artery is thicker than that of the temporal artery and tends to bend the smaller needles provided for the 10-0 monofilament nylon suture. Flow is restored by removing the clips on the recipient artery initially and the clip on the donor vessel last. Small bleeding points, if they occur, usually cease within a few minutes with light pressure from an absorbable gelatinous sponge (Gelfoam). On occasion, however, it is necessary to place an additional suture if the bleeding does not terminate with light pressure. The temporary rubber dam is removed and the dura graft is then sewn into place. The dural closure is facilitated by a separate incision in the lateral wall of dura for the entrance of the artery into the subarachnoid space. Nevertheless, a completely watertight closure is not possible because of the necessity of allowing adequate room for the occipital artery as it passes through the dural opening. Accordingly, a very tight muscle closure is necessary which, in turn, is facilitated by retaining the muscular cuff in the transverse portion of the wound and taking the patient out of the "flex position." Sutures are left in place for two weeks. The transplanted occipital artery lies deep in the wound and follows the transverse course to the point of the anastomosis. However, it is still palpable posterior to the mastoid process.

Interposition Vein Graft—The External Carotid Artery-Posterior Cerebral Artery

A subtemporal approach (Fig. 9.6) is used to expose the posterior cerebral artery. We routinely use both mannitol and cerebral spinal fluid drainage to achieve good exposure of the posterior cerebral artery so that there is a very modest amount of brain retraction. The Yasargil self-retaining retractor is essential (one blade is sufficient). The inferior aspect of the temporal lobe is covered with one large square of Surgicel before the cottonoids are placed for the brain retractor. The Surgicel is left in place and has prevented small bleeding points from developing when the cottonoid is removed from the wound. This is particularly important as 4,000 to 5,000 units of heparin given just prior to posterior cerebral artery occlusion is not reversed. Heparin is given in an effort to prevent thrombus formation in the posterior cerebral artery during the period of stagnant flow and to impede the formation of thrombus in the vein graft when flow is restored. In one case, early in the series, before we used heparin routinely, thrombus formed in the vessel during a 20-minute occlusion time. Just prior to temporary occlusion of the posterior cerebral artery the patient is also given 250 mg of pentobarbital.

The posterior cerebral artery is dissected free from the arachnoid as it courses around the peduncle (the P-2 segment of the posterior cerebral artery). The P-1 segment of the vessel is not exposed, and it is not necessary to disturb the third nerve. There is no need to identify the posterior communicating artery, which in these cases is always very small. The portion of the vessel that is isolated for temporary occlusion has been referred to by Zeal and Rhoton[41] as the anterior half of the P-2 segment. It measures approximately 25 mm long. Fortunately, in most instances, long and short circumflex thalamo-perforating vessels arise either from the P-1 segment or from the portion of the P-2 segment very close to the posterior communicating artery, and it is possible to place the first temporary clip distal to these vessels. The hippocampal, peduncular perforating, and medial posterior choroidal artery are also seen to rise most commonly from the very anterior portion of this segment. The anterior temporal artery often arises in the field of occlusion, but bleeding from this vessel can be controlled readily with the self-retaining retractor. The posterior choroidal and posterior temporal branches arise distal to the site of the anastomosis. We have found considerable variation in the distribution of these branches along the segment that has been isolated for temporary ligation. Invariably, however, one is able to select a portion of the vessel about 1.5 cm in length free of perforating vessels which is suitable for receiving the anastomosis. The posterior cerebral artery at the point of the anastomosis has appeared to be

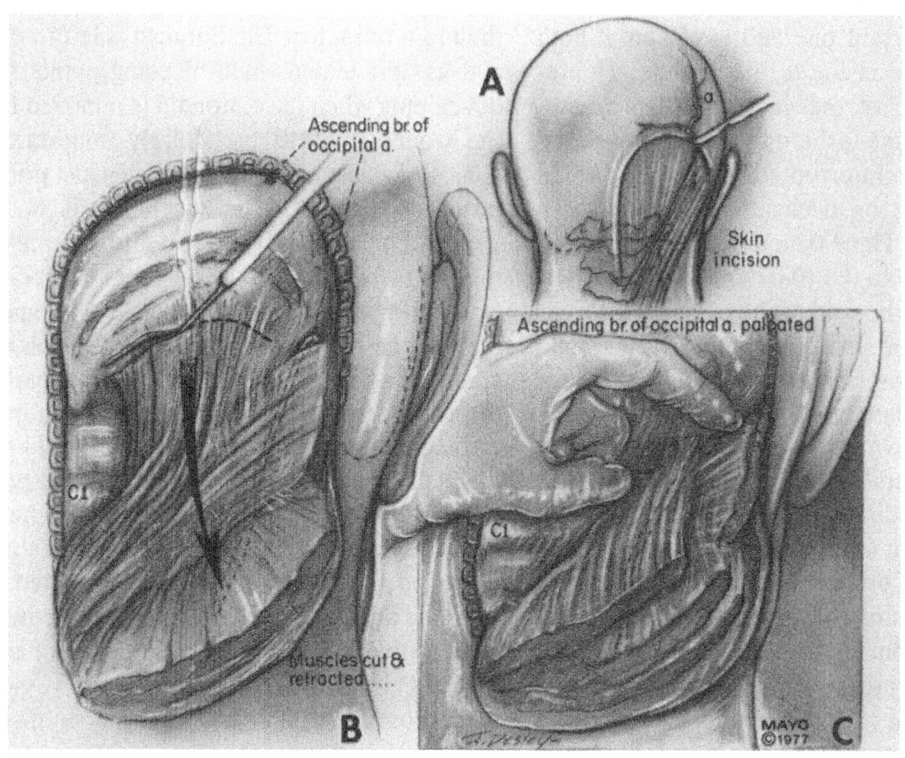
A
Ascending br. of occipital a.
Skin incision
Ascending br. of occipital a. palpated
C1
C1
Muscles cut & retracted
B
MAYO ©1977
C

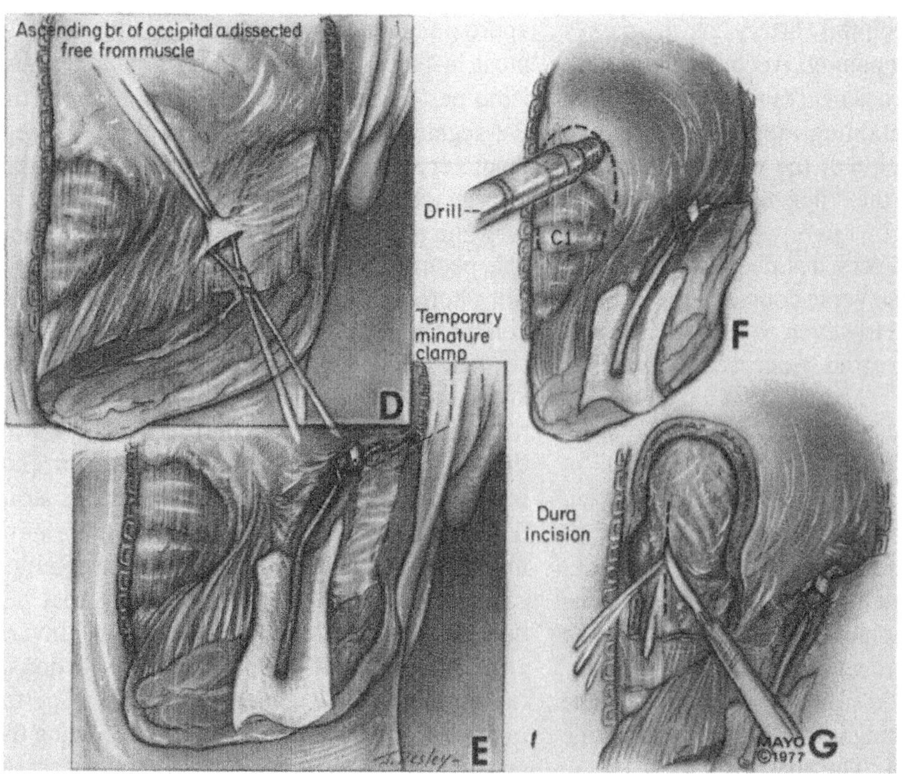
Ascending br. of occipital a. dissected free from muscle
Drill
C1
Temporary minature clamp
D
F
Dura incision
E
MAYO ©1977
G

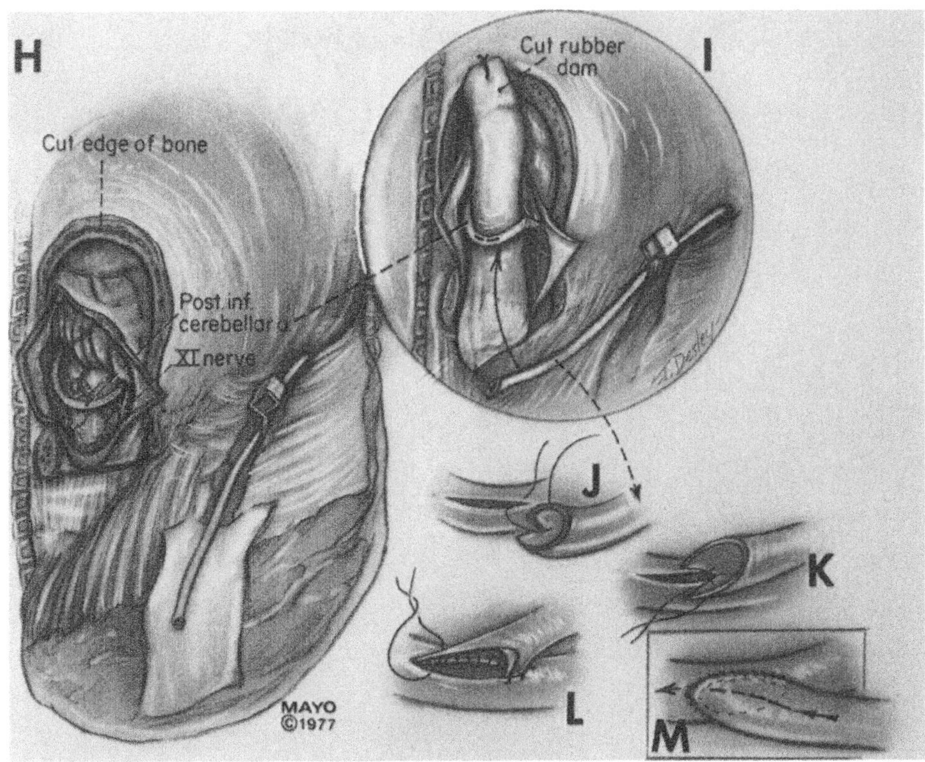

Figure 9.5. Sketch of surgery procedure. **A.** Hockey-stick skin incision is made extending above the level of superior nuchal line; **B,** deep neck muscles are cut from their insertion, leaving a cuff of tissue for closure; **C,** occipital artery is identified in the mastoid groove posterior and superior to mastoid process; **D,** occipital artery is dissected free from adjacent tissue; vessel lies deep to splenius capitis and longissimus capitis; dissection is simplified by maintaining this tissue plane; **E,** occipital artery is shown lying free in the muscle bed from which it was dissected; **F,** small unilateral suboccipital craniectomy is made, with unilateral resection of arch of C-1; **G,** dura is opened with straight incision; **H,** dura sutured to margins of craniectomy, and medullary loop of posterior inferior cerebellar artery (PICA) is identified; **I,** PICA is elevated by a temporary rubber dam; **J,** PICA is opened with a linear incision, and occipital artery is fish-mouthed; **K** and **L,** anastomosis is performed with interrupted 9-0 monofilament nylon sutures; **M,** completed anastomosis; **N,** transplanted course of occipital artery.

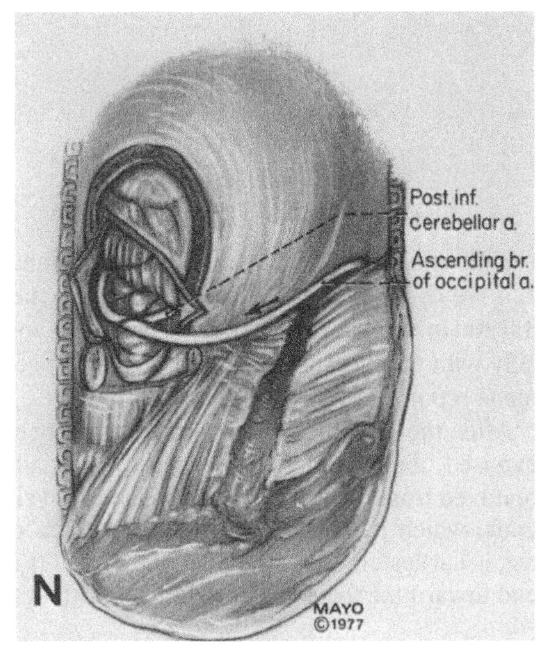

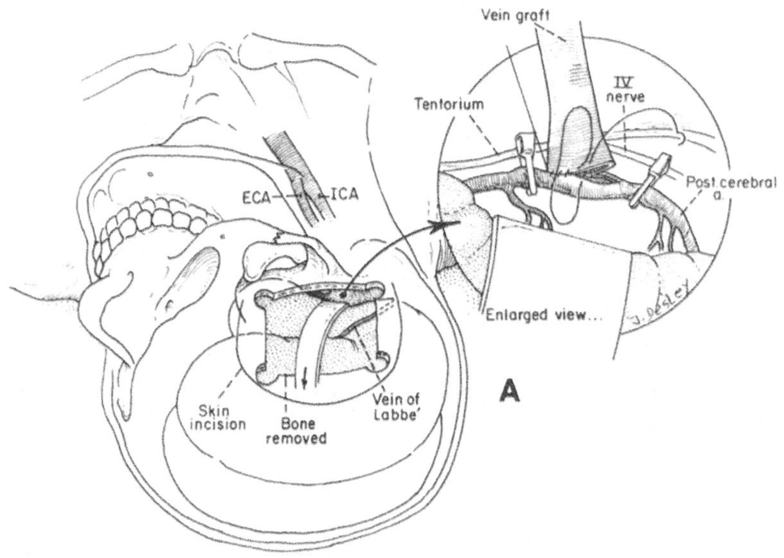

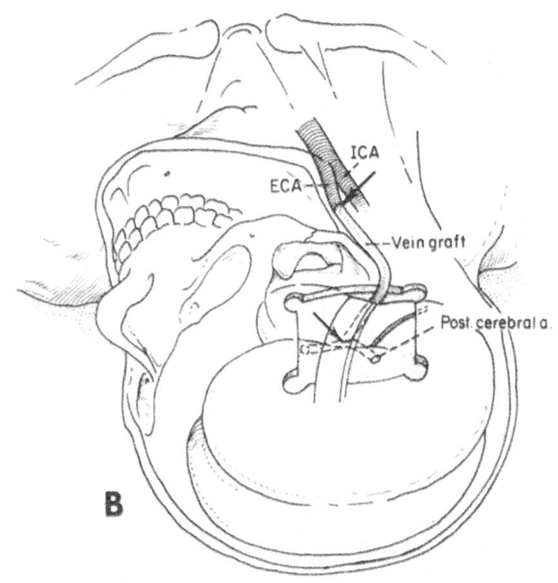

Figure 9.6. Operative sketches of the subtemporal approach currently used for exposure of the posterior cerebral artery for bypass grafting. This approach minimizes brain retraction and yet provides an adequate space for suture manipulation with a single blade of the self-retaining retractor. **B.** Diagram of the vein following completion of the proximal and distal anastomoses. The tunnel for the vein passes from the medial aspect of the temporalis muscle to the subgaleal space over the zygoma through subcutaneous tissue anterior to the ear, and then through a fascial plane deep to the parotid gland to join the external carotid artery (ECA) at the level of the digastric muscle. ICA = internal carotid artery.

slightly smaller than a middle cerebral trunk, and we estimate that the diameter approaches 3.0 mm in most instances. This compares favorably with the measured diameter in fixed specimens reported by Zeal and Rhoton.[41]

After the posterior cerebral artery has been exposed, the self-retaining retractor is partially removed from the wound, and a saphenous vein graft, which has been exposed in the thigh or leg, is harvested. The distal end of the graft (the end toward the foot) is secured firmly with ligature to a Shiley vein distender. Ice-cold heparinized saline is used to distend the graft and to identify bleeding points. With the use of a Shiley catheter having a 200-mm bulb, overdistention of the graft is prevented. This is important for if the graft is distended under too much pressure, small hemorrhages will develop in the wall of the vein, promoting thrombosis and graft failure.

A tunnel for the graft is created between the medial inferior surface of the temporalis muscle and the external carotid artery in the neck. This tunnel for the graft crosses the zygoma anterior to the ear and then follows a fascial plane deep to the parotid gland. It enters the neck at the apex of the cervical incision, which has been used to expose the external carotid artery. A thoracotomy tube is brought through this tunnel and through an opening in the temporalis muscle created just above the zygoma in such a fashion that the vein will not kink as it crosses the zygoma. The vein is then brought through the lumen of the thoractomy tube and the thoractomy tube removed. In this manner twisting and kinking of the vein is avoided. The vein is now distended with a temporary Sugita clip placed on the distal end of the vein, the end destined for anastomosis with the posterior cerebral artery. Throughout the remaining portion of the anastomotic procedure the vein is intermittently irrigated with heparinized saline through the Shiley distender. The free length of the vein graft approximates 20 to 25 cm. The distal segment of the graft is allowed to remain redundant in the middle fossa as this facilitates the placement of the vein in various positions during the intracranial anastomosis. This is an important point as it enables the surgeon to work relatively free from obstruction created by the vein itself. Cottonballs work well to pack the vein into the anterior middle fossa during the initial part of the anastomosis. Before the vein is placed in the depths of the wound for the anastomosis, its end is repaired by making a horizontal cut across the vessel proximal to the site of the temporary clamping. Depending on the size of the vein, it may either be spatulated or cut on an oblique angle. The distended saphenous vein in most instances approximates 7 mm in diameter at the site of the anastomosis.

The self-retraining retractor is then replaced, and the posterior cerebral artery temporarily occluded after barbiturates and heparin have been administered. Sugita clips are useful for this temporary occlusion. The vessel is then opened with a broken razor blade secured in a micro-holder. On occasion it has been necessary to extend the suture line with microscissors. The apex suture is placed and 7-0 prolene suture or 8-0 prolene suture cut to a length of approximately 3 cm. The final tie in the suture line is completed between the cut stump end of the first knot and the free end of the running suture so that an adequate amount of suture should be left on the knot for this final tie. We have routinely closed the medial side initially and then reversed direction of the sutures at the opposite apex of the arteriotomy using a single backhanded suture. The distal temporary clip is removed first and then the proximal temporary clip on the posterior cerebral artery is removed. There is no back bleeding out of the vein graft because of the valves. At this point the graft is thoroughly irrigated (as it has been intermittently during the procedure up to this point to prevent the entrapment of air in the lumen of the vein). The graft is then withdrawn further into the neck so that the appropriate length of the graft in the middle fossa can be measured and contoured to the shape of the middle fossa.

The external carotid artery is then doubly ligated distally and divided for the end-to-end anastomosis or if an end-to-side anastomosis is preferred, it is only temporarily ligated distally with a vessel loop. The proximal external carotid artery can easily be occluded with a McFadden clip or a small vascular clamp. The end-to-end technique employs approximately 14 interrupted 5-0 prolene sutures. The end-to-side technique uses a running 5-0 prolene suture. For the end-to-end anastomosis the vein graft is fish-mouthed; for the end-to-side anastomosis, the vein is cut on an oblique and spatulated. It is not necessary to isolate the common or internal carotid arteries for this anastomosis. It is, however, necessary to dissect the external carotid artery as far distally as possible to give adequate length to that vessel for the rotations that will be required for the placement of interrupted sutures in the end-to-end anastomosis. With greater experience in this operative procedure, we have preferred the end-to-side anastomosis of the vein to the external carotid artery and commonly use a long arteriotomy in the external carotid artery approximating 15 mm.

Subdural hygromas are such a frequent complication of this procedure that we now routinely take precautions to treat this potential complication during the initial procedure. An atrial catheter is positioned in the inferior portion of the superior vena cava using ECG localization. This catheter is threaded through the resected stump of the common facial vein in the neck and threaded through the jugular vein. It is then connected through a low-pressure Hakim valve in a tunnel posterior to the ear through a Hakim ventricular catheter placed in the subdural space.

The wounds are then closed using a dural graft. Although the author commonly uses a subgaleal drain for aneurysm cases, it is not used in this procedure as it tends to promote the development of a subgaleal hygroma.

Operative Results

Occipital to Posterior Inferior Cerebellar Artery Bypass

In the 20 patients who were disabled there were two deaths within two months from the date of the operative procedure. In both cases death resulted from a failure to provide adequate flow through the graft. In one case the graft occluded and in another the graft simply could not carry the amount of flow demanded. The remaining 18 patients were improved from the operative procedure and virtually all resumed an ambulatory status, with 10 patients having an excellent result (meaning normal function) and eight patients achieving a self-care status with no major fixed deficit other than ataxia. In the 19 patients not disabled prior to surgery, there were no deaths, but there were four occlusions probably related to an insufficient gradient across the site of the anastomosis, implying that retrospectively the operation was ill-advised. There were 15 excellent results with the patients returning to normal employment. There was no morbidity and no mortality. The four patients in whom the grafts occluded were unchanged following the surgery.

Interposition Vein Grafts

In this group 32 patients were operated on. There were 18 excellent results with patients resuming normal activities without a focal neurologic deficit and six good results in patients achieving a vast improvement in clinical symptomatology but without the resumption of normal employment or activities. One patient remained unchanged from his condition prior to surgery, with continued TIA (graft occluded). Two patients had a poor result and there were five deaths. In these seven cases of poor results or death, four were attributable to progressing strokes not altered by the operative procedure and three to graft occlusions.

Analysis of Complications

Occipital Artery to Posterior Inferior Cerebellar Artery Bypass

Our primary problems in connection with this operative procedure were related to the marginal neurologic status of these patients before surgery. Respiratory complications were frequent and usually resulted from previously impaired cranial nerve function that made swallowing and handling of secretions difficult. Accordingly, we have followed the practice of leaving a nasotracheal tube in place in all patients in whom the preoperative neurologic examination has revealed impairment in ninth and tenth nerve function.

Surgery with patients in the sitting position carries with it the potential risk of air emboli, hypotension, and convexity subdural hygromas or air. We feel, however, that these risks are well justified from the advantages achieved by this position. All patients should receive adequate blood volume replacement on a unit-for-unit basis. This helps to prevent air emboli by maintaining a high venous pressure and also avoids hypotension. These patients have areas in the brain in which autoregulation is no longer preserved and they are extraordinarily vulnerable to fluctuations in perfusion pressure and cardiac output. Accordingly, it is imperative to maintain an adequate perfusion pressure throughout the operation.

Complications such as epidural hematoma and aseptic meningitis related to blood in the subarachnoid space are not unique to this type of procedure and can be prevented with appropriate measures.

Interposition Vein Grafts

Many of the complications in this procedure have also been related to the patient's marginal preoperative neurologic function. However, there were two major types of technical complications in the series: graft occlusion and subdural hygroma. Causes for graft occlusion appeared to be related to atherosclerosis in the recipient vessel, with damage to atherosclerotic plaque from temporary clips, distal occlusions in the posterior cerebral arteries during the period of temporary occlusion (manifested by virtually no back flow from those vessels following release of the occluding clips), and technical or surgical errors in the suture lines or in procuring the saphenous vein graft. Although one cannot minimize the contribution that surgical errors or technical difficulties will make in an operation of this magnitude, we were impressed that the particular cases in which the graft became occluded were not clearly related to technical difficulties in either the proximal or distal anastomosis. One occlusion may have been attributable to overdistention of the graft in its period of preparation, as the graft became hard and difficult to palpate a freely pulsatile pulse for several days before it became occluded on the Doppler flow probe. We have concluded that intraoperative heparinization is a risk that must be accepted in these cases as it appears that the posterior cerebral artery is more likely to undergo spontaneous thrombosis with stagnant flow than is a branch of the middle cerebral artery during temporal artery to middle cerebral artery bypass grafting. We have never failed to have a back flow out of one of these vessels in the middle cerebral artery distribution during a period of 20 to even 45 minutes of temporary occlusion. It is quite possible that the reaction to ischemia in larger vessels is more sensitive than that in the smaller artery, and for this reason we strongly believe that intraoperative heparinization is necessary without reversal.

Subdural hygromas have been such a frequent complication in this series that we now routinely place a subdural atrial shunt at the time of the operation. The cause for the development of a subdural hygroma is not apparent but curiously in one patient who had both a subdural hygroma and a late graft occlusion, the subdural hygroma resolved following the late graft occlusion. We believe that the combination of a pulsating graft through a small opening in the arachnoid at the base of the brain in the area of spinal fluid flow along with a preexisting degree of cerebral atrophy predisposed these patients to this complication. Subdural hygromas are one of our most common complications after temporal artery to middle cerebral artery bypass procedures, but symptomatic subdural hygromas in this group are found in only 2% to 3% of surgically treated patients. In the group of patients with interposition vein grafts this frequency approaches 50%. In two cases the subdural hygromas became acutely symptomatic, producing a profound increase in intracranial pressure and occluding the vein graft.

A homonymous hemianopsia is a complication that one might expect to find not infrequently in this group of patients. It has proved to be relatively uncommon. Two patients had transient field defects that persisted for approximately 24 hours, and one patient with a patent graft had a permanent homonymous field defect. This latter patient did not have evidence of a venous infarction on angiography of CT scanning. Drake[10a] has previously commented on the collateral flow to the distal posterior cerebral artery.

We have had one venous infarction with an associated intracerebral hematoma in the series which required reoperation and removal of the hematoma. Four patients had isolated small hematomas in the temporal lobe which did not require surgery.

Indications for Angiography and Surgical Intervention

The patients on whom we have operated to date are either suffering from a progressing neurologic deficit or have been disabled by the frequency and severity of transient ischemic events. These are not individuals who have sustained only one or two TIAs. Patients accepted for occipital to posterior inferior cerebellar artery (PICA) bypass procedures have had either bilateral intracranial vertebral artery occlusions proximal to the origins of the PICAs or unilateral vertebral artery occlusion in tandem with a high-grade intracranial stenosis of the opposite vertebral artery. Patients accepted for interposition vein grafts between the external carotid artery and the proximal posterior cerebral artery have had a high-grade stenosis of the basilar artery or a total occlusion of that vessle. In these patients the posterior communicating arteries are invariably absent or very small so that there has been no collateral flow from the carotid system to the basilar system.

Presenting complaints have included ataxia, visual disturbances, altered mentation, and changes in sensorium with erect posture. Some patients had progressing strokes in the brainstem or cerebellum. Others had multiple TIAs not altered by anticoagulant therapy. Not one patient evaluated had only one or two TIAs of the posterior circulation. In our experience, angiograms in these patients are often normal or show only minimal large vessel disease.

Other Operative Procedures for Posterior Circulation Ischemia

The variety of atherosclerotic lesions in the posterior circulation and the unique characteristics of the frequently anomalous vasculature have made it necessary that a variety of approaches be developed for the surgical management of these cases. Although major ischemic symptomatology in the posterior circulation, as indicated above, is usually related to intracranial large vessel disease, there is a role for vertebral artery transposition procedures at the origin of the vertebral artery with rotation of the vertebral artery and anastomosis of that vessel to the common carotid artery. Similarly, interposition vein grafts between the common carotid artery and the vertebral artery have been employed as well as on-lay patch grafts of vertebral artery stenotic lesions.

We have performed intracranial vertebral endarterectomies and believe that this procedure has a definite role in selected patients who have a high-grade stenosis of the vertebral artery near the point where the vertebral artery pierces the dura to enter the posterior fossa.

Intraluminal angioplasty[35] has a role in the management of very focal stenotic lesions of the basilar artery, but it is a procedure that carries with it considerable risk and should only be used, in our judgment, if one of the other procedures cannot be employed for one reason or another. We have had two excellent results with this operation but have had three deaths.

In our experience the use of the superficial temporal artery as a pedicle donor for a bypass procedure to the posterior cerebral or superior cerebellar artery has been unsuccessful. There were seven cases operated on in this group, but only two of the seven patients maintained a good flow through the bypass graft. Typically, a good pulse was palpable over the site of entry of the vessel into the middle fossa for the first several days following the operation and then, thereafter, the pulse progressively diminished. Postoperative angiography would demonstrate patency of the graft but very little flow through the anastomosis.

Intracranial transposition procedures—side-to-side anastomosis between the posterior cerebral artery and the superior cerebellar artery—is an operative procedure that is indicated in patients who have a fetal type of circulation and a proximal lesion in the basilar or vertebral artery.[31] In the five cases operated to date there has been no morbidity and no mortality. In our experience this is perhaps the best type of bypass graft available to us. The indications for this procedure are limited but the results have been excellent.

References

1. Astrup J, Siesjö BK, Symon L: Thresholds in cerebral ischemia: the ischemic penumbra. Stroke 12:723–725, 1981
2. Astrup J, Symon L, Branston NM, et al: Cortical evoked potential and extracellular K^+ and H^+ at critical levels of brain ischemia. Stroke 8:51–57, 1977
3. Ausman JI, Lee MC, Klassen AC, et al: Stroke: what's new? Cerebral revascularization. Minn Med 59:223–227, 1976
4. Boysen G: Cerebral hemodynamics in carotid surgery. Acta Neurol Scand (Suppl) 52:1–84, 1970
5. Branston NM, Strong AJ, Symon L: Extracellular potassium activity, evoked potential and tissue blood flow: relationship during progressive ischaemia in baboon cerebral cortex. J Neurol Sci 32:305–321, 1977
6. Caplan LR, Rosenbaum AE: Role of cerebral angiography in vertebrobasilar occlusive disease. J Neurol Neurosurg Psychiatry 38:601–612, 1975
7. Caplan LR, Sergay S: Positional cerebral ischaemia. J Neurol Neurosurg Psychiatry 39:385–391, 1976
8. Cartlidge NEF, Whisnant JP, Elveback LR: Carotid and vertebral-basilar transient cerebral

ischemic attacks: a community study, Rochester, Minnesota. Mayo Clin Proc 52:117–120, 1977

9. Castaigne P, Lhermitte F, Gautier JC, et al: Arterial occlusions in the vertebrobasilar system. A study of 44 patients with post-mortem data. Brain 96:133–154, 1973
10. Crowel RM, Olsson Y, Klatzo I, et al: Temporary occlusion of the middle cerebral artery in the monkey: clinical and pathological observations. Stroke 1:439–448, 1970

10a. Drake CG: Giant intracranial aneurysms: experience with surgical treatment in 174 patients. Clin Neurosurg 26:12–95, 1979

11. Fisher CM: The arterial lesions underlying lacunes. Acta Neuropathol (Berl) 12:1–15, 1969
12. Fisher CM: Occlusion of the vertebral arteries: causing transient basilar symptoms. Arch Neurol 22:13–19, 1970
13. Fisher CM: Clinical syndromes in cerebral thrombosis, hypertensive hemorrhage, and ruptured saccular aneurysm. Clin Neurosurg 22:117–147, 1975
14. Fisher CM, Caplan LR: Basilar artery branch occlusion: a cause of pontine infarction. Neurology (Minneap) 21:900–905, 1971
15. Fisher CM, Gore I, Okabe N, et al: Atherosclerosis of the carotid and vertebral arteries—extracranial and intracranial. J Neuropathol Exp Neurol 24:455–476, 1965
16. Fisher CM, Karnes WE, Kubik CS: Lateral medullary infarction—the pattern of vascular occlusion. J Neuropathol Exp Neurol 20:323–379, 1961
17. Hanson EJ Jr, Anderson RE, Sundt TM Jr: Comparison of ^{85}krypton and ^{133}xenon cerebral blood flow measurements before, during, and following focal, incomplete ischemia in the squirrel monkey. Circ Res 36:18–26, 1975
18. Houser OW, Sundt TM Jr, Holman CB, et al: Atheromatous disease of the carotid artery: correlation of angiographic, clinical and surgical findings. J Neurosurg 41:321–331, 1974
19. Kety SS, Schmidt CF: The nitrous oxide method for the quantitative determination of cerebral blood flow in man: theory, procedure and normal values. J Clin Invest 27:476–483, 1948
20. Khodadad G: Occipital artery-posterior inferior cerebellar artery anastomosis. Surg Neurol 5:225–227, 1976
21. Khodadad G, Singh RS, Olinger CP: Possible prevention of brain stem stroke by microvascular anastomosis in the vertebrobasilar system. Stroke 8:316–321, 1977
22. Lhermitte F, Gautier JC, Derouesne C: Nature of occlusions of the middle cerebral artery. Neurology (Minneap) 20:82–88, 1970
23. Marshall J: The natural history of transient ischaemic cerebrovascular attacks. Q J Med 33:309–324, 1964
24. Reichman OH: Extracranial-intracranial arterial anastomosis, In Whisnant JP, Sandok BA (eds.): Cerebral Vascular Diseases: Ninth Conference. Grune and Stratton, New York, 1975
25. Schmiedek P, Gratzl O, Spetzler R, et al: Selection of patients for extra-intracranial artery bypass surgery based on rCBF measurements. J Neurosurg 44:303–312, 1976
26. Spetzler R, Chater N: Microvascular bypass surgery. Part 2: Physiological studies. J Neurosurg 45:508–513, 1976
27. Stein BM, McCormick W, Rodriguez JN, et al: Incidence and significance of occlusive vascular disease of the extracranial arteries as demonstrated by post-mortem angiography. Trans Am Neurol Assoc 86:60–66, 1961
28. Sundt TM Jr, Grant WC, Garcia JH: Restoration of middle cerebral artery flow in experimental infarction. J Neurosurg 31:311–322, 1969
29. Sundt TM Jr, Michenfelder JD: Focal transient cerebral ischemia in the squirrel monkey: effect on brain adenosine triphosphate and lactate levels with electrocorticographic and pathologic correlation. Circ Res 30:703–712, 1972
30. Sundt TM Jr, Piepgras DG: Occipital to posterior inferior cerebellar artery bypass surgery. J Neurosurg 48:916–928, 1978
31. Sundt TM Jr, Piepgras DG, Houser OW: Interposition saphenous vein grafts for advanced occlusive disease and large aneurysms in the posterior circulation. J Neurosurg 56:205–215, 1982
32. Sundt TM Jr, Sharbrough FW, Anderson R, et al: Cerebral blood flow measurements and electroencephalograms during carotid endarterectomy. J Neurosurg 41:310–320, 1974
33. Sundt TM Jr, Sharbrough FW, Piepgras DG, et al: Correlation of cerebral blood flow and electroencephalographic changes during carotid endarterectomy. Mayo Clin Proc 56:533–543, 1981
34. Sundt TM Jr, Siekert RG, Piepgras DG, et al: Bypass surgery for vascular disease of the carotid system. Mayo Clin Proc 51:677–692, 1976
35. Sundt TM Jr, Smith HC, Campbell JK: Transluminal angioplasty for basilar artery stenosis. Mayo Clin Proc 55:673–680, 1980
36. Sundt TM Jr, Whisnant JP, Piepgras DG, et al: Intracranial bypass grafts for vertebral-basilar ischemia. Mayo Clin Proc 53:12–18, 1978
37. Tew JM Jr: Reconstructive intracranial vascular surgery for prevention of stroke. Clin Neurosurg 22:264–280, 1975
38. Waltz AG, Sundt TM Jr: The microvasculature and microcirculation of the cerebral cortex after arterial occlusion. Brain 90:681–696, 1967

39. Yasargil MG: Diagnosis and indications for operations in cerebrovascular occlusive disease. In Yasargil MG (ed.): *Microsurgery Applied to Neurosurgery*. Theime Verlag, Stuttgart, 1969
40. Yasargil MG, Krayenbuhl HA, Jacobson JH II: Microneurosurgical arterial reconstruction. Surgery 67:221–233, 1970
41. Zeal AA, Rhoton AL Jr: Microsurgical anatomy of the posterior cerebral artery. J. Neurosurg 48: 534–559, 1978

10

The Use of Tissue Adhesives in Cerebrovascular Surgery

Hajime Handa, Sen Yamagata, and Waro Taki

Introduction

Since the application of plastic adhesives in medical therapy, several synthetic materials have been used in cerebrovascular surgery for coating and reinforcing intracranial aneurysms; embolizing arteriovenous malformations (AVM), carotid-cavernous fistulas (CCF), or intracranial aneurysms; and adhesive in experimental microvascular repair and anastomosis, etc. However, there are several precautions necessary and problems to be resolved in the clinical use of these materials. Clinical application is still controversial because long-term follow-up results are lacking as are detailed investigations of toxicity. In this chapter the experimental results and clinical use of plastic adhesives to date are reviewed, and current concepts of the therapeutic use of plastic adhesives in cerebrovascular disease are summarized.

General Conception of the Characteristics and Toxicity of Cyanoacrylate Adhesives

The plastic adhesive that has been commonly used in surgical procedures is cyanoacrylate monomer or its mixture (Fig. 10.1). There are several kinds of cyanoacrylate monomers, depending on the alkyl group of the side chain. These monomers are watery substances that are solidified by anionic polymerization under moisture or base. At that time strong adherence with living tissue occurs, although the mechanism of adherence to the living tissue surface is not well understood. In general, these cyanoacrylate adhesives, which are employed in surgery, contain additives like plasticizers, thickening agents, inhibitors, and others for the purpose of easy management and adjustment for each surgical use.

Methyl 2-Cyanoacrylate

This material, commonly called Eastman 910, contains methyl 2-cyanoacrylate monomer and plasticizer, thickening agent, and an inhibitor. It was the first material in the cyanoacrylate derivatives introduced as plastic adhesive in surgery.[10,55] However, the toxic effect of this adhesive to the neural tissue and blood vessel was reported by several investigators.* Among them, Tsuchiya et al[79] reported gliosis, cellular infiltration and neural death of the cortex when this adhesive was applied to the pia-arachnoid above the cerebral cortex. Regarding the reaction of large peripheral blood vessel to this adhesive, they also described various degrees of destruction of the adventitia and muscular

* References 24, 28, 36, 45, 79, 81, 85, 88.

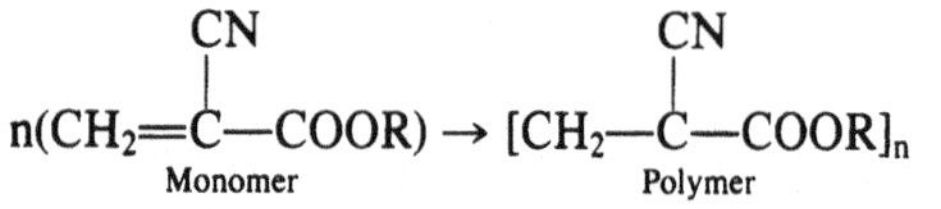

$$n(CH_2{=}\overset{\displaystyle CN}{\overset{|}{C}}{-}COOR) \rightarrow [CH_2{-}\overset{\displaystyle CN}{\overset{|}{C}}{-}COOR]_n$$

Monomer Polymer

Figure 10.1 Chemical structure of alkyl 2-cyanoacrylate. R represents alkyl grouping.

layer. Likewise, using canine arteries, Weissberg et al[28,36,81] observed necrosis of the arterial wall resulting in fusiform dilatation angiographically within 10 days after application and subsequent replacement of the necrotic areas by fibrous tissue. Concerning the marked histotoxicity and rapid fragmentation of this adhesive, Woodward et al[85] suggested that a high wetting capacity (i.e., susceptibility to enzymatic hydrolysis) of methyl 2-cyanoacrylate polymer may cause physicochemical changes resulting in the release of toxic substances and rapid dispersal of this polymer. In their studies they also reported that in comparing hexyl and decyl cyanoacrylates with methyl 2-cyanoacrylate, there was no difference in strength of adhesiveness between the three and that the heat of polymerization was less in the higher homologues of cyanoacrylates which were related to the speed of polymerization rate and regulated by the degree of monomer purity.

Ethyl 2-Cyanoacrylate

Another commonly used cyanoacrylate adhesive is ethyl 2-cyanoacrylate, known as Aron Alpha A Sankyo, which has been investigated in the middle 1960s. Since this adhesive has demonstrated less histotoxicity than methyl 2-cyanoacrylate,[12,39,90] it has been used for various surgical procedures such as closure of skin incisions, adhesion of blood vessels, repair of skull or dural defect, and coating of intracranial aneurysm. Yodh and Wright[90] reported that the ethyl 2-cyanoacrylate was far superior to methyl 2-cyanoacrylate as an aneurysm-coating agent. Likewise, Chou et al[12] reported that cats did not develop any neurologic deficit in the three-year follow-up period after the application of this adhesive to one cerebral hemisphere, and that histologically only minor changes in the brain were observed with preservation of cerebral cytoarchitecture and of the leptomeningeal vessel. Minimal reaction to the blood vessel was also noted by Ohta et al[56] and others.[34,68,73] On the other hand, there have been reports describing the toxicity of this adhesive and complications after the use of this material probably due to old ethyl 2-cyanoacrylate[13] or ethyl 2-cyanoacrylate produced by different manufacturers[19]

Isobutyl 2-Cyanoacrylate

Since this adhesive was introduced in the middle 1960s, like other cyanoacrylates it has been investigated mainly as an adhesive for vascular reconstruction.[7,47a,50,70,80] In addition this material has been recently employed as an embolizing agent because of low viscosity, instant polymerization on contact with blood, and less toxicity.[22,41] At the same time, the histotoxicity of this material injected into the blood vessel has been investigated. Zanetti and Sherman[92] found that only about 15% of the intra-arterial cyanoacrylate casted was in actual contact with the vessel endothelium. Moreover, they noted that the tissue reaction of isobutyl cyanoacrylate was mild, limited to loss of intima, and with minimal changes of the media up to three months following injection. These findings were also observed by other investigators in dogs and in humans when this kind of cyanoacrylate was used for the visceral, renal, and peripheral vessel occlusive therapy.[25,29,54,69] On the contrary, White et al[83] reported a marked response to intra-arterial isobutyl 2-cyanoacrylate in the embolization of celiac circulation of pigs. They observed chronic inflammation, foreign body giant-cell reaction, and focal disruption of internal elastic lamella in the section of medium-sized artery four to five months after embolization. In a recent study Vinster et at[79a] examined the pathology of the human AVM resected after embolization with cyanoacrylate. They observed a variable but focally chronic inflammatory reaction within the walls of the embolized AVM channels and no foreign-body giant cells in the parenchyma; they concluded that the reaction did not appear to be as profound as that reported by White et al.[83] Moreover, they based their conclusion on the clinical results of the patients, and there was no reason to believe that embolic material had lodged in vessels outside the AVM to cause significant cerebral infarcts, although silent small infarcts might have occurred without clinical sequelae.

Other Kinds of Cyanoacrylates

Since the report by Woodward et al,[85] which indicated that the histotoxicity was less in the higher homologues of cyanoacrylates, comparative studies on the histotoxicity of several kinds of cyanoacrylates in brain tissue and blood vessels have been conducted.[30,47] Lehman et al[47] compared five kinds of cyanoacrylates (methyl, ethyl, *n*-propyl, *n*-octyl, and isobutyl cyanoacrylate) to evaluate neural and vascular damage. Although a large amount of cyanoacrylate was employed in their studies, definite neural toxicity was found in all of the cyanoacrylates tested, and the relative toxicity was observed to be in the order of alkyl side chain length. Of these, only the *n*-octyl compound was found to be sufficiently nontoxic to warrant consideration in cerebrovascular surgery.

EDH-Adhesive (Biobond)

This plastic adhesive was introduced by Handa et al[32,57] as a coating material of intracranial aneurysm in 1960. Although methyl 2-cyanoacrylate has an excellent property of tissue adhesiveness, it has some disadvantages as a coating material such as less flexibility and rapid dispersal of its polymer. In order to overcome these shortcomings, synthetic rubber was blended in methyl 2-cyanoacrylate so that more flexibility and elasticity could be obtained. Moreover, polyisocyanate was added to increase the duration of the effect on brain tissue reaction. Handa et al[33] showed that there was little reaction between the film of this material and cerebral surface of dogs when the dura was closed completely after application, although infiltration of round cells, polynuclear lymphocytes, and fibroblast were observed in the subarachnoid space. Likewise, they described minimal reaction to the blood vessels, showing little proliferation of the adventitia and no damage of the media and intima after application to the dog's arteries. Concerning these minimal tissue reactions of EDH-adhesive compared with methyl 2-cyanoacrylate, they theorized that it was explained by the chemical bond between methyl 2-cyanoacrylate and nitrile rubber which was bridged by polyisocyanate; if free radicals of methyl 2-cyanoacrylate such as the CN-radical are responsible for the severe tissue reaction, they are bound with nitrile rubber and thus less toxic. Even if methyl 2-cyanoacrylate itself is responsible, only a small amount comes in contact with tissue because of a large amount of nitrile rubber. The superiority of this adhesive was also noted by other investigators.[46,72] In comparative studies of the histotoxicity of methyl 2-cyanoacrylate, silicon rubber, polyvinyl polyvinyledene chloride, EDH-adhesive, and epoxy polyamide resin, Handa et al,[33] and Tsuchiya et al[79] reported the least reaction, with EDH-adhesive showing no evidence of inflammation or cellular infiltration in the cortex or blood vessels 30 days to two to three months after application on the brain surface or the vessel wall of dogs and rabbits.

Treatment of Aneurysm with Plastic Adhesive

Although clipping and ligation of the neck of intracranial aneurysms is the ideal procedure in surgical treatment, it can not be performed in all cases because of large size, fusiform configuration of aneurysm, or inaccessibility to the neck. Among several alternative methods, one is a technique of coating and reinforcement of aneurysms (Table 10.1). This technique was first introduced by Dott[21] in 1933, who employed wrapping with muscle tissue to initiate subsequent fibrotic change. Since then, several kinds of synthetic agents had been studied for coating aneurysms such as latex,[84] polymethyl-methacrylate,[23,38] vinylchloride-vinylidenedichloride copolymer,[65] and silicone rubber.[77] Along with these materials, methyl 2-cyanoacrylate was also investigated in the early 1960s.

In 1960 Handa et al[32] designed a more suitable coating agent, EDH-adhesive, by combining methyl 2-cyanoacrylate with nitrile rubber and isocyanate to increase the flexibility and elasticity without losing the excellent adhesiveness of cyanoacrylate. This adhesive is just like glue and can be painted with a spatula in thick layers, becoming hard in five to ten minutes.

Table 10.1. Plastic adhesive for the treatment of aneurysm (I) coating material.

	Plastic adhesive	Evaluation*
Dutton et al[23] Hunter et al[38]	Polymethyl-methacrylate	Good
Selverstone & Ronis[65]	Vinylchloride-vinylidenedichloride copolymer	Poor
Handa et al[32]	EDH-adhesive (Methyl 2-cyanoacrylate + nitrile rubber + isocyanate)	Excellent
Carton et al[8] Messor et al[53]	Methyl 2-cyanoacrylate (Eastman 910)	Poor
Todd & Crue[77]	Silicon rubber	Good
Yodh & Wright[90] Chou et al[12]	Ethyl 2-cyanoacrylate (Aron Alpha)	Excellent
Yashon et al[89]	Isobutyl 2-cyanoacrylate	Good

* Evaluation is based on the examination performed by Handa et al.[33]

Employing this adhesive in 42 cases with aneurysm, Handa et al[33] reported excellent results, with no rebleeding except in one case of recurrent hemorrhage which occurred from the incompletely coated fundus of the aneurysm. This material is still in routine use in our clinic and has so far been employed to coat and reinforce aneurysms in more than 300 cases without serious complications. The superiority of this adhesive was also supported by other investigators. Follow-up results after coating aneurysms using this material was reported by Stowsad and Buhl.[71] They showed no recurrent bleeding in 10 cases that were followed up for three to eight years, although one patient died of rebleeding because of the incomplete coating.

On the other hand, Carton et al[8] used only methyl 2-cyanoacrylate in humans intracranially to repair a hole at the site of an aneurysm in 1962. It was also employed in coating aneurysms by Messer et al[53] and others.[9] However, subsequent investigations revealed the severe histotoxicity of this material. Coe et al[14] reported one clinical case where thrombosis of the aneurysm and middle cerebral artery occurred after wrapping a fusiform giant aneurysm using autogenous fascia and this adhesive, although they did not link this adhesive to the outcome. Moreover, another case where an aneurysm coated with this material ruptured three days after operation was reported by Sachs et al.[60] A more detailed description of the physical and chemical properties of various coating materials mentioned above is found in the monograph by Handa and his associates.[33]

Since the middle 1960s, another coating agent, ethyl 2-cyanoacrylate (Aron Alpha), which is characterized by rapid polymerization and complete firm adhesiveness, has come into use after experimental and clinical studies in the various surgical procedures. At present there is general agreement that the histotoxicity of this material is much less than that of methyl 2-cyanoacrylate or of other plastic adhesives, and it has been employed for coating unclippable aneurysms, especially for preventing clips from slipping.[12] However, rapid polymerization of this adhesive makes layers impossible, and its application to intracranial aneurysms is still controversial because of the potential toxicity to the surrounding neural tissue.[13,19] Moreover, among 53 aneurysms operated on using this adhesive alone for coating, or after clipping, Mazur et al[52] reported only one case of delayed thrombosis of the parent vessel after neck clipping with two clips and the adhesive. Thus, there is a danger of thrombosis of the patent vessel if a surplus amount of adhesive is applied.

Other higher homologues like isobutyl 2-cyanoacrylate were also employed as a coating agent.[89] Further investigations should be performed regarding histotoxicity with respect to age, additives, or other impurities of these coating agents.

Thus, at present, it is recommended to use

only EDH-adhesive or new ethyl 2-cyanoacrylate as a coating and reinforcement material of unclippable aneurysms. In addition, the following procedures should be performed.

1. Dissection of the aneurysm as free as possible from the neighboring structures.
2. Accurate application of coating materials.
3. Wrapping the aneurysm with oxydized cellulose to make a thick film.

Another technique for the treatment of aneurysms using plastic adhesive is the embolization of aneurysms with adhesive injected directly after craniotomy or with a detachable balloon filled with solidifying liquid agent (Table 10.2).[1b] Utilizing the direct injection technique of methyl methacrylate, Genest[27] first tried to treat the artificial aneurysm intravascularly in dogs. As an agent to occlude the surgically constructed aneurysm, isobutyl 2-cyanoacrylate was investigated by Zanetti and Sherman[92] in 1972 and by others[68a] because of low viscosity, ease of injection, instant polymerization on contact with blood, and minimal toxicity. Furthermore, this technique was applied to humans with aneurysm.[63,67]

Recent development of balloon catheter technique has made it possible to catheterize intracranial arteries, and using detachable balloon catheter, some investigators have been trying to treat intracranial aneurysms as well as AVM and carotid-cavernous sinus fistulas (CCF).[18,66,75] After catheterization the aneurysm was attempted to occlude intravascularly by a balloon inflated in the aneurysmal sac with a solidifying synthetic agent like cyanoacrylate, silicon or hydroxy methacrylate. Taki et al[75] reported one case with giant aneurysm of the middle cerebral artery which was occluded by an inflated balloon catheter filled with solidifying liquid without affecting the blood flow of parent vessel. However, from the clinical experiences using this technique, Debrun et al[18] concluded that indications for this technique should be limited because of technical difficulties, although cavernous saccular aneurysm of carotid siphon and saccular aneurysms of the C-1 and C-2 segment of the internal carotid artery could be successfully treated.

Romodanov et al[59c] recently reported the results of embolization of 119 saccular aneurysms. The embolization was performed in the chronic stage, and 108 out of 119 patients were embolized by the detached balloon with 97 good results. Seven patients had neurologic deficit and another seven patients died. In 93 patients, the aneurysm was occluded, and the patency of parent artery was preserved. In 15 patients the

Table 10.2. Plastic adhesive for the treatment of aneurysm (II) embolizing material.

	Plastic adhesive	Method
(I) Direct Injection		
Genest et al[27]	Methyl methacrylate	Direct injection
Zanetti & Sherman[92]	Isobutyl cyanoacrylate (experimental)	Direct injection
Sashin et al[63]	Isobutyl cyanoacrylate (clinical)	Direct injection by stereotaxic electronic radiographic technique
Sheptak et al[67]	Isobutyl cyanoacrylate (clinical)	Direct injection after craniotomy
Alksne & Smith[1a]	Iron powder suspended in methyl methacrylate (clinical)	Stereotactic injection
(II) Within the balloon		
Serbinenko[66]	Solidifying contrast material (clinical)	Detachable balloon catheter
Debrun et al[18]	Silicon polymer (clinical)	Detachable balloon catheter
Taki et al[75]	Hydroxyethyl methacrylate	Detachable balloon catheter

aneurysm as well as parent artery was occluded. Their good results may suggest that this treatment will be accepted as the first choice in future.

Treatment of AVM with Plastic Adhesive

Optimal therapy for the treatment of AVM is to extirpate the lesion. However, surgical treatment for the deeply seated AVM is still controversial, and the extirpation of AVM can not always be performed because of technical difficulties. To these inoperable AVMs, artificial embolization is considered to be a more effective alternative method or preoperative procedure in making the operation easier. In 1960 Luessenhop and Spence[48] attempted to occlude feeding vessels of intracranial AVM using spheric emboli made of methyl-methacrylate through a catheter placed in the common carotid artery. Since then, embolizing materials such as muscle, autologous clot, Oxycel, Gelfoam, silicone sponge, and polyvinyl alcohol were investigated, and some of them were clinically used to embolize the feeding vessels of vascular malformations.[16,46] Though it was an easy and relatively safe procedure, there was a fundamental disadvantage inherent in this method of employing the particular agents as emboli. Namely, it was impossible to embolize the small feeding vessels in AVM. To date, it is well understood that the small vessels that are not embolized will enlarge unless the shunt of the malformation is completely obliterated. To effect treatment with embolization, embolizing materials must pass into the nidus of the AVM, not merely obstruct the main feeding vessels. For this purpose, plastic liquids have been investigated as embolizing materials. Among the liquid emboli, silicone rubber was first employed, and it was injected by Sano et al[62] directly from the common carotid artery and then followed by other investigators[4e,20] (Table 10.3). As one of the liquid embolizing materials, cyanoacrylate was investigated by Zanetti and Sherman[92] in 1972 because of its characteristic reaction to blood—rapid solidification on contact. They used isobutyl 2-cyanoacrylate, which has a low viscosity, more rapid polymerization, and less toxicity than methyl or ethyl 2-cyanoacrylate in occluding the surgically constructed AV fistula in dogs. In their studies, it was demonstrated that this cyanoacrylate had a strong adhesive and a satisfactory occlusive ef-

Table 10.3. Plastic adhesive for the treatment of intracerebral AVM.

	Plastic adhesive	Method
Sano et al[62,66]	Silicon rubber (clinical)	Direct injection into the common carotid artery
Zanetti & Sherman[92]	Isobutyl cyanoacrylate (experimental)	Injection through catheter
Sashin et al[63]	Isobutyl cyanoacrylate (clinical)	Injection through the catheter placed at the intracranial feeding vessel
Serbinenko[66]	Balloon filled with solidifying contrast material (clinical)	Detached after catheterization into the intracranial feeding vessel
Debrun et al[17]	Balloon filled with silicon polymer (clinical)	Detached after catheterization into the intracranial feeding vessel
Kerber[41]	Isobutyl cyanoacrylate (clinical)	Injection through the small catheter placed at the feeding vessel
Kerber[42]	Isobutyl cyanoacrylate (clinical)	Injection through the calibrated leak balloon placed at the feeding vessel
Debrun et al[18]	Isobutyl cyanoacrylate (clinical)	Injection through the detachable graduated leak catheter placed at the feeding vessel

fect with mild tissue reaction that was limited to loss of intima with minimal changes in media subsequently. The technique was first applied to humans with AVM by Sashin et al.[63] Cromwell and Harrison[15] reported three patients with AVMs that were successfully treated by direct injection of isobutyl 2-cyanoacrylate mixed with iophendylate (Pantopaque) at craniotomy. In two of them AVM was completely resected without significant blood loss after embolization, and 30% obliteration was observed by subsequent angiography in one case. Likewise, Samson et al[60a] have reported their experience of the embolizations of the AVMs by direct injection of isobutyl 2-cyanoacrylate at craniotomy. Six of 10 patients with AVMs were treated with injection alone, and the AVM was completely obliterated in four of them. Four patients underwent the injection and immediate surgical excision of AVMs. No operative mortality and no permanent neurologic morbidity was described. In our clinic, isobutyl-2-cyanoacrylate or ethyl-cyanoacrylate mixed with iophendylate is employed. Before injecting the glue, fluoroscopic or intraoperative angiography is mandatory to ensure that the feeding artery is punctured. Depending on the size of the lesions, 0.3 to 1.0 ml of glue is injected from the feeding artery. After solidification of AVM with glue, removal of AVM becomes easy with minimum blood loss. Figure 10.2 shows successful embolization and extirpation of the left parietal AVM. Postoperatively, transient partial Gerstmann's syndrome developed, but it completely disappeared in the following seven days.

On the other hand, improvements in catheter technique[43b] and the development of various kinds of catheters have brought a superselective catheterization of intracranial vessels, making it possible to obliterate the affected vessels more accurately.[5,26,22a,74] In 1974 using a detachable balloon catheter, Serbinenko[66] reported the embolization of feeding vessels of AVM or AV fistula, and the occlusion of CCF sparing the blood flow of the internal carotid artery. The embolization of AVM with cyanoacrylate after superselective catheterization seems to be a promising technique because of the possibility of occlusion of the nidus itself.[18a,43a,49a] Application of superselective embolization with cyanoacrylate to the intracerebral AVM was first reported by Kerber.[41,43b,43c] After the experimental studies, he applied this technique to treat a patient with inoperable large occipital AVM by the injection of isobutyl 2-cyanoacrylate through a small silicone catheter. Pevsner and Doppman,[59b] using their own microballoon catheter, treated 32 patients with vascular lesions, mainly intracranial angioma. They used two kinds of embolizing materials, depending on the size of shunt and volume of shunt flow, and embolized with isobutyl 2-cyanoacrylate in 28 cases, and with silicone in 4 cases.

In their series, although there were one death and three neurologic complications, permanent in one and temporary in two, 14 patients with cerebral hemorrhage had no rebleeding after embolization and greater than 80% occlusion of the lesions was achieved in 13 (40%) of 32 cases. Likewise, Bank et al[3] have reported their clinical experience of 46 patients with intracranial AVMs or AV fistulas treated with isobutyl-2-cyanoacrylate. A total of 51 of a possible 62 feeding vessels was successfully occluded and six complications were described—catheter glued in place in three, overload edema in one, cerebral infarction in one, and intracerebral hemorrhage in three cases. Moreover, Debrun et al[18a] recently reported their 46 cases of cerebral AVM embolized with isobutyl 2-cyanoacrylate, including 13 patients managed by intraoperative embolization. In their last series, AVM was completely occluded in two of 11 cases, almost completely in one, and partially in the other cases. The catheter was glued in malformation in two cases and mild neurologic complications occurred in 4 cases, although there was no mortality.

The optimal physical and biologic characteristics of liquid polymers for catheter embolization include low viscosity, controllable polymerization, biocompatibility (lack of toxicity), sterilizability, radiopacity, prolonged shelf time and commercial availability.[59a] Cyanoacrylate partly satisfies these characteristics and currently isobutyl-2-cyanoacrylate (IBCA) has been used. Cyanoacrylate has a relatively low viscosity of 1.6 centistrokes at 25°C, iophendylate is mixed with IBCA for adjusting the polymerization time and also for making IBCA

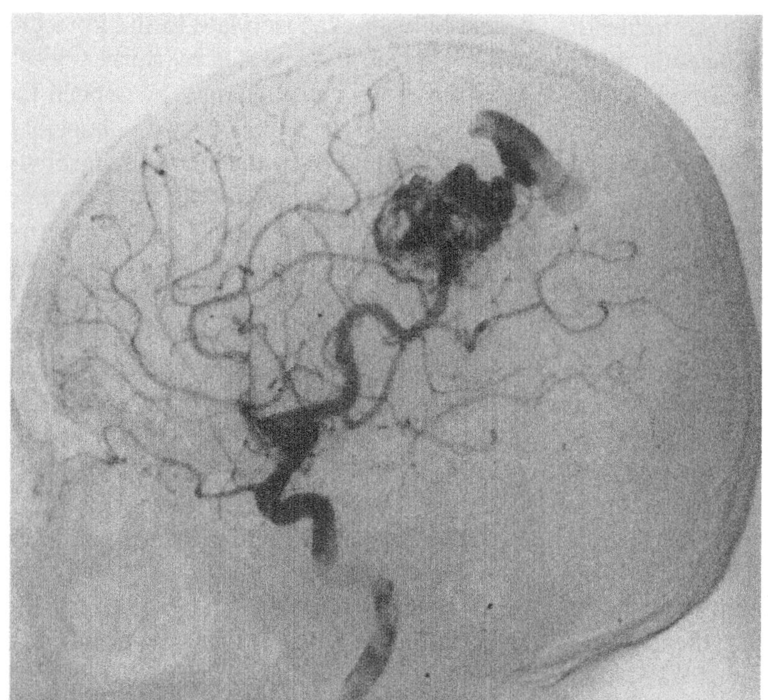

A

Figure 10.2. Intraoperative embolization of the left parietal arteriovenous malformation. **A.** Pretreatment. **B.** Posttreatment. **C.** Radiograph of the surgical specimen. The cyanoacrylate and iophendylate (Pantopaque) mixture was injected into the feeders.

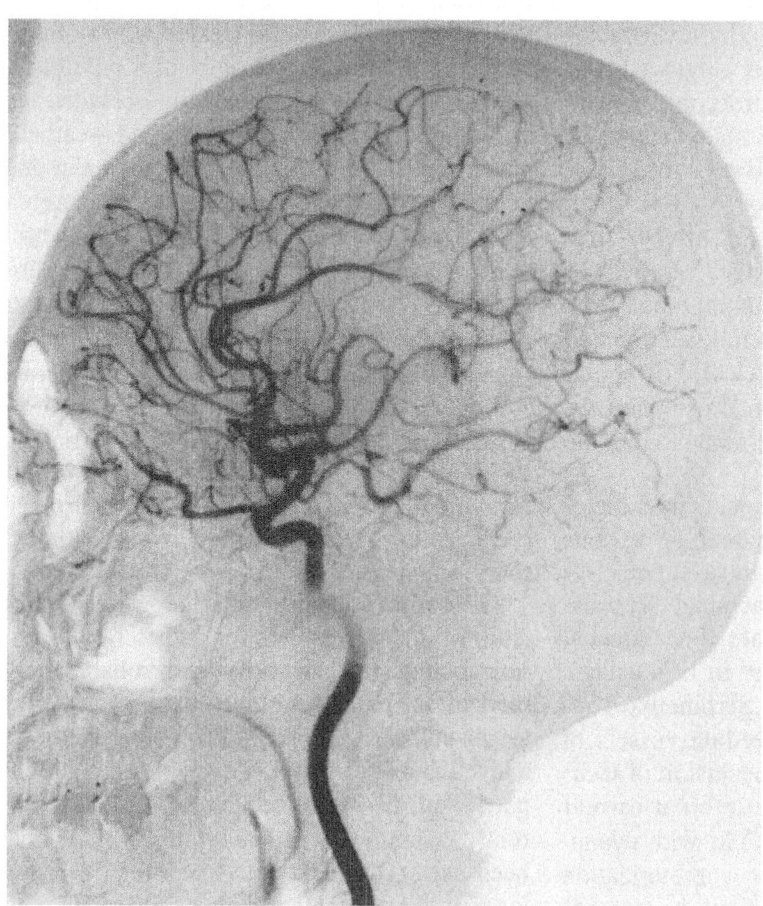

B

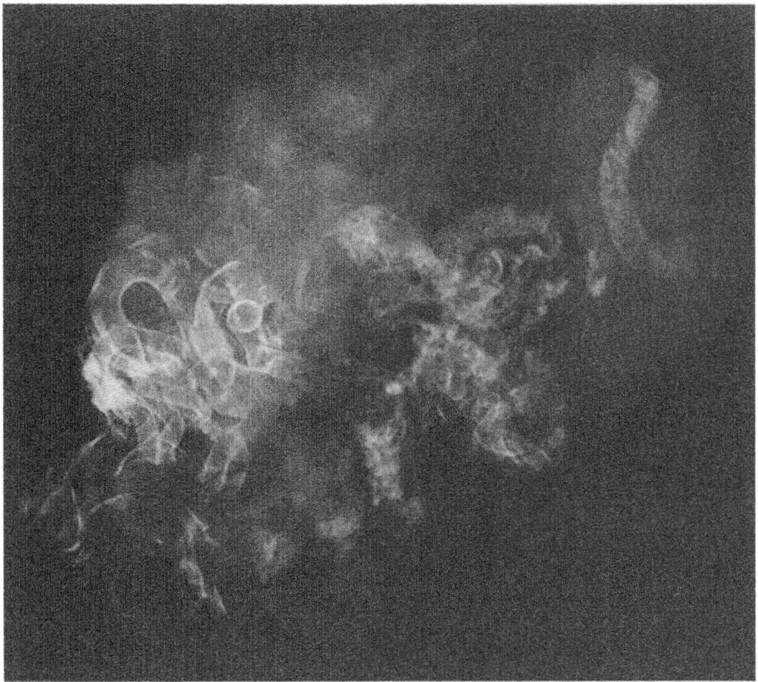

Fig. 10.2C

radiopaque. Generally 1 : 1 mixture is used. Disadvantage of Pantopaque is that it has a high viscosity, which requires high injection pressure when a large volume should be injected through the microballoon catheter. Thus there arises a risk of rupturing the balloon or intracranial artery, resulting in the undesirable occlusion of the normal proximal arteries and/or intracranial hemorrhage. The viscosity problem may be solved by using octa or decanoic acid, mild alkylacids, or a monoalkyl phosphoric acid ester solution in IBCA.[59a] For opacification of monomer milligrams amounts of either tantalum or titanium oxide in 0.1 to 0.2 ml of dispersant and a total of 0.3 to 0.5 ml of IBCA are visualized fluoroscopically and radiographically.

Although rapid polymerization time of IBCA is in good accordance with the circulation time, a balloon may be glued to the artery unless it is removed quickly. Quick withdrawal of the catheter may cause occlusion of proximal normal arteries by the glue that remained in the immaturely deflated balloon. Also, the abrupt injection may cause incomplete injection of IBCA, resulting in the insufficient embolization.

These technical difficulties are improved by the use of detachable-leak balloon catheter. Figure 10.3 shows the embolization of mixed dural pial AVM treated with detachable-leak balloon catheter. The balloon, which was glued to the feeder, was easily detached from the catheter.

Treatment of CCF with Plastic Adhesives

CCF may be divided into two discrete types—traumatic and spontaneous. Traumatic CCF has usually one or two fistula and up-to-date treatment of the detachable balloon technique.[17,58,64] After introduction of the balloon into the fistula, the balloon is inflated to fill the fistula and then is detached from the catheter with preservation of carotid blood flow.[2] For preventing a detached balloon from shrinkage, a one-way valve at the base of the balloon is used, but gradual deflation sometimes makes a false aneurysm. For complete sealing liquid plastics such as silicone, hydroxyethylmethacrylate (HEMA)[76] have been injected into the balloon. Debrun et al[17] have reported that in their 54 cases of post-traumatic CCF, 53 fistulas were obliterated in 59% of cases carotid blood flow were preserved.

A 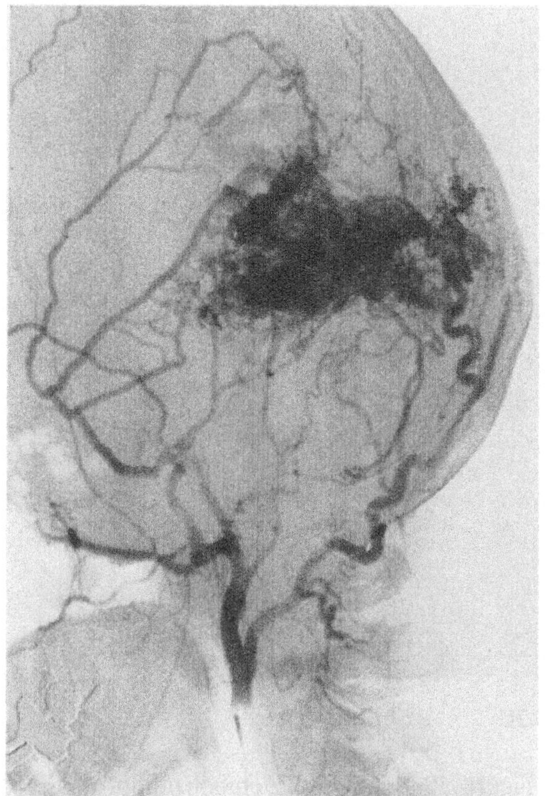

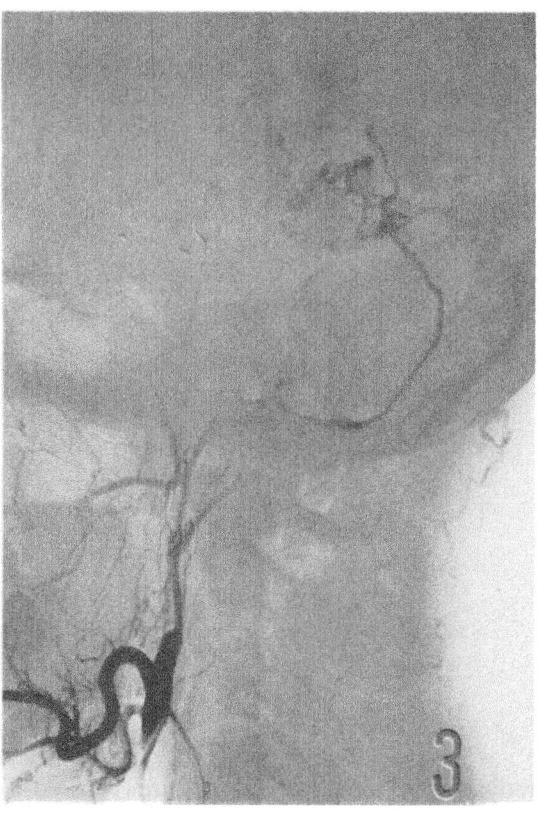 B

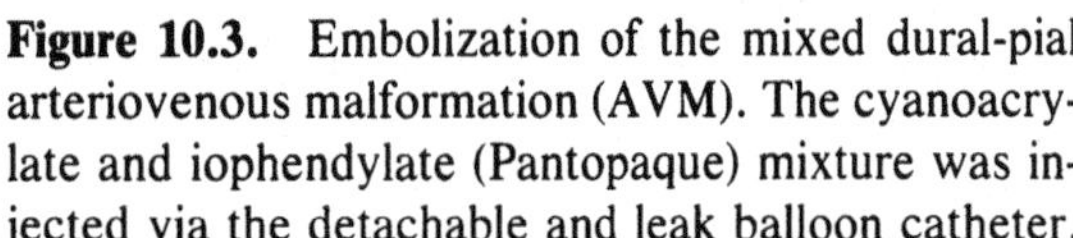

Figure 10.3. Embolization of the mixed dural-pial arteriovenous malformation (AVM). The cyanoacrylate and iophendylate (Pantopaque) mixture was injected via the detachable and leak balloon catheter. Although the balloon was glued to the feeder, it was detached from the catheter. **A.** Preembolization. **B.** Postembolization. Two small feeders still remain and will be embolized.

Some investigators use cyanoacrylate to occlude the fistula with success, through the microballoon catheter or direct injection at craniotomy[3,43a,60b]

Another type of spontaneous CCF involves many arterial sources such as internal carotid, external carotid, and vertebral artery. Among feeding arteries, the external carotid artery frequently supplies this type of fistula and is often its exclusive source of blood. These are managed by ligation or embolization, but mere embolization of the feeders hardly eradicates the lesion.

To effect the embolization, the mixture of cyanoacrylate and iophendylate is injected through a detachable leak balloon catheter. Figure 10.4 shows the embolization of spontaneous CCF treated with cyanoacrylate injection through the detachable leak balloon catheter.

Vascular Reconstruction with Plastic Adhesives

The use of tissue adhesive in vascular reconstruction was first reported by Nathan et al in 1960.[55] (Table 10.4) They considered methyl 2-cyanoacrylate as a promising reagent for the nonsuture closure of arterial incision after testing 28 synthetic adherent plastics. Carton et al[10,11] also employed this material in vessel anastomosis and repair after arteriotomy and reported the feasibility of using cyanoacrylates for suture. Since these reports, methyl 2-cyanoacrylate has been investigated as an adhesive in reconstructions of blood vessels.[31,35,37,82,] From the studies on a total of 170 linear and circumferential vascular repair in dogs using this plastic adhesive, Healey et at[35] observed that although this method had some advantages

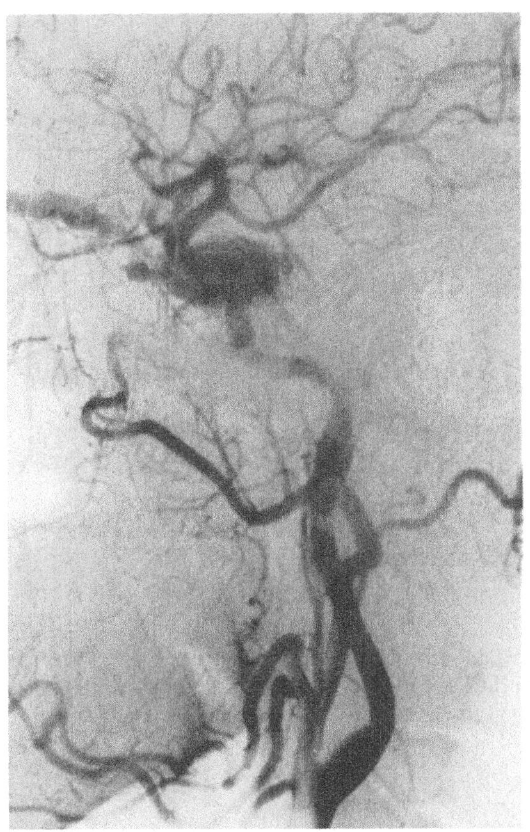

A

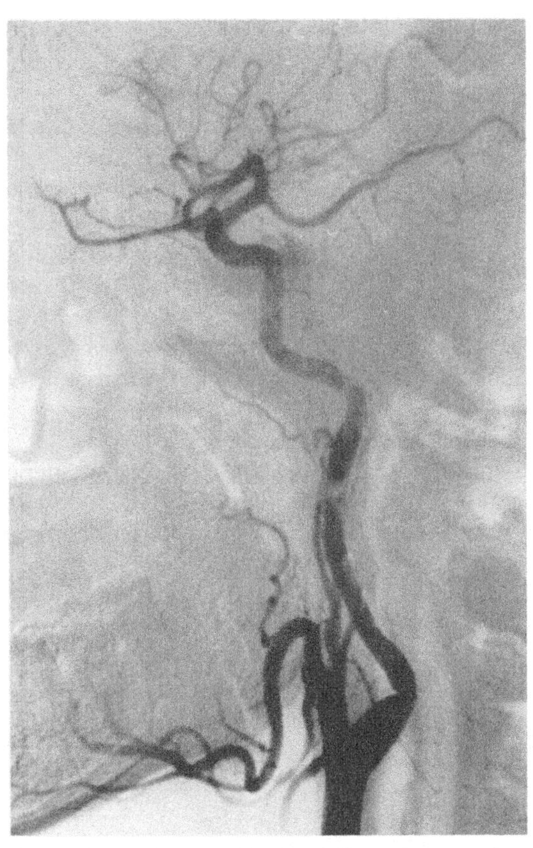

B

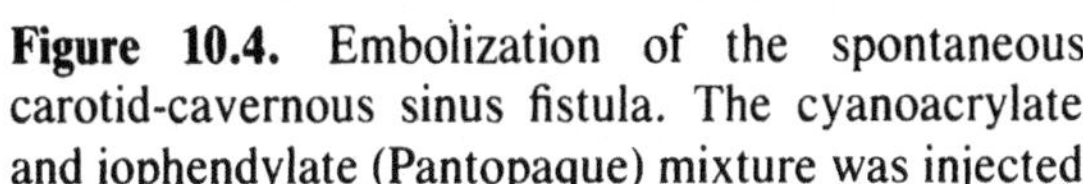

Figure 10.4. Embolization of the spontaneous carotid-cavernous sinus fistula. The cyanoacrylate and iophendylate (Pantopaque) mixture was injected via the detachable and leak balloon catheter. **A.** Preembolization. **B.** Postembolization.

like a minimal decrease in the size of lumen of the vessel anastomosed and a reduction in the time required for anastomosis without any special apparatus, certain precautions must be taken to obtain good results. If the adhesive entered the lumen of the vessel, thrombosis was inevitable, and an excessive amount of adhesive caused extended tissue reaction. Subsequent studies on this adhesive revealed severe histotoxicity, and some of the findings showed that this adhesive caused medial necrosis resulting in thrombus formation and development of aneurysm at the anastomotic site.[11,82] However, regarding thrombus formation in vessels larger than 2 mm in external diameter, technical problems in performing the anastomosis are considered the main factors, not medial necrosis. These are supported by the excellent results by Jacobson et al[40] who employed microsurgical technique and by other investigators.[10,37] Moreover, Manax et al[49] observed no late vessel occlusion or narrowing in more than 200 end-to-end and end-to-side anastomoses of various vessels in dogs when methyl 2-cyanoacrylate was applied as an adjunct after suture anastomosis. On the other hand, although fusiform or aneurysmal dilations were observed by Weissberg and Goetz,[81] and Carton et al[11] after coating or after repair of arteriotomy using this adhesive, Kessler and Carton[44] noted that it was possible to prevent anastomotic aneurysms by circumferential reinforcement with fascia and adhesive. Compared with reconstructions of the relatively large vessels, it appeared difficult to obtain a high patency rate in the anastomosis of vessels smaller than 2 mm in external diameter. Hoppenstein et al[36] reported that small arteries 0.5 to 2 mm in diameter reacted

Table 10.4. Vascular reconstruction with plastic adhesive

	Adhesive	Type of reconstruction	Vessel diameter	Combined technique	Result (follow-up)
Nathan et al[55]	M 2-C	Repair of arteriotomy	4 mm		77% (1 wk–3 mo)
Carton et al.[10]	M 2-C	E-E Anast.	4–5 mm	Flanged ring	96% (Short term)
Ohta et al[56]	E 2-C	Repair of arteriotomy			100%
		E-E Anast.	2–4 mm	Stay sutures	88% (14 d–180 d)
		E-S Anast.			100%
Jacobson et al[40]	M 2-C	E-E Anast.	3–4 mm	Stay sutures microscope	100% (12 h–6 mo)
Carson et al[7]	I B C	E-E Anast.	2–4 mm	O-Ring	91%
Souther et al[70]	I B C	E-E Anast.	1–2 mm	Stay sutures microscope	82% (1 d–42 d)
Suzuki & Onuma[73]	E 2-C	E-E Anast.	2–3 mm	Soluble splint	70% (7 d–69 d)
Shintani et al[68]	E 2-C	Repair of arteriotomy	1 mm	Stay sutures microscope	100% (2 wk) 95% (6 wk)
Crowell et al[16]	E 2-C	Repair of arteriotomy	MCA of monkey	Microscope	100% (1 yr)
Yamagata et al[87]	I P C	E-E Anast.	1 mm	Soluble tube	98% (2 wk)
Yamagata et al[86]	I P C	E-S Anast.		microscope	91% (3 mo)

M 2-C, methyl 2-cyanoacrylate; E 2-C, ethyl 2-cyanoacrylate; IBC, isobutyl 2-cyanoacrylate; IPC, isopropyl 2-cyanoacrylate; E-E Anast., end-to-end anastomosis; E-S Anast., end-to-side anastomosis; MCA, middle cerebral artery.

differently from large arteries, and thrombosis occurred in a large percentage after coating with methyl 2-cyanoacrylate. This was also pointed out by Weissberg et al[82] who obtained a poor patency rate in the end-to-side anastomosis of branches of the femoral artery 1 to 1.5 mm in external diameter.

In the middle 1960s investigation of ethyl 2-cyanoacrylate was begun in the vascular reconstruction as well as in other surgical procedures.[56,91] Because of the superiority in histotoxicity and longer maintenance of the tensile strength, methyl 2-cyanoacrylate has been replaced by this adhesive. Ohta et al[56] obtained excellent results in vessel repair using this adhesive. Likewise, successful nonsuture end-to-end anastomosis was reported by Suzuki and Onuma[73] in combination with intravascular souble splint. This adhesive was applied to microvascular surgery, which has made significant progress in recent years. Shintani et al[68] closed a 10-mm arteriotomy of arteries 0.8 to 1.5 mm in outside diameter in combination with three stay sutures and obtained a high patency rate with minimal tissue reaction, no fusiform dilatation, and satisfactory bonding property. Furthermore, this adhesive was investigated for long-term effect in intracranial microvascular repair using the middle cerebral artery of monkey, and satisfactory results were obtained by Crowell et al.[16]

On the other hand, higher homologues of cyanoacrylate were also investigated in microvascular reconstructions. Using isobutyl 2-cyanoacrylate, Weinstein et al[80] reported excellent results in the repair of 3-mm to 4-mm arteriotomy, observing moderate chronic inflammation and fibrotic changes in the adventitia and media with little evidence of necrosis. Easy microvascular end-to-end anastomosis using lyophilized dural cuff and this adhesive was reported with a relatively high patency rate by Tschop.[78] Moreover, Yamagata et al[86,87] introduced nonsuture microvascular anastomosis using isopropyl 2-cyanoacrylate and a soluble tube made of polyvinyl alcohol as an internal stent. Both end-to-end and end-to-side anastomoses were performed using common carotid arteries about 1 mm in diameter of rats, and high patency rates were reported in both types of anastomosis. Although the development of aneurysm was found in end-to-side anastomosis in their studies, it was prevented by reinforcement with the adhesive used.

Conclusion

In the surgical treatment of cerebrovascular disease, various kinds of plastic adhesives have been employed as coating agents for aneurysms and as embolizing materials for aneurysms, AVM, and CCF. In addition, plastic adhesives have been investigated for vascular reconstruction. To date, experimental and clinical results regarding some of the cyanoacrylates indicate potential usefulness and support the clinical application if they are utilized appropriately.

As a coating material for aneurysm, EDH-adhesive and ethyl 2-cyanoacrylate may be used to reinforce and coat aneurysms that are unmanageable without severe complications or in the case of unsatisfactory clipping of the neck. The use of tissue adhesive as an embolizing material seems to have great potentiality for the intravascular occlusive therapy of aneurysm, AVM, and CCF. In recent years significant progress has been made in catheters as well as in embolizing materials. However, there are still many technical problems to be resolved before clinical application: estimation of volume of tissue adhesive to be injected, possibility of passing the adhesive through the lesion and resulting in lung embolus, long-terms results of histotoxicity of plastic adhesive injected into the vessel, complexity of superselective catheterization of intracranial arteries, and others.

At present the obliteration of intracranial aneurysms with plastic adhesive by direct injection at craniotomy or after transarterial catherization is still an experimental procedure. It may be feasible some day to treat some of aneurysms with this technique, using more suitable polymerizing materials. However, the embolization of intracranial AVMs with plastic adhesive appears to be an effective method of obliterating the lesions considered to be inoperable or facilitating the surgical resection that follows, and isobutyl 2-cyanoacrylate currently seems to be the best embolizing substance. Moreover, occlusion of CCF with plastic adhesive by combining with craniotomy or by intravascular approach is considered to be the best means in some of CCFs.

The use of plastic adhesive in blood vessel reconstruction seems to have potential in the development of easier and time-saving techniques. It is obvious that such development is necessary in microvascular anastomosis, which requires a more refined technique and longer time than large-vessel anastomosis. Despite the difficulty in small-vessel anastomosis with plastic adhesive, it has been noted in a few reports that it is possible to have a high patency rate in nonsuture anastomosis of vessels less than 2 mm in external diameter employing plastic adhesive. This may be because a higher homologue of cyanoacrylate was used in anastomosis, in addition to improvements in the anastomosis technique. Although it is obvious that further investigations are necessary regarding the long-term histotoxicity of these plastic adhesives, it appears that clinical application is not as hazardous when compared with the conventional suture method[1,4,51] because necrosis of the middle layer is observed in usual suture anastomosis and the medial necrosis that occurs on application of plastic adhesive is completely replaced by strong fibrous tissue within three months.

Further investigations should be continued to develop a superior plastic adhesive and to improve the technique of the treatment with plastic adhesive. At the same time, more accurate and detailed studies about the histotoxicity of currently used cyanoacrylate adhesives are required. In future studies, age and detailed composition of each cyanoacrylate adhesive used should be described. Furthermore, comparative studies of higher homologues of cyanoacrylate adhesive should be performed because of the possibility of reducing the toxicity of the adhesive.

References

1. Acland RD, Trachtenberg L: The histopathology of small arteries following experimental microvascular anastomosis. Plast Reconstr Surg 59:868–875, 1977

1a. Alksne JF, Smith RW: Iron-acrylic compound for stereotaxic aneurysm thrombosis. J Neurosurg 47:137–141, 1977

1b. Alksne JF, Smith RW: Stereotaxic occlusion of 22 consecutive anterior communicating artery aneurysms. J Neurosurg 52:790–793, 1980

2. Bahuleyan K, Nelson LR, Peck FC Jr: Occlusion of carotid-cavernous fistula with a balloon catheter. Surg Neurol 3:283–287, 1975

3. Bank WO, Kerber CW, Cromwell LD: Treatment of intracerebral arteriovenous malformations with isobutyl 2-cyanoacrylate: Initial clinical experience. Radiology 139:609–616, 1981

3a. Bank WO, Kerber CW, Drayer BP, et al: Carotid-cavernous fistula: endarterial cyanoacrylate occlusion with preservation of carotid flow. J Neuroradiol 5:279–285, 1978

4. Baxter TJ, O'Brien BM, Henderson PN, et al: The histopathology of small vessels following microvascular repair. Br J Surg 59:617–622, 1972

4a. Berenstein A, Kricheff II: Catheter and material selection for transcatheter embolization: Technical considerations. 1. Catheters. Radiology 132:619–630, 1979

4b. Berenstein A, Kricheff II: Catheter and material selection for transcatheter embolization: Technical considerations. 2. Materials. Radiology 132:631–639, 1979

4c. Berenstein A: Flow-controlled silicone fluid embolization. AJR 134:1213–1218, 1980

5. Berenstein A: Technique of catheterization and embolization of the lenticulostriate arteries. J Neurosurg 54:783–789, 1981

6. Brooks B: The treatment of traumatic arteriovenous fistula. South Med J 23:100–106, 1930

7. Carson HS III, Allen BS Jr: Comparative studies of experimental blood vessel anastomosis using biological adhesives. South Med J 60:1331–1335, 1967

8. Carton CA, Heifetz MD, Kessler LA: Patching of intracranial internal carotid artery in man using a plstic adhesive (Eastman 910). J Neurosurg 19:887–896, 1962

9. Carton CA, Kennedy JC, Heifetz MD, et al: The use of a plastic adhesive (Methyl 2-cyanoacrylate) in the management of intracranial aneurysms and leaking cerebral vessels. A report of 15 cases. Intracranial aneurysms and subarachnoid hemorrhage: Charles C Thomas, Springfield, Ill, 1965, pp 372–440

10. Carton CA, Kessler LA, Seidenberg B, et al: Experimental studies in the surgery of small blood vessels. IV Nonsuture anastomosis of arteries and veins, using flanged ring prostheses and plastic adhesive. Surg Forum 11:238–241, 1960

11. Carton CA, Kessler LA, Seidenberg B, et al: Experimental studies in surgery of small blood vessels. II Patching of arteriotomy using a plastic adhesive. J Neurosurg 18:188–194, 1961

12. Chou SN, Oritz-Surez HL, Brown WE: Technique and material for coating aneurysms. Cli Neurosurg 21:182–193, 1974

13. Chou SN: Use of cyanoacrylate. J Neurosurg 46:266, 1977

14. Coe JE: Late thrombosis following the use of autogenous fascia and cyanoacrylate (Eastman 910) for the wrapping of an intracranial aneurysm. J Neurosurg 21: 884–886, 1964

15. Cromwell LD, Harris AB: Treatment of cerebral arteriovenous malformations. A combined neurosurgical and neuroradiological approach. J Neurosurg 52:705–708, 1980

15a. Cromwell LD, Kerber CW: Modification of cyanoacrylate for therapeutic embolization: Preliminary experience. Am J Roentgenol 132:799–801, 1979

16. Crowell RM, Morawetz RB, Jones TH, et al: Successful adhesive repair of middle cerebral arteriotomy in primates. In Microsurgery for Cerebral Ischemia. Springer-Verlag, NY, 1978, pp 166–172

17. Debrun G, Lacour P, Caron JP, et al: Inflatable and released balloon technique. Experimentation in dog—application in man. Neuroradiology 9:267–271, 1975

18. Debrun G, Lacour P, Caron JP, et al: Detachable balloon and calibrated-leak balloon technique in the treatment of cerebral vascular lesions. J Neurosurg 49: 635–649, 1978

18a. Debrun G, Vinuela F, Fox A, et al: Embolization of cerebral arteriovenous malformations with bucrylate. Experience in 46 cases. J Neurosurg 56:615–627, 1982

19. Diaz FG, Mastri AR, Chou SN: Neural and vascular tissue reaction to aneurysm-coating adhesive (ethyl 2-cyanoacrylate). Neurosurgery 3:45–49, 1978

20. Doppman J, Zapol W, Pierce J: Transcatheter embolization with a silicon rubber preparation. Invest Radiol 6:304–309, 1971

21. Dott NM: Intracranial aneurysms: cerebral arterio-radiography: surgical treatment. Edinburgh Med J 40:219–234, 1933

22. Dotter C, Goldman ML, Rösch J: Instant selective arterial occlusion with Isobutyl 2-cyanoacrylate. Radiology 114:227–230, 1975

23. Dutton JEM: Intracranial aneurysm. A new method of surgical treatment. Bri Med J 2:585–586, 1956

24. Dutton JEM, Yates PO: An experimental study of the effects of a plastic adhesive, Methyl 2-Cyanoacrylate Monomer (M 2 C-1) in various tissue. J Neurosurg 24: 876–882, 1966
25. Freeny PC, Mennemeyer R, Kidd CR, et al: Long-term radiographic-pathologic follow-up of patients treated with visceral transcatheter occlusion using isobutyl 2-cyanoacrylate (Bucrylate). Radiology 132:51–60, 1979
26. Gacs G: Catheterization and superselective angiography of the cerebral vessels. Neuroradiology 12:239–241, 1977
27. Genest AS: Experimental use of intraluminal plastics in the treatment of carotid aneurysms: Preliminary report. J Neurosurg 22:136–140, 1965
28. Goetz RH, Weissberg D, Hoppenstein R: Vascular necrosis caused by application of methyl 2-cyanoacrylate (Eastman 910 Monomer): 7-month follow up in dog. Ann Surg 163:242–248, 1966
29. Goldman ML, Freeny PC, Tallman JM, et al: Transcatheter vascular occlusion therapy with isobutyl 2-cyanoacrylate (Bucrylate) for control of massive upper-gastrointestinal bleeding. Radiology 129:41–49, 1978
30. Gottlob R, Blumel G: The toxic action of alkylcyanoacrylate adhesives of vessels. Comparative studies. J Surg Res 7:362–367, 1967
31. Hafner CD, Fogarty TJ, Cranley JJ: Nonsuture anastomosis of small arteries using a tissue adhesive. Surg Gynecol Obstet 116:417–421, 1963
32. Handa H, Ohta T, Ishikawa S, et al: Coating and reinforcing of experimental cervical aneurysms with synthetic resins and rubbers. Neurol Med Chir (Tokyo) 2:185–186, 1960
33. Handa H, Ohta T, Kamijyo Y: Encasement of intracranial aneurysms with plastic compounds. Prog Neurol Surg 3:149–192, 1969
34. Hashimoto Y, Iwata K, Koyama Y: Application of plastic adhesive to surgical field. J Ther Eng (Tokyo) 46:859–867, 1964
35. Healey JE Jr, Clark RL, Gallager HS, et al: Nonsuture repair of blood vessels. Ann Surg 155:817–825, 1962
36. Hoppenstein R, Weissberg D, Goetz RH: Fusiform dilatation and thrombosis of arteries following the application of methyl 2-cyanoacrylate (Eastman 910 monomer). J Neurosurg 23:556–564, 1965
37. Hosbein DJ, Blumenstock DA: Anastomosis of small arteries using a tissue adhesive. Surg Gynecol Obstet 118:112–114, 1964
38. Hunter CR, Mayfield FH, McBride BH, et al: Intracranial implantation of liquid plastic in the experimental animal (macaque): Possible clinical application in surgical management of intracranial aneurysms. Surg Forum 7:539–544, 1956
39. Inou T, Mori S, Mizuno K, et al: A new adhesive for vascular surgery. J Int Coll Surg 44:241–252, 1965
40. Jacobson JH II, Moody RA, Kusserow BK, et al: The tissue response to a plastic adhesive used in combination with microsurgical technique in reconstruction of small arteries. Surgery 60:379–385, 1966
41. Kerber CW: Intracranial cyanoacrylate, a new catheter therapy for arteriovenous malformations. Invest Radiol 10:536–538, 1975
42. Kerber CW: Balloon catheter with a calibrated leak. A new system for superselective angiography and occlusive therapy. Radiology 120: 547–550, 1976
43. Kerber CW, Bank WO, Cromwell LD: Cyanoacrylate occlusion of carotid-cavernous fistula with preservation of carotid artery flow. Neuroradiology 4:210–215, 1979
43a. Kerber CW, Bank WO, Cromwell LD: Calibrated leak balloon microcatheter: A device for arterial exploration and occlusive therapy. AJR 132:207–212, 1979
43b. Kerber CW: Flow-controlled therapeutic embolization: A physiologic and safe technique. AJR 134:557–561, 1980
43c. Kerber CW: Use of balloon catheters in the treatment of cranial arterial abnormalities. Stroke 11:210–216, 1980
44. Kessler LA, Carton CA: Experimental studies in surgery of small blood vessels with the use of plastic adhesive. III Prevention of aneurysmal dilatation. Surg Forum 11:403–404, 1960
45. Kline DG, Hayes GJ: An experimental evaluation of the effect of a plastic adhesive, Methyl 2-cyanoacrylate, on neural tissue. J Neurosurg 20:647–654, 1963
46. Krayenbühl H: Behandlung intrakranieller Aneurysmen mit synthetischem Klebestoff. Münch Med Wschr 106:1370–1373, 1964
46a. Kunstlinger F, Brunelle F, Chaumont P, et al: Vascular occlusive agents. AJR 136:151–156, 1981
47. Lehman RA, Hayes GJ: The toxicity of alkyl 2-cyanoacrylate tissue adhesives: Brain and blood vessels. Surgery 61:915–922, 1967
47a. Liebert W, Szymas J: Embolization of n-butyl 2-cyanoacrylate for the reconstruction of the arteries in dogs. I. Clinical evaluation. Polim Med 10:225–232, 1980
48. Luessenhop AJ, Spence WT: Artificial embolization of cerebral arteries. Report of use in a case of arteriovenous malformations. JAMA 172:1153–1155, 1960

49. Manax WG, Bloch JH, Longerbeam JK, et al: Plastic adhesive as an adjunct in suture anastomoses of small blood vessels. Surgery 54:663–666, 1963
49a. Margolis MT, Freeny PC, Kendrick MM: Cyanoacrylate occlusion of a spinal cord arteriovenous malformation. Case report. J Neurosurg 51:107–110, 1979
50. Matsumoto MT, Pani KC, Hardaway CRM, et al: A method of arterial anastomosis using cyanoacrylate tissue adhesive. Arch Surg 94:388–391, 1967
51. Maxwell GP, Szabo Z, Buncke HJ Jr: Aneurysms after microvascular anastomoses. Plast Reconstr Surg 63:824–829, 1979
52. Mazuor JB, Salager JL: Late thrombosis of middle cerebral artery following clipping and coating of aneurysms. Surg Neurol 10:131–133, 1978
53. Messer HD, Strenger L, McVeety HJ: Use of plastic adhesive for reinforcement of a ruptured intracranial aneurysm. J Neurosurg 20:360–362, 1963
54. Miller FJ, Rankin RS, Gliedman JB: Experimental internal iliac artery embolization: evaluation of low viscosity silicon rubber, isobutyl 2-cyanoacrylate, and carbon microspheres. Radiology 129:51–58, 1978
55. Nathan HS, Nachlas MM, Solomon RD, et al: Nonsuture closure of arterial incisions using a rapidly-polymerizing adhesive. Ann Surg 152:648–659, 1960
56. Ohta K, Mori S, Koike T, et al: Blood vessel repair utilizing a new plastic adhesive. Experimental and clinical studies. J Surg Res 5:453–462, 1965
57. Ohta T: Coating and reinforcement of the intracranial aneurysm with synthetic resins and rubbers. Arch Jap Chir 30:753–776, 1961
58. Peeters FL, van der Werf AJ: Detachable balloon technique in the treatment of direct carotid-cavernous fistulas Surg Neurol 14:11–19, 1980
59. Pevsner PH: Micro-balloon catheter for superselective angiography and therapeutic occlusion Am J Roentgenol 128:225–230, 1977
59a. Pevsner PH, George ED, Doppman JL: Interventional radiology polymer update: Acrylic. Neurosurgery 10:314–316, 1982
59b. Pevsner PH, Doppman JL: Therapeutic embolization with a microballoon catheter system. AJR 134:949–958, 1980
59c. Romodanov AP, Shchezlor VI: Intravascular occlusion of saccular aneurysms of the cerebral arteries by means of a detachable balloon catheter: Advances and Technical Standards in Neurosurgery, Vol 9. Springer-Verlag, 1982
60. Sachs E Jr, Erbengi A, Margolis G, et al: Fatality from ruptured intracranial aneurysm after coating with methyl 2-cyanoacrylate (Eastman 910 Monomer, M 2 C-1). Case report. J Neurosurg 24:889–891, 1966
60a. Samson D, Ditmore OM, Beyer Jr CW: Intravascular use of isobutyl 2-cyanoacrylate: Part I. Treatment of intracranial arteriovenous malformations. Neurosurgery 8:43–51, 1981
60b. Samson D, Ditmore QM, Beyer Jr CW: Intravascular use of isobutyl 2-cyanoacrylate: Part II. Treatment of carotid-cavernous fistulas. Neurosurgery 8:52–55, 1981
61. Sano H, Kanno T, Katada K, et al: Treatment of the dural AVM: Embolization using Aron Alpha. Neurol Med Chir (Tokyo) 20:845–851, 1980
62. Sano K, Jimbo M, Saito I: Artificial embolization with liquid plastic. Neurol Med Chir (Tokyo) 8:198–201, 1966
63. Sashin D, Goldman RL, Zanetti P, et al: Electronic radiography in stereotaxic thrombosis of intracranial aneurysm and catheter embolization of cerebral arteriovenous malformation. Radiology 105:359–363, 1972
64. Sekhar LN, Heros R, Kerber CW: Carotid-cavernous fistula following percutaneous retrogasserian procedure. J Neurosurg 51:700–706, 1979
65. Selverstone B, Ronis N: Coating and reinforcement of intracranial aneurysms with synthetic resins. Bull Tufts-N Engl Med Cent 4:8–12, 1958
66. Serbinenko FA: Balloon catheterization and occlusion of major vessels J Neurosurg 41:125–145, 1974
67. Sheptak PE, Zanetti PH, Susen AF: The treatment of intracranial aneurysms by injection with a tissue adhesive. Neurosurgery 1:25–29, 1977
68. Shintani A, Zervas NT, Kuwayama A: Rapid microvascular repair using plastic adhesive. Stroke 3:34–40, 1972
68a. Siqueira MG, Vieira IA, Ciliao EA, et al: Intracranial saccular aneurysms: Experimental evaluation of intravascular therapeutic procedure. Arq Neuropsiquiatr 38:24–32, 1980
69. Skjennald A, Klevmark B, Stenwig JT: Transcatheter embolization of the renal artery with bucrylate in renal carcinoma. Acta Radiol 21:215–219, 1980
70. Souther SG, Levitsky S, Roberts WC: Bucrylate tissue adhesive for microvascular anastomosis. Arch Surg 103:496–499, 1971
71. Stowsand D, Buhl K: Early and late results after coating intracranial aneurysms with biobond. Acta Neurochir (Wien) 32:73–82, 1975
72. Suger O, Tsuchiya G: Plastic coating of intracranial aneurysms with EDH-Adhesive. J Neurosurg 21:114–117, 1964
73. Suzuki J, Onuma T: A soluble internal splint for experimental vascular anastomosis. J Neurosurg 35:355–358, 1971

74. Taki W: Experimental and clinical studies on superselective angiography and embolization using balloon catheter systems. Arch Jap Chir 49:637–662, 1980
75. Taki W, Handa H, Yamagata S, et al: Balloon embolization of a giant aneurysm using a newly developed catheter. Surg Neurol 12:363–365, 1979
76. Taki W, Handa H, Yamagata S, et al: Radiopaque solidifying liquids for releasable balloon technique: A technical note. Surg Neurol 13:405–408, 1980
77. Todd EM, Crue BL Jr: The coating of aneurysms with plastic materials. In WS Field, AL Sahs (eds.): Intracranial Aneurysms and Subarachnoid Hemorrhage, Charles C Thomas, Springfield, Ill, 1965, pp 357–371
78. Tschopp HM: Small artery anastomosis using a cuff of dura mater and a tissue adhesive. Plast Reconstr Surg 55:606–611, 1975
79. Tsuchiya G, Sugar O, Yashon D, et al: Reaction of rabbit brain and peripheral vessels to plastic used in coating arterial aneurysms. J Neurosurg 28: 409–419, 1968
79a. Vinster HV, Debrun G, Kaufman JC, et al: Pathology of arteriovenous malformations embolized with isobutyl 2-cyanoacrylate. Report of two cases. J Neurosurg 55:819–825, 1981
80. Weinstein PR, Wilson CB: Nonsuture closure of small vessel arteriotomies. Surg Forum 20:447–449, 1969
81. Weissberg D, Goetz RH: Necrosis of arterial wall following application of methyl 2-cyanoacrylate. Surg Gynecol Obstet 119:1248–1252, 1964
82. Weissberg D, Schwartz P, Goetz RH: Nonsuture end-to-side anastomosis of small blood vessels. Surg Gynecol Obstet 123:341–346, 1966
83. White RI Jr, Standberg JV, Gross GS, et al: Therapeutic emoblization with long-term occluding agents and their effects on embolized tissues. Radiology 125:677–687, 1977
84. Woodhall B, Golden J: Fibroblastic stimulation of rabbit artery adventitia by marine varnish, 'krylon' and latex. Laboratory study related to the surgery of congenital cerebral aneurysm. Arch Surg 66:567–592, 1953
85. Woodward SC, Herrmann JB, Cameron JL, et al: Histotoxicity of cyanoacrylate tissue adhesive in the rat. Ann Surg 162:113–122, 1965
86. Yamagata S, Carter LP, Handa H, et al: Experimental studies in nonsuture end-to-side microvascular anastomosis. Neurol Med Chir (Tokyo) 21:701–708, 1981
87. Yamagata S, Handa H, Taki W, et al: Experimental nonsuture microvascular anastomosis using a soluble PVA tube and plastic adhesive. J Microsurg 1:208–215, 1979
88. Yashon D, Jane JA, Gordon MC, et al: Effects of methyl 2-cyanoacrylate adhesives on the somatic vessels and the central nervous system of animals. J Neurosurg 24:883–888, 1966
89. Yashon D, White RJ, Arias BA, et al: Cyanoacrylate encasement of intracranial aneurysms. Technical note J Neurosurg 34:709–713, 1971
90. Yodh SB, Wright RL: Experimental evaluation of four synthetic adhesives for possible treatment of aneurysms. J Neurosurg 26:504–510, 1967
91. Yoshimura K, Ohta K, Koike T, et al: Studies of plastic adhesives in surgery: Part II Nippon Rinsho (Tokyo) 21:563–573, 1963
92. Zanetti PH, Sherman FE: Experimental evaluation of a tissue adhesive as an agent for the treatment of aneurysms and arteriovenous anomalies. J Neurosurg 36:72–79, 1972

11

Dissection of Internal Carotid, Vertebral, and Intracranial Arteries

Robert G. Ojemann

Introduction

Dissection in the wall of the carotid, vertebral, or intracranial artery causing narrowing or occlusion of the arterial lumen or acting as a source of emboli is an established cause of cerebral ischemia 1–50. The dissection develops when blood enters the wall of the artery through a defect and forces the layers apart. The etiology of the dissection is usually designated as spontaneous or traumatic. The term spontaneous is used to indicate that no obvious precipitating injury was recognized, although pathology may be found in the arterial wall in some cases. Traumatic causes include nonpenetrating injury to the head and neck, direct injury to the vessel and percutaneous carotid angiography.

Spontaneous Dissection—Internal Carotid Artery

Pathogenesis

Dissection of the internal carotid artery begins at two sites of predilection in the internal carotid artery—just distal to the origin and between C2 and the base of the skull. The possible relationship of congenital deficits in the wall of the artery, of cystic medial necrosis, and of fibromuscular hyperplasia to the cause of the dissection has been discussed.[15,20,39]

In seven of the first 11 reported cases, the involved internal carotid artery, as well as the opposite carotid and aorta, was said to show cystic medial necrosis.[15] However, this was not found in the detailed pathologic study of a specimen removed at surgery.[26] In that case the wall of the artery showed no underlying intrinsic disease, but the muscle and elastic tissue had an irregular disorganized arrangement rather than the usual laminar pattern. Similar findings were reported in four arteries removed at operation.[14] Fibromuscular dysphasia has been associated with at least six reported cases of dissection.[35]

The question arises as to whether these are truly spontaneous dissection. Although obvious external trauma was not a factor, it is possible that other factors relate to the onset. In three cases of Fisher et al,[15] symptoms began during a period of heavy coughing. In addition, minor falls may be significant, as noted in the report by Ringel et al, where a 49-year-old male, while skiing, developed acute dissection of both internal carotid arteries and the right vertebral artery at the level of the second vertebra and of the left vertebral artery at the sixth cervical vertebra.[39] The relationship of head rotation to injury to the internal carotid artery is discussed in the section on traumatic dissections.[5,17,39,44]

It is likely that intracranial emboli from the area of the carotid dissection may be a primary cause of symptoms in many patients. This has

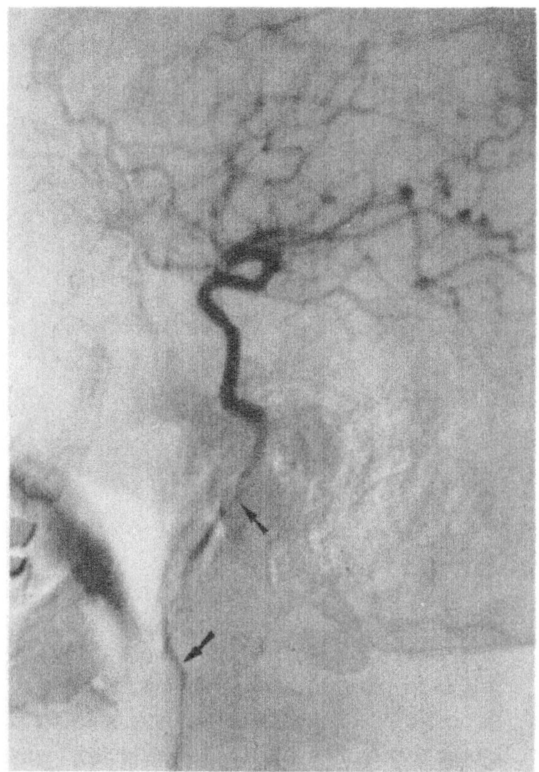

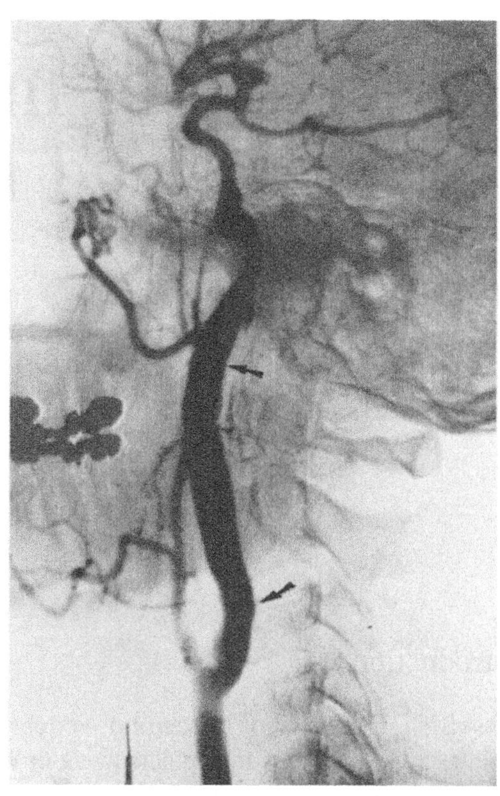

Figure 11.1. **A.** The patient, a 41-year-old housewife, presented with a fluctuating neurologic deficit. Typical angiographic appearance of internal carotid dissection is seen. Extracranial portion of the internal carotid artery shows a long, irregular string of contrast media from just above bifurcation to the base of the skull ("string sign") (*arrows*). The artery resumes normal caliber in the petrous bone. **B.** At operation, the typical enlarged bluish appearance of the artery was seen. Dissected intima and thrombus were removed by placing a Fogarty catheter in the true lumen. Postoperative angiogram shows normal restoration of bloodflow through dilated artery (*arrows*).

been demonstrated in cases of both traumatic and spontaneous dissection.[3a,13a,30,35]

Clinical Manifestations

The average age of patients with dissection is in the mid 40s, considerably younger than that of patients with stroke due to atherosclerosis.[15,20,30] Approximately two-thirds of the patients are male. Hypertension is present in only a small number.

The history of headache and unilateral facial pain followed by transient ischemic attacks (TIAs) or neurologic deficit is highly suggestive of the diagnosis, and the findings of oculosympathetic palsy add further support to this impression.[15,20,30] The pain has been described as constant and nonthrobbing but fluctuating in intensity. In some patients there is scalp tenderness.[32] The period of evolution of symptoms leading to the diagnosis is relatively short compared with patients having atherosclerosis, usually being under 10 days.[15,32]

In a report of 16 patients where the diagnosis of carotid dissection was definite or highly likely, 11 had TIAs, 10 had headache or facial pain, and 8 noted a subjective bruit.[15] At the time of the initial examination, only 3 of the 16 patients reported by Fisher et al were hemiplegic or aphasic; 4 had a slight hemiparesis or monoparesis; 6 had a normal neurologic examination except for oculosympathetic palsy (miosis and ptosis); and in 3 the examination was normal.[10] Subsequently, Mokri et al reported 5 patients who had angiographic changes suggestive of internal carotid dissection and in whom the initial clinical manifestations were unilateral head and face pain associated with ipsilateral oculosympathetic paresis.[32]

The unilateral head pain is presumably due to the direct effect of the arterial dissection on pain receptors within the wall of the artery.[32] Oculosympathetic palsy is presumed to be due to involvement of sympathetic fibers that accompany the internal carotid artery.

Angiographic Findings

Diagnosis is usually established by angiography except where complete occlusion has occurred. Characteristic findings that have been noted include a long irregular narrowing beginning above the carotid bifurcation in the neck and extending throughout much of the extracranial course of the internal carotid artery which has been called the "string sign" (Fig. 11.1A, 11.3); a distal internal carotid pouch occurring between C2 and the base of the skull (Fig. 11.2); a proximal internal carotid pouch and a double lumen.[1,14,15,19,36] Long carotid dissections may be combined with short dissection pouches (Fig. 11.3).

In the report of a single case of spontaneous carotid dissection, it was pointed out that the long stenotic segment of the cervical internal carotid artery (the "string sign") seen on angiography might be a reliable indication of carotid dissection.[36] Subsequently, 22 cases of dissection of the cervicocerebral arteries were reported, and in 16 patients angiography demonstrated a long narrow column of contrast material.[15] In another report 11 of 19 patients showed this finding.[14] The "string sign" is the result of the dissecting hemorrhage compressing the natural lumen. If differs markedly from the short stenotic lesion of atherosclerosis and rarely occurs with other types of occlusive cerebrovascular disease.[15] These long dissections usually extend to the base of the skull without entering the petrous canal, but there are exceptions. In one case the dissection involved only this portion of the artery.[19]

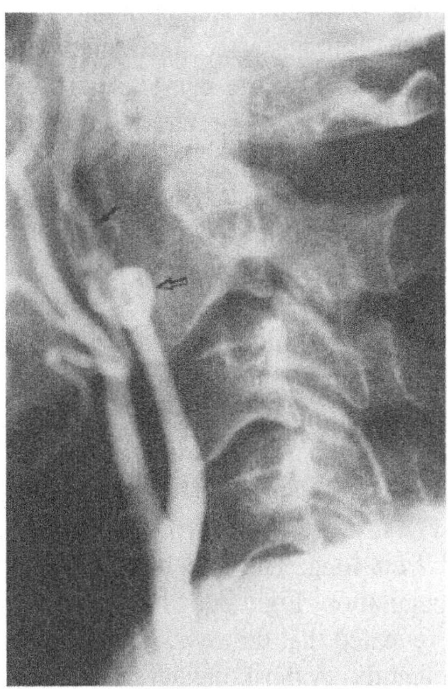

Figure 11.2. Another angiographic finding in carotid dissection is a localized aneurysmal sac or outpouching at level of C2 (*open arrow*). Just above the sac is an irregular narrowing of internal carotid artery (*black arrow*).

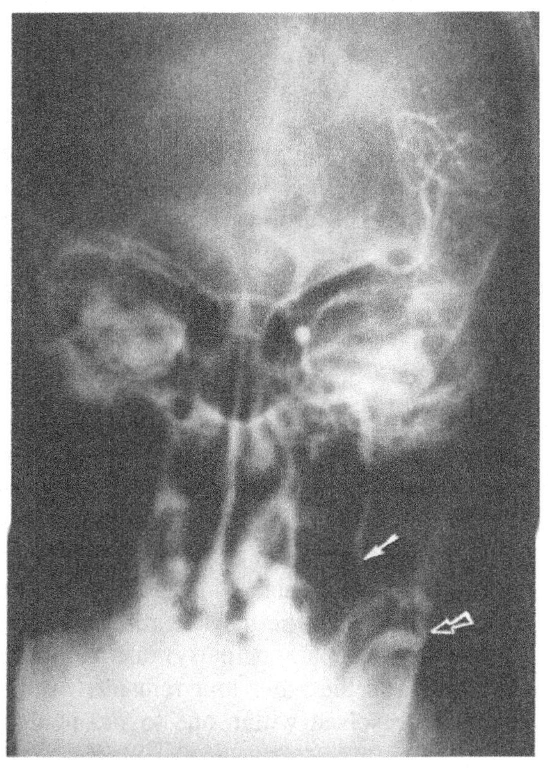

Figure 11.3. Localized aneurysmal sac (*open arrow*) in proximal internal carotid artery with the long, irregular narrowing to the base of the skull (*white arrow*). ▷

Another distinctive angiographic finding in carotid dissection is a localized aneurysmal sac or out-pouching on the cervical portion of the internal carotid artery between C2 and the base of the skull (Fig. 11.2). The case of Hardin et al[21] was proved at surgery and that of Bostrom and Liliequest[7] at autopsy. Similar pouches in the distal internal carotid artery have been described frequently in traumatic carotid dissection, and it is possible that this finding means the lesion was, in fact, traumatic in origin.[45,46]

Fisher et al in case 7, described another angiographic finding in a patient who had serial angiograms.[15] When first studied because of recent TIAs, there was a typical carotid "string sign" 7 cm long. The patient was treated with anticoagulation. Eight days later another angiogram revealed that the residual lumen had widened slightly. A third angiogram seven months later showed full restoration of the lumen. At the site of the proximal end of the previous narrowing, there was an oval-shaped sac or pouch measuring 10 × 4 mm. Possibly, the occasional puzzling, small sac of this type seen on the proximal internal carotid artery represents a healed dissection.

In some cases the internal carotid artery has become totally occluded. In these patients the occlusion usually begins 2 cm or more distal to the origin of the internal carotid artery with a gradual taper of the vessel proximal to the occlusion. There is usually no evidence of atheroma in the cases studied at operation or autopsy. However, this type of carotid occlusion is not distinctive since intracranial occlusion of the distal internal carotid artery from any cause may be associated with retrograde thrombus extending into the neck and give the same angiographic picture.

Clinical Course and Treatment

In the early reports of spontaneous dissection, a high incidence of severe neurologic deficits was noted.[36] However, with increased recognition of the problem, it has been reported that many cases will have a benign clinical course.[15,17] In five patients where the only neurologic finding was an oculosympathetic palsy, one had a major stroke and the other four remained well.[32] Headache resolved within one to six months, but the oculosympathetic palsy was still present in four of the five patients several months later. Resolution of the angiographic abnormality has been reported in several patients.[17,18,30,35]

Experience to date would indicate that those patients who are recovering from a neurologic deficit, have only TIAs or who have no cerebral neurologic symptoms can be effectively treated with anticoagulation.[12,15,17,30,31] This was illustrated in case 7 of Fisher et al.[15] The patient was treated with heparin intravenously. No more symptoms were noted, and the arterial lumen increased and became nearly normal on follow-up angiography. Two cases of dissection occurring following pregnancy have also been treated with anticoagulation with good results.[12] How long the anticoagulation should be continued has not been established, but the use of heparin for 10 to 14 days followed by warfarin sodium for at least three months seems a reasonable program. In a report of two patients, antiplatlet therapy was followed by cessation of TIAs and angiographic demonstration of resolution of occlusion.[38]

When the patient has an acute progressing or fluctuating neurologic deficit or symptoms recur despite medical therapy, surgical treatment may be indicated. Surgical treatments that have been used include endarterectomy, resection and insertion of a graft, use of a balloon catheter, carotid ligation, and STA-MCA bypass graft.

At operation the internal carotid artery is often enlarged and has a bluish appearance. This finding is characteristic for a dissection. The use of a balloon catheter at the time of operation to remove the dissected intima has been described in two cases.[35,36] The angiograms of a patient who presented with a fluctuating neurologic deficit are illustrated in Figs. 11.1A,B. Direct resection of the area of pathology followed by insertion of a graft has been described, with exposure being aided by osteotomy of the mandible.[21,48] Removal of the dissected intima and subintimal thrombus has also been done without division of the mandible by direct exposure and primary closure without a patch.[10,40] Postoperative angiography was reported to show good restoration of flow.

Bypass surgery with anastomosis of the superficial temporal artery to middle cerebral artery branch has been used in a few patients with TIAs or with severely compromised cerebral circulation due to bilateral dissection.[32]

Spontaneous Dissection—Vertebral and Intracranial Arteries

Dissection has been reported to involve the vertebral artery and all major intracranial branches. Reported dissections of intracranial arteries have been summarized in 1971[26,41], in 1977,[49] and in 1979.[1]

The middle cerebral artery has been the most frequent site of intracranial involvement reported.[26,41,43] Alexander et al listed the internal carotid, middle cerebral, and basilar arteries as the most common sites, and reports of involvement of the vertebral, posterior cerebral, and anterior cerebral arteries were also noted.[1]

Pathogenesis

Examination of the wall of the artery shows the dissection with associated thrombus to be either circumferential or eccentric. It is usually between the intima and media but may be located within either of these layers.[1,22,49]

Discussion of the pathogenesis includes consideration of trauma, congenital medical defects, atherosclerotic changes in the wall, fibromuscular dysplasia, arteritis, infection, and homocystinuria.[1,19,22,25,49] Cystic medial necrosis has rarely been found.[1] Usually, a definite cause cannot be conclusively demonstrated. In the pathologic examination of a case of middle cerebral dissection, Chang et al[11] found splitting, fraying, disintegration, and irregular thickening of the elastic lamina; but similar, although less severe, changes were seen in two other patients without dissection. Hochberg et al[22] could not trace the dissection process to any specific cause in their detailed examination of a case of middle cerebral dissection.

Clinical Manifestations

The onset of symptoms is most common in young adults.[1,26,41] The age of reported patients has ranged from 6 months to 69 years.[1] The majority of cases were between 15 and 35 years old.[26] Several reports of spontaneous middle cerebral dissection have included a number of patients under 20 years of age.[11,15,22,25] No sex predominance has been noted.

Usually frequent and severe headache is a prominent symptom.[42] A detailed analysis of clinical reports of intracranial dissection containing sufficient data revealed that 19 of 20 cases had headache, often severe, and in supratentorial dissections, localized to the side of the involved artery.[49]

The onset of neurologic symptoms is variable, but an acute severe neurologic deficit due to infarction usually develops.[26,49] One patient with a dissection of the basilar artery had symptoms from compression of the pyramidal tracts and chronic subarachnoid hemorrhage before developing severe infarction.[1] In another case an intracerebral hematoma followed rupture of the vessel, and three other reports of such cases are noted.[37]

Angiography

Angiography usually shows either a narrowed or occluded artery.[1] The unusually long segmental narrowing ("string sign") has been seen in the vertebral, middle, and posterior cerebral arteries[15,22,25] (Fig. 11.4). A double lumen has been demonstrated.[26]

Treatment

Most patients with intracranial dissection have not survived. Bypass graft has been tried in some with stenosis and direct operation when there is SAH, but the results are poor.[35]

Traumatic Dissection

Pathogenesis

Dissection of the internal carotid artery and its branches can occur following nonpenetrating injury to the head and neck, direct injury to the artery, and percutaneous carotid angiography.[13,16,27,34,43–46] Nonpenetrating injury to the head and neck may cause an intimal tear in the cervical carotid vessels. The tear may lead to the development of a localized dissection or an-

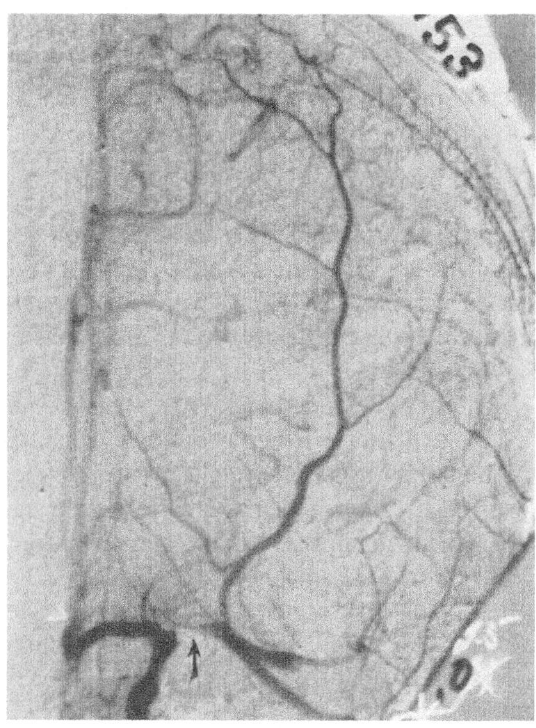

Figure 11.4. Dissection in middle cerebral artery with narrowing to a "string" for 8 mm from its origin (*arrow*). Artery then widens to normal diameter, but flow is markedly reduced in the middle cerebral territory. Large external carotid branch extends across middle cerebral artery.

eurysmal out-pouching.[11,12,21] Thrombus may be the source of cerebral emboli, and occlusion of the artery may develop.[11,50]

The most likely mechanism for production of this tear is the sudden severe stretch of the internal carotid artery over the upper cervical spine when the neck is hyperextended and laterally flexed to the opposite side.[11,12,21,50] The possible importance of atlantoid compression of the internal carotid artery was first recognized by Boldrey et al.[6] In their case 1, the patient had the onset of symptoms with head turning. Angiography showed a lesion at the C1 level and at operation (illustrated by a diagram) the gross findings were consistent with a dissection, although it was not recognized as such at the time.

The cases of intracranial dissection where trauma has been suggested have followed closed head injury without fracture.[22] Surgical trauma to the internal carotid artery during tonsillectomy and to the middle cerebral artery after ligation of an aneurysm has been reported as a cause of dissection.[45,46]

Clinical Manifestations

Traumatic dissection can produce the same picture as spontaneous dissection. The patient may present with a head injury with the initial diagnosis of cerebral concussion or contusion.

The interval between the trauma and onset of symptoms is variable. In the majority of patients symptoms occur within 24 hours of the trauma[3] however long symptom free intervals may occur. In the six cases reported by Stringer and Kelly, three developed rapid deterioration in neurologic status within three hours.[45] In one, the onset of symptoms was eight days. Another developed TIA two weeks after an accident. The last patient was well until one year after recovery from a serious head injury when he developed a stroke due to an embolus from the area of dissection and aneurysmal formation.

Symptoms in patients with intracranial dissection may be acute or delayed.[1] Hollin et al reviewed the reported cases of posttraumatic middle cerebral occlusion including those where dissection had been demonstrated at autopsy.[23] The interval between trauma and onset of symptoms varied from a few hours to several days.

Angiography

When a patient with a history of trauma develops neurologic symptoms and the computed tomography (CT) scan is normal, angiography is needed to help establish a diagnosis. It is also imperative that adequate views of both the head and the neck be obtained.

When nonpentrating trauma to the head and neck cause arterial injury, the most common angiographic finding is internal carotid occlusion 1 to 3 cm above the bifurcation.[46] However, in some patients an intimal tear leads to development of a dissection.

In all of the patients reported by Stringer and Kelly, there was evidence of angiography abnormality between C2 and the base of the skull.[45] This consisted of a localized narrowing of the vessel and/or an aneurysmal out-pouching. Another important finding was that in four of the six patients there was evidence of intracranial emboli. Follow-up angiograms were done in four of the six patients in their series. These studies showed that none of the dissections progressed to complete occlusion: one had disappeared. In three the ipsilateral false aneurysm had enlarged, and in three an aneurysmal out-pouching in the opposite, asymptomatic, internal carotid artery was seen and had not been demonstrated on the initial angiographic study. These aneurysmal sacs may remain unchanged for several years, or they may spontaneously thrombus.[45,46] In both circumstances the patient usually remains asymptomatic.

Clincial Course and Treatment

The natural history of the illness is unknown. However, the findings of Stringer and Kelly suggest that the problem may, as with spontaneous dissection, be a more benign process than originally thought.[45] All six of their patients were treated medically and had an uncomplicated course. Anticoagulation was used when emboli were demonstrated and there was no complication from this therapy. Zelenock et al[41] treated one patient with antiplatlet drugs and another with heparin and warfarin sodium and both made a good recovery. Four patients had surgery; in two the internal carotid artery was gradually occluded, one had an aneurysmorrhaphy and one an STA-MCA bypass.

References

1. Alexander CB, Burger PC, Goree JA: Dissecting aneurysms of the basilar artery in 2 patients. Stroke 10:294–298, 1979
2. Anderson RMcD, Schechter MM: A case of spontaneous dissecting aneurysm of the internal carotid artery. J Neurol Neurosurg Psychiatry 22:195–201, 1959
3. Bergguist BJ, Boone SC, Whaley RA: Traumatic dissection of the internal carotid artery treated by ECIC anastomosis. Stroke 12:73–76, 1981
4. Bigelow NH: Intracranial dissecting aneurysm. An analysis of their significance. Arch Pathol 60:271–275, 1955
5. Bladin PF: Dissecting aneurysm of carotid and vertebral arteries. Vasc Surg 8:203–223, 1974
6. Boldrey E, Maass L, Miller E: The role of atlantoid compression in the etiology of internal carotid thrombosis. J Neurosurg 13:127–139, 1956
7. Bostrom K, Liliequest B: Primary dissecting aneurysm of the extracranial part of the internal carotid and vertebral arteries. Neurology 17:170–186, 1967
8. Brice J, Cromptom MR: Spontaneous dissecting aneurysm of the cervical internal carotid artery. Br Med J 2:790–792, 1964
9. Brown OL, Armitage JL: Spontaneous dissecting aneurysms of the cervical internal carotid artery: Two case reports and a survey of the literature. Am J Roentgenol 118:648–653, 1973
10. Burklund CW: Spontaneous dissecting aneurysm of the cervical carotid artery: A report of surgical treatment in two patients. Johns Hopkins Med J 126:154–159, 1970
11. Chang V, Rewcastle NB, Harwood-Nash DCF, Norman MD: Bilateral dissecting aneurysms of the intracranial internal carotid arteries in an 8 year old boy. Neurology 25:573–570, 1975
12. Dagi RF, Beal MF, Brem S, Welch J, Ojemann RG, Poletti CE: Internal carotid artery dissection after pregnancy. (To be published)
13. Dratz H, Woodhall B: Traumatic dissecting aneurysm of left internal carotid, anterior cerebral and middle cerebral arteries. J Neuropathol Exp Neurol 6:286–291, 1947
14. Ehrenfeld WK, Wylie EJ: Spontaneous dissection of the internal carotid artery. Arch Surg 111:1294–1301, 1976
15. Fisher CM, Ojemann RG, Roberson GH: Spontaneous dissection of cervico-cerebral arteries. Can J Neurol Sci 5:9–19, 1978
16. Fleming JFR, Park AM: Dissecting aneurysms of the carotid artery following arteriography. Neurology 9:1–6, 1959
17. Friedman WA, Day AL, Quisling BG, Sypert GW, Rhoton Al Jr: Cervical carotid dissecting aneurysms. Neurosurgery 7:207–214, 1980
18. Gee W, Kaupp HA, McDonald KM, Lin FZ, Curry JL: Spontaneous dissection of the internal carotid arteries. Spontaneous resolution documented by serial ocular pneumoplathymography and angiography. Arch Surg 115:944–999, 1980
19. Giedke H, Kriebel J, Sindermann F: Dissecting aneurysm of the petrous portion of the internal carotid artery. Case report and review of previous cases. Neuroradiology 10:121–124, 1975
20. Greiner AL: Spontaneous dissecting aneurysms of the cervical internal carotid artery. Stroke 7:6
21. Hardin CA, Snodgrass RG: Dissecting aneurysms of internal carotid artery treated by fenestration and graft. Surgery 55:207–209, 1964
22. Hochberg FH, Bean CS, Fisher CM, Roberson GH: Stroke in a 16 year old girl secondary to

terminal carotid dissection. Neurology 25:725–729, 1975
23. Hollin SA, Sukoff MD, Silverstein A, Gross SW: Post-traumatic middle cerebral artery occlusion. J Neurosurg 25:526–535, 1966
24. Jentzer AA: Dissecting aneurysm of left internal carotid artery. Angiology 5:232–234, 1954
25. Johnson AC, Graves VB, Pfaff JP Jr: Dissecting aneurysm of intracranial arteries. Surg Neurol 7:49–51, 1977
26. Kunze ST, Schiefer W: Angiographic demonstration of a dissecting aneurysm of the middle cerebral artery. Neuroradiology 2:201–206, 1971
27. Lai MD, Hoffman HB, Adamkiewicz JJ: Dissecting aneurysm of internal carotid artery after non-penetrating neck injury. Case report. Acta Radiol 5:290–295, 1966
28. Liliequist B: The roentgenologic appearance of spontaneous dissecting aneurysm of the cervical internal carotid artery: Report of a case. Vasc Surg 2:223–226. 1968
29. Lloyd F, Bahnson HT: Bilateral dissecting aneurysms of the internal carotid arteries. Am J Surg 122:549–551, 1971
30. Luken MG, Ascherl GF Jr, Correll JW, Hilal SK: Spontaneous dissecting aneurysms of the extracranial internal carotid artery. Clin Neurosurg 26:353–375, 1979
31. McNeill DH Jr, Dreisbach J, Marsden RJ: Spontaneous dissection of the internal carotid artery. Arch Neurol 37:54–55, 1980
32. Mokri B, Sundt TM Jr, Houser OW: Spontaneous internal carotid dissection, hemicrania and Horner's syndrome. Arch Neurol 36:677–680, 1979
33. New PFJ, Momose KJ: Traumatic dissection of the internal carotid artery of the atlantoaxial level, secondary to non-penetrating injury. Radiology 93:41–49, 1969
34. Northcroft GB, Morgan AD: A fatal case of traumatic thrombosis of the internal carotid artery. Br J Surg 32:105–107, 1944
35. Ojemann RG, Crowell RM: Surgical Management of Cerebrovascular Disease. Williams and Wilkins, Baltimore, 1983 pp 111–121
36. Ojemann RG, Fisher CM, Rich JC: Spontaneous dissecting aneurysm of the internal carotid artery. Stroke 3:434–440, 1972
37. Pilz P, Hartjes HJ: Fibromuscular dysplasia and multiple dissecting aneurysms of intracranial arteries. A further cause of moyomoya syndrome. Stroke 7:393–398, 1976
38. Pozzati E, Gaist G, Popp M: Resolution of occlusion in spontaneously dissected carotid arteries. Report of two cases. J Neurosurg 56:857–860, 1982
39. Ringel SO, Harrison SH, Norenberg MD, Austin JH: Fibromuscular dysplasia: Multiple "spontaneous" dissecting aneurysms of the major cervical arteries. Ann Neurol 1:301–304, 1976
40. Roome NS Jr, Aberfeld DC: Spontaneous dissecting aneurysm of the internal carotid artery. Arch Neurol 34:251–252, 1977
41. Sato O, Bascom JF, Logothetis J: Intracranial dissecting aneurysm. Case report. J Neurosurg 35:483–487, 1971
42. Scott GE, Neubueger KT, Donst J: Dissecting aneurysms of intercranial arteries. Neurology (Minneap) 10:22–27, 1960
43. Sirois J, Lapointe H, Cote PE: Unusual local complication of percutaneous cerebral angiography. J Neurosurg 11:112–116, 1954
44. Spudis EV, Scharyj M, Alexander E, Martin JF: Dissecting aneurysm in the head and neck. Neurology 12:867–875, 1962
45. Stringer WL, Kelly DL: Traumatic dissections of the extracranial internal carotid artery. Neurosurgery (To be published).
46. Sullivan HG, Vines FS, Becker DP: Sequelae of indirect internal carotid injury. Radiology 109:91–98, 1973
47. Thapedi IM, Ashenhurst EM, Rozkilsky B: Spontaneous dissecting aneurysm of the internal carotid artery in the neck: Report of a case and review of the literature. Arch Neurol 23:549–554, 1970
48. Wylie EF, Ehrenfeld WK: Extracranial occlusive cerebrovascular disease. WB Saunders Co, Philadelphia, 1970, pp 48, 192
49. Yonas H, Agamanolis D, Takaoka Y, White RJ: Dissecting intracranial aneurysms. Surg Neurol 8:407–415, 1977
50. Zelencok GB, Kazmers A, Whitehouse WM Jr, Graham LM, Erlandson EE, Cronenwett JL, Lindenauer SM, Stanley JC: Extracranial internal carotid artery dissections. Noniatrogenic traumatic lesions. Arch Surg 117:425–432, 1982

Portions of this chapter are reprinted with permission from Ojemann RG, Crowell RM: Surgical Management of Cerebrovascular Disease. Williams and Wilkins, Baltimore, 1983.

12

Vertebral Artery Insufficiency and Cervical Spondylosis

Chikao Nagashima

Introduction

Because of their deep location and the protection afforded by overlying bone, surgical treatment of lesions of the vertebral arteries is a relatively recent event in the annals of medical history. It was as late as 1836 that Sanson of the Paris Faculty declared that the vertebral arteries were so hidden and inaccessible that "they were beyond the reach of surgery."[17]

It was first described by Matas that a traumatic aneurysm of upper vertebral artery was successfully operated on in July 1888.[16] In World War II Elkin and Harris were able to accumulate 10 cases of traumatic arteriovenous fistula of the vertebral artery, the largest single series, which made an outstanding contribution to the surgical history of the vertebral artery.[8]

Surgery for spondylotic vertebral artery insufficiency developed later than that for trauma of the artery. It was in 1960 that the first case of surgical treatment for spondylotic vertebral artery insufficiency was reported by Hardin et al.[12] Hardin subsequently collected 15 such cases.[11] He used *lateral* extensive exploration of the cervical spine, from C2 to C6, and removed the anterior and posterior roots of the involved transverse processes with protection of the nerve roots. Eight of his patients showed complete reversal of symptoms, and the other seven were improved. Cases treated by anterior approach reported by Gortvai in 1964[9] and Keggi et al in 1966[15] indicated the feasibility of surgical treatment through the *anterior* approach. In 1964 Jung et al reported 12 cases treated by the removal of uncal osteophytes without emphasis of the importance of periarterial fibrosis.[14] Bakay and Leslie[2] in 1965 reported two patients with anterior fusion alone, anticipating future resolution of osteophytes. Both were symptomatically and arteriographically improved. Verbiest in 1968 treated two patients by removal of the anterior root of the transverse process as well as the uncovertebral osteophyte; interbody fusion was also performed in one of these cases, both with excellent results.[34] Cloward described a double trephine technique.[6]

This author developed his techniques from observations of cadavers with displaced vertebral arteries due to severe osteophytes in the uncinate portion of the vertebrae in 1966. The ease with which those uncal osteophytes could be exposed and removed through the anterior approach with excision of the longus colli muscle lead the author to develop a simple method of uncectomy. Even after the uncectomy the vertebral artery was still kinked owing to marked perivascular fibrosis with evidence of chronic irritation of the vertebral nerves. The author therefore advocated excision of the fibrosis, including the adventitia and periarterial vertebral nerve, following unroofing of the transverse foramina at two levels above and below the interspace, so that the artery could be adequately freed and straightened. The vertebrae were not fused.

Since 1967 this method had been successfully performed in 20 consecutive cases, and the results were published in 1970.[19] Pathophysiologic responses produced by (1) reduced blood flow through the vertebral artery and by (2) electrical stimulation of the periarterial vertebral nerves as well as the stellate ganglion were subsequently investigated by the author and his associates in 1970 and 1972.[27,28] With the development of microsurgery, the author reported advantages with the use of microsurgical technique in achieving periarterial denervation in 1973.[20–22] These publications[24] and motion pictures[23] have served to popularize this operation. In 1975 Sullivan et al[33] described the first reported case of arteriographically demonstrated posterior cerebral artery occlusion with homonymous hemianopsia due secondary to embolus from a site of spondylotic vertebral artery compression. Use of decompression of the vertebral artery and periarterial stripping of fibrous ring with anterior cervical fusion resulted in restored circulation both through the vertebral and the posterior cerebral arteries. Pásztor from Hungary in 1978[29e] reported four cases totally relieved by removal of the constricting ring around the vertebral artery as well as the uncal osteophyte with the comment "this periarterial fibrotic tissue appears to play a role in the pathogenesis of symptoms." This discussion will concern itself primarily with the pathogenesis, symptoms, and diagnosis of the spondylotic vertebral artery insufficiency and surgical method employed to relieve them. Less frequently encountered, but vitally important from a treatment standpoint, are the arteriovenous fistula of the vertebral artery,[29] the arteriovenous malformation of cervical cord fed by the vertebral artery territories, and bypass procedure for treatment of vertebral artery occlusion.[29a] These lesions have also been effectively dealt with by this method.

Osteophytes Producing Vertebral Artery Compression

The term "cervical spondylosis" described chronic degenerative lesions of multiple or single cervical disks and consequent *osteophytosis* of related vertebral bodies.[4] Slow but progressive enlargement of the osteophyte may continue until it encroaches upon vital soft tissues adjacent to the spine, causing symptoms. At least three distinct and separate cervical spondylotic syndromes (Fig. 12.1) can be identified to include the following: (1) nerve root syndrome due to posterolateral or intraforaminal osteophyte, or to apophyseal osteoarthrosis encroaching on the intervertebral foramen from behind; (2) myelopathic syndrome due to marginal osteophyte compressing the spinal cord and anterior spinal arteries; and (3) vertebral neurovascular syndrome with arterial compression by the osteophyte and an irritation of the vertebral nerves. These osteophytes are classified into the following:

1. Uncovertebral or lateral osteophyte. The site of formation of the osteophyte is on the uncinate portion of the vertebrae (Fig. 12.2, C5), which in embryonic stages is the junction of the centrum and lateral masses and is also known as the neurocentral joint, Luschka's joint, and the uncovertebral joint. There is disagreement on whether this is a "true" joint or not. The osteophyte is clearly seen on plain anteroposterior spine x-ray as a lateral bony mass projecting from the vertebral bodies and compresses the vertebral artery and nerves laterally and dorsally (Figs. 12.3 and 12.4). By this type of osteophyte, narrowing of the lumen of the artery is increased by turning the head to the ispilateral side. (Fig. 12.5).
2. Apophyseal osteoarthrosis or proliferation of facet. This is less common. The site of formation of the osteophyte is on the apophyseal facets resulting in apophyseal osteoarthrosis or proliferation of the facet.[32] The disk degeneration and the apophyseal osteoarthrosis do not always occur at the same level. The latter affects the upper cervical spine predominantly (C3-4, C2-3, C4-5). Oblique projection showing the foramina is sometimes helpful in showing posterior foraminal encroachment. The vertebral artery is not displaced laterally but is displaced ventrally (Figs. 12.3, 12.4) and medially.

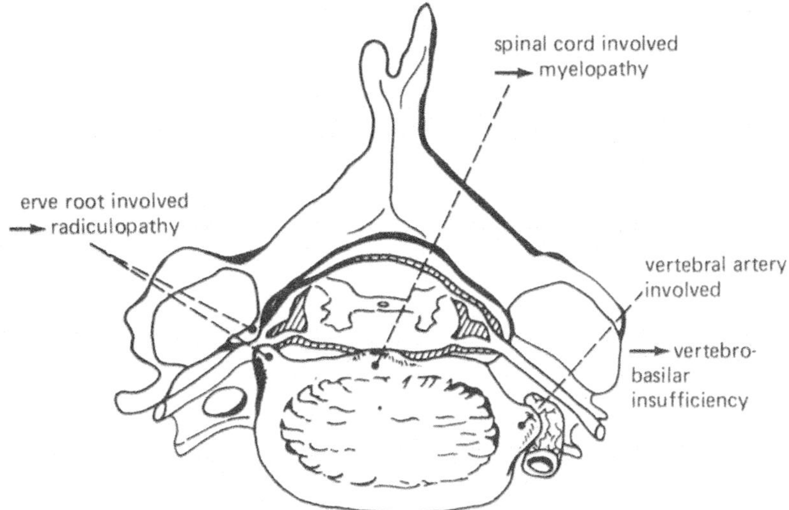

Figure 12.1. Three distinct and separate spondylotic syndromes produced by osteophytes located at various sites of vertebra. (From ref. Nagashima C[19]) with permission).

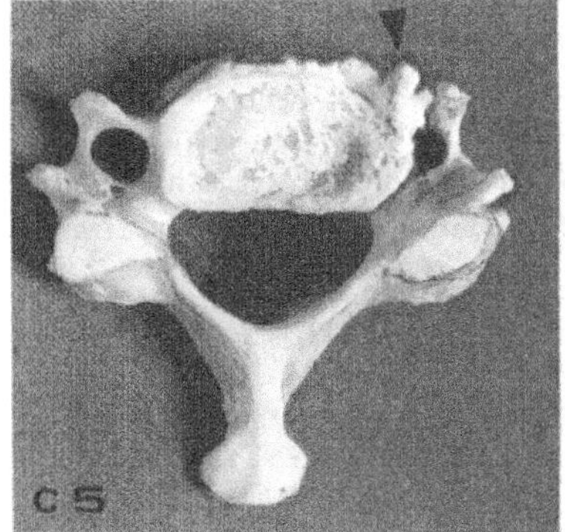

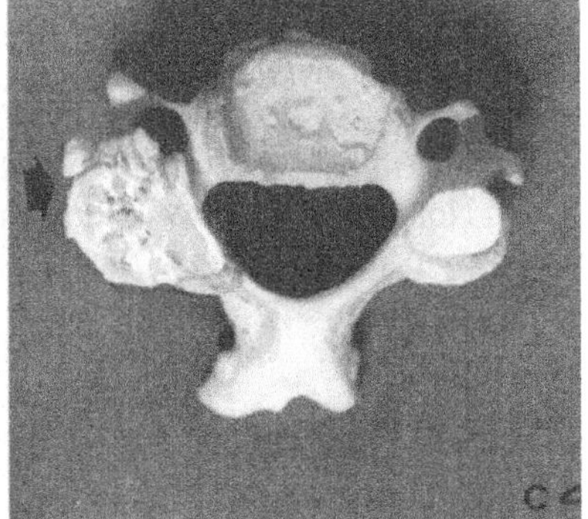

Figure 12.2. Cephalad aspects of C5 (*left*) and C4 (*right*). In C5 is shown the uncovertebral osteophyte (*small black arrowhead*) displacing vertebral artery laterally and ventrodorsally: in C4 the apophyseal osteoarthrosis (*large black arrowhead*) displacing vertebral artery dorsoventrally is shown.

Symptoms and Diagnosis

With advanced cerebrovascular atherosclerosis present, it is evident that cerebrovascular insufficiency can be precipitated by turning or hyperextending the neck. These maneuvers stretch or compress the vertebral artery and the vertebral nerves—anterior and posterior vertebral nerves—reducing vertebral blood flow and irritating the vertebral nerves. The symptoms and signs are episodic and are characterized by their reversibility in early stages. At this stage they are amenable to treatment, although repeated attacks tend to culminate in progressive irreversible damage to the brainstem, cerebellum, occipital and temporal lobes. In fact, more than 35% of patients with vertebrobasilar insufficiency developed a cerebral infarction in five years,[4b] and approximately 80% of patients with infarction of the posterior circulation experienced symptoms of vertebrobasilar insufficiency, with a mean of seven to eight weeks of symptoms prior to infarction.[8a] Early diagnosis and treatment should be stressed. The author reported the clinical data of 20 consecutive cases of this syndrome in 1970.[19a] Subsequently, 13 years of experience confirmed that many of the symptoms are apt to be misinterpreted as functional or psychosomatic in origin when the pathology is not understood and no treatment was attempted before irreversible neurologic damage develops.

The early and most common complaint is the episodes of rotatory vertigo or dizziness that occur in approximately 95% of patients with this syndrome. The dizziness was not a sensation of rotation but rather a feeling of unsteadiness, floating, lifting upward, or of sinking

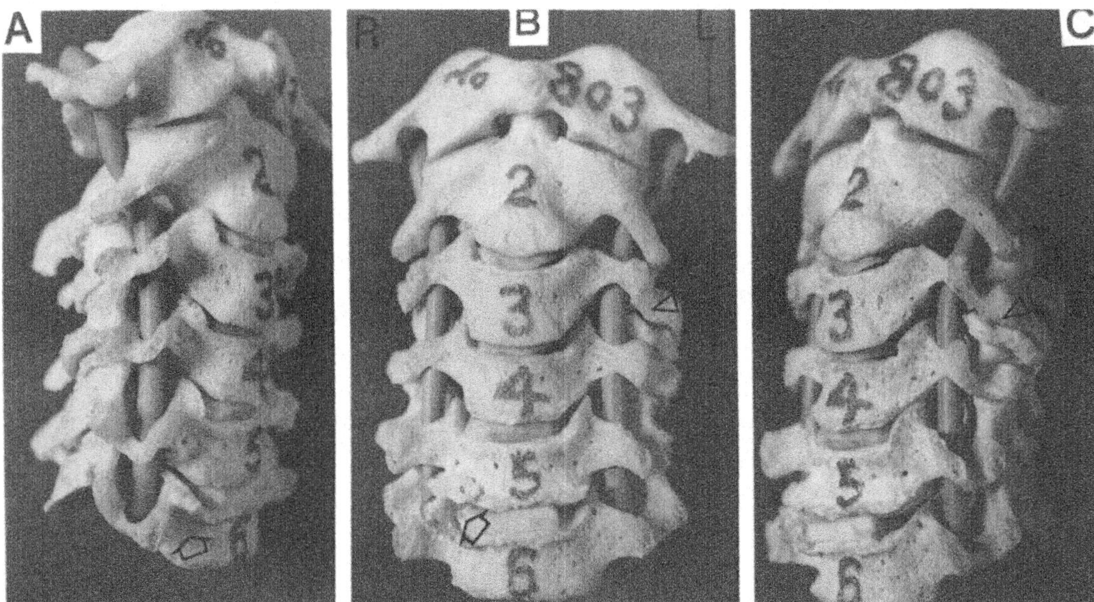

Figure 12.3. Reconstructed cervical spine by passing a Nelaton catheter through each transverse foramen, imitating the vertebral artery. **B** shows anterior aspect with uncovertebral or lateral osteophyte at C5–6 (*right, large open arrowhead*), and the apophyseal osteoarthrosis at C3–4 (*left, small open arrowhead*). Note that the uncovertebral osteophyte projects from medial to the lateral, whereas the apophyseal osteoarthrosis projects from lateral to the medial in direction. **A** shows right lateral aspect of the spine. The C5–6 uncovertebral osteophyte projects backward (*large open arrowhead*) **C** shows left lateral aspect of the spine. The C3–4 apophyseal osteoarthrosis projects ventrally from behind (*small open arrowhead*).

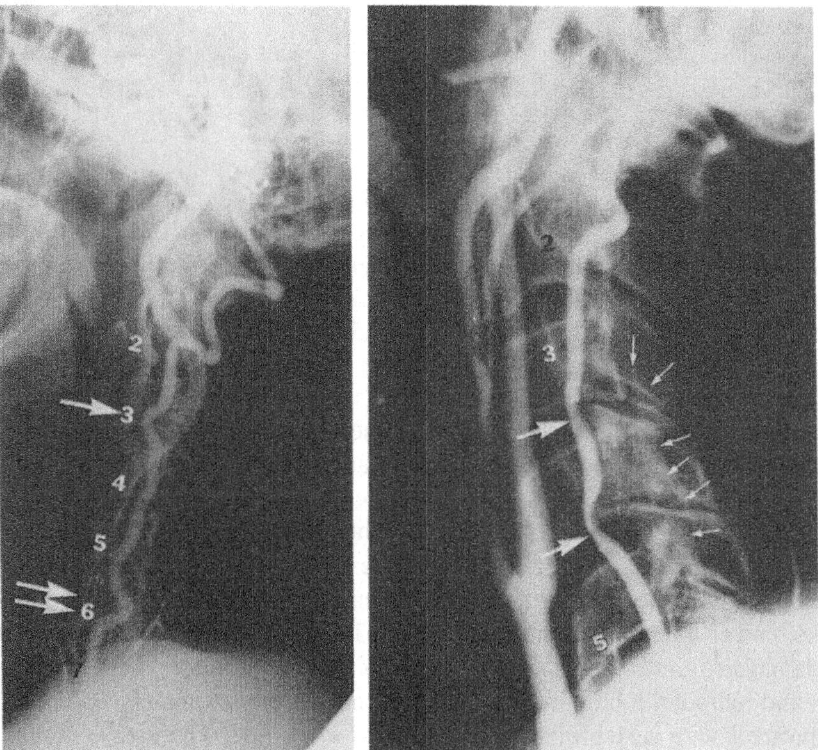

Figure 12.4. Lateral vertebral arteriograms. The artery is displaced ventrally (*single white arrows*) by dorsally-placed apophyseal osteoarthrosis; whereas the artery is displaced dorsally (*double-white-arrow*) by ventrally-placed uncovertebral osteophyte (see Figs. 12.1 and 12.2).

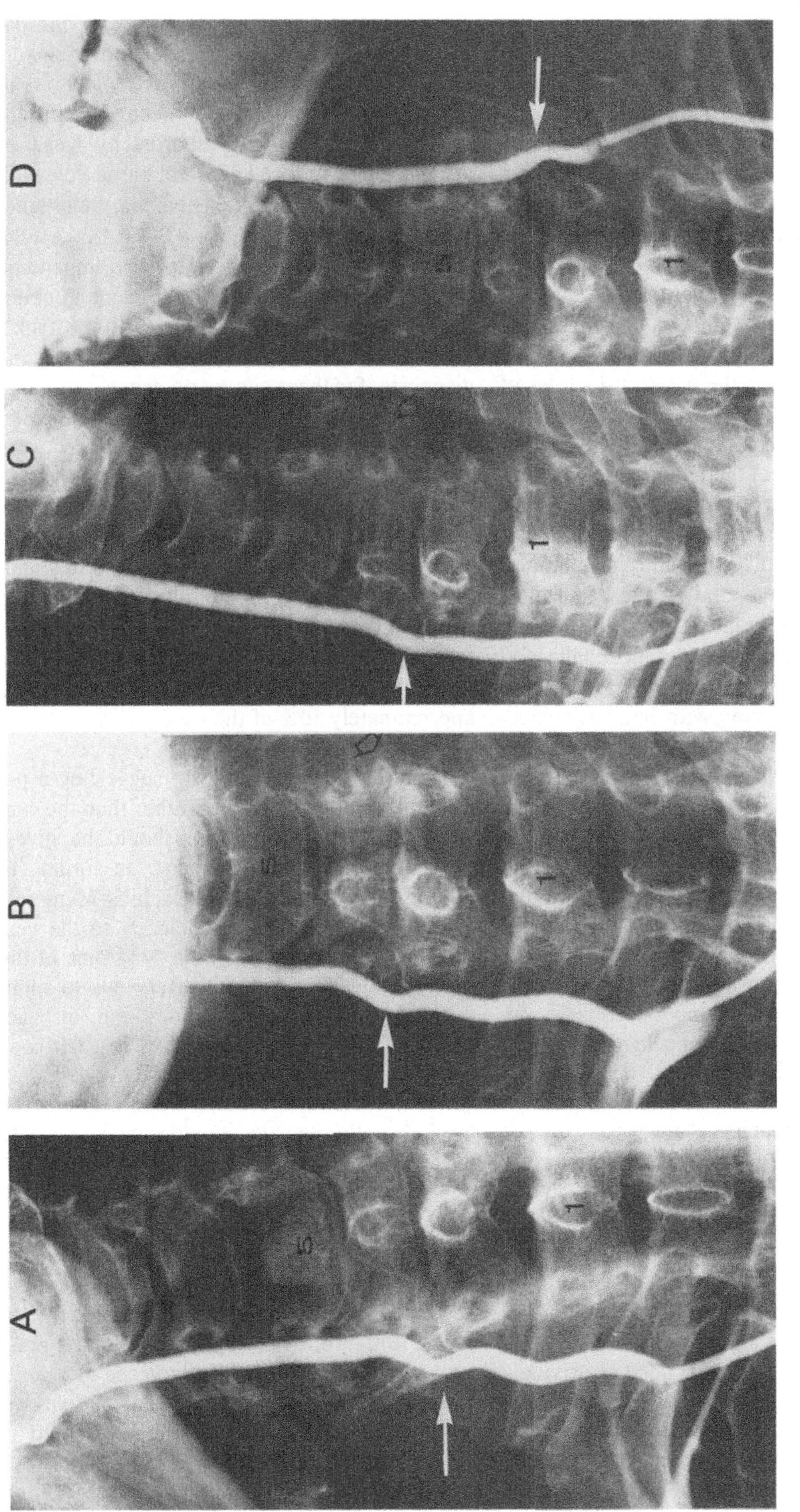

Figure 12.5. A 55-year-old male with bilateral narrowings of the vertebral arteries due to bilateral lateral osteophytes at C6–7. Right vertebral arteriograms by Seldinger technique (**A**, **B**, **C**) taken with head in neutral position, **B**, rotation to the right, **A**, and rotation to the left, **C**. Narrowing of the artery by the osteophyte (*white arrow*) is markedly increased by turning the head to the ispilateral side, **A**. *Open arrowheads* in **B** and **C** indicate C6–7 osteophyte on the left. The left arteriogram with head turned to the left also showed narrow vertebral artery compressed by the osteophyte (*white arrow*).

downward. The episodes are not merely an isolated symptom, but are frequently found in association with visual symptoms, altered consciousness, drop attack, cerebellar dysfunction, and others such as headache, motor and sensory phenomena but seldom tinnitus or auditory loss. A common association is that of vertigo resulting from pontine ischemia with blurring of vision, scintillating scotoma (either black or white, or in color), horizontal or vertical oscillopsia, macropsia or micropsia, transient amblyopia, and, less commonly, hemianopic field defects of transient type. This coincidence can be explained upon the basis of disorder of basilar system, which consists of not only the whole of the brainstem, including the diencephalon, but also much of the temporal and occipital lobes. Taking into consideration that termination of the basilar artery in the posterior cerebral arteries involves the anterior temporal arteries, posterior temporal arteries, and mesencephalic thalamic branches as well, the temporal lobe syndrome—the mesencephalic and thalamic syndrome of an elaborate kind—may also occur in association with brainstem ischemia. For instance with grand mal type of epilepsy which we frequently observe in cases of severe vertebro-basilar insufficiency, is due to centroencephalic discharges secondary to brain stem ischemia. In addition, ischemia involving temporal lobe, mesencephalon and the thalamus produces symptoms referable to the locations. Therefore, the symptoms mentioned below are combined; sensation of déjà-vu, jamais vu, depersonalization—temporal lobe symptoms, auditory or visual hallucinations—temporal lobe, occipital lobe, and the thalamus, spontaneous facial pain—thalamus. Transient global amnesia,[8b] which is thought to be due to vascular insufficiency involving the hippocampal-fornices-mammillary system,[29f] could be noted. Nagashima[25] recently observed it during the acute attack. It is characterized by a sudden loss of recent memory lasting hours and is associated with retrograde amnesia. During the attack, patients usually appear quiet and alert and are able to continue such functions as driving a car, cooking, and business activity. Psychologic amnesia should not be confused with transient amnesia. Psychologic amnesia occurs in a younger age group (under 50); falls within a clear psychologic situation, e.g., death of a loved one; and involves loss of memory for distant events of a personal nature, e.g., the patient's name, address, and telephone number. Loss of this kind of memory is extremely rare in organic disease and does not occur in transient global amnesia.[29d] EEG reported by Keggi et al,[15] indicated reduced cerebral blood flow with the patient in hyperextension and semi-erect position.

Some clouding of consciousness, impending fainting, and true syncope will occur in about two-thirds of the attacks. The "drop attack" must be considered as highly important in the diagnosis, for there can be no cause other than ischemia in the region of pyramidal decussation for the sudden fall of a patient who recovers himself as soon as he reaches the ground and then picks himself up unaided. A feature of "drop attack" is that it happens particularly in elderly females, seems to be confined to standing still and walking, more out of doors than at home, and occurs without warning. The patient falls with the knee flexed and tends to bruise the knees, the chin, or the hands.[35] This was noted approximately 10% of the cases in the author's series.

Tinnitus and auditory loss, suggesting a peripheral vestibular disorder rather than the central vestibular dysfunction, should be investigated by a neuro-otologist in order to differentiate it from vertigo such as Ménière's disease.[33a,b] Vascular insufficiency to the vestibular end-organ, seen in the syndrome of the anterior inferior cerebellar artery due to spondylotic vertebral artery compression, may accompany tinnitus and auditory loss. It was found in 5% in my series.

These episodes are elicited upon turning the head abruptly over the shoulder or when backing a car, causing embarrassment of the flow in one vertebral artery, or on extending the neck not only in looking up, but in looking horizontally while working at a desk, or on changing postures. They occur especially on arising from bed early in the morning and during micturition owing to the reflex fall in systemic blood pressure which results from an increase in vesical pressure.[35] Orthostatic hypotension is an important precipitating factor and was noted in 10% of the author's series.

Another important precipitating factor, unrelated to position or time of day, is *optic stimuli.*

The oculomotor system, including vestibular nuclei, medial longitudinal fasciculus, and ocular nuclei, is particularly sensitive to brainstem ischemia.[28] Some patients with previous attacks of dizziness or vertigo may have impairments of brainstem oculomotor control. In such instances, observation of moving objects, such as counting cars running on the street, may produce abrupt dimming, graying, or de-focusing of the eyes, followed by nausea and a faintness sensation, which causes the patient to momentarily stop what he is doing or lose his equilibrium function. Blurring is often described as a "gray-out of vision," "a sensation of looking through fog or smoke." These episodes of bilateral blurring should be differentiated from monocular blackout of vision (amaurosis fugax) associated with carotid insufficiency.[13]

Neurologic Signs

The most commonly observed neurologic signs are the positive Romberg, impaired tandem gait, and vertical or diagonal nystagmus seen through the Frenzel glass during the positioning tests of Dix and Hallpike[7] and Stenger.[30] It has been suggested that this kind of nystagmus indicates vestibular disorder of a central nature,[5,7] thus, it is very important to differentiate it from the vertigo due to a peripheral disorder of the vestibular end-organ such as Ménière's disease and the positional nystagmus of a benign paroximal type.[5,33a,33b] The Romberg's sign becomes more marked on rotating the neck. Cranial nerve paresis was noted in 30% of my series involving nerves V, VII, VIII, IX, X, and XII.

Pyramidal tract signs of hemiparesis and unilateral hyperreflexia with contralateral cranial nerve paresis of nerves VII, IX, and XII were noted, thus far, in only one patient. Alternating involvement of the motor or sensory system on one side and then the contralateral side,[18] was seen in 40% of my series. This is interpreted as due to intermittent basilar artery insufficiency. The common neurologic feature of this syndrome consists of fluctuating, transitional findings that produce the complex symptoms. In the author's experience, designations of vascular brainstem syndromes according to specific conducing arteries are inappropriate in this syndrome. However, the isolated homonymous hemianopsia of sudden onset is the hallmark of a vascular lesion in the occipital lobe, and this was to have occurred secondary to microembolus from a site of spondylotic vertebral artery compression.[33] The authors recently experienced a case of complete obstruction of one vertebral artery by large uncinate osteophyte (Fig. 12.6), owing to probable intimal injury, aggregation of platelets, and subsequent information of thrombus obliterated the lumen.[26]

It should be emphasized that objective neurologic signs in the vertebrobasilar system are the products of ischemic lesions situated in the brainstem, cerebellum, thalamus, and occipitotemporal lobes. Spondylotic vertebral artery insufficiency seldom produces fixed neurologic deficit but rather episodic symptoms without sequelae. The majority of cases (70%) do not demonstrate abnormal neurologic signs, except positive Romberg and positional nystagmus seen through the Frenzel glass. The latter is the most sensitive test in evaluating vestibular dysfunction of a central nature. As a consequence, neurologists and neurosurgeons should bear in mind that the diagnosis of spondylotic vertebral artery insufficiency must frequently be made on historical evidence and in the absence of clinical neurologic signs. Repeat and careful examinations, including nystagmus through Frenzel glass, especially during and after the attacks, may lead to correct diagnosis. The unicate osteophyte in cervical spine x-ray may be the only objective finding that substantiates the syndrome.

Cervical Radiculopathy and Myelopathy

Cervical radiculopathy due to spondylosis was noted in approximately 15%; cervical myelopathy was not encountered in my series.

Roentogenographic Investigation

The lateral bony mass protruding from the lateral aspect of the vertebral body—i.e., the uncal, uncovertebral, or lateral osteophyte—is obvious in the plain anteroposterior x-ray (Figs. 12.5, 12.6, 12.14). The most common sites of the osteophyte are between the fifth and sixth, the fourth and fifth, and the sixth and seventh cervical vertebrae. In my series, 75% of cases had unilateral, and 25% had bilateral uncinate

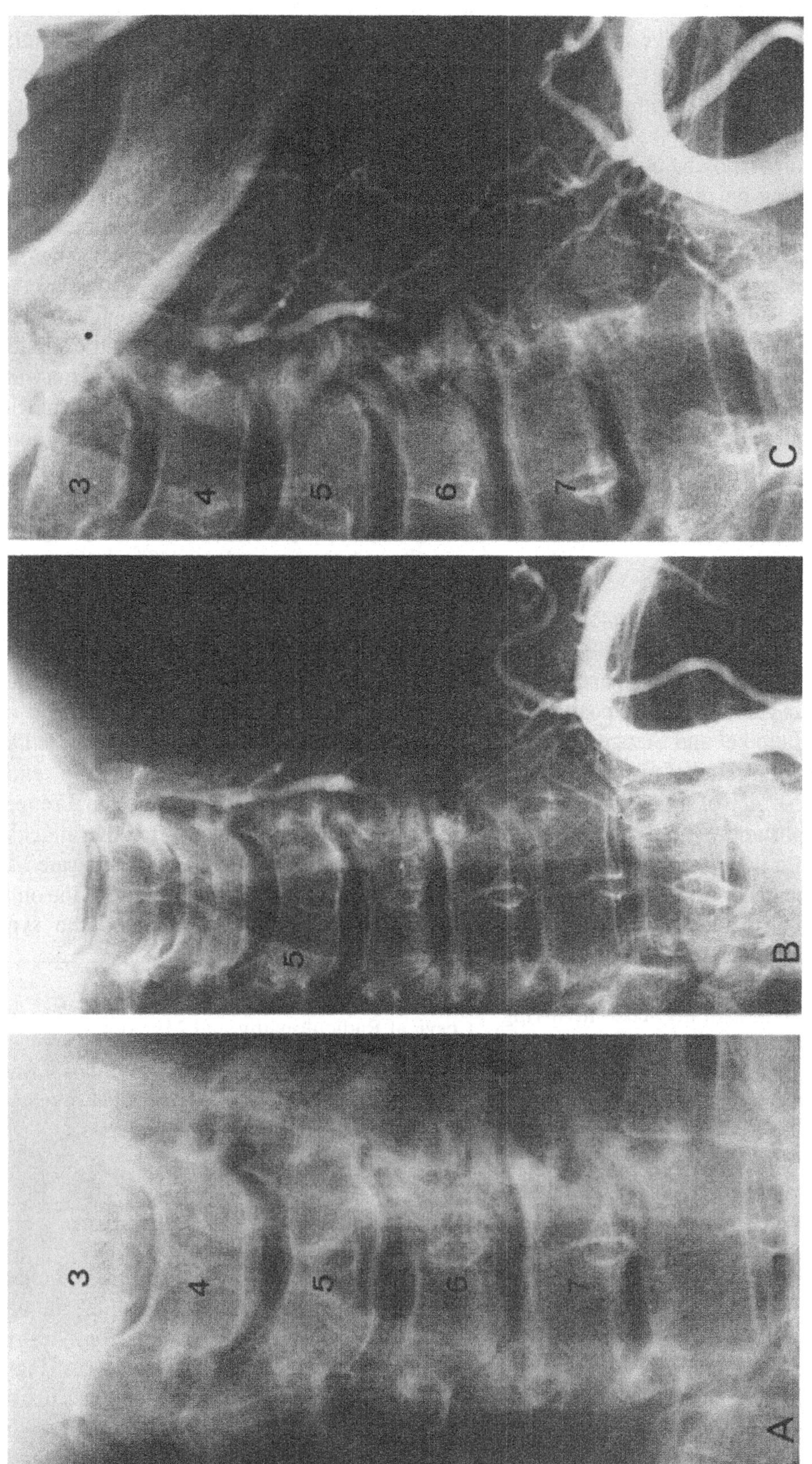

Figure 12.6. Complete obstruction of left vertebral artery with extra large uncal osteophyte at C5–6 and C6–7 in a 52-year-old female. Plain cervical spine film, **A**; *black arrows* indicate osteophytes at C5–6 and C6–7. **B** and **C** show left retrograde brachial arteriograms, indicating a complete obstruction of left vertebral artery below the level of C6. Note distal filling of the vertebral artery through collateral channels arising from branches of the thyrocervical trunk. **E, F,** and **G** also indicate distal filling of left vertebral artery in serial lateral films. **E** is taken 1.0 second, **F** is 1.5 second, and **G** is 3.0 seconds after injection. Slow filling of distal vertebral artery through collateral channels is obvious. Right vertebral artery is larger than the left and is

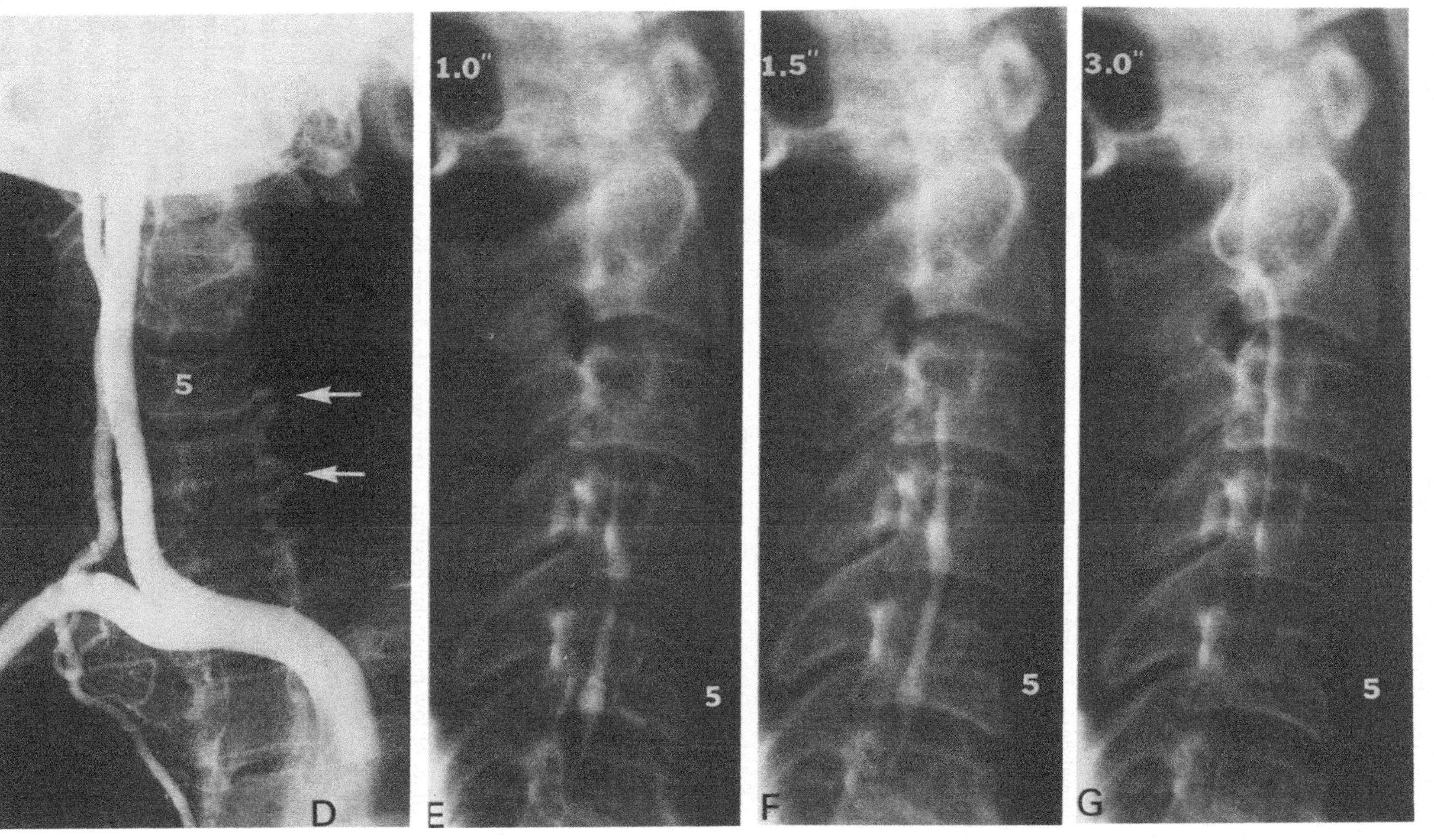

well visualized by retrograde brachial arteriogram, **D.** Again, extra-large uncal osteophytes C5–6 and C6–7 are noted (*white horizontal arrows*). It is most likely that the left vertebral artery of aortic arch origin is completely obstructed by C6–7 uncal osteophyte. (From Nagashima C, Hamaguchi, K., Iwasaki, T.[26])

osteophytes with vertebral artery compressions. Apophyseal osteoarthrosis was noted approximately in 15%. Metrizamide, Pantopaque Myodil myelography is unnecessary to verify the diagnosis and is not recommended for this syndrome.

Four-vessel arteriography, either by transfemoral Seldinger technique or by the percutaneous transbrachial retrograde technique, will demonstrate the size of the arteries and the location of the lesions. Each technique has advantages and disadvantages. The Seldinger technique permits four-vessel study in one session with a minimal dose of contrast material. However, technical difficulties will be encountered in elderly patients and in arteriosclerotic patients, with occasional serious complications resulting from wedging of the catheter in the vertebral artery, aggravating brainstem ischemia. Transbrachial retrograde arteriography poses less technical difficulties in elderly and arteriosclerotic patients and permits visualization of the brachial, subclavian, and innominate arteries. It does, however, require a large dose of contrast material. In such instances, the author routinely uses intravenous drop infusion of low-molecular dextran (Rheomacrodex) of 500 mL with steroids (dexamethasone 8 mg in adults) one day prior to and on the day of angiography. This premedication is based on the experimental study by Hammargren et al[10]. This demonstrated that the central nervous system was protected from the adverse effects of large doses of radiopaque medium. This was related to either the suspension stability of the blood, the antisludge effect of low-molecular dextran, or to the protective action of steroids on the blood-brain barrier. The medication showed good results; two cases (46-year-old female and 39-year-old male) developed vertigo and nausea immediately after injection of a 30-ml bolus of 60% iothalamate (Conray). This was encountered in 80 consecutive cases of spondylotic vertebral insufficiency (1.5%) *without* the premedication in the early stage of the author's series. After the use of premedication combined both low-molecular dextran and steroids, adverse effects have not been observed in more than 1,000 cases, even in arteriosclerotic patients.

In any case, at least six films were taken: three AP projections of the neck in hyperextension (one in plain hyperextension, one in hyperextension plus extreme rotation to the right, and one in hyperextension plus extreme rotation to the left), two projections of the neck in neutral position (one AP and one lateral), and one with a Towne projection to visualize the basilar artery and its branches (or serial lateral and Towne projections are made simultaneously with the neck in neutral position). The patient was asked if any given position had exacerbated the symptoms, and an attempt was made to simulate this position. In the retrograde brachial technique, a 30-ml bolus of 65% meglumine diatrizoate (Angiografin) was used in each injection; the left carotid arteriogram was added later.

Investigation of the carotid arterial system is as important as that of the subclavian, vertebral, and basilar arterial systems. One cannot exclude diseases in the carotid arteries as a cause of vertebrobasilar insufficiency, since these vessels are important sources of collateral blood flow through the circle of Willis into the posterior circulation.

The existence of arterial anomalies is important in evaluating the angiographic lesions of the vertebral artery, particularly if a surgical treatment is contemplated. The size of the two vertebral arteries varies considerably. Hypoplasia of one vertebral artery is common, and when present, the contralateral vessel is usually enlarged. Some of the more hypoplastic ones terminate in the neck without intracranial communication. In my series of 800 bilateral vertebral arteriograms, it was noted that the left artery was the larger in 41.9%, the right was larger in 24.6%, and both were approximately equal in 33.3%.

Visualization of the left vertebral artery by retograde brachial arteriographic technique is impossible in some patients because of anomalous origin of the vessel directly from the aortic arch in between the origins of the left subclavian and the left common carotid artery (Fig. 12.7). This variation was encountered in 6% of my series. In such instances, the Seldinger catheter should be placed between the origin of the left common carotid and the left subclavian artery, and an aortic arch study is done. Very rarely, the vertebral artery arises from the carotid bulb as a hypoglossal artery. Thus, awareness of the variations of the vertebral artery is

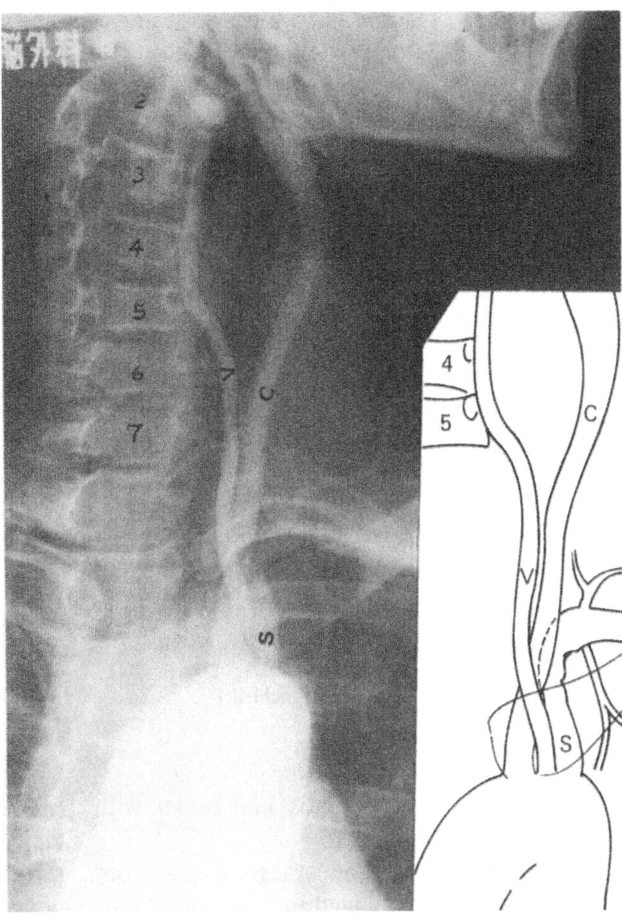

Figure 12.7. Arch aortogram showing left vertebral artery arising from arch. Note that left vertebral artery (*v*) enters into transverse foramen of C5, not into C6! *c* represents common carotid, *s*, subclavian artery.

important before significant conclusions can be drawn about total occlusion of the vessel.

As shown in Fig. 12.7, the left vertebral artery entered the transverse foramen of C5, not of C6. Although the majority of the vessel enters the C6 transverse foramen (93.6%), some enter at C5 (4.5%), C7 (1.2%), and C4 (0.7%).[1] Detailed data by Adachi[1] are shown in Table 12.1. In cases with the "aortic arch origin" of the left vertebral artery, incidence of the usual C6 entrance of the bilateral artery is low (15%), whereas unusual C7, 5, or 4 entrance of one or both arteries is high (85%). However, it should be noted that even in cases of usual "subclavian artery origin," approximately 1% (0.8% to be exact) of the cases *have unusual entrance* of one or both arteries into C4, 5, or 7 (Table 12.1). Awareness of this variation is important from a practical viewpoint. The vessel, after originating from the subclavian artery, ascends into the soft tissue of the neck. In cases of C5 or C4, the vertebral artery passes within the muscle of the longus colli before it enters into the C5 or C4 transverse foramen (Figs. 12.8, 12.9). Without this knowlege, the artery may be torn on retracting with a sharp blade or on cutting the longus colli muscle; the artery within the muscle has the same color and appearance as bundles of muscle. One should confirm the level of the entrance by lateral arteriograms (Figs. 12.8, 12.9), before surgery is contemplated.

Surgical Technique

Since the original description of this operation, the technique and general principles of the procedure have not been changed. Minor modifications, however, have been made with the development of microsurgery and more sophisticated instrumentation, which permit the procedure to

Table 12.1 Levels of entrance of the vertebral artery into the transverse foramina and sites of the origin.

Level of TF		Origins of VA		
Right	Left	Bilateral VA from SCA	Right VA from SCA Left VA from AA	Total
C4	C6	5	0	5
C6	C4	0	2	2
C5	C5	0	3	3
C5	C6	14	0	14
C4	C5	9	15	24
C5	C7	1	0	1
C6	C6	436	4	440
C6	C7	6	3	9
C7	C6	2	0	2
Total		473	27	550

Abbreviations: VA, vertebral artery; TF, transverse foramen; SCA, subclavian artery; AA, aortic arch.
Source: Adachi B.[1]

be performed more efficiently and easier with less trauma to tissues.

Endotracheal general anesthesia is used routinely. The patient is placed in the supine position with the head turned to the side opposite to the lesion. Before making the incision, it is necessary to localize by roentgenograms the interspace to be operated on. A transverse skin incision, 7 to 8 cm long, is made extending from the midline to the posterior border of the sternocleidomastoid muscle. The incision is placed in a natural wrinkle line of the neck for best cosmetic result. In cases with multiple lesions, the author previously used a longitudinal incision along the anterior border of the sternocleidomastoid muscle; however, at present time, the author does not use a longitudinal incision but rather a transverse incision of the more extensive, side to side type. The incision is made through skin, subcutaneous fat, and the platysma muscle. The skin-platysma flaps are separated from the underlying superficial cervical fascia with dissecting scissors as far as the length of the transverse incision, cephalad and caudad along the anterior margin of the sternocleidomastoid muscle. This vertical separation of the skin-platysma flaps greatly facilitates the cephalo-caudal wide exploration of the spine. The superficial cervical fascia and the areolar tissue along the anterior border of the sternocleidomastoid muscle are cut and the muscle is retracted laterally. The omohyoid muscle is next dissected along its lateral or superior margin, and the small vessels entering it are cauterized. Medial retraction of this muscle exposes the carotid sheath. The carotid artery is palpated. The plane of cleavage between the carotid sheath and the lateral border of the thyroid and larynx is separated down to the anterolateral surface of the vertebral bodies. A thin layer of prevertebral areolar tissue is grasped with tooth forceps, elevated, and incised vertically. The parallel medial margins of the longus colli muscles and the anterior longitudinal ligament covering the vertebra and the disk are ex-

Figure 12.8. Unusual entrance of right vertebral artery into C4 transverse foramen with angulation (*large white arrow*). *Small white arrows* indicate transverse process of C4. Left vertebral artery enters into C6 foramen. Vertebral arteries originated from the subclavian artery. ▷

Figure 12.9. Unusual entrance of right vertebral artery into C5 transverse foramen (*large white arrow*). Left artery enters into C6 foramen. Vertebral arteries originated from the subclavian artery. *Small white arrows* indicate transverse process of C5.

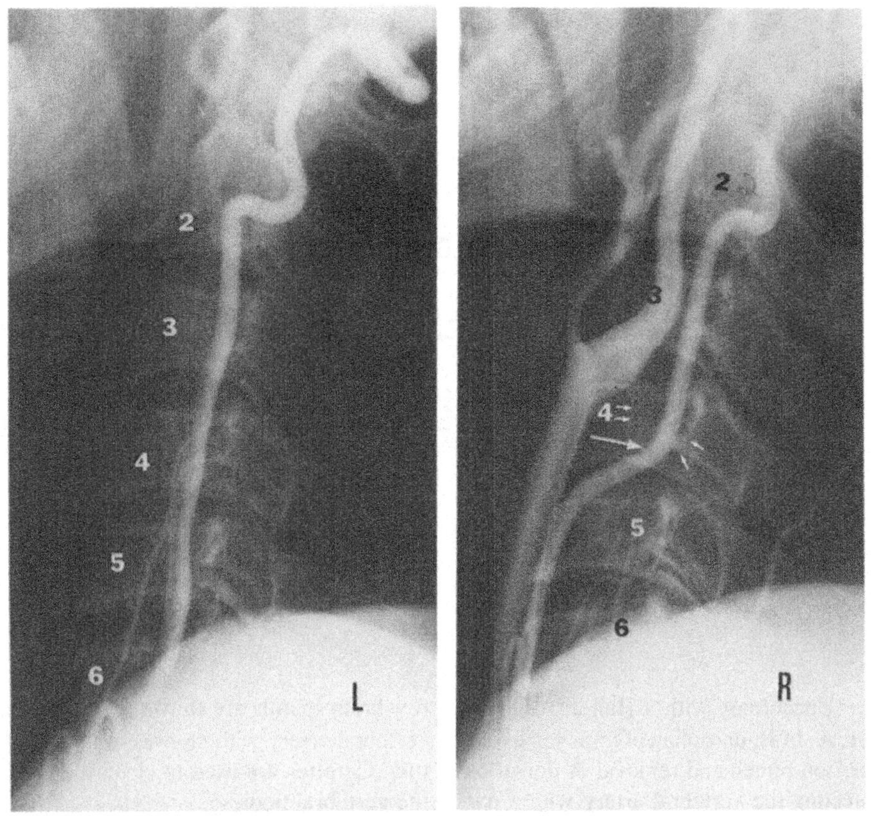

Fig. 12.8

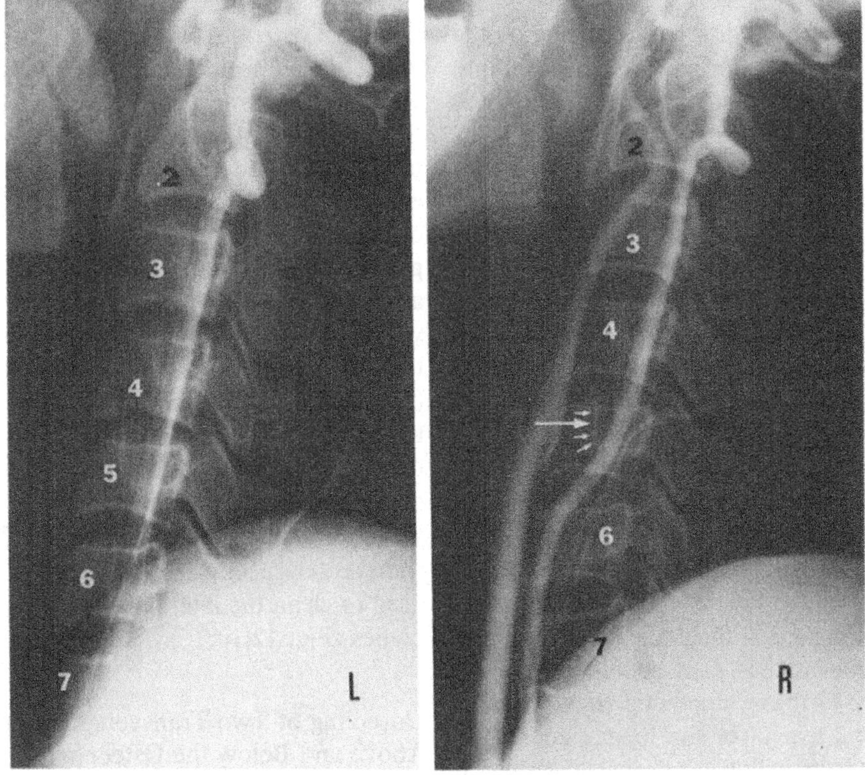

Fig. 12.9

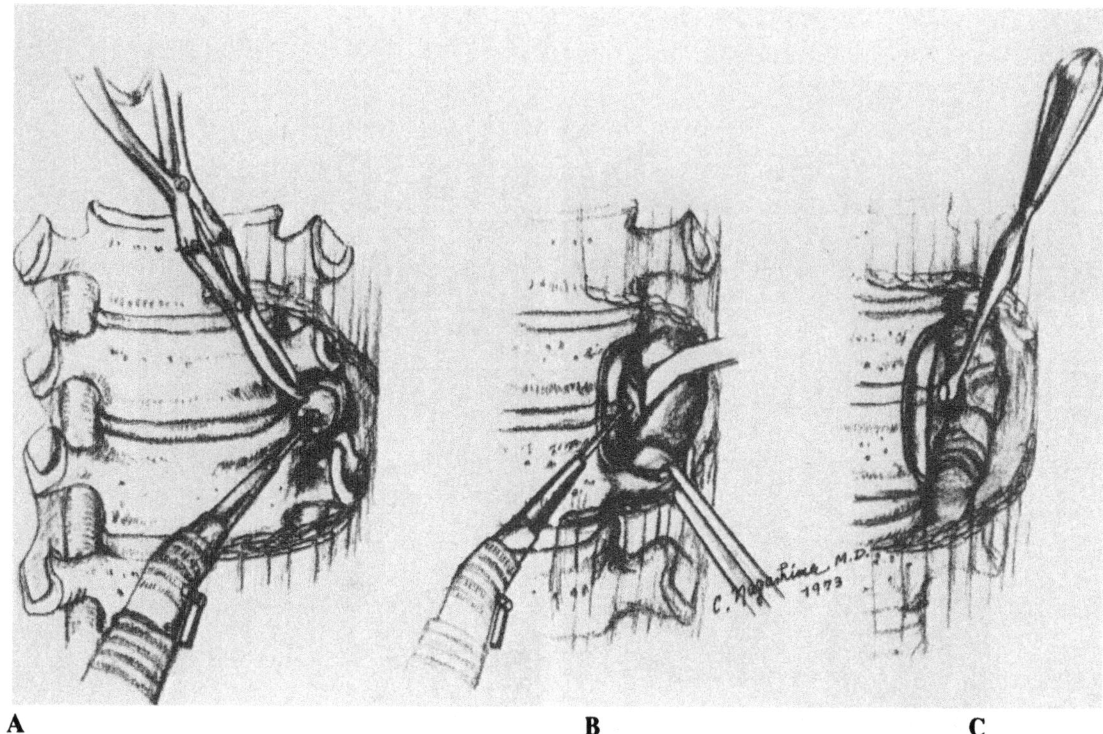

Figure 12.10. Uncectomy with a Hall air drill and Beyer rongeur, **A.** In **B,** unroofing of transverse foramen with Kerrison punch and removal of dorsal osteophyte protecting the vertebral artery with a narrow brain spatula are shown; **C** shows decompressed vertebral artery with creases remained in the adventitia. Curettes are used to clean the lateral aspect of the vertebral bodies.

posed at two or three levels, depending on the extent of the lesions. A needle is inserted into the uppermost disk, and a lateral x-ray film is made to determine the correct level.

Uncectomy With Removal of Lateral Osteophyte

Protrusion of the lateral osteophyte and transverse processes can be palpated individually through the longus colli muscle. Cloward's self-retaining retractors with blunt blades are placed both in a horizontal and vertical position, exposing the pathologic site. The longus colli muscle is cauterized along its medial margin and is separated subperiosteally from the spine on the side to be exposed. Sectioning and partial excision of the longus colli muscle greatly facilitates exposure of the uncinate portion and the transverse process. Care should be taken to avoid injury to the sympathetic trunk running on the lateral aspect of the longus colli muscle, especially in the lower cervical level, where the trunk runs closer to the muscle than in the midcervical level. Subperiosteal exposure of the uncal osteophyte is made by cutting with a long-handled scalpel and pointed No. 11 blade along the uppermost edge of the osteophyte and then exposing almost the whole aspect of the osteophyte with curettes and sharp periosteal elevator. The osteophyte is usually quite large, occupying the space in between the transverse processes above and below. This is nibbled away with the rongeur and then drilled away with an air drill. The central portion of the osteophyte is removed initially by making a hole (Fig. 12.10a) and the remainder of the osteophyte is removed with a rongeur. The uncinate portion of the vertebrae are removed by air drill up to the depth of the floor of the transverse foramen, cephalad and caudad to the transverse processes (Fig. 12.10b). Curettes are used to clean the lateral aspect of the vertebral bodies (Fig. 12.10c).

Unroofing of Two Transverse Foramina Above and Below the Osteophyte

With the excision of the longus colli muscle above and below, the transverse processes are exposed. With sharp curettes, the anterior root of the transverse process is subperiosteally exposed, including the superior and inferior margins of the transverse foramen. After the periosteum is completely separated from the bony canal, the anterior root of the transverse foramen is removed laterally to the tip of the anterior tubercle by a Kerrison punch. Two transverse foramina above and below the interspace are open.

Periarterial Stripping With Microsurgical Technique

The vertebral artery, thus freed from its compromised bony canal, appears still to be kinked owing to adhesions and perivascular fibrosis at the site where the compression had been the most severe. The periarterial stripping is best achieved by microsurgical technique (Fig. 12.11). A Zeiss microscope with a 300-mm objective lens and 12.5 × ocular lenses and magnification setting of 6 × is used. Precise margins of the thickened adventitia can be identified. (Fig. 12.13). A sharp dural hook is inserted into the thickened area of fibrosis and adventitia. This is elevated and an incision is made with a No. 15 blade knife. Through this opening, Yasagil's periosteum elevator is inserted into a cleavage plane between the adventitia and the media. Careful separation of the adventitia from the media is then accomplished by an adventitia elevator (Fig. 12.12), into which groove the tip of the bipolar coagulating forceps is introduced. The vertebral venous plexus is then coagulated by the forceps. This permits incision and excision of the thickened adventitia, including fibrosis without severe bleeding. This periarterial stripping should be performed because the periarterial fibrosis does, not only constrict and kink the artery, but also gives rise to the Barré syndrome (posterior cervical sympathetic syndrome)[3,31] owing to irritation of the periarterial vertebral nerves.

Stellate ganglionectomy is not added since marked functional differences exist between the vertebral nerve and the stellate ganglion.[27] Stimulation of the vertebral nerve produced many varieties of pupillary changes with or without ocular motion in either eye, but with headaches, or dizziness; however stimulation of the stellate ganglion produced prompt mydriasis of only the ipsilateral pupil without other eye changes, headaches, or dizziness.

Venous bleeding, if encountered, is arrested by applying, with gentle pressure, pieces of Gelfoam immersed in thrombin solution or by bipolar coagulation. The deep structures of the wound are permitted to fall together, and the platysma muscle, subcutaneous layer, and skin are closed in layers. Prior to closure, the wound is well irrigated with saline until the saline is crystal clear. The platysma muscle is closed carefully with 4-0 interrupted silk sutures to prevent a depressed scar, and the skin is apposed with subcuticular Vicryl sutures in female patients, in male patient the skin is closed with 4-0 interrupted nylon sutures. No drain is used.

Postoperative Care

The next morning patients, from their beds, are usually able to see more clearly the ceiling, the faces of the nurses, and their families. Since no interbody fusion is done, no supporting collar or restriction of neck movement is needed. Patients are encouraged to be up and around on the next day. Those who had the orthostatic hypotension preoperatively should be followed carefully. The majority of patients with preoperative orthostatic hypotension do not show it postoperatively. However, the patient who still shows orthostatic hypotension should be administered a blood pressure stabilizing drug, such as carnegine. It is recommended that these patients be encouraged in both physical and psychosomatic aspects until they regain their physical strength and their feeling of well-being with improvement of the orthostatic hypotension. As a rule, patients are ready to leave the hospital within seven days after the operation.

Criteria and Indications for Surgery

Criteria and indications for surgical treatment have been developed with 32 cases treated surgically over a period of 12 years. The present policy and recommendations are as follows:

1. Adult patient, mostly over the age of 40, with repeated attacks of vertigo or dizziness associated with signs and symptoms of vertebrobasilar insufficiency produced by rotat-

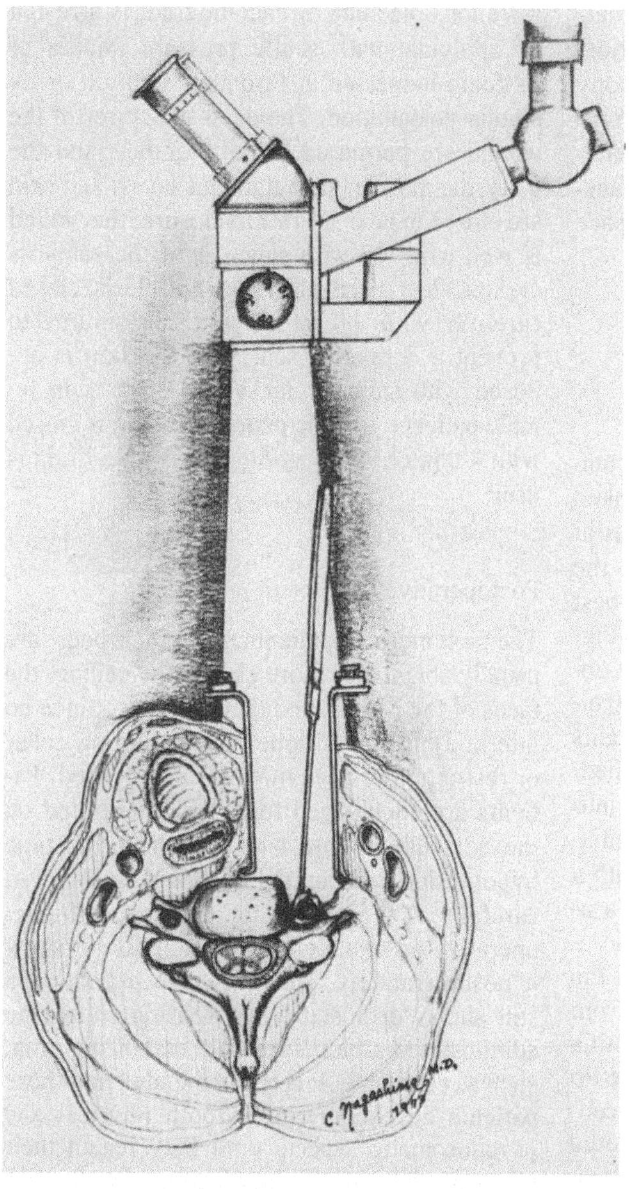

Figure 12.11. Periarterial stripping under the operating microscope. A 300-mm objective lens and 12.5 × ocular lens are used with actual magnification of 6 ×. Thickened adventitia is elevated by a sharp dural hook.

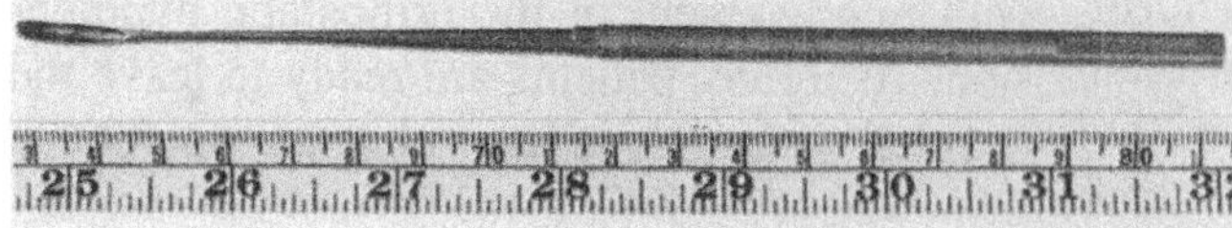

◁

Figure 12.12. Adventitia elevator designed by the author.

ing or hyperextending neck, or changing postures.

2. Uncal osteophyte(s) demonstrated in cervical plain anteroposterior x-ray.
3. Vertigo or dizziness due to vestibular disorder central in nature verified by neuro-otologic examination, i.e., it is not due to disorders of the peripheral vestibular end-organ such as Ménière disease or benign paroximal type of positional vertigo.
4. Four-vessel angiograms, including that of the subclavian, common carotid, and innominate arteries, can help determine if the spondylotic vertebral compression is the

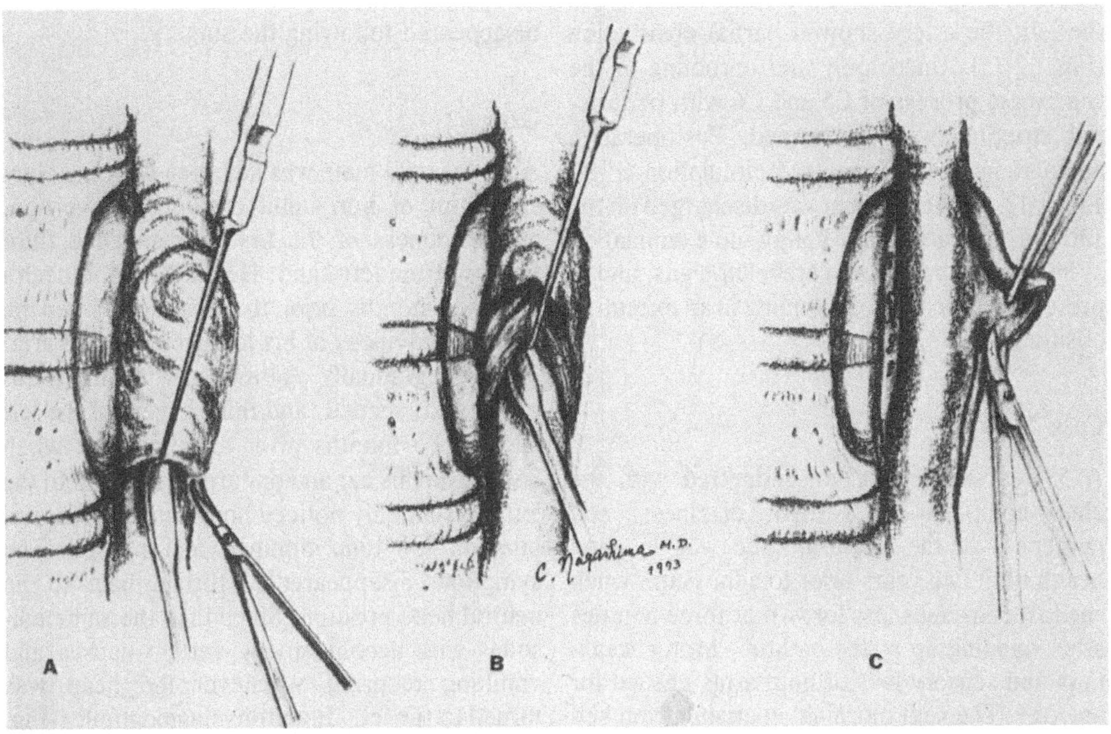

Figure 12.13. Excision of perivascular fibrosis with adventitia. In **A,** precise margin of thickened adventitia is identified and elevated by a sharp hook, and a Yasargil's periosteum elevator is inserted into a plane between adventitia and media. In **B** the adventitia is separated from the media over the anterior one-half of the entire circle of the artery. In **C** the adventitia with fibrous or fibrocartilaginous tissue is excised by Dandy scissor. Bleeding from periarterial veins are controlled by bipolar coagulation or application of pieces of Gelfoam with gentle pressure.

most causative lesion producing the present symptoms.

5. Objective neurologic findings indicating brainstem, cerebellar, occipital, and temporal lobe lesions.

Of the five criteria, 1 through 4 are the most essential and must be present for recommending surgery to the patient almost regardless of associated disease. This is because the cerebrovascular disease is usually progressive[4b,8a] associated with a poorer prognosis than the associated disease, and the repeated attacks culminate in irreversible damage in the brainstem. Patients with extensive atherosclerosis form the subclavian up to the vertebral artery in continuity, or with severe irregular narrowings of the basilar artery are not amenable to the surgical treatment.

Representative Cases

Case 1

A 53-year-old male was admitted with the chief complaint of attacks of dizziness, blurred vision, and fainting. He had been in good health until 10 years prior to admission, when while backing up his car he suddenly developed blurred vision and fainting. Similar episodes occurred once or twice a week, often on turning his head to the left or on looking upward. For five years prior to admission he felt his gait was unsteady, as if he was walking on a cloud. Neurologic examination on admission revealed cerebellar ataxia, positive Romberg's sign, down-beat vertical nystagmus seen through the Frenzel glass on positioning test of Dix-Hallpike. An uncinate osteophyte was noted at C5–6; the vertebral artery was very much compressed by the osteophyte (Fig. 12.14). On turning the head to the left, the artery showed partial obstruction (Fig. 12.15). Uncectomy and unroofing of the transverse process of C5 and C6 with periarterial stripping were performed. Postoperative angiograms showed restored circulation (Figs. 12.14, 12.15). The patient was discharged on the 10th postoperative day. Follow-up examination at five years showed no cerebellar signs, and at present he is actively continuing in an executive position.

Case 2

A 58-year-old female was admitted with the chief complaint of vertigo, dizziness, and numbness of the left arm. She was in good health until two years prior to admission, when she lost consciousness for two or three minutes after standing up in the bathtub. Motor weakness and sensory loss of both arms ensued for one day. The next morning on arising from bed she had a sudden episode of vertigo followed by nausea and vomiting but no tinnitus or hearing loss. The same attack was noted one year prior to admission upon standing up, again, from the bathtub. Her home doctor diagnosed her as "CO intoxication." The patient did not agree with the diagnosis. Numbness in the left arm developed three months prior to admission. Neurologic examination revealed a positive Romberg sign, unsteady gait with tendency to deviate to the left and signs of C6 radiculopathy on the left. Neurootological examination revealed direction-fixed horizontal nystagmus to the left side on positional and positioning tests. X-ray revealed the left uncal osteophyte at C5-6 (Fig. 12.16), and the left vertebral artery was narrowed and displaced laterally. On turning the head to the left, the kink became more severe and the lumen of the artery was markedly narrowed (Figs. 12.17, 12.18). Uncectomy and unroofing of the transverse foramina of C5 and C6 with periarterial stripping were performed. The patient was discharged on the seventh postoperative day. On the postoperative x-ray, the osteophyte was no longer visualized but an uncectomy defect was present. The angiograms showed disappearance of the narrowing (Figs. 12.16–12.18). After 10 years follow-up, the patient had no episode of dizziness or fainting and is doing well. Symptoms of C6 radiculopathy disappeared following the surgery.

Case 3

A 56-year-old male was admitted with the chief complaint of horizontal oscilloposia, vertigo, and numbness of the first, second, and third fingers of the left hand. He was in good health until six months prior to admission, when he noticed heaviness of his left shoulder and arm. This was gradually aggravated with numbness of the first, second, and third fingers of the left hand. Two months prior to admission, when backing up his car and on turning his head to the left, he suddenly noticed horizontal oscillopsia, bilateral low-tone tinnitus, and nausea. The symptoms disappeared on turning back to the neutral head position. Since then the same episodes with accompanying vertigo nausea and vomiting recurred whenever the head was turned to the left. Electronystagmography (Fig. 12.19) revealed the horizontal nystagmus lasting throughout the period of rotating the neck to the left, with some fluctuation in amplitude and frequency of the nystagmus. Nausea, oscillopsia, and vertigo occurred at the same time. Signs of left C6 radiculopathy were noted on neurologic examination. The left vertebral artery was displaced laterally and narrowed by a C6-7 osteophyte (Fig. 12.20A), which produced severe stenosis on turning the head to the left (Fig. 12.20B). In lateral view, the artery was displaced dorsally with a sharp angulation (Fig. 12.21). Following uncectomy, unroofing of C6 foramen, and periarterial stripping from C7 to C6, all symptoms disappeared. The patient was discharged on the seventh postoperative day. Periarterial tissues over the C7 transverse process such as tendons and muscles were markedly fibrotic, presumably because of tissue reaction against the osteophyte. A small piece ($1 \times 0.5 \times 1.5$ mm) of calcified material was extirpated from the muscle adjacent the osteophyte. Postoperative arteriograms showed disappearance of filling defect and sharp angulation (Figs. 12.21, 12.22). Electronystagmographs were normal. After 14 months follow-up, the patient is actively engaged in his previous job.

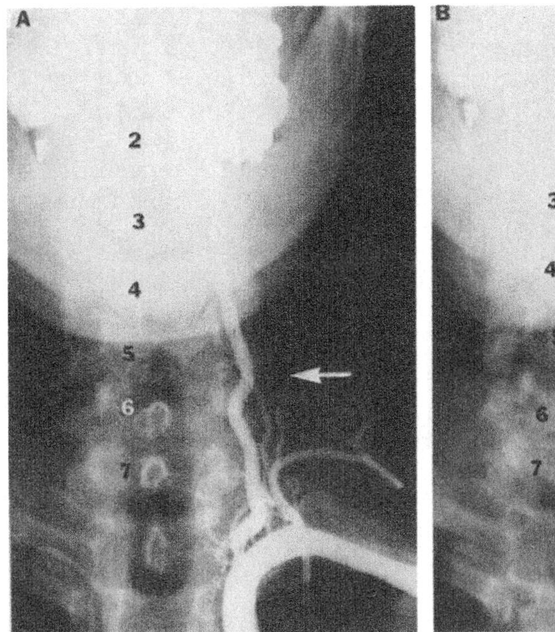

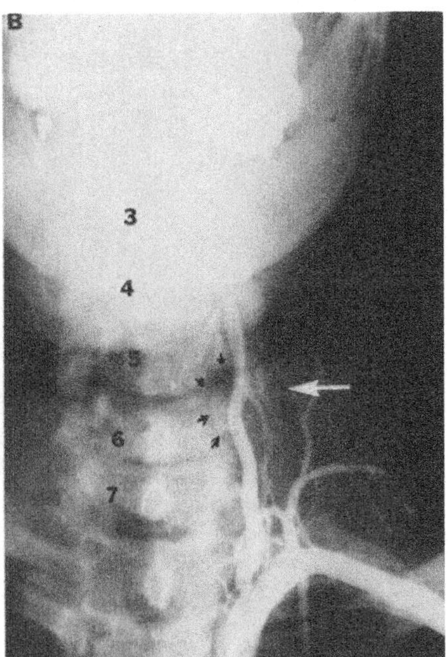

Figure 12.14. Case 1. Retrograde vertebral arteriograms taken with head in neutral position. **A.** Preoperative film shows lateral displacement and kinking of the artery at level of C5–6 (*white arrow*); **B.** postoperative film shows loss of kinking (*white arrow*). *Small black arrows* indicate uncectomy defect.

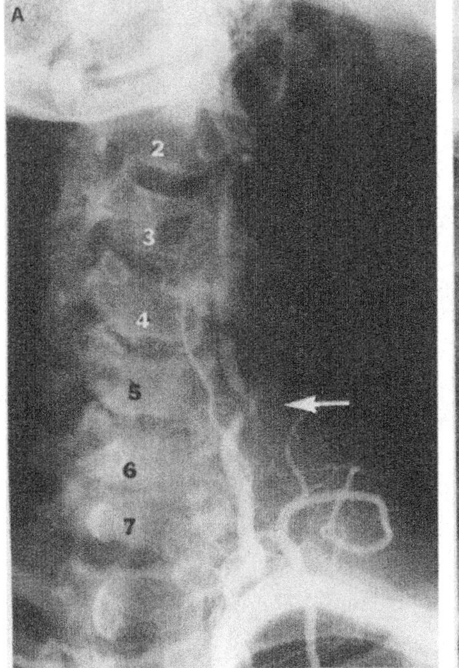

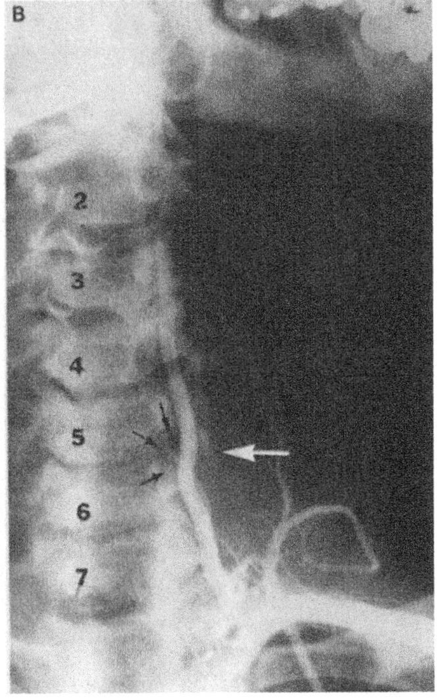

Figure 12.15. Case 1. Retrograde vertebral arteriograms taken with head rotated to the left plus hyperextension. **A.** Preoperative film shows partial obstruction of the artery at C5–6 (*white arrow*); **B.** postoperative film shows absence of artery obstruction.

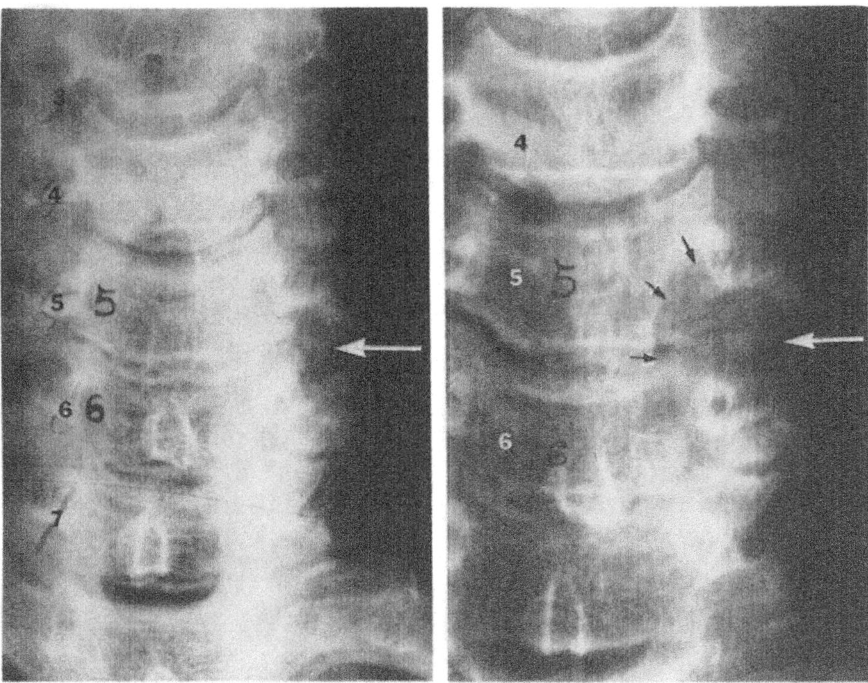

Figure 12.16. Case 2. Cervical spine films. *Left:* Preoperative film shows lateral osteophyte (*white arrow*). *Right:* Postoperative film shows uncectimy defect (*black arrows*) and complete disappearance of the lateral osteophyte.

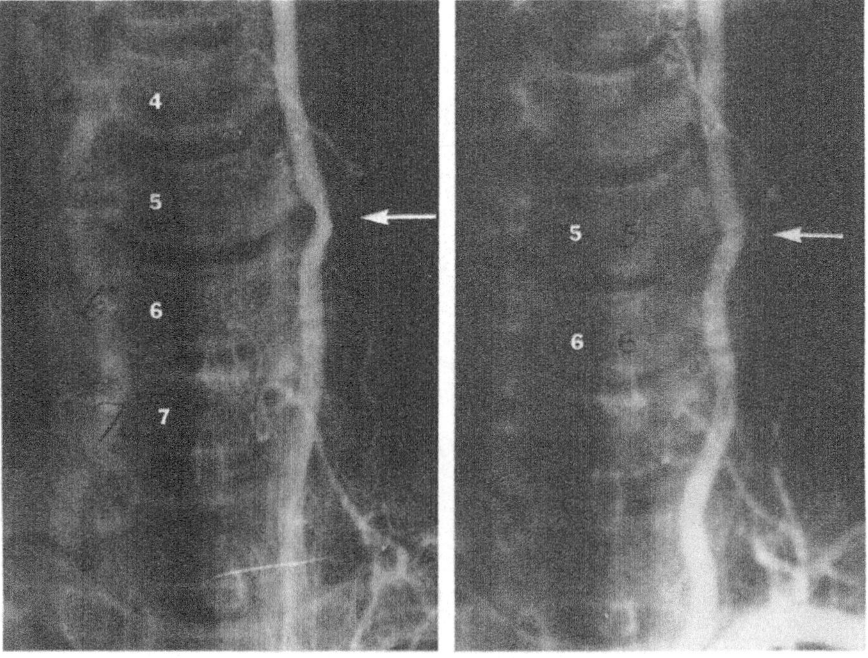

Figure 12.17. Case 2. Retrograde vertebral arteriograms taken with head in neutral position. *Left:* Preoperative film shows stenosis of the artery at level of C5–6 (*white arrow*). *Right:* Postoperative film shows absence of artery stenosis.

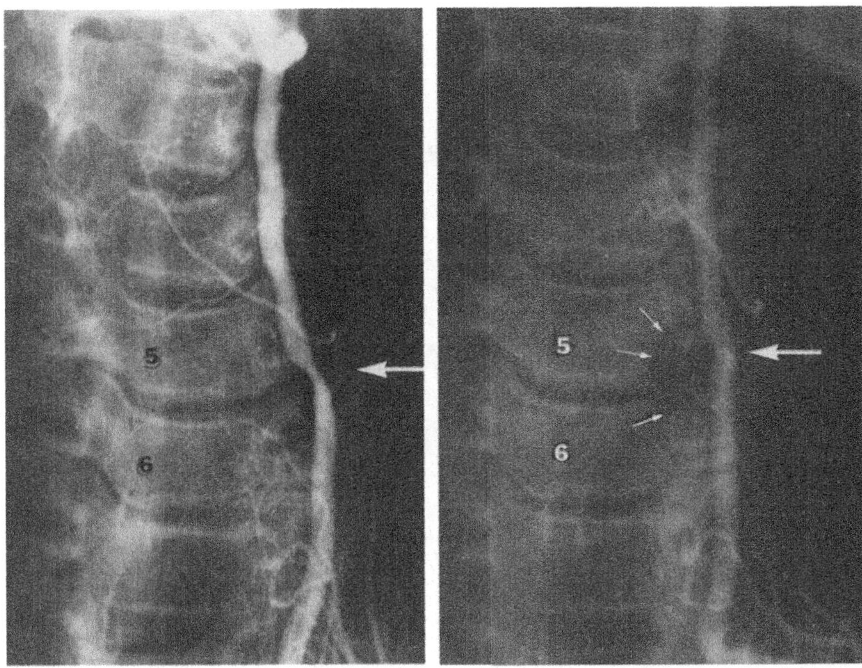

Figure 12.18. Case 2. Retrograde vertebral arteriograms taken with head in rotation to the left plus hyperextension. *Left:* Preoperative film shows marked stenosis of the artery at C5–6 (*white arrow*). *Right:* Postoperative film shows absence of artery stenosis. *Black arrows* indicate uncectomy defect.

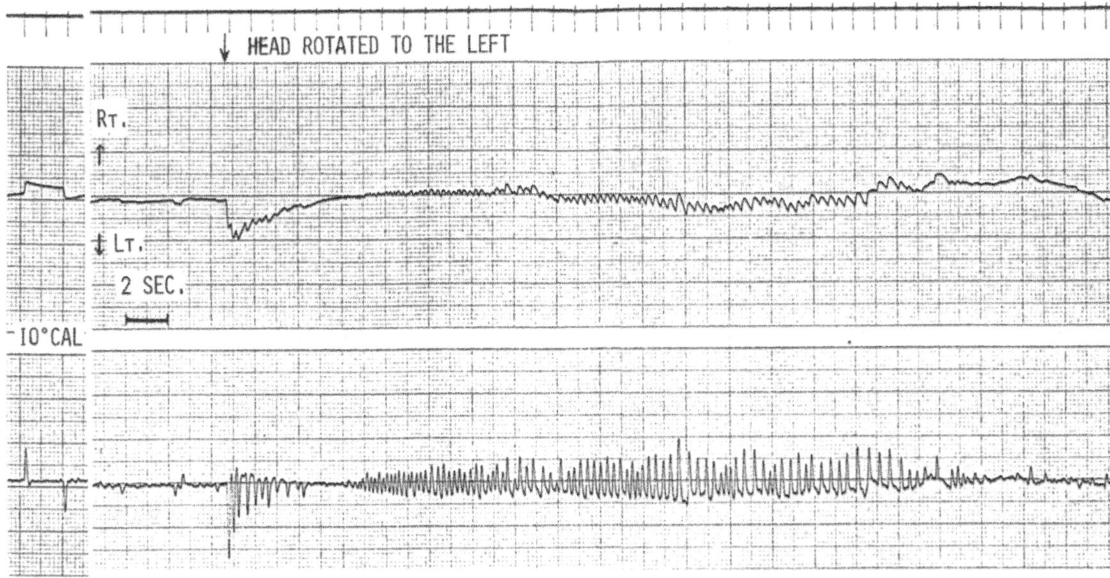

Figure 12.19. Case 3. ENG on turning head to the left. Upper trace is the ENG of horizontal component of the eye movement (time constant 3.0 ms), and the lower trace is the differentiated ENG indicating eye velocity (time constant 0.03 ms). Calibrations for 10° eye movement are shown on the left of the recording. Note horizontal nystagmus with rapid phase to the right began to appear 6.5 seconds after head turning, increased in amplitude, and lasted for about 30 seconds. This occurred repeatedly so long as on keeping the same posture and disappeared suddenly on taking neutral head position or on turning head to the right.

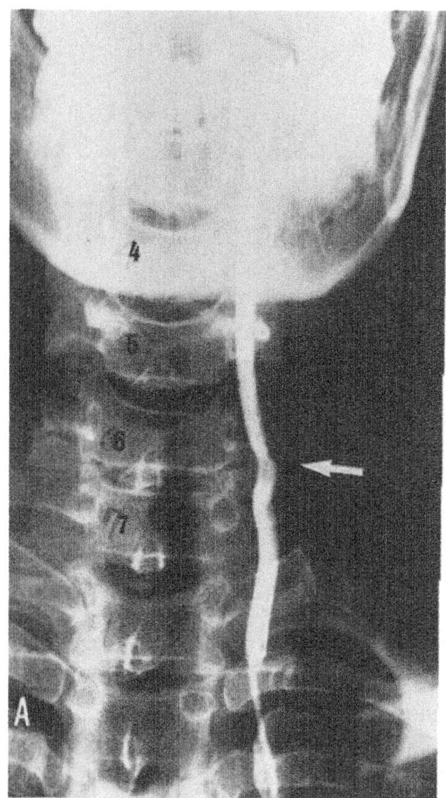

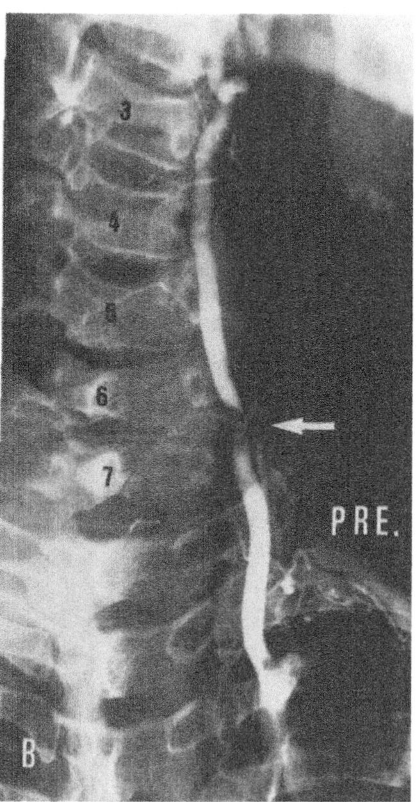

△

Figure 12.20. Case 3. Left vertebral arteriograms by Seldinger technique taken with head in neutral position, **A,** and rotation to the left, **B.** Narrowing of the artery by lateral osteophyte at C6–7 is markedly increased by turning head to the left, with the filling defect (*white arrow* in **B**). In this neck position, horizontal nystagmus with oscillopsia was elicited (see Fig. 12.19).

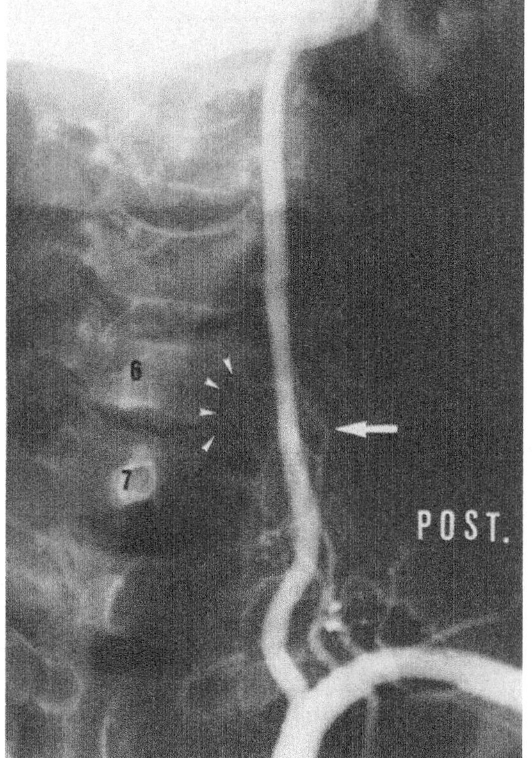

◁

Figure 12.21. Case 3. Postoperative left vertebral arteriogram through the retrograde brachial artery injection taken with the head rotated to the left. Note, disappearance of the filling defect at level of C6–7 (*large white arrow*). Compare with Fig. 12.20B. *Small arrowheads* indicate uncectomy defect. No nystagmus and no oscillopsia were elicited in this position postoperatively.

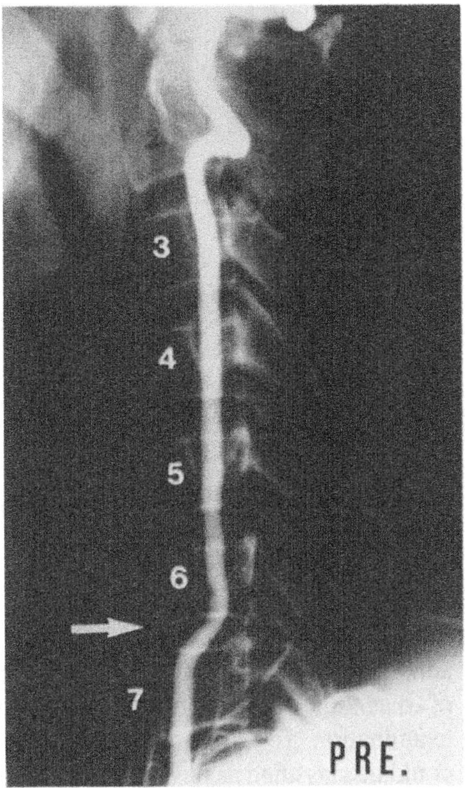

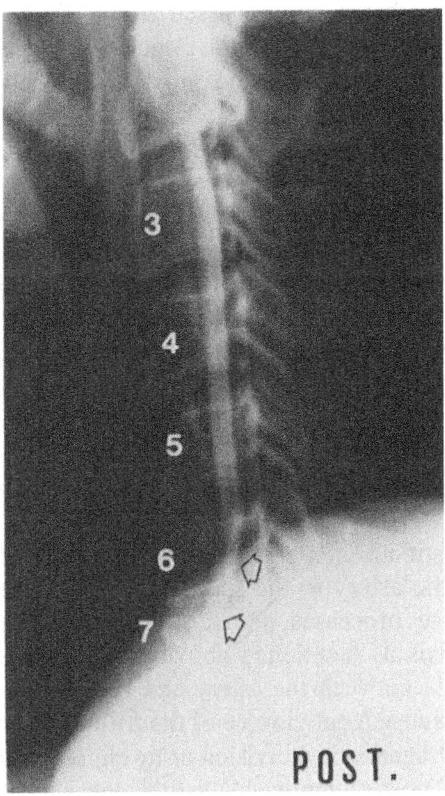

Figure 12.22. Case 3. Pre (PRE)- and postoperative (POST) lateral arteriograms. Dorsally displaced vertebral artery with sharp angulation at C6–7 (*white arrow* in PRE.) rendered gentle curvature after the operation (*open arrows* in POST.)

Application of the Technique for Other Lesions of the Vertebral Artery

The surgical technique employed for spondylotic vertebral artery insufficiency has been modified for treatment of other pathologic lesions of the vertebral artery that impair or endanger the function of the brainstem and spinal cord. These include arteriovenous (AV) fistula of the vertebral artery,[27] AV malformation of the cervical cord, and vertebro-carotid anastomosis for treatment of vertebral artery occlusion.[28]

The present unroofing technique of the transverse foramen provides extensive exposure of the vertebral artery. The artery is best freed from the bony canal by separation of the periosteum on the floor of the transverse foramen. A heavy silk ligature can be passed between the floor of the foramen and the posterior aspect of the artery. The radicular branch originating from the vertebral artery should be clipped and divided. Care should be taken not to damage the roots. They are behind the artery and extend obliquely near the tip of the anterior tubercle. The use of conventional electrocoagulation near the tip of the anterior tubercle often results in abrupt muscle contraction of the arm and damage to the root. If bleeding is encountered in this area, accurate bipolar coagulation of the bleeding point with fine bipolar forceps is preferable.

Both in AV fistula and in AVM, the site of pathology is frequently located behind the artery. The isolation of the vertebral artery should be started one or two levels below the lesion. Following removal of the anterior roots of the transverse processes, the periosteum is elevated from the transverse foramen either by curved sharp curettes or a fine periosteal elevator. The vertebral veins remain intact covered with the periosteum. After complete elevation of the artery from the floor of the transverse foramen, a heavy silk is passed around the artery, which permits temporary occlusion of the vessel if required. On looking for the feeding artery to the AVM, the author prefers to use the less cumbersome ×3 or ×2 magnifying glass and fiberoptic light. The feeder frequently is located in the space between two transverse processes above and below and is distended, permitting embolization of the AVM. Careful separation of the feeder from the root and the vein is essential for ligating, clipping the feeder, and embolization of the AVM. If the feeder is torn, temporally clipping the vertebral artery proximal and distal to the feeder greatly diminishes the bleeding and permits closure of the feeder.

The fistulous communication is often located behind the artery in the space in between the transverse processes above and below. The same steps as mentioned above may disclose the fistula between the artery and vein, which permits subsequent closure of the fistula either by direct ligation and division or by clipping. In cases of posttraumatic AV fistula, the site of pathology is often covered with scar tissue, which obscures the lesion. Meticulous and careful separation is imperative to avoid unexpected profuse bleeding. In such instances, the intact portion of the vertebral artery, proximal and distal to the lesion, should be explored first. Temporary clipping with aneurysm clips is advisable.

Vertebro-carotid anastomosis in cases of proximal vertebral artery occlusion is easier to treat than the AV fistula or the AVM. A free segment of the artery 3 or 4 cm distal from the site of occlusion provides enough room to accomplish anastomosis directly to the external carotid, or indirectly to the common carotid artery with use of autogenous saphenous vein graft. Temporary clipping of the vertebral artery by this technique is also useful on removal of vascular tumors in the neck.

Surgical Results and Postoperative Long-Term Management

The author has performed this operation in 32 patients during the past 14 years. The object of all surgical procedures is to restore blood flow within the vertebral artery, to prevent future recurrence of ischemic attacks, and to avoid of cerebral infarction. Good results require early diagnosis. Tables 12.2 and 12.3 show that in this series "excellent" results were achieved in 87.5% of the patients at the time of discharge; however, 14 years' follow-up examination revealed that only about 80% could be classified as having excellent results. It is important to mention that although those under "good" show only a 5.7% worsening in the follow-up, the intermittent symptom itself was not mild but required medication. Although the operation causes no untoward effect on cerebral circulation and provides blood flow within the vertebral artery, it did not result in long-lasting cures. Although osteophytes, irritation of vertebral nerves, and factors causing damage to the intima were eliminated after the operation, dysautoregulation and, normal variation remained unchanged (Fig. 12.23). "Normal" variation is no longer normal when the brain perfused by the variant vessel is ischemic.[4a] Ischemia,[15a,17a,b] diabetes,[3a] aging,[29b,36] and long-

Table 12.2. Result at time of discharge of 32 patients.

Result	No. of patients	Percentage
Excellent	28	87.5
Good	4	12.5
Same	0	0
Poor	0	0

Excellent, total relief of symptoms; good, relief of some or all symptoms but intermittent discomfort continuing; same, postoperative condition the same as preoperative; worse, symptom increased or new symptoms present.

Table 12.3. Final status when last seen in follow-up examination of 22 patients.

Result	No. of patients	Percentage
Excellent	18	81.8
Good	4	18.2
Same	0	0
Poor	0	0

Result criteria defined in Table 12.2.

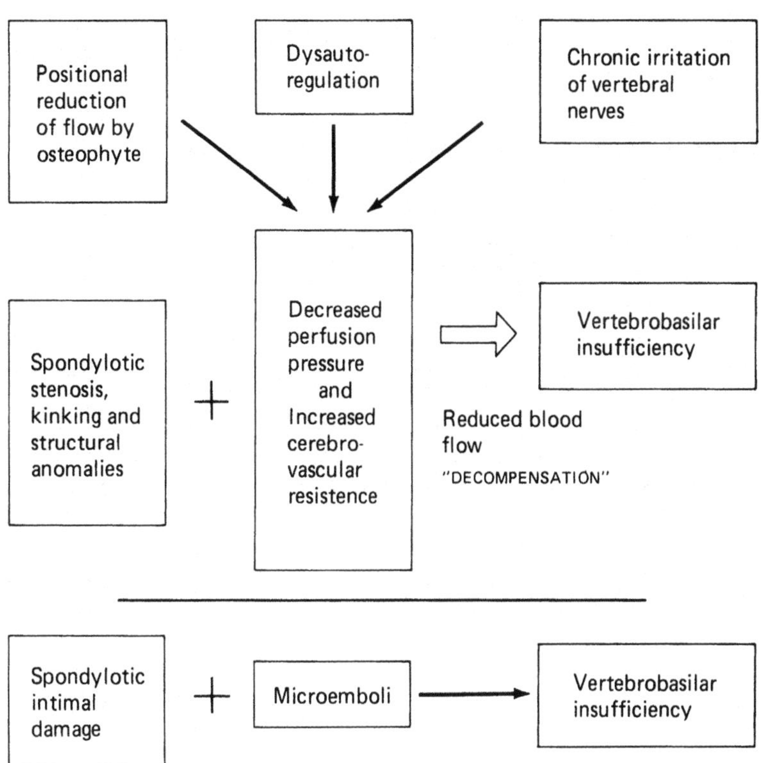

Figure 12.23. Pathogenesis of vertebrobasilar insufficiency due to spondylosis. Two principal mechanisms are shown: (1) decompensation of posterior circulation owing to critically decreased flow and (2) liberation of microemboli from mural thrombus secondarily to spondylotic intimal damage. Chronic irritation of the vertebral nerves (sympathetic nerves with communicating rami to somatosensory fibers) may give rise to nuchal dull ache, dysequilibrium, and vasospasm owing to long-standing, excessive impulses.

standing vertebrobasilar insufficiency[29c] may result in loss of autoregulation so that mild hypotension causes critically reduced blood flow as shown in Fig. 12.23 ("decomposition"), with subsequent profound ischemia.

In this author's series the only postoperative complication was a spontaneous pneumothorax secondary to ruptured emphysematous blebs or bullae of the right lung in a 66-year-old male. The collapsed lung expanded after one week, and the patient made an excellent recovery. Follow-up results were delivered from questionnaires or reexaminations in outpatient clinics, and results were obtained in 22 patients. Of 32 cases, six elderly patients died of unrelated diseases such as malignant neoplasma, myocardiac infarction, traffic accident, hypertensive intracerebral hemorrhage, and suicide. No correspondence was obtainable in four cases. In cases evaluated as "good" in the postoperative group (Table 12.3), there were patients who had had orthostatic hypotension, hypertension, atrophy in the occipital lobe, in the cerebellum on computed tomography (CT)-scan, psychotic instability due to social maladaptation, and diabetes, all requiring both medical and psychologic care. Although follow-up arteriograms of 20 cases showed virtual absence of stenosis or obstruction even on rotating the neck, three showed elongated tortuous basilar artery with an irregular lumen, which may require intracranial vascular surgery[6b] in the future.

It should be emphasized that other factors such as polycythemia, cardiac arrythmia, seizures, multiple sclerosis, hypoglycemia, hyperglycemia, and over-aggressive antihypertensive therapy may seriously contribute to the outcome. Postoperative long-term management in cooperation with the neurologist, hematologist, geriatric specialist, cardiologist, psychiatrist, and neurosurgeon are of importance. Once more it should be stressed that symptoms are transient and reversible in the early stage. Both medical and surgical treatment, should be started before irreversible lesions in the central nervous system are produced.

References

1. Adachi B: Das Arteriensystem der Japaner. Maruzen Co, Kyoto, 1928, p 147
2. Bakay L, Leslie EV: Surgical treatment of vertebral artery insufficiency caused by cervical spondylosis J Neurosurg 23:596–602, 1965

3. Barré M: Sur un syndrome sympathetique cervical postérieur et sa cause frequent: l' arthrite cervical. Rev Neurol 33:1246–1248, 1926
3a. Bentsen N, Larsen B, Lassen NA: Chronically impaired autoregulation of cerebral blood flow in lon-term diabetics. Stroke 6:497–502, 1975
4. Brooker AEW, Barter RW: Cervical spondylosis. A clinical study with comparative radiology. Brain 88:925–936, 1965
4a. Carney AL: Vertebral artery surgery: Historical development, basic concept of brain hemodynamics, and clinical experience of 102 cases. Adv Neurol 30:249–282, 1981
4b. Cartilige NEF, Whisnant JP, Elveback LR: Carotid and vertebral basilar transient cerebral ischemic attacks. Mayo Clin Proc 52:117–120, 1977
5. Cawthorne T: Positional nystagmus. Ann Otol Rhinol Laryngol 63:481–490, 1954
6. Cloward RB: Treatment of lesion of the cervical spine by anerior surgical approach. In Austin G (ed.): The Spinal Cord. Charles C Thomas, Springfield, Illinois, 1972, p 396
6a. Corkill G, French BN, Michas C, et al: External carotid-vertebral artery anastomosis for vertebrobasilar insufficiency. Surg Neurol 7:109–115, 1977
6b. de los Reyes RA, Ausman IJ, Diaz FG, et al: The surgical treatment of vertebrobasilar insufficiency. Acta Neurochir 68:203–216, 1983
7. Dix MR, Hallpike CS: The pathology, syptomatology and diagnosis of certain common disorders of the vestibular system. Ann Otol Rhinol Laryngol 61:986–1016, 1951
8. Elkin DC, Harris MH: Arteriovenous aneurysm of the vertebral vessels. Report of ten cases. Ann Surg 124:934–951, 1946
8a. Fischer CM: Clinical syndromes in cerebral thrombosis, hypertensive hemorrhage, and ruptured saccular aneurysm. Clin Neurosurg 22:117–147, 1975
8b. Fischer CM, Adams RD: The transient global amnesia syndrome. Acta Neurol Scand [Suppl] 9,40:7–82, 1964
8c. Giroux JC: Vertebral artery compression by cervical osteophytes. Adv Otorhinolaryngol 28:111–117, 1982
9. Gortvai P: Insufficiency of vertebral artery treated by decompression of its cervical part. Br Med J 2:233–234, 1964
10. Hammargren LL, Geise AW, French LA: Protection against cerebral damage from intracarotid injection of hypaque in animals. J Neurosurg 23:418–424, 1965
11. Hardin CA: Vertebral artery insufficiency produced by cervical osteoarthritic spurs. Arch Surg. 90:629–633, 1965
12. Hardin CA, Williamson WP, Streegmann AT: Vertebral artery insufficiency produced by cervical osteoarthritic spurs. Neurology 10:855–858, 1960
13. Hoyt WF: Ocular symptoms and signs. In Wylie EJ, Ehzenfeld WK (eds.): Extracranial occlusive cerebrovascular disease—Diagnosis and Management. WS Saunders Co, Philadelphia, London, Toronto, 1970, p 9
14. Jung A, Vierling JP, Safaoui A: Douze cas d'arthrose cervicale inférrieure. Leur traitement chirurgical par abord antérieur avec ouverture du trou transversaire et uncusectomie. Press Medical 72:3367–3372, 1964
15. Keggi KJ, Granger DP, Southwick WO: Vertebral artery insufficiency secondary to trauma and osteoarthritis of cervical spine. Yale J Biol Med 38:471–478, 1966
15b. Lou HC, Lassen NA, Friis-Hansen B. Impaired autoregulation of cerebral blood flow in the distressed newborn infant. J Pediatr 94:118–121, 1979
16. Matas R: Traumatism and traumatic aneurysms of the vertebral artery and their surgical treatment. Report of a cured case. Ann Surg 18:477–521, 1893
17. Matas R: Discussion of paper of Elkin and Harris. Ann Surg 124:950–951, 1946
17a. McHenry LC Jr, West JW, Cooper ES, et al: Cerebral autoregulation in man. Stroke 5:695–706, 1974
17b. Meyer JS, Naritomi H, Sakai F, et al: Regional cerebral blood flow, diachesis and steal after stroke. Neurol Res 1:101–119
18. Millikan CH, Siekert RG: Studies in cerebrovascular disease. I. The syndrome of intermittent insufficiency of the basilar arterial system. Proc Staff Meet Mayo Clin 30:61–68, 1955
19. Nagashima, C: Cervical spondylosis and neurological syndrome. Rinsho-Shinkei-gaku 6:613–614, 1966
19a. Nagashima C: Surgical treatment of vertebral artery insufficiency caused by cervical spondylosis. J Neurosurg 32:512–521, 1970
20. Nagashima C: Microsurgery in treatment of spondylotic vertebral artery insufficiency. Kyoto International Symposium of Microneurosurgery, October 14–15, Kyoto, Japan, 1973
21. Nagashima C: Microsurgical treatment of spondylotic vertebral artery insufficiency. Neurol Surg (Jpn) 1:337–344, 1973
22. Nagashima C: Surgical treatment of spondylotic vertebral artery insufficiency. Excerpta Medica International Congress Series, (V International Congress of Neurological Surgery. Tokyo, 1973) No 293, Paper 204, 1973
23. Nagashima C: Microsurgery in treatment of

spondylotic vertebral artery insufficiency. 42nd Annual Meeting of American Association of Neurological Surgeons. St Louis, 1974
24. Nagashima, C: Microchirurgisches Operationsverfahren bei zervikaler spondylogener Insuffizienz der Arteria vertebralis. HNO-Praxis 7, Georg Thieme, Leipzig, 1982, pp 40–48
25. Nagashima C: Transient global amnesia syndrome in a patient with spohdylotic vertebral artery insufficiency. (in preparation)
26. Nagashima C, Hamaguchi K, Iwasaki T: Vertebral artery obstruction due to cervical spondylosis. (in preparation)
27. Nagashima C, Iwama K: Electrical stimulation of the stellate ganglion and the vertebral nerve. J Neurosurg. 36:756–762, 1972
28. Nagashima C, Iwama K, Miki Y: Effects of temporary occlusion of a vertebral artery on the human vestibular system. J Neurosurg 33:388–394, 1970
29. Nagashima C, Iwasaki T, Kawanuma S: Traumatic arteriovenous fistula of the vertebral artery with spinal cord symptoms. J Neurosurg 46:681–687, 1977
29a. Nagashima C, Ueno A: Carotid-vertebral anastomosis; and alteranate technique for repair of obstruction and insufficiency of the vertebral artery. Brain Nerve (Jpn) 22:1125–1138, 1970
29b. Naritomi H, Meyer JS, Sakai F, et al: Effects of advancing age on regional cerebral blood flow. Arch Neurol 36:410–416, 1979
29c. Naritomi H, Sakai F, Meyer JS: Pathogenesis of transient ischemic attacks within the vertebrobasilar system. Arch Neurol 36:121–128.
29d. Patten BM: Transient global amnesia syndrome. JAMA 217:690–691, 1971
29e. Pásztor E: Decompression of vertebral artery in cases of cervical spondylosis. Surg Neurol 9:371–377, 1978
29f. Steinmetz EF, Vroom FQ: Transient global amnesia. Neurology 22:1193–1200, 1972
30. Stenger HH: Ueber Lagenystagmus unter den besonderen Bluecksichtung der gegenlaefigen transitorischen Provocations-nystagmus bei Lagewechsel in der Sagittalebene. Arch Ohren-Nasen-Kehlkopfh 168:220–268, 1955
31. Stewart DY: Current concepts of the "Barré syndrome" or the "posterior cervical sympathetic syndrome." Clin Orthop 24:40–48, 1962
32. Stoops WL, King RB: Neural complication of cervical spondylosis, their response to laminectomy and foramenotomy. J Neurosurg 19:986–999, 1962
33. Sullivan HG, Harbison JW, Vines FS, et al: Embolic posterior cerebral artery occlusion secondary to spondylitic vertebral artery compression. J Neurosurg 43:618–622, 1975
33a. Troost, T: Dizziness and vertigo in vertebrobasilar disease. Part I: Peripheral and systemic causes of dizziness. Stroke 11:301–303, 1980
33b. Troost T: Dizziness and vertigo in vertebrobasilar disease. Part II: Central causes and vertebrobasilar disease. Stroke 11:413–415, 1980
34. Verbiest H: A lateral approach to the cervical spine: technique and indications. J Neurosurg 28:191–203, 1968
35. Williams D: Syndromes associated with carotid and vertebro-basilar insufficiency. In Gillespie JA (ed.): Extracranial Cerebrovascular Disease. Butterworth, London, 1969, pp 37–44
36. Wollner L, McCarthy ST, Doper NDW et al: Failure of cerebral autoregulation in the elderly. Br Med J 8:1117–1118, 1979

13

"Moyamoya" Disease: Clinical Review and Surgical Treatment

Yasuhiro Yonekawa, Takehiko Okuno, and Hajime Handa

Introduction

"Moyamoya" disease was previously considered confined to Japan, but recently a number of cases have been diagnosed in other areas, including Europe and North America. In Japan there has been confusion about this disease, particularly during the early period following its discovery. The purpose of this paper is to clarify aspects of this disease and its treatment and to report the results of recent clinical investigation.

History

In 1955 at the 14th Annual Meeting of the Japanese Neurosurgical Society, Shimizu and Takeuchi presented a case report that was published two years later as a case of bilateral hypoplasia of the internal carotid artery.[71] Today that case is considered to be Moyamoya disease. The 29-year-old patient suffered from visual disturbance and hemiconvulsive seizures since 10 years of age and became blind at the age of 20. Carotid angiography revealed bilateral complete occlusions of the internal carotid arteries. A biopsy of the ascending pharyngeal artery was performed and a slight proliferative change of the intima and media was seen. The occlusion was considered to be congenital hypoplasia and different from usual atheromatous occlusion of the internal carotid artery. Similar case reports were subsequently published by various authors.[31,33,48,66] In 1960, Kudo[31] focused on the type of collateral circulation in this disease and stated in his report the following:

> The blood supply in the bilateral occlusion of the internal carotid artery of this disease depends mainly upon the vertebro-basilar system, but completely abnormal vasculatures, for example, meningeal arteries contribute to the supply of anterior half of the cerebrum, without the usual angiographical pattern of the anterior, middle and posterior cerebral arteries. Our three cases of bilateral occlusion of the internal carotid artery revealed quite different intraarterial anastomotic type from that reported by Meyer and Van der Ecken and have thus proposed interesting themes for further investigation.

He advocated the concept of occlusion of the circle of Willis in this disease.

For this disease a variety of names were suggested, including "cerebral juxtabasilar teleangiectasia," "cerebral arterial rete," "rete mirabile," "cerebral basal rete mirabile," and "Moyamoya" disease ("Moyamoya" indicating puff of smoke) by Suzuki.[65] Nowadays Moyamoya disease or spontaneous occlusion of the circle of Willis are most frequently used.

At the 25th Annual Meeting of the Japanese Neurosurgical Society in 1966, Kudo, as president of the society, focused on the disease as a special theme for discussion, and the proceedings were published in 1967.[32]

In 1977 a research committee on this disease, directed by Gotoh, was organized and sponsored by the Ministry of Welfare and Health of Japan (MWHJ). Extensive investigation was systematically organized in various fields, including epidemiology, pathophysiology, clinical aspects, and pathology. This project is still under investigation but is currently directed by Handa (1984). About 752 cases were registered up to the end of 1981, and a precise analysis has been published in the annual report of the research committee.[11]

In the United States and Europe the disease has been only rarely reported. The cases reported by Weidner[76] and Leed[36] occurred in Japanese patients, but following the report of Taveras[73] in 1969, Moyamoya disease is now known to occur in whites and in blacks as well. In 1974 Picard summarized the status of worldwide outbreak of the disease.[56]

Etiology

The etiology of Moyamoya disease is unknown, and it has been debated whether the disease is acquired or congenital. Similarity of angiographic findings to those of embryonal brain, symmetrical abnormal vasculature, frequent existence of abnormal vasculature without remarkable stenosis of the internal carotid artery, and frequent intrafamilial occurrence would support the congenital theory. Suzuki et al and other investigators considered the etiology to be due to the participation of the immune mechanism, as tonsillitis was frequently encountered in the anamnesis of the patient or from other reasons.[44,65] They regarded the histological findings in the vessels to be similar to the chronic inflammatory changes observed in polyarteritis or Kawasaki disease. The role of the sympathetic nerves was also emphasized along with the inflammatory process.[63] However, a lack of other positive inflammatory findings, both histologically and biochemically, opposes this view. An autoimmune process has also been implicated,[81] but inability to identify immune complexes as described in the section on epidemiology seems to refute this concept.

Epidemiology

Cases of Moyamoya disease are much more frequently encountered in Japan than in other areas, but they have been reported sporadically all over the world.* No special regional predilection within Japan has been reported. This was confirmed in our series as well as in the cooperative study of MHWJ.[11] Incidence seems to be less than one patient per 100,000 persons a year. A female dominance[39] has also been shown in our series (1 : 1.8) and in the cooperative study of MHWJ (1 : 1.3).[11]

There appears to be two definite peaks of incidence: at childhood (around 3 years old) and in the third decade of life. The majority of cases were hospitalized within two years from the onset of the disease.

There is also some evidence[2] of a familial tendency in our series. In the above-mentioned cooperative study of MHWJ, 13 out of 147 families showed a familial tendency,[11] with parent-child occurrence being most frequent, followed by sibling cases. However, a special type of heredity has not been identified so far.

In the same study, human leukocyte antigen (HLA) was investigated in 43 cases, and a remarkable difference in antigen type between juvenile and adult cases was observed. Among HLAs, an increase of HLA-B40 in children under 10 years of age and of HLA-Bw54(22) in children over 11 years of age has been reported.[62] Further investigation and more precise analysis of HLA are required in order to draw more concrete conclusion. In relation to this study, immune complex was investigated in six juvenile cases in our series using the methods of Clq binding examination and Raji cell radioimmunoassay, but we were unable to identify any immune complexes.[18]

Clinical Symptoms and Signs

There are no specific symptoms or signs related to this disease. The various clinical manifesta-

* References 7–9, 12, 13, 19, 20, 21, 25, 30, 39, 53, 57, 58, 75, 83.

Table 13.1. Symptomatology of Moyamoya disease (our series).

	Children (N = 31)	Adults (N = 15)
TIA	29	4
Motor paresis	22	8
Speech disturbance	2	7
Visual disturbance	5	1
Convulsion	5	4
Mental retardation	6	0
Headache	7	8
Vomiting	2	4
Unconsciousness	1	8
Involuntary movement	1	2
Psychoorganic syndrome	3	6

Table 13.2. Clinical types of Moyamoya disease (cooperative study of MHWJ).

	Children	Adults	Total
Hemorrhage	7(5%)	152(65%)	159(41%)
Completed stroke	61(39%)	43(18%)	104(27%)
TIA	61(39%)	15(6%)	76(19%)
Seizure	22(14%)	13(6%)	35(9%)
Others	4(3%)	11(5%)	15(4%)
Total	153	234	389

tions are generally caused by cerebrovascular accident, ischemia, or hemorrhage, and occasionally by epilepsy (Tables 13.1 and 13.2). In juvenile cases the ischemic type is dominant (87% of our series, 78% of cases of the cooperative study[49]). Different kinds of deficits are encountered in ischemic cases. They are sometimes so progressive that cortical blindness, motor aphasia, or even a vegetative state are observed within several years despite intensive treatment.[61] They are usually preceded by transient ischemic attacks (TIAs) or reversible ischemic neurologic deficites (RINDs). This transient weakness or paresis could be provoked by some condition of hyperventilation such as blowing wind instruments, blowing something hot to cool it, or crying. It is considered to be induced by decreased $PaCO_2$ and, therefore, by decreased cerebral blood flow (CBF). Ischemic deterioration is often precipitated by infection of the upper respiratory tract. Mental retardation is reported to be found in about half of the patients.[55,65] In adult cases the hemorrhagic type is more prevalent,[35,41] appearing in 41% of our cases and in 65% of cases of the cooperative study. Predominance of the hemorrhagic type is noticed especially in females (Fig. 13.2). Previously, subarachnoid hemorrhage was considered to be the major type of bleeding, but ven-

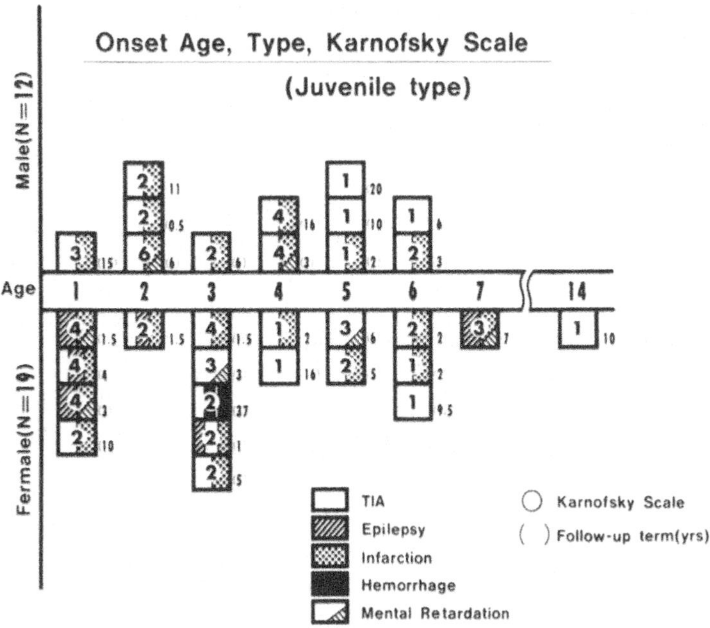

Figure 13.1. Follow-up study of Moyamoya disease (juvenile cases).

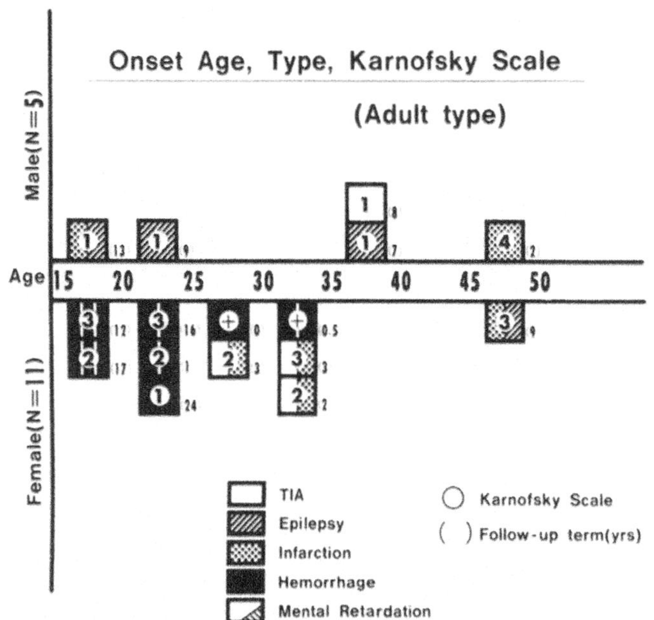

Figure 13.2. Follow-up study of Moyamoya disease (adult cases).

tricular hemorrhage seems to be more common, judging from computed tomography (CT)[70] and autopsy findings.[72] Four of our eight adult patients with bleeding had recurrent bleeding at an interval from several days to more than 10 years. One of them initially showed ischemia and bled 31 years later.

Fatal outcomes have been frequently encountered in cases of massive bleeding. For example, in the series of Tanaka, 20 out of 22 autopsied cases had bleeding.[72]

Vagueness still surrounds the natural history of the disease and whether the juvenile type and the adult type can be considered to belong to the same disease entity is problematic. Our series demonstrated that clinical manifestations do not always remain the same but are interchangeable (Figs. 13.1 and 13.2). The pathologic process appears to be active through to the age of 10, when it is considered to have stabilized. Cases with the onset under 4 years of age seem to have relatively bad Karnofsky scale and, hence, bad functional prognosis.[18] Cases with TIAs of relatively late onset in juvenile type seemingly have a better prognosis.

Pathology

The first autopsy case was reported by Maki and Nakata in 1965.[38] It was that of a 9-year-old child who died of hemorrhage. They enumerated the following important findings:

1. Narrowing of main trunks of the intracranial skull base arteries
2. Many abnormal small vessels originating from the circle of Willis
3. Undifferentiated small arteries and veins in the subarachnoid space and in the cerebral parenchyma
4. Secondary parenchymatous changes such as infarction and necrosis encountered in the temporal and occipital lobes.

Later, autopsy cases were reported by various authors,[3,23,37,51,52] including Handa et al,[16] Suzuki et al,[67] Tanaka et al,[72] and Hosoda et al.[24] Most autopsy cases revealed death due to intracranial hemorrhage. Previously it was considered that the bleeding originated from ruptured cortical "Moyamoya" vessels. However, accumulated autopsy reports and the development of CT scan revealed intraventricular hemorrhage originating from the ventricular wall, basal ganglia, or thalamus to be the major source of bleeding.

The following are considered to be the main causes of bleeding[72]:

1. Rupture of dilated and stressed perforating arteries

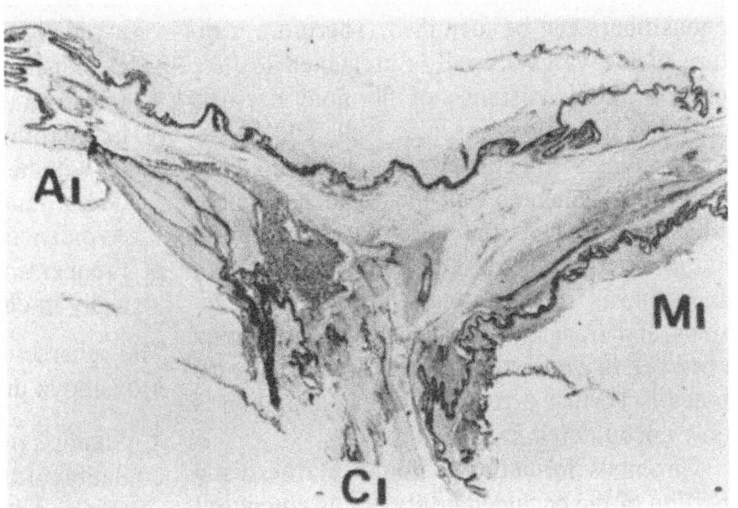

Figure 13.3. Histology of a main artery constricting the circle of Willis. Note the remarkable intimal thickening. (Courtesy of Prof. Tanaka.)

2. Fibrinoid necrosis of arterial wall in the basal ganglia
3. Rupture of microaneurysms in the periventricular region, especially around the superior-lateral wall of the lateral ventricles.

Severe stenosis at the carotid fork has been reported to be due to concentric lamellar intimal thickening by cellular fibrous tissue[3] (Fig. 13.3). In juvenile cases the lamellar structure is not so clear despite a high degree of intimal thickening, although it is frequently observed in adult cases. The latter finding is most conspicuous in the more peripheral arteries such as the anterior cerebral artery and middle cerebral artery, in both juvenile and adult cases. The internal elastic lamina is frequently partly stratified whereas the tunica media and adventitia are usually normal.

Pathologic changes in the perforating arteries of Moyamoya can be classified into three types: stenosis, dilatation, and mixed. In the first, the lumen is stenosed by fibrous tissue and by proliferation and winding of the internal elastic lamina (Fig. 13.4). Fibrosis of the tunica media and proliferation of elastic fibers are typical findings, which may be regared as elastofibrosis. Sometimes organized thrombus occludes the vascular lumen. Dilated vessels have a thinned vascular wall with preservation of the

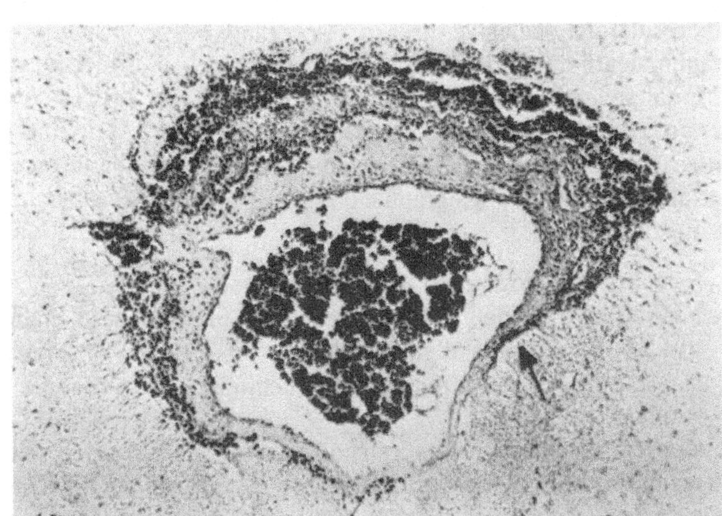

Figure 13.4. Histology of a perforating artery. Note the thinning of the vascular wall (*arrow*) with preservation of the internal elastic lamina. (Courtesy of Prof. Tanaka.)

elastic lamina, but in extreme cases only collagenous fibers can be identified. Therefore, rupture of the vascular wall is presumed to take place without existence of fibrinoid necrosis covering the whole vascular wall. Old hematoma cavities sometimes contain ruptured artery with fragmented wall and organized lumen, which may indicate the possibility of rerupture of the vessel. In the mixed group with dilatation and stenosis in perforating arteries, stenotic lesions and fragmentation of the elastic lamina observed in perforating arteries are usually also noted in cortical arteries, whereas dilatation is only encountered in limited cases.

Thrombus formation is found at the distal portion of the occluded artery and is composed of either white thrombus consisting mainly of platelets or of fibrin thrombus, or mixed thrombus. This thrombus does not play an essential role in the etiology of Moyamoya disease, but is considered to participate in the progress of the disease and in the development of cerebral ischemia.[3,24]

Clinical Examination

No remarkable findings are found in the laboratory data.[65]

Angiography

Cerebral angiography is indispensable in the diagnosis of this disease, but it should be performed with great care. The complication rate is considered to be higher than in the more usual atherosclerotic occlusive disease. A postangiographic death due to infarction occurred in our hospital several years ago. Considerable numbers of complications have not been published hitherto. The following measures have been undertaken to prevent angiographic complications in our department:

1. Selective angiography with Seldinger's method by a trained hand. Unnecessary intravascular wedging of the catheter, especially at the internal carotid artery, should be avoided.
2. General anesthesia in children and infants to maintain hemodynamics and stable blood gases.
3. Intraoperative hypotension should be avoided so that an intravenous drip is always established even in adult cases.
4. Intraoperative administration of low molecular dextran and frequent irrigation of catheter with heparin saline to prevent clot formation around the catheter.
5. Avoidance of preoperative dehydration.
6. Preoperative administration of steroid, especially in children.

The characteristic angiographic findings of Moyamoya disease are as follows:

1. Stenosis or occlusion beginning at the termination of the intracranial internal carotid artery and also at the origin of the anterior and middle cerebral arteries.
2. Abnormal vascular network in the region of the basal ganglia.
3. Above-mentioned findings symmetrical on both sides.
4. Transdural anastomosis ("rete mirable").

Findings 1 through 3 of the above are included in the diagnostic criteria of Moyamoya disease proposed by the research committee of MHWJ[11] (Table 13.3).

Suzuki et al classified progression of the disease into six phases, according to angiographic findings[66]:

1. Stenosis of the intracranial bifurcation of the internal carotid artery.
2. First appearance of Moyamoya (dilatation of the intracerebral arteries).
3. Increasing of Moyamoya (disappearing process of the middle and anterior cerebral arteries).
4. Finer formation of Moyamoya (disappearing process of the posterior cerebral arteries).
5. Shrinking of Moyamoya (disappearance of the intracerebral arteries).
6. Disappearance of Moyamoya and collateral circulations only from the external carotid system.

These changes have, however, not always been observed in our series, nor in others, although some remarkable changes such as the progression of stenosis in the main trunks and decreased visualization of cortical arteries were noticed in accordance with progression of symptoms, especially in juvenile cases (Fig.

Table 13.3. Guidelines for the diagnosis of Moyamoya disease proposed by the MHWJ research committee on spontaneous occlusion of the circle of Wills.

I. Age of onset varies but is rather prevalent in youths and in females.
  a. Symptoms and type of progression vary, namely, asymptomatic type or type of transient or fixed neurologic deficits of slight or severe degree can exist.
  b. Cerebral ischemia is observed usually in the juvenile case and hemorrhage in the adult case.
  c. In juvenile cases hemiparesis, monoparesis, sensory disturbance, involuntary movement, headache, convulsion would appear with recurrence, sometimes alternating the side. Mental retardation and fixed neurologic deficits are also observed. Hemorrhagic type is rare.
  d. In adult cases symptoms similar to those observed in juvenile cases may appear, but most of them have sudden onset of intraventricular, subarachnoid, or intracerebral hemorrhage. Recovery from bleeding with or without fixed deficits is the usual course, but direct mortality is also observed in severe cases.

II. Angiography is indispensable for the diagnosis, with the following findings observed and recognized bilaterally:
  a. Stenosis or occlusion at the terminal portion of the intracranial internal carotid artery (ICA) and/or at the proximal portion of the anterior cerebral artery (ACA) and/or the middle cerebral artery (MCA).
  b. Abnormal Moyamoya vessels in the vicinity of the above mentioned areas in the arterial phase.

III. Etiology is unknown and basic disease is ruled out.

IV. The following pathologic findings are helpful for diagnosis.
  a. Intimal thickening and resulting stenosis or occlusion are observed around the intracranial terminal portion of the ICA usually bilaterally. They are sometimes associated with lipoid degeneration.
  b. In the main arteries (ACA, MCA, PCOM) of the circle of Willis, various degrees of stenoses and occlusions are observed in association with intimal fibrous thickening, winding of the internal elastic lamina, and thinning of the tunica media.
  c. Many tiny vascular channels (perforators and anastomatic branches) are observed around the circle of Willis.
  d. Small vessels of conglomerated networks are observed in the pia mater.

Diagnostic criteria will be divided into two groups. Autopsy cases without angiography will be investigated separately in reference to IV.
  1. Definite diagnosis fulfills all of the findings described in II and III simultaneously.
  2. Probable diagnosis fails to fulfill the criteria (b) in II but fulfills the other criteria mentioned under definite diagnosis.

13.5). Abnormal networks named Moyamoya in the region of basal ganglia are considered to function as collateral pathways (intraparenchymatous anastomosis) to the cortical arteries.

In addition to this type of collateral circulation in the basal ganglia, "ethmoidal Moyamoya" or "Moyamoya-like" network in the frontobasal region may also be visualized (Fig. 13.6). In our series some juvenile cases revealed this type of Moyamoya, which is considered to function as a collateral pathway to the forebrain via the ethmoid sinus through branches of the internal maxillary artery.

Transdural anastomosis termed "rete mirabile" (but this is not true rete mirabile) is abundant[17,50] and may also be named "vault Moyamoya."[29] The contributing arteries to this anastomosis are as follows: anterior falcal artery, middle meningeal artery, ethmoidal arteries, occipital artery, tentorial artery, and superficial temporal arteries. Of these, the first three are considered to be main contributing arteries. According to Kodama et al,[29] the appearance of "vault Moyamoya" seems to be confined to specific localities, of which there are nine in juvenile cases and six in adults. These transdural anastomoses are also considered to play a significant role as collateral pathways.

From the surgical point of view, cortical arteries deserve more attention. Territory of the middle cerebral artery (MCA) might be divided into two (or three) segments—i.e., the candelabra (anterior part) and the rest, including the angular artery and the posterior temporal artery (posterior part). About half of our Moyamoya cases revealed nonvisualization of the posterior

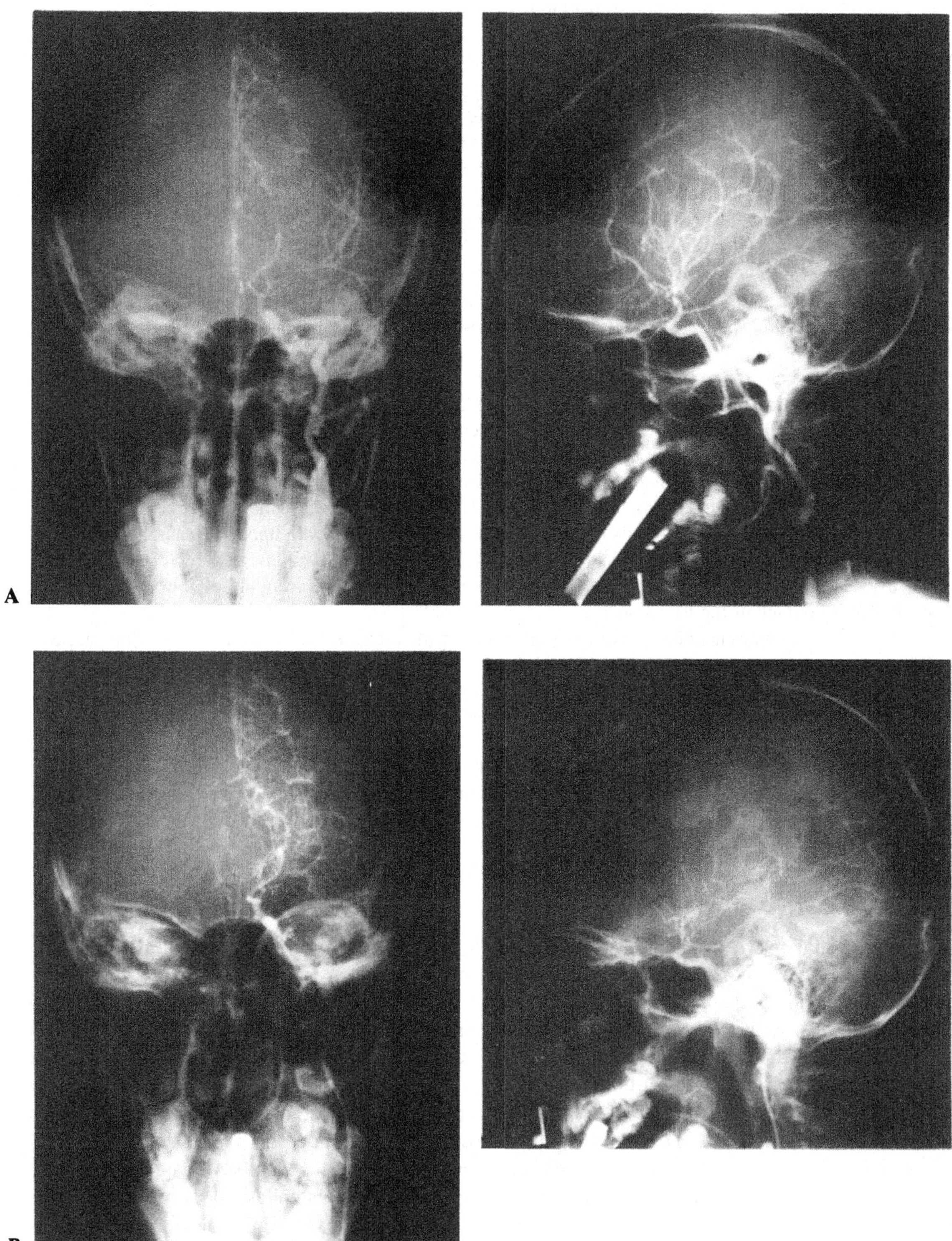

Figure 13.5. **A.** An 8-year-old girl with typical angiographic findings but with preservation of the main arteries. **B.** Seven months later the patient was readmitted because of progression of ischemic symptoms on the nonoperated side. The angiography revealed nonvisualization of the MCA.

part of the MCA. Table 13.4 indicates angiographic nonvisualization of the cortical arteries. In our juvenile cases the entire territory of the MCA and the posterior cerebral artery (PCA) seems to be more involved than that in the adult cases.

The vertebrobasilar system has been reported to be involved rather rarely in this disease.[64,65] In our department there have been two juvenile cases in which the trunk of the basilar artery occluded completely (Fig. 13.7). Scarceness of collateral circulation due to nonvisualization of the cortical artery seems to be closely related with CT findings (low-density areas).

Aneurysms in combination with Moyamoya disease have been frequently reported.[1,6,47,52,78] Three types of aneurysms seem to occur with Moyamoya disease: (1) There are the aneurysms at the usual sites, namely the circle of Willis; (2) There are aneurysms of the peripheral arteries such as the posterior choroidal artery, the anterior choroidal artery, and Heubner's artery; and (3) there are aneurysms localized in the area of Moyamoya vessels. The last two have been reported to be false aneurysms, in view of their location and form and in view of their histological examination with lack of aneurysmal wall. But the true aneurysm with aneurysmal wall might also be included. Aneurysms of all these three groups might rupture and are considered to be one of the probable origins of cerebral hemorrhage.

CT Scan

Approximately 40% of the ischemic type of Moyamoya disease is reported to have normal CT finding.[11] Positive CT scan findings of Moyamoya disease in the ischemic type after Handa et al and others[5,14,15,43,69] are as follows:

1. Low-density areas (LDA) confined to cerebral cortex and subcortex.
2. Dilated cerebral sulci and fissures.
3. Slight ventricular dilatation. LDAs are not usually observed in the basal ganglia, in contrast with acute infantile hemiplegia and/or atherosclerotic occlusive disease.

In our series LDAs in children have been more frequently observed in PCA territory than in the other territory. This seems to be related to the scarceness of the collateral supply through the affected PCA (Table 13.5).

In the hemorrhagic type, high-density area

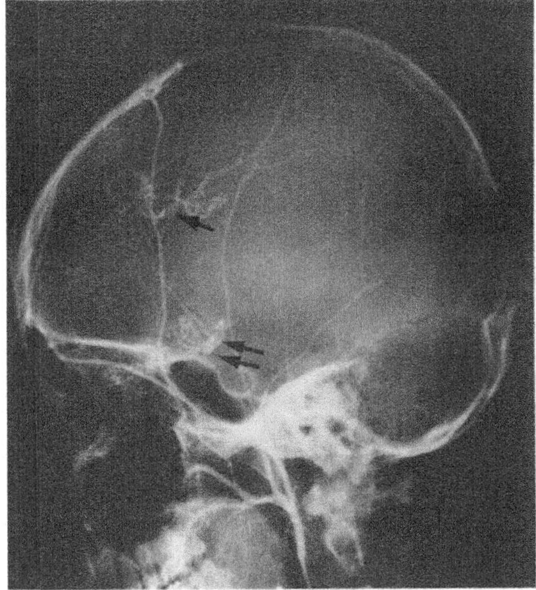

Figure 13.6. A case with transdural anastomosis "vault Moyamoya" (*single arrow*) and the ethmoidal Moyamoya (*double arrows*) well visualized.

Table 13.4. Angiographic nonvisualization of the cortical arteries.

		Adults (N = 13)	Children (N = 18)
ACA		38%	30%
MCA	anterior + posterior	15%	46%
MCA	posterior	65%	49%
PCA		4%	47%

ACA, anterior cerebral artery; PCA, posterior cerebral artery; MCA, middle cerebral artery.

Table 13.5 Angiographic findings of PCA and CT findings.

	Normal CT	Abnormal CT	PCA territory
Normal PCA			
Children	2	4	3
Adults	3	5	0
Abnormal PCA			
Children	1	12	8
Adults	1	3	1

PCA, posterior cerebral artery.

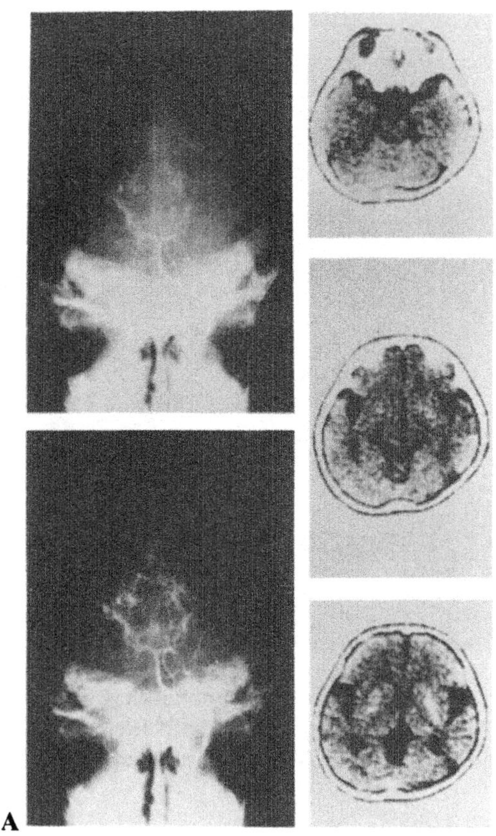

Figure 13.7. **A.** This 2-year-old female was admitted with the diagnosis of Moyamoya disease, having TIAs and CT scan and vertebral angiogram as indicated. **B.** Bypass procedure was postponed because of recurrent viral infections such as mumps and varicella. Seven months later she was admitted again with completed stroke with tetraparesis and visual disturbance. CT scan revealed an extensive infarction, and vertebral angiography showed a complete occlusion of the basilar artery.

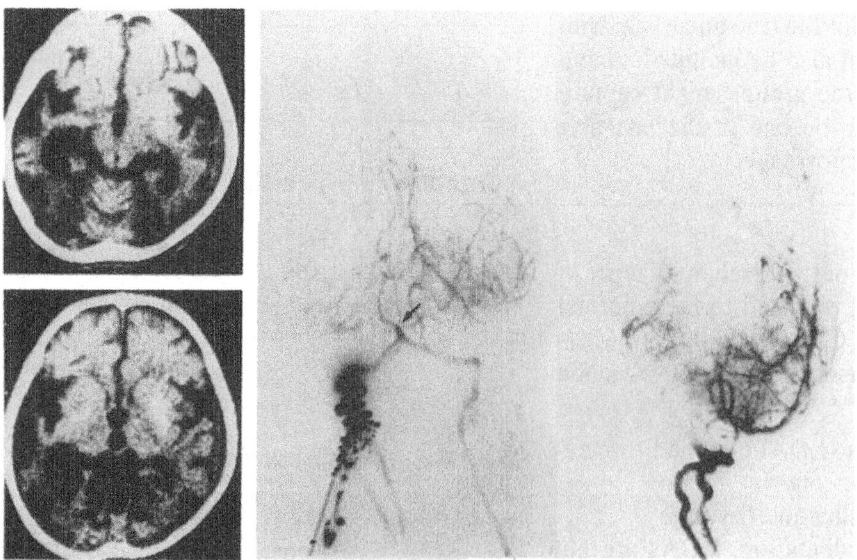

(HDA) may be observed in the basal ganglia, ventricular system, subcortex, and cortex, in that order of frequency.[11]

Enhancement of Moyamoya vessels in the basal ganglia on contrast study is often observed, but this finding is considered to be unreliable in predicting the existence of the disease. Although these are all nonspecific findings, attempts are being made to use the CT scan as a screening test in combination with newer methods such as the dynamic CT scan, which seems to be very promising.

Typical findings of Moyamoya disease on dynamic CT scan are as follows:

1. Appearance of abnormal vasculature in the basal ganglia.
2. Delayed dye filling in the territory of the MCA.
3. Wash-out delay of the above-mentioned filling.

As dynamic CT scan is less invasive compared with angiography, this method can be used as a screening test and an indicator of effectiveness of the revascularization procedure for Moyamoya disease (Fig. 13.8).

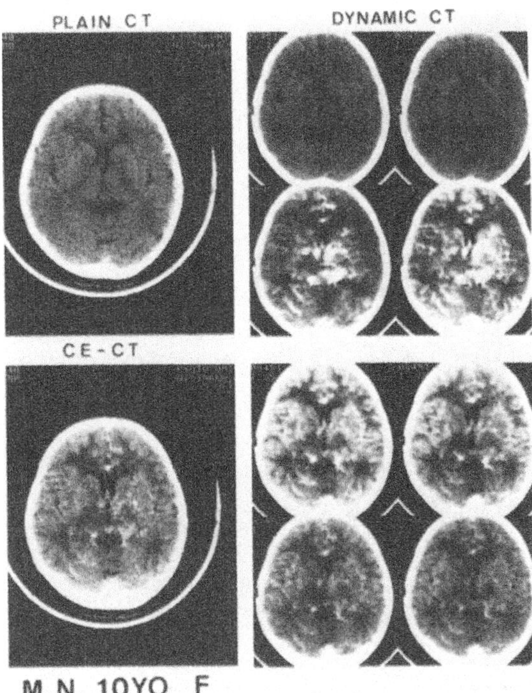

Figure 13.8. A case of Moyamoya disease. The dynamic CT scan indicates the vascular network markedly. This visualization of Moyamoya could not be obtained with the usual contrast study of CT scan.

CBF Measurement

Regional CBF measurement by intracarotid injection[74] has methodological weaknesses owing to the carotid occlusion or high degree of stenosis found in this disease. There is also the danger of ischemic complications. To overcome these difficulties, we have introduced the xenon 133 inhalation system of Cerebrograph® (Novo Co. Ltd.) for the measurement of rCBF. Applying 9 to 13 detectors on both sides, respectively, rCBF based on the method of Obrist is calculated using the Hewlett Packard 9845 S calculator system.

To evaluate and compare the rCBFs of the grey matter, we use F1 or ISI values. Decreased response to $PaCO_2$ changes,[74] postoperative increases of rCBF, and postoperative changes in the rCBF distribution were confirmed in our series. The disadvantages of this method are as follows:

1. Extracranial contamination may occur, especially in the frontal and temporal basal portions, owing to mucous membranes and temporal muscles.
2. Difficulty in placing the detectors in the same position as in the previous examination in order to compare exact local differences.
3. Infants and patients with tracheostomies are not suitable for this method.

Further attempts will be made to measure rCBF in three dimensions with xenon-enhanced CT, photon-emission CT, and positron-emission CT to evaluate hemodynamic and metabolic changes. Krypton 81m-emission CT study also has proved advantageous in revealing the peculiar hemodynamics of Moyamoya disease. The vertebral artery was revealed to supply some significant collateral flow to the territory of the internal carotid artery in this disease (Fig. 13.9).

A relatively invasive method using argon and mass spectrometry based on Fick's principle seems to be very effective in measuring CBF and related metabolic parameters of Moyamoya disease. Reduced CBF at the superficial part of the brain and reduced cerebral metabolic rate of oxygen ($CMRO_2$) have been reported.[42]

Doppler Sonography

Doppler sonography is well known as one of the most useful methods for detecting extracranial stenoocclusive lesions noninvasively. We have registered the change of flow pattern of Moyamoya disease pre-, intra- and postoperatively.[46]

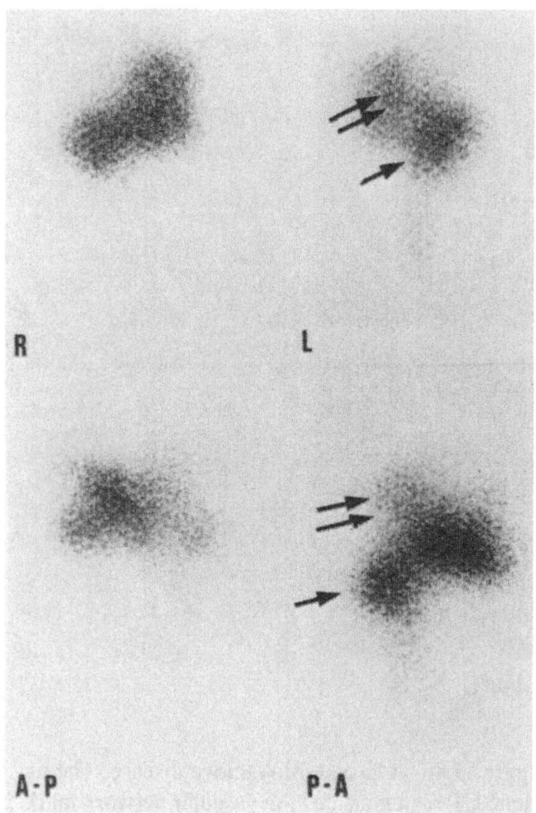

Figure 13.9. An adult case of Moyamoya disease. ^{81m}Kr-emission reveals significant collateral circulation from the left vertebral artery to the cerebrum. *Single arrow* indicates cerebellar hemisphere and *double arrow* indicates supratentorial structures.

The special flow patterns in Moyamoya disease are as follows:

1. Decreased or absent flow in the cervical portion of the internal carotid artery on both sides.
2. Flow pattern changes of the external carotid artery, especially of the superficial temporal artery into the pattern of the internal carotid artery. This finding is well correlated with the angiographic findings of "rete mirabile" through transdural anastomosis.

A method of visualizing stenotic sites with color displays by scanning Doppler flow signals has become available recently.

Electroencephalogram

Abnormal EEG findings in Moyamoya disease are nonspecific. EEG shows low voltage or slow waves with or without an asymmetry.[28,48,55] They are related to permanent ischemic changes or transient hemodynamic changes due to $PaCO_2$ variation. Yoshii et al[82] summarized EEG changes in Moyamoya disease as follows:

1. Abnormal EEG changes are frequently observed in juvenile cases but are less common in adult cases.
2. Diffuse and/or bilateral slow waves are observed usually as abnormal waves and occasionally as spike waves.
3. "Build up" appearance of delta waves during hyperventilation and "re-build up" appearance of polymorphous slow waves a few minutes after hyperventilation (Fig. 13.10) are considered characteristic in juvenile cases. Although quite often related with TIAs, these appearances are observed less frequently in adult cases. Photic stimulation has usually no effect on EEG.

Other kinds of examinations such as SER (somatosensory-evoked response) deserve to be mentioned. SER reflects the neuronal function in somatosensory centrifugal pathways. Abnormality of SER is reported to be better correlated to clinical fixed neurologic deficits than to CT findings. By contrast, ABR (auditory brainstem response) is reported to reveal no abnormality in Moyamoya disease except for patients with vertebrobasilar occlusion (Fig. 13.11).

Diagnosis

Diagnostic criteria for Moyamoya disease have been proposed by the research committee of MWHJ, as described in Table 13.3.

The following differential diagnoses should be taken into consideration:

1. Atherosclerotic occlusive disease. Occlusive processes are observed mainly at the cervical bifurcation followed by the carotid siphon. They do not usually reach the carotid fork, therefore blood supply from the vertebrobasilar system via the posterior communicating artery is usually present, without Moyamoya vessel formation. The CT findings are also different: LDAs are observed in the basal ganglia as well as in the cortex and subcortex, whereas LDAs in Moyamoya dis-

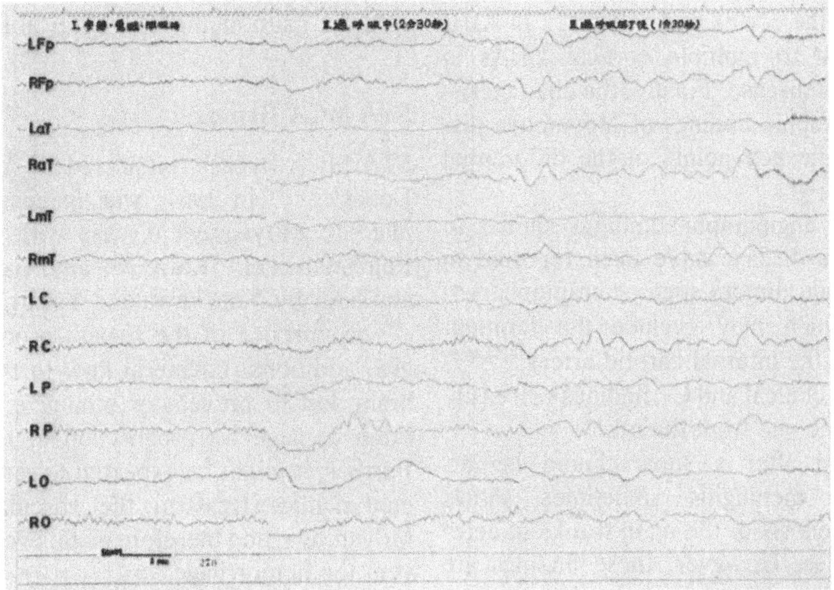

Figure 13.10. EEG in a 10-year-old girl. I. At rest. Note a marked asymmetry. The left hemisphere shows low voltage. The background activity is alpha waves of 8–10 cps mixed with 7 cps theta waves in the right hemisphere. II. During hyperventilation. There is marked buildup in the right parietal area. III. 90 seconds after the end of hyperventilation. Note the delta waves over the right hemisphere.

ease are confined in the cortex and subcortex and are frequently multiple. Probable cases, according to criteria of the research committee of MWHJ, particularly those with unilateral lesion, should be followed up carefully as an unfinished or incomplete type.

2. Acute infantile hemiplegia (AIH). Sudden onset of hemiplegia is characteristically observed in both diseases; however, preceding reversible ischemic episodes are frequently observed in Moyamoya disease, but not in AIH. They can be also differentiated on CT

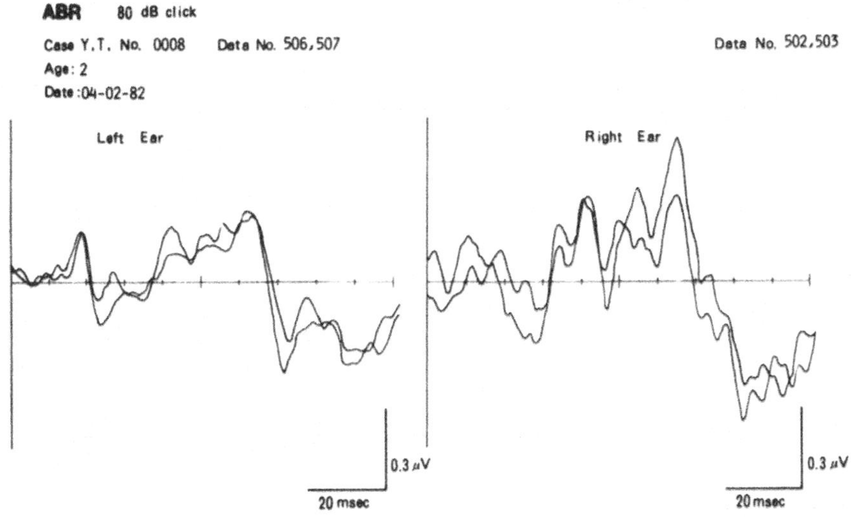

Figure 13.11. ABR of the patient with occlusion of the basilar artery described in Fig. 13.7. Note the prolonged latency of the V wave.

findings; LDAs appear in the basal ganglia as well as in the cortex and subcortex in AIH, in contrast to multiple cortical LDAs in Moyamoya disease. Finally, the characteristic angiographic findings of Moyamoya disease are the key points of the differential diagnosis.
3. Confusing angiographic findings similar to Moyamoya disease have been reported in certain brain tumors such as craniopharyngioma, which may occlude the terminal portion of the internal carotid artery.[4,34,45,60] However, clinical and CT findings will easily differentiate one from the other.
4. Vasospasm after a subarachnoid hemorrhage or meningitis sometimes shows marked stenosis of the main trunks of cerebral arteries. However, these findings are usually transient and improve after a time. The clinical manifestations are also usually different.

Treatment

Medical Treatment

Although no effective specific treatment has been reported hitherto, steroids are considered effective in certain cases, especially in cases with involuntary movements and in the active phase of recurrent ischemic attacks. The mechanism of their effectiveness is unknown, although influences on vasculitis, edema, and CBF have all been presumed.

Acetylsalicylic acid (ASA) may also be prescribed, as platelets are considered to play an important role in the progressive thrombotic occlusions of the main vascular trunk in Moyamoya disease.[24]

Other symptomatic medication for bleeding, epilepsy, and headache will not be mentioned here.

Surgical Treatment

Superficial temporal artery-middle cerebral artery (STA/MCA) bypass, encephalomyosynangiosis (EMS), omentum transplantation, and stellate ganglionectomy can be enumerated. And for the hemorrhagic group, ventricular drainage and hematoma evacuation are considered the main methods of surgical treatment.

STA-MCA Bypass

STA-MCA bypass, pioneered by Yasargil and Donaghy[77,79] in 1967, was independently applied to Moyamoya disease with success by Reichman et al,[59] Karasawa and Kikuchi et al,[27] and later by Yonekawa and Yasargil.[79]

The purpose of the bypass procedure is to give additional collateral flow to the ischemic brain and to prevent or minimize irreversible brain damage on progression of the disease. Further, it might be expected to reduce the hemodynamic stress to the vascular network Moyamoya, and therefore might eventually prevent the hemorrhage.

It was Professor Krayenbuhl during the international symposium of EC/IC bypass in 1976 who told the author (YY) to pay attention to Dr. Tew's skepticism regarding the application of the bypass procedure to the treatment of Moyamoya disease. Dr. Peerless was also skeptical, as cases of complication with postoperative hemiplegia, despite patent bypass, had been recorded. Professor Suzuki was also of the same opinion and that seemed to be the reason that he resorted to the cervical sympathectomy as the surgical treatment of this disease.[68]

From bitter experiences with ischemic complications in our earlier series, we investigated the hemodynamic changes before and after bypass procedures with various monitoring parameters, e.g., measurement of the intra-arterial pressure (IAP) of the MCA, Doppler sonography, power EEG, etc.

To avoid complications when performing the revascularization procedure, the following should be considered:

1. Suitable cortical arteries of about 1 mm in diameter may be few, despite extensive craniotomy, or may be hidden relatively deep in the sulci. There may be a rich supply of small branches to the cortex, making preparation of a cortical branch for bypass difficult. If a suitable cortical branch cannot be found, EMS or omentum transplantation should be considered as the revascularization procedure.
2. The middle meningeal artery and frontal

branches of the STA should be preserved as far as possible when performing craniotomy in cases where marked transdural anastomosis is observed, or when Doppler sonography reveals the pattern of the internal carotid artery in these arteries. These transdural anastomoses make an important contribution to collateral circulation.

3. In combination with STA-MCA bypass, EMS or the double bypass (one is for the candelabra and the other for the angular artery) may be applied to prevent harmful changes in blood flow and its distribution, which, in some cases, have been recorded by CBF measurement and angiography following bypass.
4. Intraoperative hypotension should be carefully avoided, as the collateral circulation through basal Moyamoya and rete mirable appears to be critical in cases with active ischemia, and hypotension might lead to ischemic complication. The IAP of the cortical arteries is extremely low in comparison with cerebrovascular occlusive disease of atherosclerotic origin. Intraoperative Doppler sonography may reveal a weak flow signal even when a suitable recipient artery is present on the cortex.
5. Hyperventilation or a low $PaCO_2$ level should be also avoided. Collateral pathways are affected by low $PaCO_2$, increasing the danger of ischemic complications. Furthermore, with the brain shrinkage due to hyperventilation and CSF drainage after opening of the arachnoid, a considerable volume of the air will remain in the subdural space after craniotomy closure. This might induce delicate hemodynamic changes. Subgaleal or epidural drainage with negative pressure also is considered to reduce CBF. As a rule, we use halothane anesthesia and maintain the $PaCO_2$ above 40 mmHg so that sufficient CBF and expansion of the brain can be accomplished.
6. The duration of clamping of the MCA during anastomotic procedure should be as short as possible, because of the complicated mode of collateral circulation. Prolonged clamping might induce a cardinal decrease of rCBF. Power EEG revealed marked decrease of fast waves toward the end of the clamping in certain cases.
7. Steroids are used routinely, as in tumor surgery for the reasons mentioned in the section on medical treatment.

Encephalomyosynangiosis (EMS)

This type of operation was first reported by Henschen in 1950.[22] His intention was to divert blood flow from the external carotid artery into the internal carotid system by applying temporal muscle to the brain surface of a patient with bilateral internal carotid stenosis. This method has since been revived and applied to Moyamoya disease by Karasawa and Kikuchi et al.[26] It is felt that new vascularization via temporal muscle takes place much more effectively in juvenile cases than in adult cases and when the arachnoidea has been opened extensively. EMS was thus routinely performed in our juvenile series—EMS alone when suitable recipient arteries could not be found or EMS in combination with usual STA-MCA bypass to prevent the ischemic complication due to change of blood flow distribution after the STA-MCA bypass alone.

Omentum Transplant

Pedicled omental application has been investigated and evaluated as an effective treatment for lymphedema of the upper extremity after radical mastectomy,[10] ischemia of the lower extremity, postirradiation carotid rupture after radical neck surgery, and cerebral ischemia. Autogenous-free graft transplant of the greater omentum has been performed, for example, in a patient with extensive scalp defect in plastic surgery. The capability of fluid absorption and vascularization by the transplanted greater omentum was reevaluated by Yonekawa and Yasargil.[80] The method has been described in detail elsewhere. Omentum is considered to have a much greater potential to vascularize ischemic tissues than muscle. We have applied this method to two juvenile cases with success. However, this method has two disadvantages in comparison with EMS: it is technically difficult, and it needs laparotomy. Both of our cases were boys and no suitable recipient artery could be found. The method of pedicled omentum transposition on the brain surface reported by Goldsmith has been performed frequently in

China and is reported to be effective for cerebral ischemia but seems to need further precise evaluation.

Other Methods

Durapexia (Tsubokawa) and duraencephalosynanjiosis (Matsushima[40]) belong to the same category of operation as EMS, namely, introduction of external carotid flow into the internal carotid system via newly developed vascularization. Perivascular sympathectomy combined with superior cervical ganglionectomy was advocated by Suzuki et al[68] to improve CBF, but this method has not been widely acknowledged as a method of improving CBF permanently.

Ventricular drainage for intraventricular hemorrhage and evacuation of intracerebral hematoma for the hemorrhagic type of this disease will not be mentioned here.

Results of Our Operative Treatment

A summary of our operated cases are listed in Table 13.6. Twenty children and 11 adults un-

Table 13.6. Clinical summary of operated cases.

	Patient	Age		Onset age	Manifestation	Operation	Results
(a) Juvenile type							
1	TK	10	F	5	lt rt TIAs, MR	lt rt STA-MCA	NIA
2	AS	13	F	3	lt rt TIAs, MR	lt rt STA-MCA	NIA
3	OA	8	F	6	rt lt TIAs, rt Cs	lt rt STA-MCA	NIA
4	SK	5	M	4	rt lt TIAs, lt rt CS	lt STA-MCA + rt OM	NIA
5	OS	6	M	2	rt lt TIAs	rt STA-MCA + lt OM	rt worse, lt NIA
6	NT	4	F	3	rt lt TIAs, rt lt CS	rt lt STA-MCA	NIA
7	WY	6	M	2	rt lt TIAs, rt lt CS	lt STA-MCA	worse (m.h.)
8	KK	7	F	6	rt lt TIAs, rt Cs	lt rt STA-MCA	decreased TIAs
9	KR	7	F	3	lt rt TIAs, lt rt CS	lt rt STA-MCA	NIA
10	TK	7	M	5	rt lt TIA, rt CS	lt rt STA-MCA	NIA
11	KN	2	M	2	Epi, rt CS	rt STA-MCA	NIA
12	AH	6	F	4	rt TIAs	rt STA-MCA	NIA
13	SM	12	M	6	lt TIAs	lt STA-MCA	NIA
14	HK	3	F	2	lt TIAs, Epi CS	lt STA-MCA	lt NIA, rt TIAs
15	YJ	10	F	1	rt TIAs, lt TIAs, rt CS	rt STA-MCA	rt NIA, lt TIAs
16	NM	9	F	4	rt TIA, rt CS	rt STA-MCA	NIA
17	FK	8	F	3	lt TIA, lt CS	lt STA-MCA	NIA
18	TY	2	F	1	Epi, lt rt TIA, lt rt CS	rt EMS	NIA
19	KA	4	F	3	Epi, lt TIAs, lt CS	lt STA-MCA	NIA
20	TF	9	M	6	rt TIAs, rt CS	rt STA-MCA	NIA
(b) Adult type							
21	DA	30	F	28	SAH	lt STA-MCA	NSAH
22	HN	38	F	17	SAHs	lt rt STA-MCA	NSAH
23	FM	27	F	26	lt TIAs, lt CS	lt STA-MCA	NIA
24	UK	37	F	35	lt rt TIAs, lt rt CSs	lt STA-MCA, rt EMS	NIA
25	NJ	39	M	39	Epi, TIA, lt CS	lt STA-MCA	NIA
26	ES	39	M	36	lt TIAs	lt STA-MCA	NIA
27	AM	34	F	3	lt TIAs, SAH	lt STA-MCA	SAH NIA
28	TY	28	F	21	Epi, lt CS	lt STA-MCA	NIA
29	HY	23	F	25	SAH	lt STA-MCA	NSAH
30	KK	49	M	49	CSs	lt rt STA-MCA	NIA
31	TM	35	F	33	lt TIA	lt rt STA-MCA	NIA

NIA, no ischemic attacks; CS, completed stroke; Epi, epilepsy; m.h., malignant hyperthermia; NSAH, so subarachnoid hemorrhage.

derwent surgical treatment through the end of 1982. The follow-up term varies from one month to six years. About half of them received surgical treatment on both sides. Most of the surgery was the STA-MCA bypass with or without combination EMS. EMS without bypass was performed only in two cases because no proper recipient artery could be found. For the same reason omental transplant was performed in two cases. A double bypass, one for the candelabra the other for the angular or posterior temporal artery, without EMS was performed because of hemodynamic considerations. A second operation of the bypass on both sides was performed approximately two to three months after the first operation, when the delicate hemodynamics of Moyamoya disease were considered to have stabilized. There were two cases in which postoperative neurologic deterioration persisted for more than three weeks—case 7, where a malignant hyperthermia was detected just at the beginning of the operation, and case 5, where newly developed ischemia occurred. In five cases new LDAs appeared postoperatively, which are discussed later. They were connected with transient or permanent neurologic deficits. TIAs were sometimes observed on the contralateral side of the bypassed brain (cases 15, 16). Recurrence of ventricular hemorrhage was noticed in case 27, in which the STA-MCA bypass was constructed five years before on the left side.

From the results listed in Table 13.6, it has been felt that revascularization procedure could prevent or minimize the progression of cerebral ischemia from the clinical point of view. The results coincide well with the report of Karasawa et al.[27] Whether this procedure does reduce the chance of bleeding remains to be studied.

Angiography

Follow-up angiography, which is usually performed after two months, could not be performed for various reasons in two out of the early 30 STA-MCA bypasses. Of these two cases, one had a patent bypass and the other was occluded, as assessed by Doppler sonography. The patency rate thus was more than 95%. Visualization of cortical MCAs also occurred in cases where EMS alone was performed (Fig. 13.12). Other findings, such as dilatation of deep muscular arteries, dural arteries, and arteriolar or capillary blushes, indirectly indicate the contribution of these vessels as collateral pathways. These "blushes" may originate from vasa vasorum and periadventitial vessels preserved at the time of STA dissection. In contrast to the postoperative angiographic findings of occlusive atherosclerotic occlusive disease, visualization of the entire territory of the MCA through STA-MCA bypass was infrequent in advanced Moyamoya disease. In a few cases flow pattern within the territory of the MCA changed remarkably postoperatively. Figure 13.13 indicates a case in our earlier series in which the posterior part of the MCA was clearly visualized though the bypass, while the anterior part, which had been opacified by the preoperative internal carotid angiography, was visualized neither via the bypass nor via the internal carotid artery. Postoperative CT scan revealed a new LDA accordingly associated with temporary deterioration of neurologic deficits.

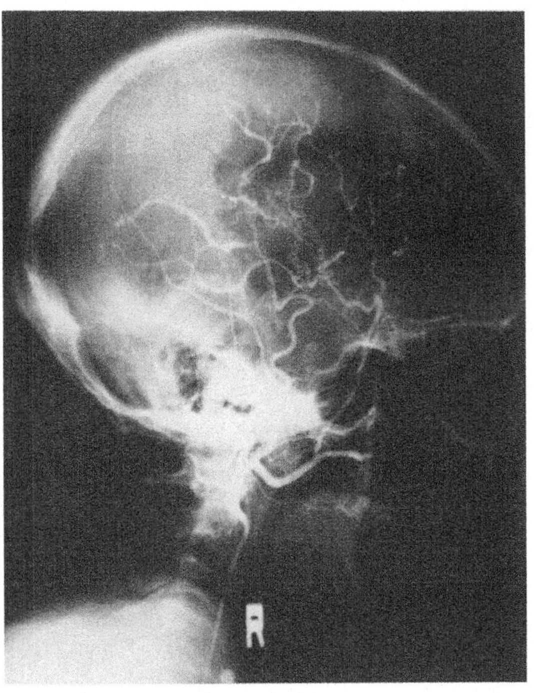

Figure 13.12. A case with EMS. Note dilated muscular artery and visualization of the MCA.

A reduction of Moyamoya after the revascularization procedure has been reported by

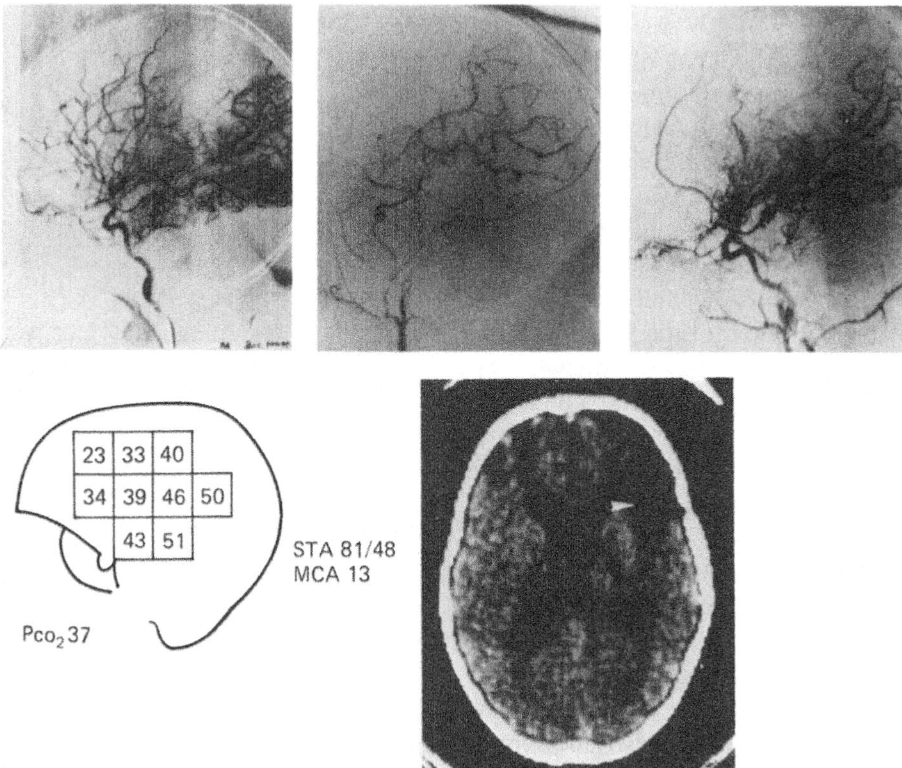

Figure 13.13. A 4-year-old girl. Left internal carotid angiography (CAG) revealed well-visualized arteries of the candelabra, whereas the angular artery and posterior temporal artery are not visualized (*left*). Postoperative angiography displayed good visualization of the posterior part of the MCA through the bypass (*middle*) and the selective internal CAG displayed a nonvisualization of the whole MCA. Postoperative CT scan revealed a new LDA accordingly.

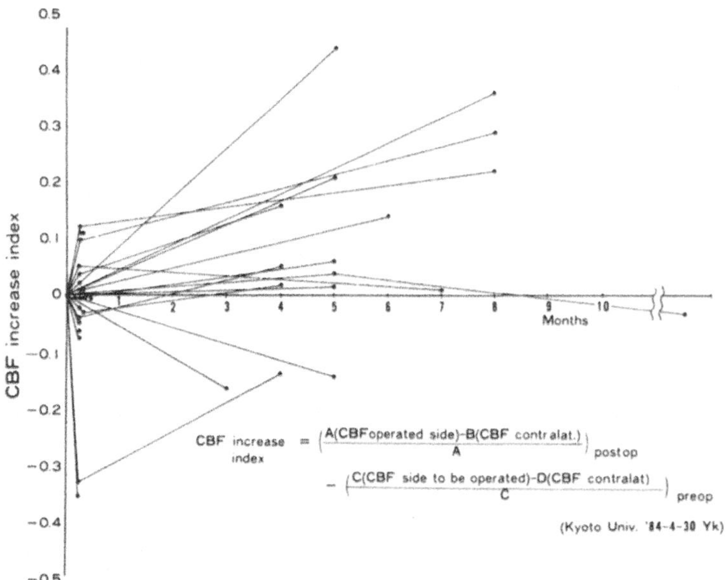

Figure 13.14. CBF measured and time course.

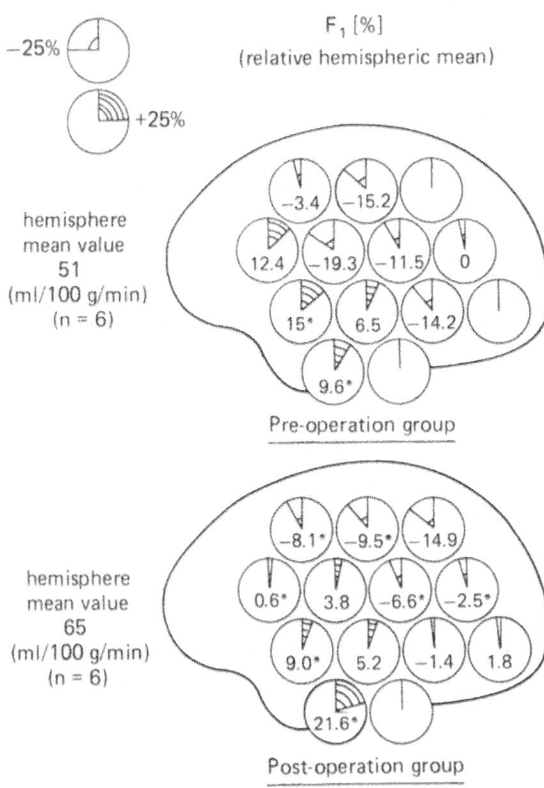

Figure 13.15. Change of the blood flow distribution.

Karasawa et al.[27] However, we could confirm marked reduction of Moyamoya in only two cases by follow-up angiography at two months, and further observations on this matter are required.

rCBF Measurement

Preoperative and postoperative rCBF was measured for a total of 70 times on the surgically treated patients, and their findings can be summarized as follows:

1. Symptomatic side revealed reduced CBF as compared with asymptomatic side in 80% of cases.
2. Paradoxical response (CBF decrease) to 5% CO_2 inhalation in 40% of cases irrespectively operated or not operated.
3. Decreased CBF on the operated side at one week in 60% of the series.
4. Better distribution of rCBF and increased CBF on the operated side at several months in 80% of cases (Fig. 13.14).

Plain comparison of pre- and postoperative CBF was difficult to evaluate so that CBF increase index was introduced as shown in Fig. 13.14.

Positron CT scan was performed in 4 cases and their findings can be summarized as follows:

1. More extensive region of decreased CBF as compared with LDA in the usual CT scan.
2. Either no response or a scarce response to CO_2 loading in CBF, oxygen extraction fraction (OEF), or $CMRO_2$; but cerebral blood volume (CBV) responded to CO_2 loading whether there was surgery or not (Fig. 13.16).

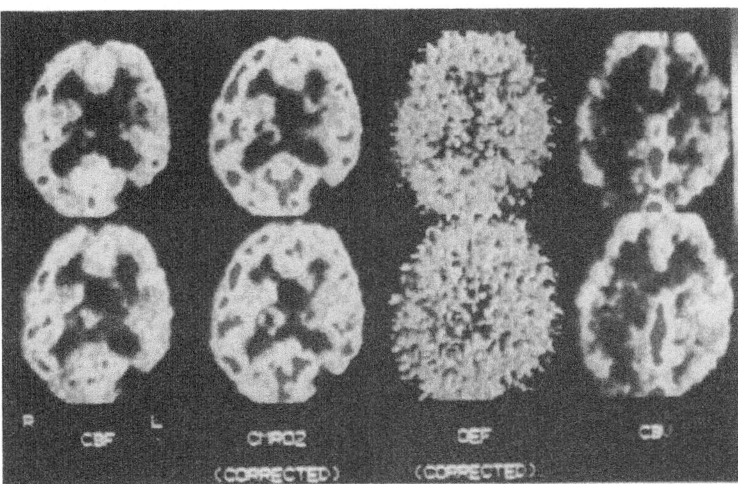

Figure 13.16. Positron CT image of a patient with Moyamoya disease already operated upon. * *Upper row*; control, *lower row*; CO_2 loading. Note no response to CO_2 loading in CBF, OEF, $CMRO_2$ but CBV did respond. (Courtesy of Prof. Torizuka)

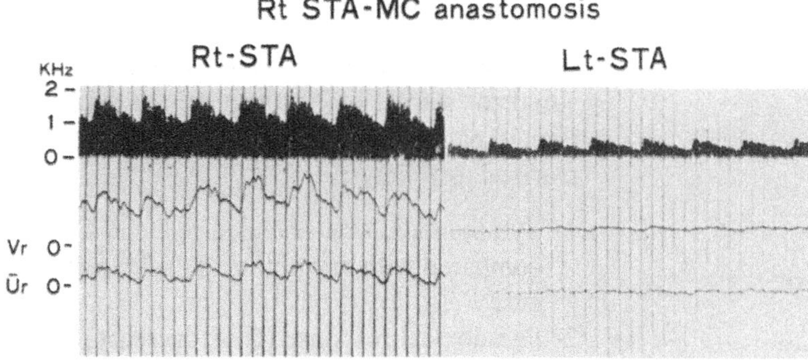

Figure 13.17. Postoperative Doppler sonography of the STA. Note the marked increase of flow volume and the different flow pattern on the right side as compared with the left.

Doppler Sonography

The flow pattern of the internal carotid artery in branches of the external carotid artery has frequently been observed in Moyamoya disease preoperatively and correlated well with the angiographic findings of transdural anastomoses.

Postoperative patency of the STA-MCA bypass by Doppler sonography (Fig. 13.17) was assessed from the following findings[46]:

1. Marked increase of STA blood flow as the donor artery in comparison with preoperative findings.
2. Marked difference in the flow volume compared with unoperated side.
3. A flow pattern change of the STA to that of the internal carotid artery.

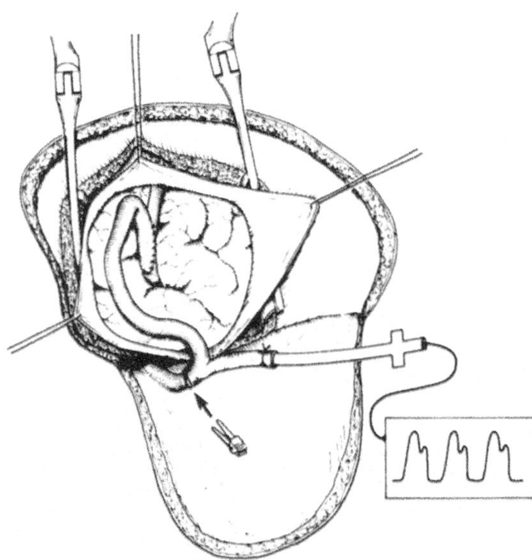

Figure 13.18. Method of measurement of the IAP after completion of a STA-MCA bypass.

These changes could be observed more or less in accordance with angiographic patency. Remarkable improvement of blood flow through the STA could be observed only in half of our series with angiographically confirmed patency. This is in good contrast with constant marked postoperative increase of the STA flow in atherosclerotic occlusions as mentioned previously.[46]

Intraoperative Doppler sonography revealed absent or weak flow signals in cortical arteries in almost half of our cases, indicating decreased cortical flow.

IAP Measurement

The method of IAP measurement was reported elsewhere[79] and is illustrated in Fig. 13.18. It is considered to reflect cortical flow and the capacity of the collateral circulation. As shown in Fig. 13.19, IAP in Moyamoya disease was far lower than in the usual cerebrovascular occlusive lesion of atherosclerotic origin and may be below the theoretical opening pressure of 10 mm Hg. Again these findings indicate decreased cortical flow in Moyamoya disease.

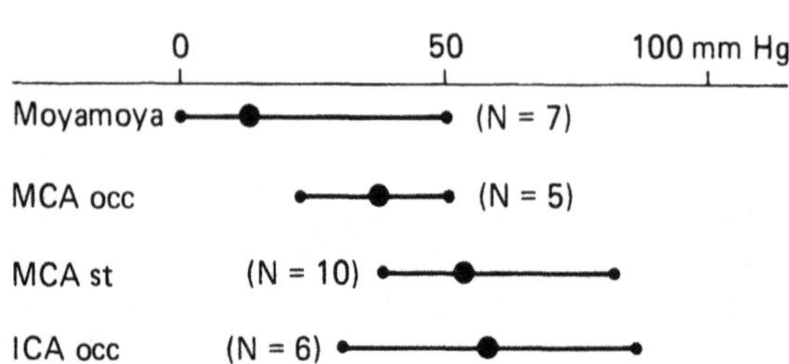

Figure 13.19. IAP in various cerebrovascular occlusive disease. Note the low IAP in Moyamoya disease. The larger *closed circles* indicate mean values.

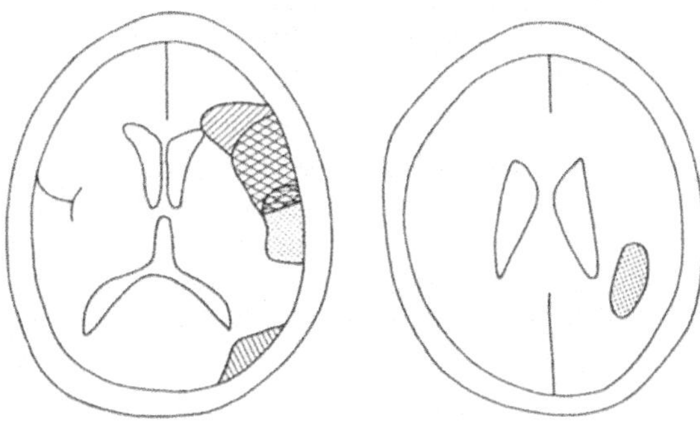

Figure 13.20. Postoperative LDAs appeared in various parts of the brain.

CT Scanning

The postoperative appearance of a new LDA was noticed in five cases, four were juveniles and one was an adult (Fig. 13.20). In the four juveniles a case of malignant hyperthermia was included, as mentioned above. The other three cases revealed one watershed-type and two wedge-shaped types in the frontal region, respectively, despite patent bypasses. The latter two LDAs seem to have resulted either from change of blood flow distribution following bypass construction or from temporary occlusion of the cortical artery during the anastomotic procedure.

Dynamic CT scan was performed in 11 cases pre- and postoperatively. All of them revealed improved hemodynamics in the postoperative scan as their criteria were mentioned previously.

Conclusion

It is now more than 20 years since Moyamoya disease was discovered in Japan. At first it was considered to be confined to Japan, but was later diagnosed in Europe and North America as well. The etiology is unknown.

The angiographic findings are characteristic, classically revealing symmetrical stenoses or occlusions of both carotid forks, associated with abnormal vascular network, called Moyamoya, in the basal ganglia.

In the juvenile type, cerebral ischemia is the typical clinical presentation, whereas cerebral hemorrhage predominates in the adult type. One-third of cases have been reported to show progressive deterioration. Although no definite effective treatment has been found hitherto, surgical therapy to augment collateral circulation seems to be promising.

However, in our early series of the juvenile type, complications have been occasionally encountered because of lack of knowledge about the precarious perioperative hemodynamic situation. Regarding cerebral hemodynamics peculiar to this disease, we have proposed several measures to prevent ischemic complications.

Acknowledgment

This work is partly sponsored by the research committee on spontaneous occlusion of the circle of Willis, Ministry of Health and Welfare, Japan.

The authors are deeply indebted to Dr. Moritake and Dr. Taki, and to the staffs of the Department of Neurosurgery, Kyoto University, for their valuable help. We also thank Mrs. Kuwagata and Miss Murai for their help in typing the manuscript and Dr. Stevens for his help in correcting the English.

References

1. Adams HP Jr, Kassell NF: Intracranial saccular aneurysm and moyamoya disease. Stroke 10:174–179, 1979
2. Austin JH, Sters JC: Familial hypoplasia of both internal carotid arteries. Arch Neurol 24:1–10, 1971
3. Carlson CB, Harvey FH, Loop J: Progressive alternating hemiplegia in early childhood with basal arterial stenosis and telangiectasia (moyamoya syndrome). Neurology 23:734–744, 1973
4. Debrun G, Sauvergrain J, Aicardi J, et al: Moyamoya, a nonspecific radiological syndrome. Neuroradiology 8:242–244, 1975
5. Fujiwara S, Kodama N, Sakurai Y, Hori S: CT scan in moyamoya disease of children. Brain Dev (Tokyo) 10:446–451, 1978
6. Furuse S, Matsumoto S, Tanaka Y, et al: Moyamoya disease associated with a false aneurysm. Neurol Surg (Japan) 10:1005–1012, 1982
7. Galligioni F, Andrioli GC, et al: Hypoplasia of the internal carotid artery associated with cerebral pseudoangiomatosis—Report of 4 cases. Am J Roentgenol 112:251–262, 1971
8. Gold AP, Carter S: Acute hemiplegia of infancy

and childhood. Ped Clin North Am 23:413–433, 1976
9. Goldberg HJ: "Moyamoya" associated with peripheral vascular occlusive disease. Arch Dis Child 49:964–966, 1974
10. Goldsmith HS, De Los Santos R, Beattie EJ Jr: Relief of chronic lymphedema by omental transposition. Ann Surg 196:572–585, 1967
11. Gotoh F (ed.): Annual Report (1981) of the research committee on spontaneous occlusion of the circle of Willis ("Moyamoya" disease). Ministry of Health and Welfare, Japan, 1982
12. Halonen H, Halonen V, et al: Occlusive disease of intracranial main arteries with collateral networks in children. Neuropadiatrie 4:187–206, 1973
13. Handa J, Handa H: Progressive cerebral arterial occlusive disease: Analysis of 27 cases. Neuroradiology 3:119–133, 1974
14. Handa J, Handa H, Nakano Y, Okuno T: Computed tomography in moyamoya: Analysis of 16 cases. Comput Tomogr 1:165–174, 1977
15. Handa J, Nakano Y, Okuno T, et al: Computerized tomography in Moyamoya syndrome. Surg Neurol 7:315–319, 1977
16. Handa H, Tani K, Kajikawa H, Sato K, Yamashita J, Osaka K, Haebara H, Tamegai M, Kyogoku M: Clinicopathological study on an adult case with cerebral arterial rete. Brain Nerve (Tokyo) 21:181–191, 1969
17. Handa J, Waga S, Handa H: Dural-cortical arterial anastomosis as a collateral channel in carotid occlusive disease. Clin Radiol 22:302–307, 1971
18. Handa H, Yonekawa Y, Suda K, et al: Postoperative appearance of newly developed LDA on CT scan. Research on the immune complex. In Gotoh (ed.): Annual report (1981) of the research committee on spontaneous occlusion of the circle of Willis. MHWJ, pp 124–130
19. Harwood-Nash DC, Fita CR: Neuroradiology in infants and children. CV Mosby, Saint Louis, 1976, pp 948–955
20. Harwood-Nash DC, McDonald P. Argent W: Cerebral arterial disease in children. Am J Roentgenol 3:672–686, 1971
21. Hately W, Shapiro R: Carotid rete mirabile—An unusual example associated with diffuse bilateral cerebral telangiectasia. Clin Radiol 20:32–35, 1969
22. Henschen C: Operative Ravascularization des zirkulatorisch geschadigten Gehirns durch Auflage gestielten Muskellappen (Encephalo-myo-synangiose). Langerbecks Arch Klin Chir 264:392–401, 1950
23. Hirakawa A, Kowada M, Fukasawa H, et al: Cerebrovascular Moyamoya disease—A case report and review of 12 autopsy cases in Japan. Brain Nerve (Tokyo) 26:1215–1225, 1974
24. Hosoda Y: A pathomorphological analysis of so called "Spontaneous occlusion of the circle of Willis" (cerebrovascular "Moyamoya" disease). Brain Nerve (Tokyo) 26:471–481, 1974
25. Iraci G, Martin G, et al: Further observations on the so called "Japanese cerebrovascular disease." Am J Roentogenol 115:35–38, 1972
26. Karasawa J, Kikuchi H, Furuse S: A surgical treatment of "Moyamoya" disease. Encephalo-myosynangiosis. Neurol Med Chir (Tokyo) 17:29–37, 1977
27. Karasawa J, Kikuchi H, Furuse S, et al: Treatment of moyamoya disease with STA-MCA anastomosis. J Neurosurg 49:679–688, 1978
28. Kodama N, Aoki Y, Hiraga H, et al: Electroencephalographic findings in children with Moyamoya disease. Arch Neurol 36:16–19, 1979
29. Kodama N, Fujiwara S, Horie Y, et al: Transdural anastomosis in moyamoya disease- vault moyamoya-, Neurol Surg (Tokyo) 8:729–737, 1980
30. Krayenbuehl HA: The moyamoya syndrome and the neurosurgeon. Surg Neurol 4:353–360, 1975
31. Kudo T: Occlusion of the internal carotid artery and the type of recovery of cerebral blood circulation. Clin Neurol (Tokyo) 1:199–200, 1960
32. Kudo T: General Aspects. In Kudo T (ed.): A disease with abnormal intracranial vascular networks. Spontaneous occlusion of the circle of Willis (in Japanese). Igaku Shoin, Ltd., (Tokyo), Japan 1967, pp 1–31
33. Kudo T: Spontaneous occlusion of the circle of Willis. A disease apparently confined to Japanese. Neurology 18: 485–496, 1968
34. Lee KF, Hodes PhJ: Intracranial ischemic lesions. Radiol Clin North Am 5:363–393, 1967
35. Lee KLK, Cheung EMT: Moyamoya disease as a cause of subarachnoid hemorrhage in Chinese. Brain 96:623–628, 1973
36. Leed NK, Abott KH: Collateral circulation in cerebrovascular occlusive disease in childhood via rete mirabile and perforating branches of anterior chorioidal and posterior cerebral arteries. Radiology 85:628–634, 1965
37. Mabuchi A, Tanabe H, Fujikawa Y, et al: An autopsy case of the abnormal network of the intracranial artery—Congenital dysplasia of the cerebral artery. Brain Nerve (Tokyo) 25:1759–1765, 1973
38. Maki Y, Nakata Y: Autopsy of a case with an anomalous hemangioma of the internal carotid artery at the skull base. Brain Nerve (Tokyo) 17:764–766, 1965
39. Maki Y, Nakata Y, et al: Clinical and radioisoto-

pic follow-up study "Moyamoya." Child's Brain 2:257–271, 1976

40. Matsushima Y, Fukai N, Tanaka K, et al: A new surgical treatment of Moyamoya disease in children. A preliminary report. Surg Neurol 15:313–320. 1981
41. Meriwether RP, Barnett HJM, Echolos DH: Moyamoya disease as a cause of subarachnoid hemorrhage in a Negro patient. J Neurosurg 44:620–622, 1976
42. Mitsugi T, Kikuchi H, Karasawa J, et al: Evaluation of CBF studies, changes of CBF and cerebral metabolism after surgical treatment in "Moyamoya" disease. In Kawafuchi J (ed.): Proceedings of the 10th Japanese conference on surgery of cerebral stroke. Neuronsha (Tokyo) 1981, pp 323–327
43. Miyasaka K, Takei H, Nakagawa Y, et al: A disease showing "Moyamoya" vascular networks in base of brain: Evaluation of angiography and cranial computer tomography. Brain Nerve (Tokyo) 30:1083–1091, 1978
44. Miyazaki M, Takeshiro A, Sugawa M, et al: Aortitis syndrome associated with so-called intracranial "moyamoya" phenomenon. Case report. Neurol Med (Tokyo) 12:53–58, 1980
45. Mori K, Takeuchi J, Ishikawa M, et al: Occlusion arteriopathy and brain tumor. J Neurosurg 49:22–35, 1978
46. Mortitake K, Handa H, Yonekawa Y, et al: Ultrasonic Doppler assessment of hemodynamics in superficial temporal artery middle cerebral artery anastomosis. Surg Neurol 13:249–257, 1980
47. Nagamine Y, Takahashi S, Sonobe M: Multiple intracranial aneurysms associated with moyamoya disease. Case report. J Neurosurg 54:673–676, 1981
48. Nishimoto A, Takeuchi S: Abnormal cerebrovascular network related to the internal carotid arteries. J Neurosurg 29:255–260, 1968
49. Nishimoto A, Ueda K, Onbe H: Cooperative study on Moyamoya disease in Japan. In Kawafuchi J: Proceedings of the 10th Japanese conference on surgery of cerebral stroke. Neurosha (Tokyo) 1981, pp 53–58
50. Numagnchi Y, Balsys R, Marc JA, et al: Some observations in progressive arterial occlusions in children and young adolescents (Moyamoya disease). Surg Neurol 6:283–300, 1976
51. Ogawa Y, Hosoda Y, Matsuyama H: An autopsy case of occlusion of the circle of Willis in a child. Brain Nerve (Tokyo) 26:483–487, 1974
52. Ohashi T, Ueda K, Mizukawa N, et al: Autopsy cases of Moyamoya disease. Brain Nerve (Tokyo) 27:1017–1027, 1975
53. Ohno K, Fujimoto T, Komatsu K, et al: Spontaneous successive occlusion of the circle of Willis with the growth of abnormal vascular networks at the base of brain. In relation to the pathogenesis of so-called "Moyamoya" disease. Brain Nerve (Tokyo) 29:37–43, 1971
54. Okamoto J, Mukai K, Kashihara M, et al: A case of atypical Moyamoya disease with or ruptured aneurysm on Moyamoya vessel. Neurol Surg (Tokyo) 10:897–903, 1982
55. Okuno T, Hojo H, Nakano Y, et al: Clinical analysis and computed tomography of cerebrovascular Moyamoya disease in childhood. Ann Paediatr Jpn (Tokyo) 23:175–187, 1977
56. Picard L, Levesque M, Crouzet G, et al: The moyamoya syndrome. J Neuroradiol 1:47–54, 1974
57. Poor GY, Gacs GY: The so-called "Moyamoya" disease. J Neurol Neurosurg Psychiatry 37:370–377, 1974
58. Prensky AL, Davis DO: Obstruction of major cerebral vessels in early childhood without neurological signs. Neurology 20:945–953, 1970
59. Reichman OH, Anderson RE, Roberts TC, et al: The treatment of intracranial occlusive cerebrovascular disease by STA-Cortical MCA anastomosis. In Handa (ed.): Microneurosurgery. Igaku Shoin Ltd., Tokyo, 1975, pp 31–46
60. Rosengreen K: Moya-Moya vessels collateral arteries of the basal ganglia. Malignant occlusion of the anterior cerebral arteries. Acta Radiol Diagn 15:145–151, 1974
61. Schrager GO, Cohen SJ, Vigman MP: Acute hemiplegia and cortical blindness due to Moya Moya disease: Report of a case in a child with Down's syndrome. Pediatrica 60:33–37, 1977
62. Sekiguchi S, Kobayashi K, Hattori M, et al: HLA antigen in spontaneous occlusion of the circle of Willis. In Gotoh F (ed.): Annual report (1979) of the research committee on spontaneous occlusion of the circle of Willis. MHWJ, pp 76–78
63. Suzuki J, Kodama N, Fujiwara S, et al: Research on the etiology of "Moyamoya" disease. (First report). In Gotoh F (ed.): Annual Report (1981) of the research committee on the circle of Willis. MHWJ, pp 21–34
64. Suzuki J, Kodama N, Mineura K: Mechanism of symptomatic occurrence in cerebrovascular Moyamoya disease. Brain Nerve (Tokyo) 28:459–470, 1976
65. Suzuki J, Takaku A: Cerebrovascular "Moyamoya" disease. Disease showing abnormal net like vessels in base of brain. Arch Neurol 20:288–299, 1969
66. Suzuki J, Takaku A, Asahi M: The disease showing the abnormal vascular network at the

base of brain, particulary found in Japan. Brain Nerve (Tokyo) 18:897–907, 1966

67. Suzuki J, Takaku A, Fukasawa H: Cerebrovascular "Moyamoya" disease among Japanese, on study of a autopsy case in Kudo T (ed.): A disease with abnormal intracranial vascular networks. Igaku shoin Ltd., Tokyo, 1967, pp 97–104
68. Suzuki J, Takaku A, Kodama N, et al: An attempt to treat cerebrovascular "Moyamoya" disease in children. Child's Brain 1:193–206, 1975
69. Takahashi M, Miyauchi T, Kowada M: Computed tomography of Moyamoya disease: Demonstration of occluded arteries and collateral vessels as important diagnostic signs. Radiology 134:671–676, 1980
70. Takahashi M, Saito Y, Konno K: Intraventicular hemorrhage in childhood Moyamoya disease. J Comput Assist Tomogr 4:117–120, 1980
71. Takeuchi K, Shimizu K: Hypoplasia of the bilateral internal carotid arteries. Brain and Nerve (Tokyo) 9:37–43, 1957
72. Tanaka K, Oka K, Yamashita M: Intracranial and systemic vascular lesions and intracranial hemorrhage in spontaneous occlusion of the circle of Willis. In Gotoh F (ed.): Annual report (1981) of the research committee on spontaneous occlusion of the circle of Willis. MHWJ pp 86–98
73. Taveras JM: Multiple progressive intracranial arterial occlusion: A syndrome of children and young adults. Am J Roentgenol 106:235–268, 1969
74. Uemura K, Yamaguchi K, Kojima S, et al: Regional cerebral blood flow on cerebrovascular "Moyamoya" disease. Brain Nerve (Tokyo) 27:385–393, 1975
75. Urbanek H, Farkova H, et al: Nishimoto-Takeuchi-Kudo disease. J Neurol Neurosurg 33:671–673, 1970
76. Weidner W, Harafee W, Markham C: Intracranial collateral circulation via leptomeningeal and rete mirabile anastomosis. Neurol 15:39–48, 1965
77. Yasargil MG: Microsurgery applied to neurosurgery. Thieme, Stuttgart, 1969
78. Yasargil MG, Smith RD: Association of middle cerebral anomalies with saccular aneurysms and Moyamoya disease. Surg Neurol 6:37–43, 1976
79. Yonekawa Y, Yasargil MG: Arterial extracranial intracranial anastomosis, Technical and clinical aspects. Results. In Krayenbuhl H (ed.): Advances and technical standards of neurosurgery. Vol 3. Springer, Wien, 1976, pp 47–78
80. Yonekawa Y, Yasargil MG: Brain vascularization by transplanted omentum. A possible treatment of cerebral ischemia. Neurosurgery 1:256–257, 1977
81. Yonemitsu T, Kasai N, Fujiwara S, et al: Research on the etiology of "Moyamoya" disease (Second Report). In Gotoh F (ed.): Annual Report (1982) of the research committee on the spontaneous occlusion of the circle of Willis. MHWJ, pp 131–144
82. Yoshii N, Kudo T: Electroencephalographical study on occlusion of the Willis arterial ring. Clin Neurol (Tokyo) 8:301–310, 1968; Brain Nerve (Tokyo) 29:33–38, 1977
83. Zulch KJ, Dreesbach HA, Echbach O: Occlusion of the middle cerebral artery with the formation of an abnormal arterial collateral system-moyamoya type-23 months later. Neuroradiology 7:19–24, 1974

14

Cerebral Arteritis

Bennett M. Derby and Humberto M. Cravioto

Introduction

This chapter is a clinical-anatomic survery of forms of identifiable "vasculitis" of the brain, with emphasis on entities involving the angiographically visible cerebral circulation. Processes involving tiny vascular channels that are not radiologically detectable are included to provide comprehensive coverage of inflammatory disease of intracranial vessels. As the categorization of a clinical problem as an "arteritis" stems in chief from cerebral arteriographic appearances of segmental irregularity, this chapter also includes known causes of radiologically visible vascular wall changes, some of them only in part inflammatory, so as to provide a differential diagnosis. The discussion is arranged in broad areas of pathogenesis.

Definition

The term "arteritis" is perhaps not the most precise anatomic word for this chapter heading since inflammation may simultaneously involve capillaries and veins as well as arteries. The inclusive term, vasculitis, is accurate but has been customarily used in the literature for dermal entities, with which this discussion is not involved. The alternative term, angiitis, is correct histologically and is most preferable even though it is infrequently used clinically. The overall designation of arteritis remains convenient in common usage and readily understood. This discussion will deal not only with true inflammatory conditions, but with anything that can give the clinical and angiographic appearance of a primary arterial wall disease and thus mimic arteritis.

Anatomic Correlation

Arteries can be subdivided according to their distribution as well as their size. Arteries branching directly from the aorta (e.g., carotid) are primary branches, and the branches of the carotid at its bifurcation are secondary branches. These are extradural. Subdivision into the named cerebral arteries creates tertiary branches (e.g., middle cerebral artery), which are intradural and invested by the leptomeninx. This chapter deals mainly with tertiary arteries and their branches. In this situation the role of a primary process in the arachnoid secondarily affecting the contained vessels must always be considered. Certain processes that affect the carotid arteries in the neck are also considered because they frequently produce cerebral pathology, can be diagnosed radiologically, and are potentially surgically approachable.

The nomenclature of artery size is based fundamentally on whether they are chiefly elastic (conducting; primary and secondary), chiefly muscular (distributing; tertiary and onward), or tiny (end-flow regulation; arteriole). The intradural and intracerebral arteries vary from those elsewhere in having much less muscularis, rare vasa vasorum, and no external elastica, and are more liable to wall damage. A simpler classification into large, medium, and small arteries has much practical value. Large and medium arteries are primary and secondary branches rich in elastic tissue. Past the internal carotid and vertebrobasilar trunks, arteries are small. At the point where optic magnification is required for visualization, 100 μm in diameter (14 red blood cell diameters in tissue section), the vessel is an arteriole. Branches that penetrate cerebral substance have become arterioles. Several forms of arteritis involve small arteries visible on arteriography and arterioles not seen on arteriography.

As the circulation schema proceeds to the smallest arteriole, capillary, venule, and small vein, different diseases come to bear. As the vessel character changes and diameter becomes smaller, the known primary inflammatory diseases operating at this level tend to spare small arteries and are no longer visible on angiography. Histologic vessel wall involvement is no longer restricted to the arterial side, but frequently involves venules and small veins as well as smallest arterioles and capillaries, meriting the inclusive anatomic designation of angiitis. It is doubtful that a purely venous primary inflammatory disease exists.

To further distinguish the various forms of angiitis beyond the size and location of the vessel involved, many histologic factors are taken into consideration. These include identification of which one or more layers of the vessel wall are predominantly affected; assessment of the character of the cells in the exudate (polymorphonuclear leukocytes, eosinophils, mononuclear cells, Langhans' or foreign body multinucleated giant cells, epithelioid cells); search for the type of necrosis and whether fibrinoid is present; determination of fragmentation and destruction of elastica; and staging of the development of the lesion (acute, subacute, chronic, healed or mixed).

Angiographic Correlation

Irregularity with narrowing and alternating dilatation of the caliber of a small artery lumen in an arteriogram confirms the presence of arterial disease but cannot determine whether focal wall thickening is necrotic and cannot distinguish whether the layer involved is (1) subendothelial, (2) intramural, or (3) adventitial with intrinsic compression. Yet each of these loci is primarily involved in widely varying diseases: From subintimal atherosclerosis through periarteritis to granulomatous meningitis, the arteriographic appearances may be similar. The diagnosis of an "arteritis" has been frequently loosely applied to angiographic segmental flow column abnormality without supporting information regarding inflammatory processes. The presence of total branch occlusion on arteriogram likewise cannot differentiate between embolic tamponade, lumen closure from vessel wall thickening, or thrombosis over a mural lesion. Arteriographic appearance does not give primary information as whether the arteries are primarily involved by a vascular disease, or whether the arteries are only secondarily affected by a nonvascular disease.

Inferential diagnostic probabilities may emerge from the finding of one or more unilateral or bilateral lesions, but are not formed solely on the appearance of an individual narrowed or blocked lesion on an x-ray film. In contrast, highly focal ectasia of small arteries directly demonstrates out-pocketing of mural segments due to necrosis or reactive atony of the vessel wall, permitting probable narrowing of the diagnostic spectrum to exclude processes that do not necrotize small arteries. It is worth emphasizing that cerebral angiography is vastly more illuminating as to the presence, number, and distribution—if not the type—of tertiary lesions than is the customary histopathologic study of the brain.

Clinical Correlation

Primary cerebrovascular inflammatory diseases can be broadly viewed in two groups. Those involving arteries visible on arteriography and capable of producing focal neurologic deficit are the arteritides. A clinical stroke-like syndrome of hemiparesis, with or without hemianopia, hemisensory findings, and aphasia may be expected. Arteriographic lesions may be more numerous and widespread than expected from clinical deficit.

Those diseases involving the microscopic

vasculature of small arterioles, capillaries, and venules, below the threshold of arteriography, are the angiitides. These, in general, produce only microcirculatory disorders of obtundation or seizures, without focal neurologic findings. A focal aggregate of many tiny lesions, particularly in a strategic area such as the brainstem, may, however, produce focal deficit.

Both groups infrequently may excite a sudden hemisphere stroke syndrome from secondary thrombosis or hemorrhage, but customarily evolve in a continuingly active progressive or stepwise manner. In the production of clinical deficit, edema undoubtedly may contribute but mass effect and increased intracranial pressure do not occur.

Angiitides do not involve cerebral vessels alone. These diseases are systemic and are invariably accompanied by concomitant prominent clinical constitutional and laboratory manifestations. Granulomatous angiitis is the exception. Adequate diagnosis perforce includes attention to blood count, muscle enzymes, liver function, and renal testing, as well as a complete history and examination directed at body systems and the skin. Liver and muscle biopsies are often appropriate. Granulomatous angiitis, lupus erythematosus, and Behçet's disease so constantly involve the leptomeninges with shedding of lymphocytes and a protein leak in the cerebrospinal fluid that lumbar puncture is an essential. The diagnosis of an undetermined cerebral arteritis rests directly on tissue diagnosis. The opportunity to view small arteries under the dissecting microscope and take cerebral biopsy is paramount should occasion arise to evacuate a hematoma, clip an aneurysm, do an air study, or place a shunt. Repeated arteriography after an interval may show evanescence of previous abnormalities, indicating a one-phase disease and thus excluding polyphasic arteritis, which is a continuing disease process.

Infectious Arteritis

Bacterial and Fungal Infection

The wall of cerebral arteries may be directly involved by hematogenous lodgement of infectious organisms or from contiguous invasion from infected leptomeninges. In any infection, either or both routes may operate; therefore, the distinction outlined below may at times be artificial. Under certain circumstances tertiary artery mural infection permits focal enlargement into gross aneurysm which may produce a singular clinical picture.

Meningitis

Since the cerebral arteries run through the arachnoid and its sleeves, they are continuously at risk for direct extension of infection through adventitia into the media. The result may be focal change in caliber alone, or occlusion. Subclinical focal arachnoid hemorrhage from leakage or hemorrhagic infarction from occlusion may occur ("red meningitis") due to necrosis of the vessel wall. In theory, the longer the duration of unchecked meningitis, the more likely is arterial involvement, but arteriographic study of acute bacterial meningitis has commonly shown arteritis. In autopsy material the histologic findings of arteritis are most frequently seen in the more chronic group of treated bacterial meningitis, especially in tuberculous meningitis.[14] This takes the form of endarteritis obliterans in which the elastic and medial coats are intact, although infiltrated by mononuclear cells, and subintimal proliferation of connective tissue without inflammatory cells progressively narrows the lumen (Fig. 14.1). Although the discrepancy from arteriography may, in part, be due to the limitations of autopsy sampling, there is a real basis for accepting dynamic reaction of cerebral arteries in acute meningitis with segmental spasm and/or atony, from purely irritative effect. Arteritis shown by arteriography has been described in every variety of meningitis, from acute bacterial to the chronic infectious processes caused by low-grade bacteria, fungi, and syphilis.[52,85]

In the chronic infectious meningitides there may be little evidence of a systemic disease in the patient prior to abrupt focal neurologic deficit. A prototype is meningovascular syphilis, announcing as a stroke-like syndrome in which an arteritis from subclinical meningitis may not be an early consideration when the patient is first seen. This is never a problem if lumbar puncture is routinely done in any and all neurologic problems without increased intracranial pressure, since the pleocytosis and elevated protein will be immediately revealed, and a positive serologic test for syphilis (STS) or posi-

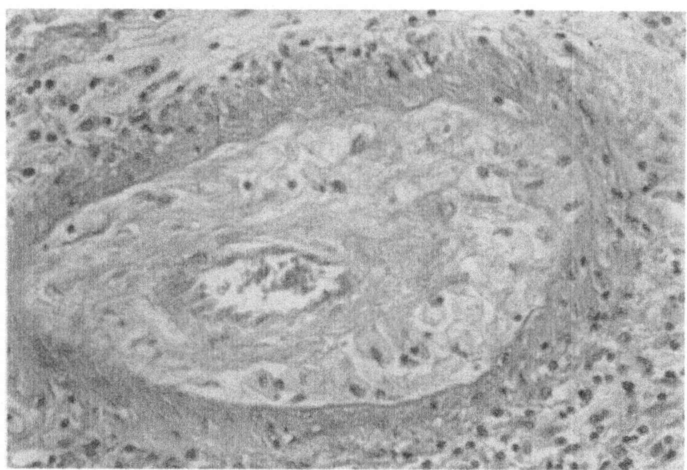

Figure 14.1. Tuberculous endarteritis in meningitis. The lumen is 80% narrowed by subintimal fibroplasia. The media and adventitia are infiltrated by mononuclear cells. H&E ×900.

tive fungus culture will follow. In neurologic lues, caution is necessary in the diagnosis of menningovascular syphilis. There is no primary cerebral vascular arteritis. The vessels are always involved secondary to the basic meningeal process, revealed by CSF study, including STS. A stroke syndrome and a positive STS in peripheral blood constitutes no evidence for luetic arteritis.

Septicemia and Fungemia

Although this may coexist with meningitis, focal necrosis of arterioles may also occur in the absence of meningitis, leading to multiple intracerebral and subarachnoid hemorrhage. In bacterial infection this is classically and most frequently seen with staphylococcal septicemia in which the clinical picture of cerebral disease may even dominate the systemic disease. The minute size of the arterioles involved and the macroscopic hemorrhage that sometimes follows often obscure the precise points of origin. The process is one of acute embolization with formation of multiple intracerebral microabscesses ("metastatic encephalitis") and a widespread necrotizing arteriolitis probably due to a direct bacterial invasion and necrosis of the vessel wall. The acuity of the disease and the fragility of the arteriole involved do not allow healing, and aneurysm formation does not occur.[30] Bacterial arteriolitis without aneurysm is the cause of intracranial hemorrhage in a small percentage of large surveys.[92,114a,140] Histologic study of some of these cases has shown focal

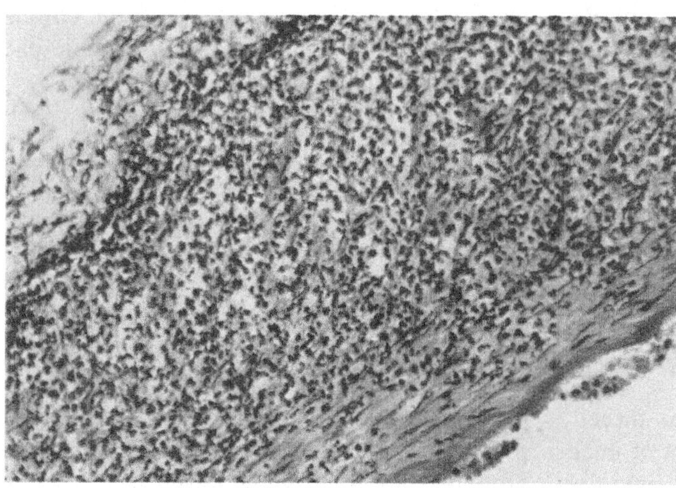

Figure 14.2. Acute carotid arteritis. Architecture of the entire wall is severely disrupted, with edema and polymorphonuclear leukocyte infiltrate throughout. H&E ×900

necrosis of arterioles below the level of ordinary radiographic visualization. Typically seen in model fashion with the fulminant acute staphylococcal septicemias and rarely with acute meningococcemia, the same subarteriographic process at the smallest arteriolar level occurs from time to time in less peracute bacteremias, in which early rupture without aneurysm also occurs.

In disseminated fungal disease widespread invasion of cerebral substance occurs via the bloodstream and, as with any meningoencephalitis, may come to involve arteries and arterioles. Peculiarly, only two organisms show great preference for such vessels. *Aspergillus* regularly causes multiple intracerebral hemorrhage as well as hemorrhagic infarction. The specific invasion of arterioles is easily demonstrated microscopically[61] and creates vivid brain hemorrhage[22]. The collective group causing the so-called phycomycoses (mucormycosis) may occasionally be widespread but typically begin as a craniofacial focus, erode directly into subfrontal lobe, and extend intraluminally throughout the parenchymal arterioles and into the extra-axial carotid arterial system.[29,127]

Mycotic Aneurysm

When the wall of an artery with well-formed coats above the size of an arteriole is invaded by bacteria, there is frequently a sequence of acute inflammatory necrosis, loosening of the wall, and reparative fibrosis. With persistence of the organism, the sequence may be repeated and simultaneous, or the process may heal. There may be thinning of a portion of the wall which undergoes progressive enlargement, going beyond segmental dilatation into formation of a fibrous sac (aneurysm), the diameter of which equals or exceeds that of the parent artery. This may heal, or rupture at variable intervals.

Vasa vasorum do not exist beyond the basal trunk (secondary) arteries. The usual route of mural infection is septic thrombus impacted in the lumen of tertiary arteries or their branches. The resultant stepwise formation of an aneurysm requires an organism of lesser virulence as well as an arteriographically visible artery. In contrast to necrotizing arteriolitis, intracerebral mycotic aneurysm occurs later in the course of bacteremic infection, which is almost invariably an endocarditis. The clinical sequence of impaction of a septic thrombus leading to a cerebral infarction, and the later appearance of aneurysm with rupture, has been documented.[82] Cases are also recorded apparently resulting from meningitis alone, without invasion from the bloodstream.[131] These aneurysms are distributed distally in the tertiary artery circulation, not at the circle of Willis, in keeping with the widespread distribution of the bacteria.

Mycotic aneurysm is discussed elsewhere as a surgical entity. It is likely that many heal without rupture, as a natural event. Multiple arterial fibrocalcification from such healing has been observed.[123] Even after rupture of mycotic aneurysms demonstrated arteriographically, healing has occurred after successful treatment with antibiotics, as shown by interval angiography.[13] Clearly, however, failure of an aneurysm to resolve may leave risk of rupture without regard to infectious activity. Interestingly, tertiary artery "mycotic" aneurysm does not seem to occur with the true mycoses.

Mycotic aneurysm also occurs in the intracavernous portion of the internal carotid artery, secondary to thrombophlebitis of the cavernous sinus,[131] bacteremia,[117] or *Penicillium* infection of orbit and sinuses[101] with obstructive orbital phlegmon and ophthalmoplegia. Cervical carotid artery mycotic aneurysm also occurs.[73]

Carotid Arteritis

The wall of the internal carotid artery may become inflamed at any point from common bifurcation in the neck to the point of entry through dura, but rarely has been associated with cerebral manifestations. Hematogenous mycotic aneurysm has been referred to above. The present grouping is arranged to catalogue other known or suggested causes of carotid arteritis.

Acute Necrotizing Arteritis. Occlusion of the internal carotid artery due to severe acute necrotizing panarteritis was seen on two occasions in young male individuals 29 and 33 years of age.[31] Pathologically, there was extensive necrosis, infiltration of the entire vessel wall by acute inflammatory cells, and acute thrombosis of the lumen (Fig. 14.2). There were no eosinophils. The process was limited exclusively to a portion of one internal carotid artery in one case and in the other case also affected a segment of a middle cerebral artery on the same side as that of the occluded carotid artery. This arteritis and thrombosis caused extensive cerebral infarction, cerebral edema, and death in a few days in both cases. Although an infectious organism could possibly have been responsible for this type of arteritis, the diagnosis was made only at autopsy and no organisms were found. None of the arteries or veins in other organs were affected. The process was primary within the arterial wall and not due to an adjacent or systemic focus of infection. These cases are not paralleled in the literature. Occurring in adults, they do not bear on the early childhood disorder discussed below.

Adjacent Infection. Any wound infection in the neck may involve the carotid artery. Innominate-carotid erosion is seen following radical neck dissection and tracheostomy, but mechanical and irradiation treatment factors may play a role in the inflammation of the vessel wall in addition to infection or independently. More direct are the cases of carotid erosion from staphylococcal infection of Crutchfield clamp ligation sites.[84] Pharyngomaxillary (lateral pharyngeal; parapharyngeal) space infection of dental origin can surround and infect the internal carotid at the level of the throat, but clinical neurologic effects are poorly documented. Similarly, cervical adenitis and tonsillitis have been thought to have an influence on the function of the carotid artery, deep beneath another sheath, but a demonstration of carotid wall infection has not been shown. Acute expansion of a carotid artery aneurysm of other cause may produce an acute inflammatory reaction of the wall.[79]

Infantile-Childhood Hemiplegia. The cause of this dramatic, acute hemiplegia in a young child is baffling and simply not identified. It commonly but far from always occurs in a setting of upper respiratory infection or other systemic febrile infectious disease.[11,71] Whereas some authors have concluded that inflammation of the carotid artery from dental, tonsil, lymph node, or retropharyngeal infection is the causative factor,[11] others have found no carotid artery inflammatory process.[71] The view of an infectious cause in the neck seems minimized by the predilection for supraclinoid carotid occlusion, where one is demonstrated at all, and the absence of arterial occlusion in many cases.[71] In isolated instances arteriographic and tissue change, reported as arteritic,[118] are not clearly separable from the result of acute bland thrombus formation. Unique individual reports, such as that of early childhood acute hemiplegia with proved Coxsackie A9 infection and pleocytosis, cast weight toward focal encephalitis within the dura rather than an extracranial carotid inflammatory lesion in the neck. There is a dearth of pathologic material to define this problem further, since death and surgical specimens are rare.

Viral Encephalitis

Viral encephalitis secondarily involves only microscopic vessels not visible angiographically. Tissue changes are those of hyperemia and neuronal, or neuronal plus neuropil necrosis, in which a simple reactive microscopic perivenular and meningeal mononuclear infiltrate occur. There is no involvement of larger vessels and an angiitis cannot be said to occur.

Herpes Simplex Encephalitis

This infection is transneural and not vascular in its inception; virus moves through the olfactory filaments and nerves to primarily attack the limbic subfrontal-temporal tissues. The virus produces extensive nonspecific necrosis of blood vessels as well as brain parenchyma. Although not a primary vasculitis, the lesion is characterized by mass effect, often more on one side than the other, with secondary displacement of arteries.[20,38] The brain tissue necrosis is usually hemorrhagic, and red blood cells in the cerebrospinal fluid are common.

Zoster Ophthalmicus

Varicella-zoster encephalitis is more common following trigeminal root shingles than shingles in other dermatomes. Of a total of 63 cases reported,[3,104,114a] 20% began as zoster of one of the three roots of the fifth cranial nerve, a number wholly out of proportion to the remaining total of 31 sensory craniospinal roots and in keeping with the proximate intracranial location. In 44 cases of zoster in all locations without clinical meningitis, Barham-Carter[9] found pleocytosis in 14. Ten of these 14 (70%) were in the first branch of the trigeminal nerve. Against this background, the occurrence of zoster ophthalmicus with contralateral hemiplegia, although rare, has become a bona fide entity.[1] Abnormal arteriograms have been reported in some of these cases. Vessel changes in the case of Kolodny et al[81] were due to granulomatous angiitis. In a case of acute hemiplegia in a 7-year-old boy with stasis and narrowing of left middle cerebral artery branches, zoster ophthalmicus with healing had occurred half a year before, and the cerebrospinal fluid was acellular. A carotid siphon stenosis with right amaurosis fugax and subsequent opposite hemiparesis and aphasia was described in a 73-year-old man with right zoster ophthalmicus two weeks before and a normal cerebrospinal fluid.[58] In another case biopsied temporal arteritis with ischemic optic neuropathy, without arteriography, was suggested as somehow associated with ophthalmic zoster that had cleared five weeks before.[136]

Although contralateral hemiplegia with pleocytosis may occur concomitant with zoster ophthalmicus as part of a localized brainstem encephalitis adjacent to root entry zone, it is due to zonal mesencephalitis with nonspecific viral necrosis of microscopic vessels and tissue alike. There is no arteritis visible arteriographically, and the reported instances of abnormal angiograms or arteritis reviewed above were due to other disease processes.

Primary Inflammation of Unknown Cause

Connective Tissue Disease

This group of diseases primarily affects collagen structures and logically may involve intracerebral blood vessel walls.[56,122] A rich yield of clinical stroke syndromes and abnormal cerebral arteriograms might theoretically be anticipated in this group of diseases, yet few have been described.[36] These lesions do not causatively affect the carotid-vertebral arteries and do not commonly affect cerebral arteries of requisite caliber for gross infarction. Cerebral lesions may not be present at all. Although these entities are grouped together customarily as having a common collagen-vascular pathogenesis, each in fact involves a different size and type of vessel, and the neuropathology and neurologic manifestations are thus widely varying.

The classification used below has regard to morphology, and to processes that involve the brain vessels. Immune complex disease for the most part, as identified in shunt nephritis, leprosy, bacterial endocarditis, and quartan malaria, does not provoke cerebral lesions. Henoch-Schönlein purpura and anaphylaxis do not produce a specific vascular neuropathology. Dermatomyositis, acute rheumatic fever, scleroderma, Sjogren's syndrome, and relapsing polychondritis do not involve cerebral vessels.

Periarteritis (Polyarteritis) Nodosa

This is the classic form of arteritis, affecting medium and small distributing arteries, characterized by nodular aneurysmal formation at arterial branch points which may be visible in the viscera. The basic lesion is panmural segmental necrosis in which fibrin or fibrin products are present in the muscular media, and the elastic layer is destroyed. Diffuse infiltration by polymorphonuclear leukocytes and large mononuclear cells of all layers of the artery is most marked in the adventitia (Fig. 14.3). Acute, subacute, healing, and healed lesions exist side by side. The respiratory system is spared, eosinophilia is virtually absent, and there are no giant cells, in contrast to Wegener's granulomatosis, which will be considered later. In all cases other organs are predominantly affected, and in 50% the peripheral nerves are involved. Although the frequency of neurologic symptoms in periarteritis is often tabulated in clinical reviews, cerebral syndromes specifically related to active periarteritic involvement are not separable from those that are the results of other causes, such as arteriosclerosis or encephalopathy from hypertension or uremia. Cerebral vascular and parenchymal tissue findings presented in pathologic summaries have not specifically considered their location and type in relation to the presence and character of neurologic symptoms and signs.[4,62,109] Ferris[51] stated that many times cerebral arteriography showed nothing.

In patients with periarteritis other pathologic processes also may be at work. A "healed" cebral arterial lesion of periarteritis may be in-

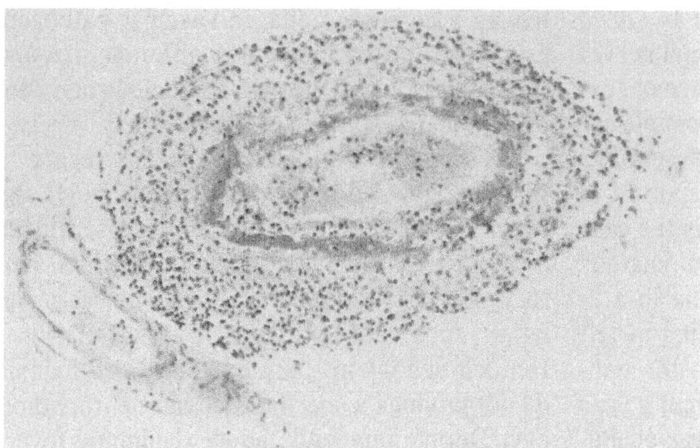

Figure 14.3. Periarteritis nodosa, leptomeningeal artery. Intimal denudation, necrosis of the media with fibrin impregnation, and loosening of adventitia are accompanied by dense mononuclear infiltrate. H&E ×40.

distinguishable from fibrous atherosclerosis, from an organized thromboembolic occlusion, or from a hypertensive fibrinoid lesion. Periarteritis develops in an age range in which coincidental cerebral infarction due to atherosclerosis is not uncommon. Where cerebral arterial lesions are directly related to periarteritis, the carotid and basilar trunks have not usually been involved, the basal circle arterial branches are variably involved, and the parenchymal branches are those that are most often involved. The arterial lesions are usually asymptomatic unless thrombosis with resultant infarction occurs, or hemorrhage as a result of mural necrosis, dissection, or rupture takes place. Although small aneurysms at bifurcation points of arteries are classic in the viscera, a satisfactory pathologic or radiologic demonstration of intracerebral aneurysm formation due to classic periarteritis has not been presented. If this actually occurs, it must be very unusual. The only statement made in the literature is that common cerebral angiographic findings are those of focal and diffuse narrowing of small- and medium-sized arteries with multiple occlusions. Yet, this is made without histopathologic verification or any description of associated clinical findings.[51] From the available information it is probable that a significant number of patients with periarteritis may develop lesions in cerebral arteries that could be demonstrable by arteriography but without developing specific neurologic syndromes. When cerebral symptoms do occur, the tissue loss and arteriogram must be analyzed in terms of the sizes and the sites of arterial lesions found, weighing the relative roles of

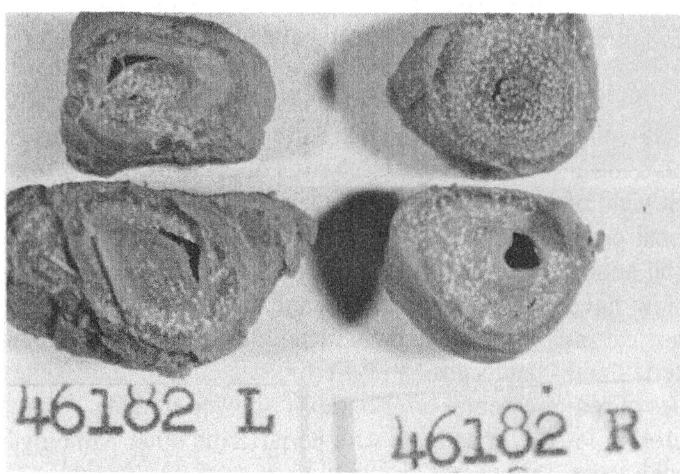

Figure 14.4. Temporal arteritis. Gross specimen. In bilateral cross sections massive eccentric thickening of the wall narrows or occludes the lumen.

hypertension and atherosclerosis as well as histologically verifiable periarteritis. Despite many years of clinical neurologic description and interest in this area, the magnitude of the contribution of intracerebral periarteritis to clinical manifestations remains unknown.

There have been but few autopsy-proven cases in which a cerebral arterial lesion has been specifically due to periarteritis nodosa. In one brief study cerebral hemispheric and brainstem vascular syndromes were recorded in 19 of 114 patients.[54] Autopsies on six with cerebral hemiparesis revealed infarction in five and hemorrhage in one. Although histologic changes of arteritis in the cerebral arteries were described in all six cases, the presence or absence of these changes in the territory of supply of the clinically involved artery was not indicated, and no correlation with hypertension or cerebral atherosclerosis was made. The neuropathologic findings in cases without neurologic manifestations were also not mentioned. The absence of necrotizing angiitis in the brain at autopsy despite many sections, in the face of multiple lesions in the viscera, has been a consistent experience at the Massachusetts General Hospital.[24] Whether polyarteritis nodosa can be truly recognized angiographically awaits good neuropathologic corroboration.

Wegener's Granulomatosis

This form of arteritis is separable from the "classic" disease due to predominant involvement of the respiratory tract,[47] although both forms show a severe systemic necrotizing angiitis.[46] Synonyms include polyarteritis with respiratory granuloma and allergic granulomatosis.

Allergic granulomatosis (Churg-Strauss) and Wegener's granulomatosis are here considered together as variants of respiratory periarteritis, a view established by Rose and Spencer.[114b] Each may be considered a separate entity, although the overlap is considerable since there is frequent paranasal sinus involvement in allergic granulomatosis, and pulmonary disease with eosinophilia is common in Wegener's granulomatosis.

In addition to arterial necrosis, these forms of respiratory periarteritis are marked by granuloma formation with giant cells at times extravascular, and more or less extensive eosinophilic infiltrates with variable blood eosinophilia. Immune-complex-mediated glomerular deposits and immune complexes are absent in most cases.[25]

Involvement of the central nervous system is rare, probably the same as in periarteritis nodosa, but the true frequency is difficult to estimate because few reports separate classic periarteritis from respiratory polyarteritis, and because clinical and neuropathologic correlation are rarely drawn. In one case there was histologic necrotizing arteritis of an anterior cerebral artery branch with both occlusion and focal subarachnoid hemorrhage which had been asymptomatic. In life the only neurologic symptoms had been due to hypertensive encephalopathy, which correlated with hypertensive fibrinoid arteriolitis and microinfarctions which were present.[37] In the accompanying tabulation of 104 cases reviewed from the literature, however, it is not clear how many had cerebral arteritis determined by tissue study, or whether the 8% incidence of intracranial hemorrhage and thrombosis was nonspecific or associated with arteritis. There was no attempt to correlate exact clinical manifestations with specific neuropathology, and arteriography was not discussed. Multiple stenoses and ectasias of branch arteries on bicarotid arteriography and small-caliber arteritis of the brain at autopsy were reported as temporal arteritis[72] and presented as such in a review.[51] General autopsy was incomplete. Because of the patient's age (56 years), absence of optic nerve involvement, normal external carotid tree on both sides, and the presence of necrotizing sinusitis, this was actually most likely Wegener's granulomatosis. Cerebral angiography in a young male with rhinitis, pleuritis, eosinophilia, pulmonary aneurysms, and cerebral infarction disclosed multiple branch-point aneurysms, but there was no tissue study.[87] Subsequently this case was shown to be an example of the multiple aneurysm formation due to embolic atrial myxoma.[88] In a review of 18 cases of Wegener's granulomatosis[47] only one had a cerebral deficit and this was the patient originally reported by Drachman 10 years before.[37] In one fulminating case with death resulting from florid visceral vasculitis, showing multiple scattered cerebral hemorrhages, just 20 days after the first symptoms, there were no inflammatory changes in the brain vessels.[17] Autopsy of a case with hypertension and renal failure, complicated by proptotic ophthalmoplegia, peripheral facial palsy, and foot drop but no central nervous system deficit, showed lacunar infarction in the brain and focal necrotizing granuloma of many arterioles.[55] Bicarotid arteriography had been negative. A more current report[93] again reviewed neurologic complications in Wegener's and autopsy findings in a nonhypertensive man who expired with hemorrhage in one caudate head. Microphotographs of an indeterminate vessel with a branch point, adjacent to the hemorrhage, showed changes hard to separate from those due to the necrosis of hematoma compression and to the necrosis of choroid plexus from the opposite side with unequivocal necrotizing inflammation of an arteriole. The total review of the scanty information available on Wegener's granuloma and the central nervous system speaks for infrequent clinical involvement and for more prevalent asymptomatic cerebral arteriolar necrosis. As in classic periarteritis, the arteriolar necrosis and lacunar infarctions are difficult or impossible to separate from those induced by hypertension.

Circulating Immune Complex Necrotizing Vasculitis

Immune complex deposition undoubtedly participates in many of the vasculitides, most prominently lupus and periarteritis nodosa, but direct causative correlation is not as yet generally available.[46] In one very well-defined group of patients, however, in whom hepatitis was followed by hepatitis B antigenemia, far-flung vasculitis occurred characterized by multiorgan involvement, including the brain. In one series of 39 patients,[39] three showed central nervous system involvement characterized by diffuse encephalopathy with normal cerebrospinal fluid in two and a left hemisphere syndrome in one, with a cerebrospinal fluid protein of 93 mg/dL. Cerebral arteriography and tissue study were not done. The ages of the patients with cerebral involvement cannot be discerned. In another series of nine patients[116b] one had a diffuse encephalopathy, one had no specific cerebral symptoms, and another had a right hemisphere deficit in the age range of 49 to 67 years. Arteriography was not done, but autopsy study was available in all. Fibrin thrombi were deposited without wall change in 20 to 30 μm arterioles in one case; "vasculitis," neither described nor depicted, was found in the second who had had no neurologic symptoms; and an undescribed "vasculitis" with multiple gross basal ganglion infarcts and multiple microinfarcts was found in the third. The impression is gained from muscle, liver, and mesentery photographs that this was an arteriolitis similar to, if not actual, periarteritis nodosa below the level of arteriographic resolution. Many of the patients in both series had mononeuritis multiplex. There has been similar vasculitis complicating the course of lymphoproliferative disorders, as reviewed in a report of arteritis complicating four cases of hairy-cell leukemia,[45] three of whom had no neurologic symptoms and one of whom had seizures. All had received transfusions but in none was hepatitis B antigen detected. Test findings in the only patient studied for immune complexes were positive. Temporal artery aneurysms were present in two patients, a radial artery aneurysm in one, and leg ischemia requiring amputation in another. Necrosis of arteries with wall destruction and mixed polymorphonuclear-mononuclear infiltrate was shown in four biopsies and in the leg specimen. In a group of 40 patients with mixed cryoglobulinemia and cutaneous vasculitis with palpable purpura, 60% of whom had serologic evidence of prior infection with hepatitis B virus, visceral periarteritis was shown in nine cases at autopsy. Neuropathy due to vasculitis was present in four. Only one patient, with no neurologic symptoms, showed CNS involvement at postmortem.[60]

In these groups of patients a primary process is complicated by necrotizing vasculitis. Whether the mechanism is defined as arising from viral, tumor, or other antigen, the resulting picture is virtual periarteritis nodosa. The question is open as to whether an identical clinicopathologic picture in these groups and the classic disease is produced by different mechanisms, or whether a parallel mechanism operates in the classic disease and merely has yet to be demonstrated.

Systemic Lupus Erythematosus (SLE)

In this disease the distinctive visceral microscopic findings of renal arteriolar wireloop lesions and "onion-skinning" of splenic arterioles have no counterpart in the brain. Cerebral hematoxylin bodies have been recorded only twice, both within the muscularis of parenchymal arterioles. In one, no clinical or pathologic details were given,[48] and in the other no neurologic disease was apparent prior to death from acute cerebral hemorrhage with microscopic "pervascular inflammation."[63] Thus, the anatomic activity of antibodies to nuclear antigen in the brain is very rare and limited to vessels, in striking contrast to the visceral nodes, valves, and myocardium as well as arterioles, in which hematoxylin bodies are frequent in most autopsied cases.[144] "LE cells" from circulating blood were present on a fresh brain smear taken at craniotomy from an area of hemorrhagic infarction.[99] Gamma globulin deposits were found in the vascular choroid plexus in two cases,[5] but there were no deposits in multiple samples of brain tissue. Microscopic neuropathology showed no significant changes in one, in whom a confusional state had cleared overnight on steroid reduction one year before death from pneumonia. There were no changes referable to lupus in the other with scattered microinfarcts attributed to prolonged and profound terminal hypotension; confusion on admission was associated with very high fever and a normal cerebrospinal fluid. In the CSF immune complexes have been detected,[65] and low levels of the fourth component of complement have been found[73,110] in patients with SLE and clinical CNS involvement. The clinical correlation has been imperfect, the usual CSF findings are not recorded, there has been no tissue study, and the role of blood-CSF protein equilibration has not been fully defined. Circulating plasma DNA has been associated with CNS involvement and systemic vasculitis in SLE,[124] but it seemed likely that the neurologic group exhibited this finding by virtue of underlying vascular disease, and circulating DNA may be a result rather than a clue to the cause of widespread vascular tissue damage. In summary of all these reports, there is no evidence of immune-mediated damage to CNS tissue itself, but rather of primary damage to vessels body-wide.

The characteristic neuropathologic picture is multifocal microscopic parenchymal necrosis and vascular changes limited to small arterioles, reflecting a diffuse microcirculatory disorder. The small size of involved vessels is consonant with the pathogenesis suggested above of vascular immune complex deposits, but a specific lupus vasculitis has never been shown. In their definitive study Johnson and Richardson[77] meticulously reviewed the literature, described the neuropathologic lesions in 24 patients, and presented a balanced synthesis of their findings. The majority of neurologic symptoms, seizures, and transient brainstem deficits were associated with microinfarcts and at times microhemorrhages. There were relatively few vascular lesions compared with the number of tissue lesions. The chief change was necrosis in smallest arterioles, well below the threshold of arteriography. Fibrin thrombi were infrequent. Only four cases showed no findings and these were free of neurologic symptoms. The CSF in one-half of patients in their review showed a protein elevated above 50 mg/dL and more than 5 lymphocytes/mm^3 were found in one half. The clinical-pathologic correlation was high: three-fourths of patients with SLE had had both neurologic manifestations and neuropathologic findings by the time the disease had run its course at death.

The chances of specific neurologic involvement earlier in the course of SLE, however, is less. The specificity of correlation is further tempered by taking into account the recognized complications of SLE, which include the nonstructural cerebral effects of steroid therapy, water and electrolyte change, renal failure, and the tissue effects of hypertension and opportunistic cerebral tuberculosis,[63] zoster meningoencephalitis,[50] cryptococcosis,[110] and nocardiosis and toxoplasmosis.[126] The picture is compounded by the occurrence of another form of serositis in SLE, aseptic meningitis.[19,110] In one review it was concluded that in as many as 50% of patients with lesions of the nervous system at autopsy, only half have had neurologic symptoms ascribable to SLE.[59]

There are no lesions of large arterioles or arteries. There may be intracerebral hemorrhage, at times associated with thrombocytopenia or hypertension. Gross cerebral infarction from carotid occlusion does not occur in SLE. Rarely, larger infarcts may result from aggregation of small infarcts. Gross hemorrhagic cerebral infarct was described at craniotomy in a young woman in whom arteriography had shown neither occlusion nor arteritis and in whom the surgical tissue showed fibrinoid angiitis.[99] Arteriographic large-vessel occlusion is cited by Ferris[51] without documentation or pathologic verification. In this same presentation cerebral arteriograms were contributed by P.F.J. New on an unpublished case with multiple aneurysms. New relates that in this case seen by him a quarter of a century ago, autopsy was done and the diagnosis of SLE made, but the details could not be retrieved.[102] The case remains unique. In another case in which no clinical information is given, arteriography did show occlusion of a middle cerebral artery.[50] Although hemiparesis is listed in the clinical literature, these publications never achieve requisite clinical, radiologic, CSF or tissue correlation so that no statement is usually possible as to whether or why a stroke syndrome is due to SLE. It is clear that an arteriographic cerebral arteritis has never been reported.

Giant-Cell Arteritis

This process, affecting arteries of medium to large caliber throughout the body, may chiefly affect the aorta or the extradural carotid arterial tree. At both loci the histologic findings are the same: inflammatory edematous disruption of the media, destruction of the elastica, and a foreign body giant-cell reaction. Fibrinoid necrosis is absent, but foci of coagulation necrosis may be seen. Giant-cell arteritis has two forms.

Aortic Arch Syndrome. The first is typically seen in young adults who present with an arch syndrome. Although initially known as Takayasu's disease, aortic giant-cell arteritis is by no means limited to females, Orientals, or the young. Futhermore, a number of etiologies may yield the same aortic pathology. Stroke syndromes that are the result of aortic giant-cell arteritis are produced by involvement of the origins of vessels supplying the cerebrum. They are invariably accompanied by and often preceded by clinical signs referable to the noncerebral distribution of arch branches. These include decreased pulses in the arms and facial atrophy. The involved vessels have large lumens; obstructive symptoms are the result of thrombosis produced by the arteritis. The arteritic process may extend for some distance along the branches of the arch, leading to a large overlap in the anatomic involvement of the aortic and extracranial carotid forms of the disease. The descending aorta is also often involved. Aortic dissection and renal hypertension are common features.

Temporal Arteritis. The second form occurs in and after middle age. Medium and small arteries are involved, most prominently those supplying the scalp and the optic nerves. The classic symptoms of headache and visual deficit provide the usual designation, temporal arteritis. Other clinical indicators of diminished external carotid artery blood flow may exist, such as claudication on mastication or infarction of the scalp or tongue. Despite the clinical emphasis on ocular and scalp symptoms, arteries throughout the body are almost always involved. The aorta shows changes in one-half of the affected patients at postmortem. This active, diffuse arteritis, causing a high erythrocyte sedimentation rate and often changes in serum proteins and enzymes, is also frequently manifested by constitutional symptoms of malaise, myalgia, and arthralgia. Because of the smaller lumens of the involved arteries in this variant of giant-cell arteritis, there is often diminished flow due to the mural inflammatory changes alone, without secondary thrombus formation. Therefore, the process may frequently be reversed by steriod therapy. The wall of the artery is grossly thickened, narrowing the lumen and palpable on clinical examination (Fig. 14.4). The walls of the carotid and vertebral arteries are almost invariably affected on histologic study,[143] but being of larger caliber they do not become occluded without secondary thrombosis. Thus, involvement of these vessels is usually asymptomatic. Inclusion of the external carotid artery in angiographic studies can show the focal ectasia of temporal arteritis with magnification.[8]

The intracranial arteries are strikingly spared. This finding could be correlated with the absence of a significant external elastic lamella in the smaller cerebral arteries. Cerebral lesions are therefore uncommon in this disease, occurring in 10% or less in autopsy series and rarely in clinical reports. Stroke when seen usually occurs as a late event long after other typical phenomena have appeared; cerebral infarction due to atherosclerosis is common in patients in the usual age range of temporal arteritis. Even in the presence of active arteritis, no concrete connection need necessarily exist between the arteritic process and a cerebral episode. One case illustrated in a review[51] as an example of intracranial arterial involvement in temporal arteritis was actually a case of Wegener's granulomatosis and is discussed here earlier.

Rheumatoid Arthritis

Although vasculitis and serosal involvement are not rare elsewhere, only very exceptionally does severe rheumatiod disease evolve an intracerebral and leptomeningeal arteriolar fibrinoid necrotizing vasculitis[113a] producing small to minute cerebral infarcts or, rarely, intracerebral hemorrhage.[141] This may or may not be associated with so-called dural nodules. The clinical picture is one of diffuse dysfunction. One case in our material showed plastic admixture of dural granuloma, meningeal fibrosis and arteriolitis, and penetrant cortical arteriolitis of the cerebral convexities. Arteriographic study is not reported, but the meningeal vessels would be of visualizable size.

Degos' Disease

A proportion of patients with malignant atrophic papulosis, a very rare disorder that universally shows cutaneous infarcts and ischemic gastrointestinal lesions, sooner or later in the course undergo multiple small cerebral infarctions. Cerebral arteriography shows occlusive changes in multiple distal branches of the cerebral arteries, and fibrinoid necrosis of media and subintimal fibrosis are seen in the cerebral arterioles and small arteries.[26]

Cogan Syndrome

Originally viewed as an isolated peripheral association of interstitial keratitis and vestibuloauditory deficit, this syndrome has emerged as a focal expression of a sytemic vasculitis with central neurologic problems in up to one-half of patients.[12] Available histologic reports are meager, suggesting a periarteritis of arterioles. Cerebral arteriography has not been reported.

Tolosa-Hunt Syndrome

This is a characteristic clinical constellation centering on the region of the orbital apex, superior orbital fissure, and anterior cavernous sinus of unknown etiology, which has gradually been defined in recent years. It involves nonspecific connective tissue inflammatory proliferation with vascular involvement. Careful observation over a period of years by a neurosurgeon delineated a subacute, interrupted, stepwise evolution of unilateral orbital pain, ophthalmoplegia, variable first-division trigeminal sensory deficit, optic neuropathy (three cases), and replaceable proptosis.[74] CSF and arteriography were negative in all these cases, and no tissue was available. However, a case study by Tolosa reported in 1954 was reviewed and photographed in which there had been arteriographic narrowing of the carotid siphon just distal to cavernous sinus at autopsy, showing wrapping of the intracavernous carotid and investment of adjacent cranial nerves by granulation tissue which did not obstruct the venous sinus and involved only the subjacent adventitia of carotid artery. This was conceived as an intracavernous carotid periarteritis by Hunt. A detailed analysis of a single case published by Lakke[83] the following year incorporated an extensive literature review which showed that this type of case had been reported for a century. In his case, carotid arteriography was negative, but at craniotomy the lateral wall of cavernous sinus and dura of lesser sphenoid wing and superior orbital fissure were covered by granulation tissue. CSF had shown nine white blood cells with a normal protein. Lakke considered the process a primary focal pachymeningitis and thought that reducible exophthalmos was due to ophthalmoplegia. Presumably because the optic nerve was spared in his case, Lakke chose to pinpoint the neurologic involvement to the superior orbital fissure as had Collier in 1921. In a subsequent review of 22 cases of "painful ophthalmoplegia" in which all known causes including acute cavernous sinus thrombosis had been excluded, orbital congestion and response to corticosteroid therapy were features.[96] CSF study was negative. Three showed optic nerve involvement. Arteriography showed irregular narrowing of the intracavernous portion of carotid in one case. There was no tissue study. It was concluded from involvement of the optic nerve that the lesion was not confined to superior orbital fissure or anterior cavernous sinus, yet absence of mechanical proptosis or mechanical limitation of eye movement excluded the posterior orbit. The picture was enlarged by demonstration of occlusion of ophthalmic veins and variable nonfilling of the cavernous sinus on orbital phlebography in eight cases of ophthalmoplegia of ill-defined cause localized to the retroorbital region.[16] Three had optic nerve involvement and one a facial palsy. The carotid siphon was narrowed in one case at arteriography. In another 25-year-old case of retroorbital pain, stepwise ophthalmoplegia, and optic nerve deficit responding to steroid therapy, orbital phlebography showed occlusion of the superior ophthalmic vein and nonopacification of the cavernous sinus.[135] Another case with facial palsy showed negative arteriography but a narrowing of the ophthalmic vein and poor filling of the cavernous sinus on the same side on venography.[132]

The assembled information points to a localization primarily in the retroorbital region which extends into anterior cavernous sinus and can occlude the flow of ophthalmic veins and within cavernous sinus. The invested intracavernous carotid may be narrowed or irregularly altered. Cranial nerves of ocular motion are invariably involved, and the first trigeminal branch and optic nerve are commonly but variably involved. The process appears one of connective tissue inflammation. The meninges, not at this immediate location, seem spared for the most part. However, pleocytosis in the case of Lakke[83] and allusions to speculated syphilis and tuberculosis in literature reviews leave this question open. Involvement of the more removed second branch of trigeminal and seventh nerve in some cases indicates that the process may spread. Interestingly, the pupil is spared and in several cases there has been interval involvement of the second-fifth cranial nerves on the opposite side. The entire picture of spotty (abrupt yet evolving), migrating, and recurrent deficit limited to supratentorial peripheral cranial nerves is consonant with abnormalities on vascular contrast studies and at rare tissue biopsy showing a disorder broadly in the connective-tissue disorders.

Granulomatous Angiitis with Predilection for the CNS

This is a rare entity that is given special and separate consideration because, although the blood vessel is the seat of the disease, the involvement is uniquely virtually limited to the nervous system. Infrequent scattered microscopic findings in other organs are only rarely found and primary-secondary arteries are excluded. It consists of an inflammatory and giant-cell reaction prominently involving small arteries, arterioles, and frequently veins. First grouped together by Cravioto and Feigin,[32] this disease was later correlated in reviews by Kolodny et al,[81] who included four of their own cases, and by Nurick et al,[105] who presented two further cases. A brief clinical profile of 26 cases was constructed by Vincent.[138]

Although the clinical course is punctuated in the majority of patients by new cerebral signs, the course in at least half is protracted over many months. Unlike the other primary vasculitides (with the exception of lupus erythematosus), in almost all patients there is pleocytosis and elevated protein content in the CSF. One of our cases had an acute cerebellar hemorrhage, diagnosed in surgical material and later confirmed at autopsy. Arteriographic findings in four cases[18,113,138] have shown small artery occlusion, an irregular lumen from segmental stenosis, and aneurysmal beading.

The separation of this disease as a discrete clinico-pathologic entity rests on the prominent inflammation of veins, restriction to tertiary arterial branches sparing basal medium and extradural arteries, confinement to the nervous system, and frequent protein leak and mononuclear cells in the CSF. Nonetheless, careful reviews, such as that of Jellinger[76] who reported five cases, have included disease of other type. Two of these cases in late life, which heavily involved the aorta and primary branches and spared the intradural tertiary circulation, must be reclassified as giant-cell arteritis, particularly since temporal artery biopsy in one was positive and optic atrophy was present in the other. Attempts to implicate virus or immune complex disorders in the pathogenesis of genuine granulomatosis angiitis[76] must first rely on accurate anatomic categorization of the disorder. Secondly, one review suggesting a viral cause did not distinguish between herpesvirus and zoster infections.[138]

Sarcoidosis

This chronic inflammatory disease of ill-defined origin primarily involves the somatic viscera, yet uncommonly involves brain with parenchymal and meningeal granulomata. Although not well known, direct involvement of the walls of small cerebral arteries and arterioles, of the caliber of perforating branches, is frequent.[69] No lesions are observed in the secondary cerebral arteries. The process is invasion of the arterial wall by epithelioid aggregates with disruption of media and internal elastica, which may grow into the lumen causing blockade. Microinfarcts may be present. In one case of Herring and Urich widespread acute inflammatory fibrinoid necrosis affected many arteries with an appearance closely resembling periarteritis nodosa.[69]

Acute Hemorrhagic Leukoencephalopathy

This dramatic disorder is the only noninfectious one discussed in which mass effect customarily occurs. As a swiftly evolving diffuse and focal hemispheric syndrome with pressure occurring in a febrile prodrome, it often requires assessment for brain abscess. Arteriography reveals bowing and stretching of arteries and veins that are normal, but distal branch occlusion on the side of hemisphere swelling may occur.[91] In discussion at a clinico-pathologic conference one case was recalled by P.F.J. New in which cerebral angiography had revealed a number of vessels "with an abnormal appearance that could have been interpreted as neoplastic in origin," but the abnormality was not specified.[20] New has recalled that although mass effect and hypervascularity with staining were present, there was no irregularity of the lumina of individual vessels.[102] Resulting correspondence related another case in which arteriography had showed displacement of arteries but no change in configuration of the media and no pathologic vessels.[41] The brain shows petechial swelling of hemisphere central white matter, worse on one side than the other, with microscopic vascular necrosis, fibrinous exudate, hemorrhage, and neutrophilic infiltrate centering on tiny precapillary arterioles, indeterminate, or postcapillary venules.[67] An immune mechanism seems obvious, but the pathogenesis is undemonstrated.

Behçet's Disease

In this chronic disease with relapsing febrile episodes of iritis, orogenital ulceration, synovitis, and thrombophlebitis, a meningoencephalitis with varying encephalopathy, intracranial hypertension, and cranial nerve or parenchymal deficit occur at one point or another in up to one-quarter of patients, usually a few years after the onset of the general process, and itself may be remitting.[27] Of 38 patients with neurologic involvement, the CSF showed pleocytosis in 80% and elevated protein in two-thirds.[116a] The common underlying histopathologic lesion in all organs involved is perivascular infiltrate with lymphocytes and histiocytes. As an inflammatory vasculitis with multiple system involvement, Behçet's disease requires distinction from the primary collagen diseases. It differs in the specific mucous membrane lesions, in invariable fever, and in the regular and recurrent CNS episodes. Neuropathologic material is scant but confirms chronic meningitis and scattered microfocal ischemic necrosis. The vessels involved are smallest arteries and arterioles in which the adventitia is mildly proliferated amidst mild perivascular round cell infiltrate, but the media and intima are intact[129]; or cuffing is only around venules and capillaries, and of no degree more than can be explained by necrosis, and not in itself sufficient to give evidence of primary inflammation.[98] Therefore, in the brain a visible arteritis is variable at best and adventitial rather than medial, raising the point that this may reflect simple secondary investment by leptomeningeal chronic inflammation. Although technically a meningoencephalitis, the descriptions of parenchymal tissue loss are those of microinfarcts or small gross infarcts rather than inflammatory liquefaction. This tallies with the suddenness of focal deficit in two-thirds of cases[116a] and implies a dynamic arteritis not well shown at autopsy study.

Differential Diagnosis

Tertiary cerebral arteries can be involved in a myriad of diseases, only rarely in part inflammatory yet all of them on occasion requiring differentiation from the two major groups of angiitis described above. Two proposed vascular processes in the literature do not have foundation to merit inclusion as discrete diseases of cerebral arteries. Buerger's disease, or so-called thromboangiitis obliterans, is an entity not separable from atherosclerotic thromboembolic disease. Stroke occurring in young women while on oral contraceptives has no recognized cerebral vascular pathology, and there have been no distinctive arteriographic changes. The dynamic attenuation of arteries in subarachnoid hemorrhage, discussed elsewhere, and ergotism, are not reviewed.

Vascular

Segmental Tertiary Atherosclerosis

Ordinarily, atherosclerotic involvement of tertiary arteries is a common finding, easily recognized by its eccentricity and circumscription and by the associated atherosclerosis of extracranial neck arteries and circle of Willis. A variety in which convexity tertiary artery branches are involved in a widespread and severe manner, and in which primary neck and secondary intradural arteries are only slightly involved, has been known to pathologists but only recently emphasized to radiologists.[80] Stimulated by a case considered as cerebral vasculitis on clinical and arteriographic grounds, and even treated with corticosteroid, three further cases were located in file review, and a total of four were reviewed with autopsy, arteriogram, and clinical correlation. Diffuse stenoses and beading characterized the films, and corresponding segmental concentric and eccentric plaque formation in leptomeningeal arteries was demonstrated on neuropathologic study. All patients were hypertensive and half diabetic, a correlation earlier known with "small artery" atherosclerosis.

Moya-Moya Disease

This is characterized by an arteriographic ("hazy" or "misty") appearance of lenticulostriate and thalmoperforant collateral arterial enlargement and increased flow consequent on obliteration of the supraclinoid carotid. The abnormal hypertropic vessels may even be seen on computed tomography (CT) scan.[33] Not identified as an arteritis, the primary process begins in the infantile age range.[145] Progressive occlusions and stenoses occur with sequential multifocal cerebral infarction in the young. Subarachnoid hemorrhage from the collaterals occurs in adult years.[133] This seems to have first been documented by Fisher in cases of American infantile hemiplegia surviving to adult years.[53] The importance of the process rests on angiographic recognition of long-standing collateralization as a clue to acute infarction or subarachnoid hemorrhage and excluding arteritis. Pathologic study has offered no insight into the original insult, which may be prenatal.[145]

Multiple Embolism

This has reference to basic cardiac mural, atrial or valvar thrombus material, showering in a bicarotid distribution. The material often lodges in subarteriogram-sized vessels, or is singular or unilateral on arteriography, or shows only cut-offs and offers no problem in diagnosis. The emboli rapidly break up and are gone, and/or dynamic spasm relents, on interval films. Nonetheless multiple emboli on some occasions may simulate an "arteritis" picture. Current interest in embolism from a "floppy" mitral valve has shown this to be a more common source than realized. Echocardiography is indicated in younger patients with a stroke syndrome or those with recurrent episodes, just as for myxoma (see below). Taken together with cardiologic assessment, grounds for mitral valve excision provide cure. The association between prolapsed mitral valve and cerebral emboli is well worked out clinically, but the precise frequency of incidence in all patients with prolapsed valve is unknown, and thus far no case has come to autopsy.[10,64]

Cholesterol Embolization

A pseudoarteritis appearance is much more apt to occur with the arterio-arterial particulate emboli of chemical nature in atheromatous emboli. The usual source is an ulcerated atherosclerotic plaque close to the origin of the internal carotid artery, discharging spontaneously at repeated intervals, provoking new, organizing, and healed tertiary and tertiary branch lesions. The process may be directly visualized in the retina in some cases. Retrograde aortic embolization, from descending aorta to carotids, was described with the clamping, turbulence, and fragmentation of atheromatous material associated with surgery on the thoracic aorta,[66] with retrograde aortic perfusion during cardiac surgery,[111] and with a retrograde femoral-aortic arch catheter angiogram.[23] Similar traumatic release of pultaceous, cholesterol-rich material has occurred during direct neck carotid puncture for cerebral angiography. In the spontaneous carotid variety atherosclerosis is severe and diffuse, and cholesterol emboli are commonly found in viscera of the lower half of the body from spontaneous discharge of atheromatous sludge and fragments from distal aorta.[121] In the "lower half" syndrome of dissemination in the distribution of the descending aorta outflow, cutaneous necrosis, nodules, and muscle pain simulating clinical periarteritis or polymyositis have directed attention to the chemical irritant effect of impacted cholesterol crystals on the artery wall. In contrast to simple organization of emboli of bland thrombus material, cholesterol in small arteries evokes necrosis, sometimes even fibrinoid necrosis, giant-cell reaction, and vivid fibrosis,[2] which is indeed periarteritis but due to local factors rather than systemic inflammatory disease.

Hypertensive Fibrinoid Arteritis

Recognized as distinct from miscellaneous thickenings of cerebral arterioles by Feigin and Prose[49] by virtue of the fibrin impregnation of the entire wall, the similarity to the segmental mural necrosis of periarteritis and the mild inflammatory reaction made the designation of an arteritis apt. There is no confusion with periarteritis nodosa or its variants which involve arteries and which have an outspoken inflammatory reaction. Plasma exudation into mural tissue alteration (fibrinoid necrosis) is not itself diagnostic of any single disease. In hypertension the lesion is not related to the severity, but rather to the duration of the elevated blood pressure. It is this lesion that is felt to precede and underlie the development of the minute aneurysmal sacs in central grey, dentate, and median pontine regions, which are the source of hypertensive intracerebral hemorrhage.[113b] Although these miliary microaneurysms can be seen on autopsy injection study and with magnification views on arteriography, the initial lesion itself cannot.

Thrombotic Thrombocytopenic Purpura

A form of generalized noninflammatory intraluminal coagulation occlusion of microscopic small arterioles and capillaries by fibrin and platelet material, clinical and tissue involvement of the brain is usual.[1a,119] The manifestations are overtly systemic, and the neurology is generally one of diffuse dysfunction at a vascular level below arteriographic visualization. Marantic (nonbacterial thrombotic) endocarditis with cerebral emboli may unusually complicate the disorder[137] and large vessel thrombosis infrequently occurs. In a review of 168 cases Silverstein found that hemiparesis had occurred in a quarter.[119] A single arteriogram report showed multiple occlusions of left anterior and middle cerebral artery branches in a 17-year-old girl with right hemiparesis prior to massive intracerebral hemorrhage, who did not have bland valve thrombi.[21] Thus, although a micro-occlusive disease, small cerebral artery thrombi due more often to intravascular aggregation than to embolism may nonetheless occur.

Fibromuscular Dysplasia

This unique process of alternating zones of muscular hyperplasia and fibrous attenuation frequently involves the internal carotid artery, with or without involvement of renal or other visceral arteries, imparting in its full development a "string of beads," "loose stocking," or corrugated aneurysmal out-pouching appearance to the dye column on arteriography. Single ring-shaped or tubular carotid stenoses may also occur. Subintimal dissection with abrupt, linear tapering on arteriography is seen. The process almost always involves both carotids, spares the bifurcation, may involve the vertebral arteries, occurs over the age of 40 with few exceptions, and occurs in a ratio of 5:2 in women. There is an astonishingly high rate (40%) of associated intracranial aneurysm in large series,[94,107] and subarachnoid hemorrhage is a regular feature of this disease. Yet the intracranial carotid and middle cerebral artery origin are uncommonly radiologically involved (in less than 10%). Intracranial involvement does not occur without the typical, above-bifurcation, $C_{1\text{-}2}$ level carotid lesion. The importance for this review is the recognition that lesions in secondary arteries may occur, but their nature may be diagnosed with certainty from the extracranial carotid portion of the arteriogram and that subarachnoid spasm, or carotid dissection extending intracranially, may occur. Segmental beading of intracranial vessels without extracranial involvement has been proposed in correspondence as due to fibromuscular hyperplasia,[44,95] but the evidence is concretely against this. Intracranial involvement of trunk arteries was shown at autopsy in one case[94] but had not been visible on arteriography in life, which demonstrated the diagnostic carotid lesions. As a result of the carotid involvement limited to neck, this is a surgically remediable disorder.[43]

Amyloid Angiopathy

Cerebral focal amyloid deposition in senile plaques and in cortical arterioles has been known for decades. Recently recognized is amyloid deposition in tertiary arteries and branches in leptomeninges involving arteries of a size visible on arteriography. Although such films have not been published, one large clinicopathologic review of 23 cases[106] and another detailed tissue study of two cases[114] illustrate the process and emphasize the association with multiple microinfarction and with major nonhypertensive intracerebral hemorrhage in the elderly.

Acromegaly

Fusiform segmental dilatation, elongation, and kinking of intradural basilar, carotid, and middle cerebral arteries were documented in a series of Hatam and Greitz[68] and were considered due to ectasia of the artery wall. This change exists in parallel with similar alterations of the colic and iliofemoral arterial systems.

Tumor

Focal Encasement

Extension of cerebral tumor to, around, and within tertiary arteries with radiographic localized dilatation and a "shaggy" appearance may be seen with gliomas and metastases and with reticulum cell sarcoma.[86]

Neoplastic "Meningitis"

When tumor is diffuse, with widespread tertiary artery irregularities and without focal mass, meningeal spread tantamount to a meningitis exists. This may be seen with primary or metastatic lymphoma, classically with metastatic carcinoma or sarcoma, with the common meningeal seeding of pineal dysgerminoma and cerebellar medulloblastoma, and rarely with anaplastic astrocytoma. As with focal encasement, tissue involvement is chiefly adventitial, by extension from the arachnoid.

Myxoma

In any left-sided cardiac tumor, as with mural thrombus, single carotid embolism may occur with blockade infarction, seen, for example, with the rare atrial sarcoma.[78] The myxoma occupies an important position, however, because it has been discovered with increasing frequency. Atrial myxoma is to be considered with echocardiography in all repetitive cerebral episodes and in a single stroke syndrome in the young. Differential diagnosis of arteritis occurs because emboli are relatively small and usually multiple and because, in addition to infarction, local tumor growth at the embolic site acts as an implant, causing small artery wall dissolution with multiple aneurysm or arteriographic "blush" formation. Myxomatous emboli may cause central retinal artery occlusion,[75] or particulate matter may be seen in retinal arterioles.[134] An ill-explained constitutional reaction occurs composed of fever, anemia, elevated sedimentation rate, and altered serum proteins, similar to bacterial endocarditis.[125] The overall picture, including cerebral arteriography, may be so striking as to faithfully mimic systemic periarteritis as in the case originally reported by Leonhardt et al.[87] Only later was echocardiography performed and the true nature of the disorder discerned.[88] Although it might be questioned whether the multiple cerebrovascular implants temper an otherwise logical cure by cardiac surgery for removal of the primary atrial myxoma, none of a series of 35 patients had subsequent neurologic events in long-term follow-up.[115]

Arteriography shows dramatic numerous dilatations, fusiform or saccular, with some showing surrounding hyperemic blushing in the arterial phase, in the distal portions of tertiary cerebral arteries. Arteriographic and pathologic correlation by Price et al[112] and New et al[103] established mucoid myxoma impaction, erosion of artery wall, and focal enlargement of the vessel. The arteriographic findings continue to be confirmed.[33,125] The combination of repeated embolism, systemic reaction, and focal arterial wall enlargement with containment is similar to mycotic aneurysm but massive hemorrhage surprisingly does not usually occur, although multiple hemorrhagic infarcts are common. The diagnosis is revealed or excluded by echocardiography.

Diffuse *mucin embolization* was described by Deck and Lee[35] to cerebral small arteries and arterioles from multiple bony metastases of breast carcinoma. The profuse intra-arterial mucin was accompanied by fat droplets and the mechanism was compared to fat embolism. Tumor product, but not tumor cells, was present in the emboli, and artery walls were neither invaded nor reactive at autopsy study following an acute, 11-day course.

Angioendotheliosis

In this curious and very rare condition, neoplastic proliferation of endothelial cells occurs within the lumen of arterioles, capillaries, and venules of the brain, producing profound subacutely evolving diffuse cerebral dysfunction on which focal findings may become superimposed due to multifocal infarction. Not an angiosarcoma, since wall invasion, new vascular channel formation, and mass do not occur, the disease is a remarkable example of tumor spread and nutrition wholly within the bloodstream. The microscopic size of the vessels precludes radiologic identification, and bicarotid angiography in two cases was normal.[128] There may or may not be lymphocytes and elevated protein in the cerebrospinal fluid, but in one case with a borderline protein of 54 mg/DL, the gamma globulin content was elevated to 33 percent of the total.[113c] Intravascular proliferation may be found at autopsy in other organs or be restricted to the brain alone as in the case of Bots[15] and of one in our own material. In our case there were intravascular coagulation deposits limited to the areas of tumor and of no clinical significance.

Physicochemical

This admittedly miscellaneous group shares one feature in common: necrosis and/or inflammation and fibrosis of the tertiary artery wall.

Radiation

Although it is reasonable to mention irradiation, with known capacity for microcirculatory damage, as a cause of tertiary artery wall damage,[51] the evidence is poor for intracranial vessels of this size. At the convexity meningeal level radiologic narrowing or occlusion in the irradiated segment, but not elsewhere is no arteritis. Moreover, the effects of tumor growth and/or necrosis are the same. What is clear is the long-delayed acellular fibrosis and stenosis of major trunks at the base, such as at middle cerebral artery origin,[34] or at carotid siphon,[100] and in the neck[89,100] where surgical repair is feasible.

Ascending Arachnoiditis

This describes the slowly progressive idiosyncratic chronic productive inflammatory reaction seen rarely after spinal anesthesia and pantopaque myelography. With long survival the process occasionally reaches posterior fossa. All meningeal vessels are entrapped in the plastic arachnoid fibrosis and undergo severe adventitial reaction, medial hyalinization, and subintimal fibrosis with narrowing ("irritant" proliferative endarteritis) and secondary production of infarction. Should vertebral arteriography be performed, arterial wall abnormality would be likely perhaps even before symptoms have appeared.

Keratin Meningitis

During operation on epidermoid cyst or craniopharyngioma, should cyst fluid escape into the meninges a very acute inflammatory reaction occurs far out of proportion to that which occurs with blood and necrotic brain debris, owing to the chemical irritant effect of keratin. During the acute and resolving phases, tertiary arteries react as with any acute meningitis. A potential for chronic leptomeningeal fibrosis with encased vessels exists.

Plastic Monomer

For the unresectable aneurysm, this has been one mode of therapy in which the swiftly hardening plastic offers mechanical barrier support. The material, however, is highly irritant and produces arterial wall necrosis and panmural fibrosis. This is not a problem at the site of application in which fibrosing cicatrical closure is desirable, and such changes at the point of earlier aneurysmal rupture could also be interpreted as in part due to the wall damage from the rupture. In one unpublished case in our material, however, monomer was applied at a locus that at autopsy study months later contained no aneurysm. At that site as well as at arteries of distant circle of Willis and opposite middle cerebral artery trunk, there was profound fibrous replacement of media with rare giant cells, dissolution of internal elastica, and stenosing subintimal fibrosis. It was concluded that monomer after topical application seeps into the surrounding arachnoid space and produces chemical necrotizing arteritis of secondary and tertiary arteries.

Drug Arteritis

The initial description by Citron et al[28] of necrotizing angiitis associated with drug abuse demonstrated unequivocal histopathologic periarteritis in medium and small visceral arteries, linked the common agent as amphetamine, and assumed a systemic pharmacologic toxic effect. In two of four autopsies intracerebral arterial involvement was briefly mentioned without detail or depiction as profound alterations in pontine arterioles in one and in arteries of the cerebrum, brainstem, and cerebellum of the other, with cerebellar hemorrhage and multiple infarction. The arterial changes illustrated in viscera were eccentric destruction of wall with aneurysm formation, medial fibrosis, subintimal proliferation, and luminal narrowing with thrombosis. A companion paper from the same institution[114c] focussed on the cerebral circulation, showing impressive arteriograms with numerous and diffuse segmental sausages, beading, blocks, narrowing, smudging, and slow flow in 14 cases. Interval arteriography in one case at three weeks showed improvement in beading and focal constrictions; blocks remained. Unfortunately, the three microphotographs of vessels in two cases purporting to show arteritis and thrombosis did not: two pictures were of veins, and one was of a deep paired microscopic arteriole and venule. All showed nonspecific findings encountered routinely in postmortem material and of an age (hemosiderin, concretions, and extravascular cholesterol clefts with fibrosis) admittedly unconnected with acute deaths of a few days' duration. This was unconvincing, and the absence of drug arteritis in extensive New York City Medical Examiner material[7] left much doubt as to what was being encountered.

In the ensuing years the aggregate of acceptable individual radiographic case reports of cerebral drug arteritis as well as the original reports have established the following: (1) multiple drugs, chiefly heroin and LSD, have been implicated, and there is no unique role for amphetamine; (2) all cases have taken the drug intravenously; (3) arteriograms have uniformly shown overt tertiary and widespread segmental narrowing and ectasia; (4) patients may be asymptomatic; and (5) microscopy is required for autopsy detection. Inasmuch as main-line introduction of drug substance must traverse the venous return and lung filter before ejection from left heart, it was theoretically difficult to entertain an arterial embolic inflammation from an extremity vein portal. This view, however, seriously underestimated the amount of material injected and overlooked the multiple particulate nature, rather than solution, of the injected crushed tablets and "filler" (talc, starch). The missing link was ushered in by the observations of Atlee[6] and fully confirmed by Pare et al[108]: the majority of intravenous users seen acutely have particles or crystals within their retinal arterioles, primarily at endflow around the macula, occasionally with retinal hemorrhage. In the series of Pare et al[108] retinoscopy was more sensitive than chest film or pulmonary functions in detection. What has not been done is to correlate detailed retinoscopy, chest films, and pulmonary function with arteriography in users with neurological disorder. Neuropathology is still lacking. Two points are manifest, one being that the amount and type of injected substance is perfectly adequate to saturate the pulmonary filtration trap and enter the intracranial circulation, as seen in the retinal arterioles representing carotid flow. The second is that crystalline nondissolved drug, whether methadone, heroin, LSD, or amphetamine, and admixed material such as talc or starch, do provoke a necrotizing granulomatous and fibrosing response in small artery walls just as described above for cholesterol. It now appears that drug arteritis, rather than a systemic pharmacotoxic process, is one of microembolic irritative panarteritis. With the creation of multiple acute aneurysmal defects in the thin walls of small cerebral arteries, it is not surprising that parenchymal or subarachnoid hemorrhage may occur in drug arteritis.[28,42]

Not understood are the rare examples in the young of carotid occlusion in the neck[120] or siphon[90] following *oral* ingestion of LSD. These reports suggest a vasoconstrictive effect in view of the close similarity of LSD to methergyside, both derivatives of ergot alkaloids, although carotid arteriography in one case[90] on the opposite side three days after onset was normal. Equally mysterious was cerebral infarction with negative carotid arteriogram following heroin sniffing.[70] In any event, in none of these three was arteritis present.

Oxalosis

In this rare, primarily inherited disease, crystalline deposits occur within the muscular media of arteries and, together with subintimal fibrotic reaction, distort the lumen. This process may be accelerated by hemodialysis and has been recorded in systemic arteriography. In one case with hemiparesis before treatment for renal failure, carotid and vertebral angiography were done disclosing irregular narrowing of external and internal carotid arteries with very severe narrowing of the supraclinoid portions of both intradural carotid arteries and smooth narrowing of the left vertebral artery at the foramen magnum. Autopsy confirmed heavy deposition of oxalate distending the media in the supraclinoid left carotid artery.[130]

Homocystinuria

This is another rare, inherited metabolic disease due to cystathionine synthase deficiency with the production of connective tissue defects whose precise pathogenesis is not known and with excretion of highly abnormal amounts of homocystine, which provides the basis for diagnosis. The clinical syndrome includes mental deficiency, rarely severe, in at least one-half of cases, inferior ectopia lentis, bony abnormalities, and widespread and premature arterial and venous thrombus formation. Cerebral infarction, not rarely multiple, occurs typically in the teen-age years associated with carotid artery disease which extends intradurally and into parenchymal arterioles. Apart from the effects of organization of thrombus, there is a primary subintimal and medial fibrous thickening with splitting of muscular media and fraying of elastica, producing a literal unique form of arteriosclerosis. Cerebral arteriograms are not published but those of aortic distribution show corrugation in addition to occlusions. The neuropathology of cerebral infarction and arterial change is presented in several publications.[40,57,142] Colored illustrations of the arterial wall in homocystinuria is provided by McKusick's group,[116] who caution that arteriography and specifically cerebral arteriography are contraindicated because of increase in thrombus formation, with worsening of clinical deficit.[97]

Concluding Remarks

Information on involvement of the cerebral arteries in inflammatory and other similar processes has been surveyed to correlate the clinical manifestations, arteriographic identification, and tissue findings. Much of the literature on angiitis of the nervous system has been derived from arteriographic description alone with little or no clinical data, making it impossible to assess the data in a conclusive manner. Similarly, there is a dearth of tissue study, and, when this is available, it is at times lacking in neurology and neuropathology orientation. The lack of specific description of actual vessel size and type can be frustrating. Accordingly, clinical-arteriographic-pathologic correlation is scant.

The potential for cerebral vascular surgery is remote with these arterial processes, which, by definition, are diffuse, but their proper recognition is essential when the clinical presentation is focal. Segmental accessible lesions amenable to resection have been itemized, including carotid diseases such as fibromuscular dysplasia and postradiation stenosis, cardiac myxoma, and symptomatic persistent cerebral mycotic aneurysm.

Acknowledgment

This chapter would not have been possible without the continued and meticulous manuscript efforts of Marion W. Jones. The assistance of Irene Lovas and the Medical Library Center of New York in assembling references is much appreciated.

References

1. Acers TE: Herpes zoster ophthalmicus with contralateral hemiplegia. Arch Ophth 71:371–376, 1964

1a. Adams RD, Cammermeyer J, Fitzgerald PJ: The neuropathological aspects of thrombocytic acroangiothrombosis. A clinico-anatomic study of generalized platelet thrombosis. J Neurol Neurosurg Psychiatry 11:27–43, 1948

2. Anderson WH: Necrotizing angiitis associated with embolization of cholesterol. Am J Clin Pathol 43:65–71, 1965
3. Applebaum E, Kreps I, Sunshine A: Herpes zoster encephalitis. Am J Med 32:25–31, 1962
4. Arkin A: A clinical and pathological study of periarteritis nodosa. A report of five cases, one histologically healed. Am J Pathol 6:402–425, 1930
5. Atkins CJ, Kondon JJ, Quismario FP, Friou GJ: The choroid plexus in systemic lupus erythermatosus. Ann Intern Med 76:65–72, 1972
6. Atlee WE: Talc and cornstarch emboli in eyes of drug users. JAMA 219:49–51, 1972
7. Baden MM: Angiitis in drug abusers. N Engl J Med 284:111–112, 1971
8. Baker HL: The clinical usefulness of magnification cerebral angiography. Radiology 98:587–594, 1971
9. Barham-Carter A: Investigation into the effects of aureomycin and chloramphenicol in herpes zoster. Br Med J 1:987–991, 1951
10. Barnett HJM, Boughner DR, Taylor DW, Cooper PE, Kostuk WJ, Nichol PM: Further evidence relating mitral-valve prolapse to cerebral ischemic events. N Engl J Med 302:139–144, 1980
11. Bickerstaff ER: Etiology of acute hemiplegia of childhood. Br Med J 2:82–87, 1964
12. Bicknell JM, Holland JV: Neurologic manifestations of Cogan syndrome. Neurology 28:278–281, 1978
13. Bingham WF: Treatment of mycotic intracranial aneurysms. J Neurosurg 46:428–437, 1977
14. Blackwood W, Corsellis JAN: Greenfield's Neuropathology. Third Ed. Edward Arnold, London, 1976
15. Bots GTAM: Angioendotheliomatosis of the central nervous system. Acta Neuropath 28:75–78, 1974
16. Brismar G, Brismar J: Thrombosis of the intraorbital veins and cavernous sinus. Acta Radiol. 18:145–153, 1977
17. Budzilovich GN, Wilens SL: Fulminating Wegener's granulomatosis. Arch Pathol 70:653–660, 1960
18. Burger PC, Burch JG, Vogel FS: Granulomatous angiitis. An unusual etiology of stroke. Stroke 8:29–35, 1977
19. Canoso JJ, Cohen AS: Aseptic meningitis in systemic lupus erythematosus. Arthritis Rheum 18:369–374, 1975
20. Case Records of the Massachusetts General Hospital: N Engl J Med 271:1313–1320, 1964
21. Case Records of the Massachusetts General Hospital: N Engl J Med 275:1125–1133, 1966
22. Case Records of the Massachusetts General Hospital: N Engl J Med 276:1369–1377, 1967
23. Case Records of the Massachusetts General Hospital: N Engl J Med 277:648–655, 1967
24. Case Records of the Massachusetts General Hospital: N Engl J Med 300:243–252, 1979
25. Case Records of the Massachusetts General Hospital: N Engl J Med 300:1378–1385, 1979
26. Case Records of the Massachusetts General Hospital: N Engl J Med 303:1103–1111, 1980
27. Chajek T, Fainaru M: Behcet's disease. Report of 41 cases and a review of the literature. Medicine 54:179–196, 1975
28. Citron BP, Halpern M, McCarron M, Lundberg GD, McCormick R, Pincus IJ, Tatter D, Haverback BJ: Necrotizing angiitis associated with drug abuse. N Engl J Med 283:1003–1011, 1970
29. Courery WR, New PFJ, Price DL: Angiographic manifestations of craniofacial phycomycosis. Report of three cases. Radiology 103:329–334, 1972
30. Courville CB: Essentials of Neuropathology. San Lucas Press, Los Angeles, 1953
31. Cravioto H: Angiitides of the nervous system. In Wolman BB: International Encyclopedia of Psychiatry, Psychology, Psychoanalysis and Neurology. Vol II. Aesculapius, New York, 1977
32. Cravioto H, Feigin I: Noninfectious granulomatous angiitis with a predilection for the nervous system. Neurology 9:599–609, 1959
33. Damasio H, Seabra-Gomes R, Damasio AR, Antunes JL: Multiple cerebral aneurysms and cardiac myxoma. Arch Neurol 32:269–270, 1975
34. Darmody WR, Thomas LM, Gurdjian ES: Postirradiation vascular insufficiency syndrome. Case report. Neurology 17:1190–1192, 1967
35. Deck JHN, Lee MA: Mucin embolism to cerebral arteries: A fatal complication of carcinoma of the breast. Can J Neurol Sci 5:327–330, 1978

37. Derby BM: Importance of collagen diseases in the production of strokes. Curr Concepts Cerebrovasc Dis 11:9–13, 1976
37. Drachman DA: Neurological complications of Wegener's granulomatosis. Arch Neurol 8:145–155, 1963
38. Drachman DA, Adams RD: Herpes simplex and acute inclusion body encephalitis. Arch Neurol 7:45–63, 1962
39. Duffy J, Lidsky MD, Sharp JT, Davis JS, Person DA, Hollinger FB, Min K: Polyarthritis, polyarteritis and Hepatitis B. Medicine 55:19–37, 1976
40. Dunn HG, Perry TL, Dolman CL: Homocystinuria. A recently discovered cause of mental defect and cerebrovascular thrombosis. Neurology 16:407–420, 1966
41. Ebels E: Necrotizing leukoencephalopathy. N Engl J Med 272:864, 1965
42. Edwards KR: Hemorrhagic complications of cerebral arteritis. Arch Neurol 34:549–552, 1977
43. Ehrenfeld WK, Wylie EJ: Fibromuscular dysplasia of the internal carotid artery. Surgical management. Arch Surg 109:676–681, 1974
44. Elias WS: Intracranial fibromuscular hyperplasia. JAMA 218:254, 1971
45. Elkon KB, Hughes GRV, Catovsky D, Clauvel JP, Dumont J, Seligmann M, Tannenbaum H, Esdaile J: Hairy-cell leukemia with polyarteritis nodosa. Lancet 2:280–282, 1979
46. Fauci AS, Haynes BF, Katz P: The spectrum of vasculitis. Clinical, pathological, immunologic and therapeutic considerations. Ann Intern Med 89:660–676, 1978
47. Fauci AS, Wolff SM: Wegener's granulomatosis: Studies in eighteen patients and a review of the literature. Medicine 52:535–561, 1973
48. Feigin I, Prose P: Some uncommon forms of cerebral vascular disease. J Mount Sinai Hosp 24:838–848, 1957
49. Feigin I, Prose P: Hypertensive fibrinoid arteritis of the brain and gross cerebral hemorrhage. A form of "hyalinosis". Arch Neurol 1:98–110, 1959
50. Feinglass EJ, Arnett FC, Dorsch CA, Zizic TM, Stevens MB: Neuropsychiatric manifestations of systemic lupus erythematosus: Diagnosis, clinical spectrum, and relationship to other features of the disease. Medicine 55:323–339, 1976
51. Ferris EJ: Arteritis. Chapter 84. In Newton TH, Potts DG: Radiology of the Skull and Brain. CV Mosby, St Louis, 1974
52. Ferris EJ, Levine HL: Cerebral arteritis: classification. Radiology 109:327–341, 1973
53. Fisher CM: Early-life carotid-artery occlusion associated with late intracranial hemorrhage. Observations on the ischemic pathogenesis of mantle sclerosis. Lab Invest 8:680–700, 1959
54. Ford RG, Siekert RG: Central nervous system manifestations of periarteritis nodosa. Neurology 15:114–122, 1965
55. Fred HL, Lynch EC, Greenberg SD, Gonzalez-Angulo A: A patient with Wegener's granulomatosis exhibiting unusual clinical and morphologic features. Am J Med 37:311–319, 1964
56. Gardner DL: Pathology of the Connective Tissue Diseases. Williams & Wilkins, Baltimore, 1965
57. Gibson JB, Carson NAJ, Neill DW: Pathological findings in homocystinuria. J Clin Pathol 17:427–437, 1964
58. Gilbert GJ: Herpes zoster ophthalmicus and delayed contralateral hemiparesis. JAMA 229:302–304, 1974
59. Glaser GH: Collagen diseases and the nervous system. Med Clin North Am 47:1475–1494, 1963
60. Gorevic PD, Kassab HJ, Levo Y, Kohn R, Meltzer M, Prose P, Franklin EC: Mixed cryoglobulinemia: Clinical aspects and long-term follow-up of 40 patients. Am J Med 69:287–308, 1980
61. Grcevic N, Matthews WF: Pathologic changes in acute disseminated Aspergillosis. Particularly involvement of the central nervous system. Am J Clin Pathol 32:536–551, 1959
62. Griffith GC, Vural IL: Polyarteritis nodosa. A correlation of clinical and postmortem findings in seventeen cases. Circulation 3:481–490, 1951
63. Hadler NM, Gerwin RD, Frank MM, Whitaker JN, Baker M, Decker JL: The fourth component of complement in the cerebrospinal fluid in systemic lupus erythematosus. Arthritis Rheum 16:507–521, 1973
64. Hanson MR, Conomy JP, Hodgman JR: Brain events associated with mitral valve prolapse. Stroke 11:499–506, 1980
65. Harbeck RJ: DNA antibodies and DNA: Anti-DNA complexes in cerebrospinal fluid of patients with SLE. Arthritis Rheum 16:552, 1973
66. Harris LS, Kennedy JH: Atheromatous cerebral embolism: Complication of surgery of the thoracic aorta. Ann Thorac Surg 4:319–326, 1967
67. Hart MN, Earle KM: Hemorrhagic and perivenous encephalitis: A clinical-pathological review of 38 cases. J Neurol Neurosurg Psychiatry 38:585–591, 1975
68. Hatam A, Greitz KT: Ectasia of cerebral arteries in acromegaly. Acta Radiol (Diagn) 12:410–418, 1972
69. Herring AB, Urich H: Sarcoidosis of the cen-

tral nervous system. J Neurol Sci 9:405–422, 1969

70. Herskowitz A, Gross E: Cerebral infarction associated with heroin sniffing. South Med J 66:783–784, 1973
71. Hilal SK, Solomon GE, Gold AP, Carter S: Primary cerebral arterial occlusive disease in children. I. Acute acquired hemiplegia. Radiology 99:71–86, 1971
72. Hinck VC, Carter CC, Rippey JG: Giant cell (cranial) arteritis. A case with angiographic abnormalities. Am J Roent 92:769–775, 1964
73. Howell HS, Baburao T, Graziano J: Mycotic cervical carotid aneurysm. Surgery 81:357–359, 1977
74. Hunt WE, Meagher JN, LeFever HE, Zeman W: Painful ophthalmoplegia. Its relation to indolent inflammation of the cavernous sinus. Neurology 11:56–62, 1961
75. Jampol LM, Wong AS, Albert DM: Atrial myxoma and central retinal artery occlusion. Am J Ophth al mol 75:242–249, 1973
76. Jellinger K: Giant cell granulomatous angiitis of the central nervous system. J Neurol 215:175–190, 1977
77. Johnson RT, Richardson EP: Neurological manifestations of systemic lupus erythematosus: A clinical-pathological study of 24 cases and review of the literature. Medicine 47:337–369, 1968
78. Joynt RJ, Zimmerman G, Khalifeh R: Cerebral emboli from cardiac tumors. Arch Neurol 12:84–91, 1965
79. Kim U, Friedman EW, Werther LJ, Jacobson JH: Carotid artery aneurysm associated with nonbacterial suppurative arteritis. Arch Surg 106:865–867, 1973
80. Knopman DS, Anderson DC, Mastri A, Larson D: Leptomeningeal artery atherosclerosis visualized by angiography: Clinical correlates. Stroke 9:262–266, 1978
81. Kolodny EA, Rebeiz JJ, Caviness VS, Richardson EP Jr: Granulomatous angiitis of the central nervous system. Arch Neurol 19:510–524, 1968
82. Laguna J, Derby BM, Chase R: *Cardiobacterium hominis* endocarditis with cerebral mycotic aneurysm. Arch Neurol 33:638–639, 1975
83. Lakke JPWF: Superior orbital fissure syndrome. Report of a case caused by local pachymeningitis. Arch Neurol 7:289–300, 1962
84. Lee JF, Tindall GT: Arterial erosion and hemorrhage during graded carotid ligation with the Crutchfield clamp. J Neurosurg 27:52–55, 1967
85. Leeds NE, Goldberg HI: Angiographic manifestations in cerebral inflammatory disease. Radiology 98:595–604, 1971
86. Leeds NE, Rosenblat R: Arterial wall irregularities in intracranial neoplasms. The shaggy vessel brought into focus. Radiology 103:121–124, 1972
87. Leonhardt ETG, Jakobson H, Ringqvist OTA: Angiographic and clinicophysiologic investigation of a case of polyarteritis nodosa. Am J Med 53:242–256, 1972
88. Leonhardt ETG, Kullenberg KPG: Bilateral atrial myxomas with multiple arterial aneurysms—A syndrome mimicking polyarteritis nodosa. Am J Med 62:792–794, 1977
89. Levinson SA, Close MB, Ehrenfeld WK, Stoney RJ: Carotid artery occlusive disease following external cervical irradiation. Arch Surg 107:395–397, 1973
90. Lieberman AN, Bloom W, Kishore PS, Lin JP: Carotid artery occlusion following ingestion of LSD. Stroke 5:213–215, 1974
91. Litel G, Ehni G: Acute hemorrhagic leucoencephalitis. Treatment with corticosteroids and dehydrating agents. J Neurosurg 33:445–452, 1970
92. Locksley HB, Sahs AL, Sandler R: Subarachnoid hemorrhage unrelated to intracranial aneurysm and A-V malformation. A study of associated diseases and prognosis. Section III. Report on the cooperative study of intracranial aneurysms and subarachnoid hemorrhage. J Neurosurg 24:1034–1056, 1966
93. Lucas FV, Benjamin SP, Steinberg MC: Cerebral vasculitis in Wegener's granulomatosis. Cleve Clin Q 43:275–281, 1976
94. Manelfe C, Clarisse J, Fredy D, Andre JM, Crouzet G: Fibromuscular dysplasia of the cervicocephalic arteries. Report of 70 cases. J Neuroradiol 1:149–231, 1974
95. Massey EW, Reader A: Cerebral vasculitis. Arch Neurol 36:321, 1979
96. Mathew NT, Chandy J: Painful ophthalmoplegia. J Neurol Sci 11:243–256, 1970
97. McKusick VA: Heritable Disorders of Connective Tissue. Fourth Ed St. Louis, CV Mosby, 1972
98. McMenemy WH, Lawrence BJ: Encephalomyelopathy in Behcet's disease. A report of necropsy findings in two cases. Lancet 2:353–358, 1957
99. Meagher JN, McCoy F, Rossel C: Disseminated lupus erythematosus simulating intracranial mass lesion. Report of an unusual case. Neurology 11:862–865, 1961
100. Momose KJ, New PFJ: Non-atheromatous stenosis and occlusion of the internal carotid artery and its main branches. Am J Roent 118:550–566, 1973

101. Morriss FH, Spock A: Intracranial aneurysm secondary to mycotic orbital and sinus infection. Am J Dis Child 119:357–362, 1970
102. New PFJ: Personal correspondence.
103. New PFJ, Price DL, Carter B: Cerebral angiography in cardiac myxoma. Correlation of angiographic and histopathological findings. Radiology 96:335–345, 1970
104. Norris FH, Leonards R, Calanchini PR, Calder CD: Herpes-zoster meningoencephalitis. J Infect Dis 122:335–338, 1970
105. Nurick S, Blackwood W, Mair WGP: Giant cell granulomatous angiitis of the central nervous system, Brain 95:133–142, 1972
106. Okazaki H, Reagan TJ, Campbell RJ: Clinicopathological studies of primary cerebral amyloid angiopathy. Mayo Clin Proc 54:22–31, 1979
107. Osborn AG, Anderson RE: Angiographic spectrum of cervical and intracranial fibromuscular dysplasia. Stroke 8:617–626, 1977
108. Pare JAP, Fraser RG, Hogg JC, Howlett JG, Murphy SB: Pulmonary mainline granulomatosis: Talcosis of intravenous methadone abuse. Medicine 58:229–239, 1979
109. Parker HL, Kernohan JW: The central nervous system in periarteritis nodosa. Mayo Clin Proc 24:43–48, 1949
110. Petz LD, Sharp GC, Cooper NR, Irvin WS: Serum and cerebral spinal fluid complement and serum autoantibodies in systemic lupus erythematosus. Medicine 50:259–275, 1971
111. Price DL, Harris J: Cholesterol emboli in cerebral arteries as a complication of retrograde aortic perfusion during cardiac surgery. Neurology 20:1209–1214, 1970
112. Price DL, Harris JL, New PFJ, Cantu RC: Cardiac myxoma. A clinicopathologic and angiographic study. Arch Neurol 23:558–567, 1970
113. Rajjoub RK, Wood JH, Ommaya AK: Granulomatous angiitis of the brain: A successfully treated case. Neurology 27:588–591, 1977
113a. Ramos M, Mandybur TI. Cerebral vasculitis in rheumatoid artheritis. Arch Neurol 32:271–275, 1975
113b. Ransohoff J, Derby B, Kricheff I: Spontaneous intracerebral hemorrhage. Clin Neurosurg 18:247–266, 1971
113c. Reinglass JL, Muller J, Wissman S, Wellman H: Central nervous system angioendotheliosis. A treatable multiple infarct dementia. Stroke 8:218–221, 1977
114. Rengachary SS, Racela LS, Watanabe I, Abdou N: Neurosurgical and immunological implications of primary cerebral amyloid (congophilic) angiopathy. Neurosurgery 7:1–8, 1980
114a. Rose FC, Brett EM, Burston J: Zoster encephalomyelitis. Arch Neurol 11:155–172, 1964
114b. Rose GA, Spencer H: Polyarteritis nodosa. Quart J Med 26:43–82, 1957
114c. Rumbaugh CL, Bergeron RT, Fang HCH, McCormick R: Cerebral angiographic changes in the drug abuse patient. Radiol 101:335–344, 1971
114d. Russell DS: The pathology of spontaneous intracranial haemorrhage. Proc Roy Soc Med 47:689–704, 1954
115. Sandok BA, von Estorff I, Giuliani ER: Subsequent neurological events in patients with atrial myxoma. Ann Neurol 8:305–307, 1980
116. Schimke RN, McKusick VA, Huang T, Pollack AD: Homocystinuria. Studies of 20 families with 38 affected members. JAMA 193:711–719, 1965
116a. Schotland DL, Wolf SM, White HH, Dubin HV: Neurologic aspects of Behcet's disease. Case report and review of the literature. Am J Med 34:544–553, 1963
116b. Sergent JS, Lockshin MD, Christian CL, Gocke DJ: Vasculitis with hepatitis B antigenemia: long-term observation in nine patients. Medicine 55:1–18, 1976
117. Shibuya S, Igarashi S, Amo T, Sato H, Fukumitsu T: Mycotic aneurysms of the internal carotid artery. Case report. J Neurosurg 44:105–108, 1976
118. Shillito J: Carotid arteritis: A cause of hemiplegia in childhood. J Neurosurg 21:540–551, 1964
119. Silverstein A: Thrombotic thrombocytopenic purpura. The initial neurological manifestations. Arch Neurol 18:358–362, 1968
120. Sobel J, Espinas OE, Friedman SA: Carotid artery obstruction following LSD capsule ingestion. Arch Intern Med 127:290–291, 1971
121. Soloway HB, Aronson SM: Atheromatous emboli to central nervous system. Report of 16 cases. Arch Neurol 11:657–666, 1964
122. Stehbens WE: Pathology of the Cerebral Blood Vessels CV Mosby, St Louis, 1972
123. Stehbens WE, Mustapha RM: Atypical calcification of enlarged terminal branches of the middle cerebral artery. Arch Neurol 29:282–284, 1973
124. Steinman CR: Circulating DNA in systemic lupus erythematosus. Association with central nervous system involvement and systemic vasculitis. Am J Med 67:429–434, 1979
125. Steinmetz EF, Calanchini PR, Aguilar MJ: Left atrial myxoma as a neurological problem: A case report and review. Stroke 4:451–458, 1973
126. Stewart G, Basten A: Lupus erythomatosus

and brain scanning. Ann Intern Med 83:733–734, 1975

127. Straatsma BR, Zimmerman LE, Gass JDM: Phycomycosis. A clinicopathologic study of fifty-one cases. Lab Invest 11:963–985, 1962
128. Strouth JC, Donahue S, Ross A, Aldred A: Neoplastic angioendotheliosis. Neurology 15:644–648, 1965
129. Strouth JC, Dyken M: Encephalopathy of Behcet's disease. Report of a case. Neurology 14:794–805, 1964
130. Sunday MT, Haughton VM: Carotid and vertebral changes with primary calcium oxalosis. Neuroradiology 12:99–102, 1976
131. Suwanwela C, Suwanwela N, Charuchinda S, Hongsaprabhas C: Intracranial mycotic aneurysms of extravascular origin. J Neurosurg 36:552–59, 1972
132. Swerdlow B: Tolosa Hunt syndrome: A case with associated facial nerve palsy. Ann Neurol 8:542–543, 1980
133. Takahashi M, Miyauchi T, Kowada M: Computed tomography of Moyamoya disease: Demonstration of occluded arteries and collateral vessels as important diagnostic signs. Radiology 134:671–676, 1980
134. Tipton BK, Robertson JT, Robertson JH: Embolism to the central nervous system from cardiac myxoma. Report of two cases. J Neurosurg 47:937–940, 1977
135. Van Dalen JTW, Bleeker GM: The Tolosa Hunt syndrome. Doc Ophthalmol 44:167–172, 1977
136. Victor DI, Green WR: Temporal artery biopsy in herpes zoster ophthalmicus with delayed arteritis. Am J Ophthal mol 82:628–630, 1976
137. Vilanova JR, Norenberg MD, Stuard ID: Thrombotic thrombocytopenic purpura. NY State J Med 75:2246–2248, 1975
138. Vincent FM: Granulomatous angiitis. N Engl J Med 296:452, 1977
139. Walker RJ, Gammal TE, Allen MB: Cranial arteritis associated with herpes zoster. Case report with angiographic findings. Radiology 107:109–110, 1973
140. Walton JN: Subarachnoid Hemorrhage. E&S Livingstone, London, 1956
141. Watson P, Fekete J, Deck J: Central nervous system vasculitis in rheumatoid arthritis. Can J Neurol Sci 4:269–272, 1977
142. White HH, Rowland LP, Araki S, Thompson HL, Cowen D: Homocystinuria. Arch Neurol 13:455–470, 1965
143. Wilkinson IMS, Russell RWR: Arteries of the head and neck in giant cell arteritis: A pathological study to show the pattern of arterial involvement. Arch Neurol 27:378–391, 1972
144. Worthington JW, Baggenstoss AH, Hargraves MM: Significance of hematoxylin bodies in the necropsy diagnosis of systemic lupus erythematosus. Am J Pathol 35:955–969, 1959
145. Yamada H, Nakamura S, Kageyama N: Moyamoya disease in monovular twins. Case report. J Neurosurg 53:109–112, 1980

Index

Lightning Source UK Ltd.
Milton Keynes UK
UKOW07f0252160716

278535UK00002B/5/P

9 781461 295327